Prebiotics and Probiotics in Human Milk

Prebiotics and Probiotics in Human Milk

Origins and Functions of Milk-Borne Oligosaccharides and Bacteria

Michelle K. McGuire

Mark A. McGuire

Lars Bode

ELSEVIER

AMSTERDAM • BOSTON • HEIDELBERG • LONDON
NEW YORK • OXFORD • PARIS • SAN DIEGO
SAN FRANCISCO • SINGAPORE • SYDNEY • TOKYO

Academic Press is an imprint of Elsevier

Academic Press is an imprint of Elsevier
125 London Wall, London EC2Y 5AS, United Kingdom
525 B Street, Suite 1800, San Diego, CA 92101-4495, United States
50 Hampshire Street, 5th Floor, Cambridge, MA 02139, United States
The Boulevard, Langford Lane, Kidlington, Oxford OX5 1GB, United Kingdom

Library of Congress Cataloging-in-Publication Data
A catalog record for this book is available from the Library of Congress

British Library Cataloguing in Publication Data
A catalogue record for this book is available from the British Library

ISBN: 978-0-12-802725-7

For information on all Academic Press publications
visit our website at https://www.elsevier.com/

Publisher: Nikki Levy
Acquisition Editor: Megan Ball
Editorial Project Manager: Jaclyn Truesdell
Production Project Manager: Nicky Carter
Designer: Victoria Pearson

Typeset by TNQ Books and Journals

Contents

Contributors

Joeri Beauprez
Inbiose NV, Ghent, Belgium

Lars Bode
University of California, San Diego, La Jolla, CA, United States

Sarah Brooker
University of Idaho, Moscow, ID, United States

Raul Cabrera-Rubio
Institute of Agrochemistry and Food Technology-National Research Council (IATA-CSIC), Valencia, Spain; TEAGASC Food Research Centre, Cork, Ireland

Stewart Campbell
CordenPharma International, Inc., Woburn, MA, United States

Maria Carmen Collado
Institute of Agrochemistry and Food Technology-National Research Council (IATA-CSIC), Valencia, Spain

Sarah S. Comstock
Michigan State University, East Lansing, MI, United States

Richard D. Cummings
Harvard Medical School, Boston, MA, United States

Sharon M. Donovan
University of Illinois, Urbana, IL, United States

Heinz Egge
(Formerly) Institute of Physiological Chemistry, University of Bonn, Bonn, Germany

Elloise du Toit
University of Cape Town, Cape Town, South Africa

Leonides Fernández
Complutense University of Madrid, Madrid, Spain

James A. Foster
University of Idaho, Moscow, ID, United States

Richard Furneaux
Victoria University of Wellington, Lower Hutt, New Zealand

Izaskun Garcia-Mantrana
Institute of Agrochemistry and Food Technology-National Research Council (IATA-CSIC), Valencia, Spain

Carlos Gómez-Gallego
University of Murcia, Murcia, Spain; University of Turku, Turku, Finland

Esther Jimenez
ProbiSearch, SL. Tres cantos, Madrid, Spain; Universidad Complutense de Madrid, Madrid, Spain

Akira Kobata
The Noguchi Institute, Tokyo, Japan

Clemens Kunz
Institute of Nutritional Science, Justus-Liebig University Giessen, Giessen, Germany

Mark A. McGuire
University of Idaho, Moscow, ID, United States

Michelle K. McGuire
Washington State University, Pullman, WA, United States

Courtney L. Meehan
Washington State University, Pullman, WA, United States

Michael Messer
The University of Sydney, Sydney, NSW, Australia

Álex Mira
Complutense University of Madrid, Madrid, Spain

Ardythe L. Morrow
Perinatal Institute Cincinnati Children's Hospital Medical Center, Cincinnati, OH, United States

Andrew Muscroft-Taylor
University of Canterbury, Christchurch, New Zealand

Olav T. Oftedal
Smithsonian Environmental Research Center, Edgewater, MD, United States

Juan M. Rodríguez
Complutense University of Madrid, Madrid, Spain; Center for Advanced Research in Public Health (CSISP), Valencia, Spain

Silvia Rudloff
Justus-Liebig University Giessen, Giessen, Germany; Institute of Nutritional Science, Justus-Liebig University Giessen, Giessen, Germany

David A. Sela
University of Massachusetts, Amherst, MA, United States; University of Massachusetts Medical School, Worcester, MA, United States

Seppo Salminen
University of Turku, Turku, Finland

David F. Smith
Emory University School of Medicine, Atlanta, GA, United States

Tadasu Urashima
Obihiro University of Agriculture and Veterinary Medicine, Obihiro, Hokkaido, Japan

Janet E. Williams
University of Idaho, Moscow, ID, United States

Ying Yu
Perinatal Institute Cincinnati Children's Hospital Medical Center, Cincinnati, OH, United States

Preface

Human milk is arguably the only food genuinely "designed" to be consumed exclusively and extensively by humans, at least during infancy, when poor nutrition can lead to both acute and chronic health disparities. As such, understanding the synthesis and composition of human milk should be a primary focus for the entire field of human nutrition. Yet, and albeit decades of research, surprisingly little is known about this important topic, and much of what is known is based on animal literature and outdated analytical techniques. This fact is easily illustrated, for example, by studying the myriad volumes of the Institute of Medicine (IOM)'s Dietary Intake Reference series — each of which describes how human milk composition was used to estimate Adequate Intake (AI) levels during infancy for each of the micronutrients and macronutrients. Take riboflavin, for example; this AI for infants (IOM, 1998) was derived largely from a 25-year-old study characterizing riboflavin content of milk produced by only five women (Roughead and McCormick, 1990), and it is noteworthy that the published article describing this study tells us nothing about how the milk samples were collected. And riboflavin is far from the only nutrient for which this incredibly little amount of data were used to estimate infant requirements and/or make recommendations for AI. Surely the research community can do better! After all, understanding human milk composition is critical not only for basic science but also for establishing industry standards and public health policy in terms of how and with what healthy and unhealthy babies should be nourished.

Our interest in creating this first-ever book concerning two components of human milk (oligosaccharides and bacteria) was driven largely by our intense desire to create an allied community of experts in this field whose collective goal is to not only relatively quickly characterize oligosaccharide and bacterial concentrations in milk but also understand their origin and/or synthesis, variation, and effects on both maternal and infant health. Indeed, human milk oligosaccharides (HMOs) and the human milk microbiome (HMM) are considered by many to be today's "hot topics" in human milk and lactation, and we are just beginning to scratch the surface in terms of understanding how they get into milk, what regulates their concentrations and profiles, and how they impact maternal and infant health and disease. We are convinced that not only are they important but they are also likely intimately linked in terms of their presence and function. Our genuine desire in creating this book was that it would move this complex and connected area of research forward as efficiently and collaboratively as possible. Hence, together we made a commitment to spearhead and edit the book you are now holding in your hands, and we hope that you find it useful in this regard.

Long gone are the days when a handful of laboratories around the world worked independently on a particular scientific problem, only to learn of each other's work at an annual meeting or when a new article was published. Instead, we are all now connected via a keystroke and a quick PubMed search. It is our hope that this connectedness, combined with a common goal to understand human milk composition, will result in an unprecedented rate of knowledge acquisition in terms of HMOs and HMM and that this knowledge will be quickly leveraged by both industry and policy experts wishing to use it to promote and improve infant health around the world. We see a very bright future for research in human milk and lactation (clearly, standing on the shoulders of giants who have gone before us) and encourage all who are involved in this noble pursuit to reevaluate what we know *and (importantly) do not know* about human milk synthesis and composition. It is our shared vision not only that will this book be the first of many editions related to HMOs and HMM but also that other researchers collectively consider spearheading the creation of similar books that provide state-of-the-science overviews of other classes of milk-borne compounds such as the proteins, lipids, vitamins, minerals, hormones, and immune factors. These books should also include detailed information on how best to collect a representative milk sample for the particular component of interest and the various and evolving techniques available for their analyses. Surely we can do better than promoting dietary intake goals for infants on estimations of the composition of milk produced by five women over two decades ago!

Michelle K. McGuire
Mark A. McGuire
Lars Bode

REFERENCES

Institute of Medicine, 1998. Dietary Reference Intakes for Thiamin, Riboflavin, Niacin, Vitamin B6, Folate, Vitamin B12, Pantothenic Acid, Biotin, and Choline. National Academy of Sciences, Food and Nutrition Board, Washington, DC.

Roughead, Z.K., McCormick, D.B., November 1990. Flavin composition of human milk. American Journal of Clinical Nutrition 52 (5), 854–857.

SECTION

A

Background, Structures, Synthesis, and Analysis

CHAPTER

From Bifidus Factor to Human Milk Oligosaccharides: A Historical Perspective on Complex Sugars in Milk

1

Clemens Kunz[1], **Heinz Egge**[2]

[1]*Institute of Nutritional Science, Justus-Liebig University Giessen, Giessen, Germany;* [2]*(Formerly) Institute of Physiological Chemistry, University of Bonn, Bonn, Germany*

1. BACKGROUND

1.1 DISCOVERY OF THE IMPORTANCE OF MICROORGANISMS FOR HEALTH AND DISEASE AND PIONEERS IN THIS RESEARCH AREA

The health situation around the turn of the 19th century was characterized by an alarmingly high mortality rate ranging from 20% to 30% in the first year of life. Infants were fed pure carbohydrates, processed food, and mixtures of milk and cereals with or without added meat, or they were given native animals' milk (Nützenadel, 2010). One of the first infant formulas consisting of modified bovine milk was developed by Justus von Liebig (1803–70) for his daughter's children and the monograph "Soup for Infants" ("Kindersuppe") published in 1864 (Liebig, 1866). It was based on the use of milk and cereals. This soup for infants led to many others also producing infant formula to improve the overall health of infants. It was Liebig who provided a scientific basis for nutritional investigations in this area of research through his technical and analytical innovations. However, at the beginning the alternative products to human milk were not very successful. This is not surprising as it was possible only later, when scientific innovations were available; was possible only later, when scientific innovations were available to perform the first balance studies (Carl von Voit, 1881), to analyze nitrogen by the method developed by Johann Kjeldahl (1883) and to determine the energy content of food (Max Rubner, 1889).

A major breakthrough for infant survival was the discovery of microorganisms and their importance to health and, at the same time, the observation that milk carbohydrates play an important role for the growth of these microorganisms. Pioneering microbiological work has been done by Theodor Escherich, one of the most

Prebiotics and Probiotics in Human Milk. http://dx.doi.org/10.1016/B978-0-12-802725-7.00001-4

respected pediatricians in Europe at that time (Table 1.1) (Weirich and Hoffmann, 2005). In 1886, Escherich had published a monograph on the relationship between intestinal bacteria and the physiology of digestion in the infant (Escherich, 1886). This research had established him as the leading bacteriologist in pediatrics.

"Pediatrics" was just beginning to develop into an independent medical field, and in Europe (e.g., in Vienna, Graz, Zurich, Berlin and Munich), the first pediatrics professorships and chairs were established and were held by internationally esteemed personalities, among them Adalbert Czerny, the author of the textbook *Des Kindes Ernährung* (*The Child's Nutrition*) which became for a long time one of the leading books in this area. The tremendous impact of this book in pediatrics at that time was summarized in 1933 in a Festschrift by Heinrich F. Helmholtz in the *Journal of Pediatrics* as follows: "[…] this work is a bible. […] At a time when pediatrics in America was still in its swaddling clothes, German masters took us into their clinics as students and by their inspiration and training played a part in the development of pediatrics in America of which they may feel proud" (Helmholtz, 1933).

Breastfeeding was not considered as a matter of importance and, therefore, not recommended. However, pediatricians observed that the mortality risk would decrease dramatically if the infants were breastfed: the mortality rate was 7 times higher for bottle-fed compared to breastfed infants (Nützenadel, 2010). The better survival of breastfed infants was obviously linked to a significantly higher resistance to various diseases, including infectious diarrhea. Henri Tissier of the Pasteur Institute in Paris tried to compare the intestinal microbiota of breastfed infants with that of infants fed bovine milk (Tissier, 1900). At the same time, Moro in Heidelberg independently found a unique predominance of *Lactobacilli*, later

Table 1.1 Theodor Escherich—A Pioneer in Pediatrics and Microbiology

- 1857–1911
- Graz (Austria), Würzburg, Munich (Germany)
- Pediatrician
- Most important bacteriologist
- Monograph 1886 "Die Darmbakterien des Säuglings und ihre Beziehung zur Physiologie der Verdauung" ("Infants' gut bacteria and their relation to the physiology of digestion")

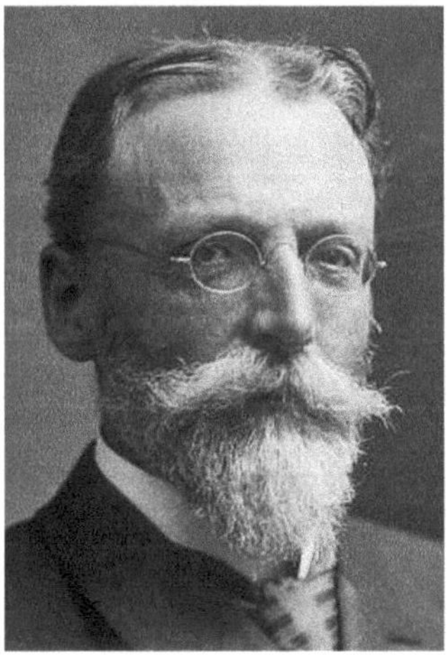

Photograph reproduced with permission from the Österreichische Nationalbibliothek ÖNB (Austrian National Library).

called *Bifidobacteria*, in the feces of breastfed infants (Weirich and Hoffmann, 2005; Moro, 1900). Moro, who was born in 1874 in Slovenia (Table 1.2), studied in Graz and started his pediatrics career in the laboratory of Escherich, who held the first chair of pediatrics in Graz. In 1900, Moro presented the first bacteriological characterization of *Lactobacillus acidophilus* (Moro, 1900). He attracted worldwide attention in various fields, such as for developing a simple percutaneous skin test for tuberculosis, which was used until the 1960s, and for recommending a carrot soup as treatment for children with diarrhea (Weirich and Hoffmann, 2005). Being a student of Escherich explains Moro's strong interest in bacteria and their importance for infant health.

Fig. 1.1 demonstrates the intimate link between basic and applied research around 1900, showing Escherich at his last lecture with Moro (left) giving an injection to an animal, while Meinhard von Pfaundler, another renowned pediatrician, was examining a child (Weirich and Hoffmann, 2005).

Being fascinated by Escherich's success in the field of bacteriology (among others), it was mainly Moro who stimulated research to find the growth factors of microorganisms in milk. In particular, Paul György, another student of Moro, was inspired by these ideas (Table 1.3).

György was a pediatrician with a strong interest in the basic sciences, especially in the field of nutrition in general and nutrition of children and adolescents in particular (Barness et al, 1979). From the beginning, he had promoted the benefit of breastfeeding for infants, although at that time those recommendations were not very popular. György was born on April 7, 1893. Shortly after World War I, he joined the group of Ernst Moro in Heidelberg. Therefore, it is not surprising that György had all

Table 1.2 Ernst Moro—A Pioneer in Pediatrics

- 1874–1951
- Graz (Austria), Heidelberg (Germany)
- Student of Theodor Escherich
- Pioneer investigator in pediatrics in various areas
- Among the founders of pediatric science in Germany
- Around 1900: Moro and Tissier (Pasteur Institute in Paris) found a unique predominance of *Bifidobacteria* in the stool of breastfed infants

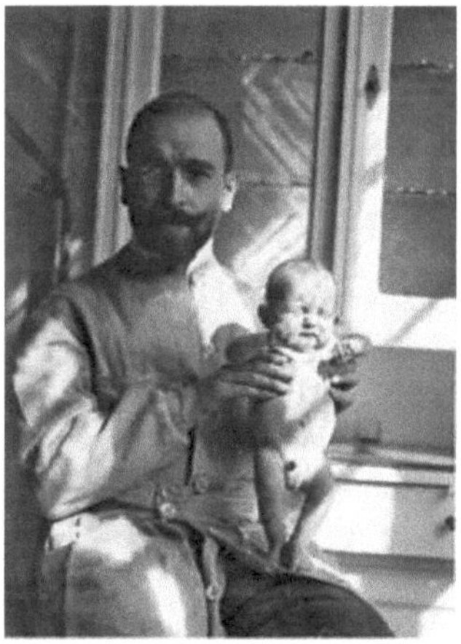

Photograph with kind permission from Springer Science and Business media; Weirich and Hoffmann, 2005.

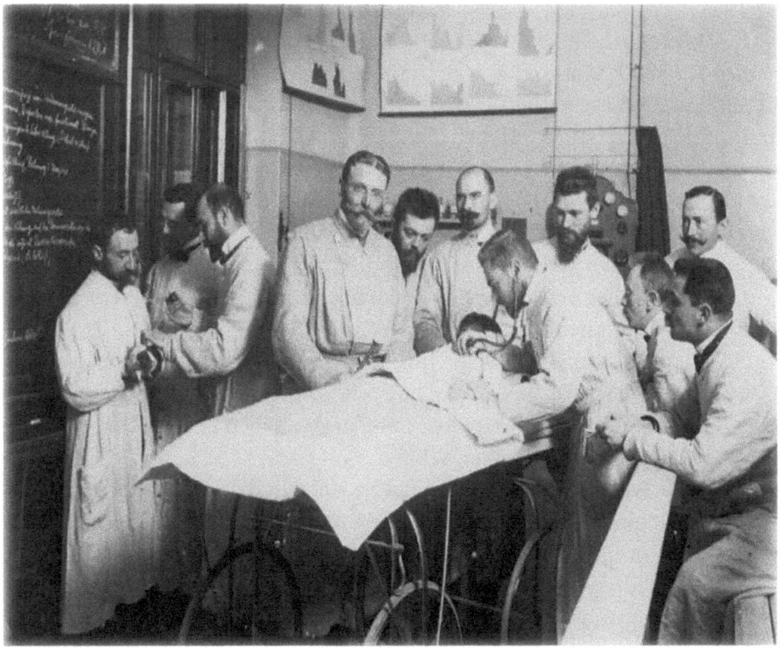

FIGURE 1.1

Escherich around 1900 at his last lecture with Moro on the left giving an injection to an animal while Meinhard von Pfaundler, another renowned pediatrician, was examining a child.

Photograph with kind permission from Springer Science and Business Media; (Weirich and Hoffmann, 2005)

Table 1.3 Paul György—A Pioneer in Pediatrics

- 1893–1976
- Pediatrician
- Budapest (Hungary), Heidelberg (Germany), Cambridge (UK), Cleveland, Ohio, and Pennsylvania (USA)
- Student of Moro
- Suporb combination of excellent investigator, sympathetic clinician, and demanding teacher; a gloriously bombastic, colorful, emphatic ward-round teacher (Barness et al., 1979)
- Great contributions to the discovery of B vitamins
- Pioneering work on the "bifidus factor" in human milk

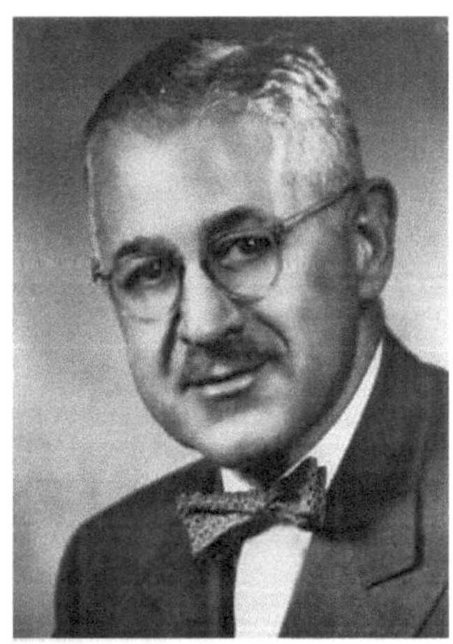

Photograph reproduced with permission from Barness, L.A., Tomarelli, R.M., Györgi, P., 1979. 1893–1976. A biographical sketch. Journal of Nutrition 109, 17–23.

his life been engaged in research on the intestinal microbiota and its relevance for the health of breastfed infants. Due to the Nazi regime, György had to leave Germany in 1933. Via Cambridge (England) he finally came to Cleveland in the United States and later went to Pennsylvania (Barness et al, 1979). As will be shown later, it was a very successful collaboration between P. György and R. Kuhn that led to the discovery of the "bifidus factor" in human milk and to the first identification of human milk oligosaccharides (HMOs) being responsible for this biological effect.

2. PHYSIOLOGICAL OBSERVATIONS AS BACKGROUND TO HMO RESEARCH

There were two parallel routes of research on carbohydrates and later on HMOs, one based on physicochemical, the other on nutritional observations (Montreuil, 1992). Table 1.4 shows important research investigations from around 1900 until the 1980s.

Very early, a not-yet-specified fraction was detected in human milk that could not be found in bovine milk. In 1888, Eschbach was the first to discover that animal milk and human milk do not contain that type of lactose, which is typically found in bovine milk (cited in Montreuil, 1992). He observed that in both types of milk a mixture of various forms of lactose with different properties exists. His conclusion was that bovine milk contained the most homogeneous type of lactose, whereas the lactose in human milk was the most heterogeneous. Then, Deniges found that the types of lactose found in human milk and bovine milk were identical but that human milk contained a carbohydrate fraction still to be identified (Montreuil, 1992).

In 1926, it was Herbert Schönfeld who significantly contributed to research in the field of growth factors in human milk by proving that the "bifidus factor" was heat resistant and contained in the nonprotein fraction of milk (Schönfeld, 1926). Schönfeld, after very careful investigations, drew the conclusion that this "bifidus factor" was most likely a vitamin, as those were just being discovered at the time.

Around 1930 in Lille (France), Michel Polonowski and Albert Lespagnol established a method to isolate the so-far-unknown carbohydrate fraction. They called this fraction, which was insoluble in methanol, "gynolactose" (Polonowski and Lespagnol, 1929, 1931). The authors themselves, however, pointed out that

Table 1.4 Milestones in Milk Carbohydrate Research

Around 1900
- Observations: different fecal compositions of breastfed and bottle-fed infants
- First indications that difference is linked to milk composition
- First description of microorganisms and their importance for health

Around 1930
- Characterization of the first individual HMO

1950–80s
- Further identification of HMOs and functional studies
- Biochemical interest due to similar epitopes on blood and tumor cells
- Intensive work on growth factors for microorganisms and antiadhesive and anti-inflammatory properties

this "gynolactose" was not homogeneous but consisted of various components. They also found that nitrogen was an essential component of the hexosamines and that this "gynolactose" showed a very strong bial reaction. As we know today, this reaction was due to the presence of *N*-acetylneuraminic acid, not yet known then. Later, Polonowski and Lespagnol, together with Montreuil, applied two-dimensional paper chromatography for the first time and identified the first two fucosyllactoses (2'-fucosyllactose and 3-fucosyllactose) in the fraction that had been previously uncharacterized (Polonowski and Montreuil, 1954).

Jean Montreuil was a charismatic personality of the sciences and one of the pioneers in the field of carbohydrates and glycoconjugates. In addition to other important discoveries, he proposed that all *N*-glycans have the same core, to which various branches are attached, which he named "antennae" to suggest their mobility and potential recognition roles (Bratosil and Mignon, 2011). After having built molecular models, he proposed interconvertible conformations, and he first coined the terms "Y" and "T" conformations, later called "bird" or "umbrella" conformations. These original studies on the structures of glycoconjugates have stimulated many researchers to study the biological roles for complex carbohyrates in health and disease.

It was Montreuil's ambition to specify the structures of this complex "gynolactose" mixture in more detail (Montreuil, 1960; see also later), though he did not realize that he would strongly compete with Richard Kuhn by doing so. Concurrent research work in Heidelberg by Kuhn and coworkers and by Montreuil and his team in Lille led to the first clear description of HMOs, namely of 2′- and 3-fucosyllactose and difucosyllactose and to the identification of lacto-*N*-tetraose, lacto-*N*-fucopentaose I and II, difucosyllactose, and many others (Kuhn and Baer, 1956; Kuhn, 1957, 1958; Montreuil, 1960; Grimmonprez and Montreuil, 1977).

3. CLOSE COLLABORATION BETWEEN RICHARD KUHN AND PAUL GYÖRGY

Research activities in the field of HMOs were then continued by Jean Montreuil with L. Grimmonprez, G. Strecker, J.M. Wieruszeski and others, Richard Kuhn and his many coworkers, Viktor Ginsburgh, Akira Kobata, Heinz Egge, and many others.

Kuhn himself already had numerous publications together with his coworkers Bär, Brossmer, and Gaue identifying various oligosaccharides (Table 1.5) (for reviews, see Montreuil, 1992; Wiegandt and Egge, 1970; Egge, 1992; Kobata, 2003). The starting point of Kuhn's work on glycolipids in general and of HMO research in particular completely differed from that of Polonowski, Lespagnol, and Montreuil. In the 1950s, Kuhn and György started their impressive cooperation on HMOs. György, in Philadelphia since 1936, contacted Kuhn and thus, about 30 years after the beginning of their joint research on lactoflavines in Heidelberg, the two research groups renewed their cooperation (Table 1.6). They started to investigate the importance of human milk in comparison to bovine milk

Table 1.5 Richard Kuhn—A Pioneer in Chemistry and in HMO Research

- 1900–67
- Wien, Munich, Zürich, Heidelberg
- Chemist, background in organic, physical, and analytical chemistry combined with strong interest in biological functions
- Structure/function studies of molecules with characteristic carbon-carbon double bonds (polyenes, flavins, vitamins, etc.)
- 1936 Nobel Prize in Chemistry (vitamins, carotinoids)
- Director at the age of 28 of the Kaiser Wilhelm Institute for Medical Research, Heidelberg (Germany)
- Impressive series of publications on glycolipids and human milk sugars together with H. Bär, R. Brossmer, A. Gauhe, F. Zilliken, H. Egge, and many others

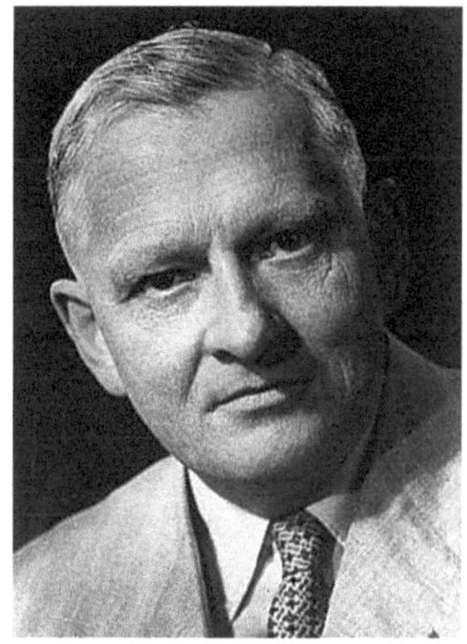

Photograph reproduced with permission from the Österreichische Nationalbibliothek ÖNB (Austrian National Library).

Table 1.6 Major Discoveries by Collaborations Between Paul György and Richard Kuhn

- In Heidelberg (1930)
- Discovery of B vitamins
- Characterization of HMO structures in combination with functional studies

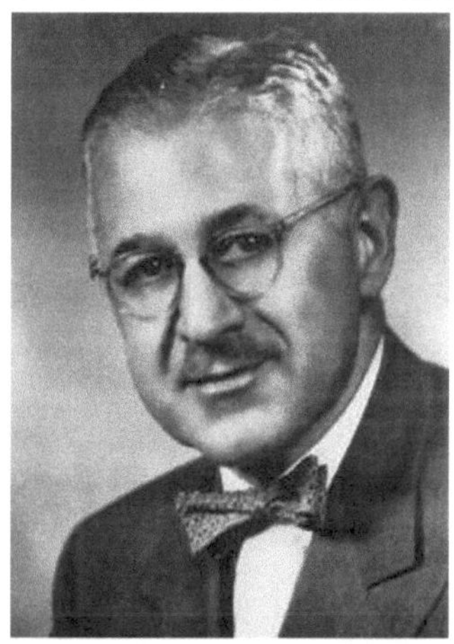

- In Heidelberg and Philadelphia (1950)
- Structure/function studies characterizing growth factors for *Bifidobacteria* (*L. bifidus*)

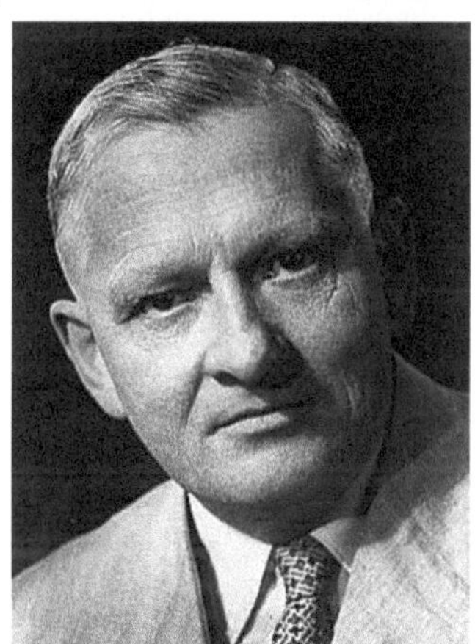

Photographs reproduced with permission from Barness, L.A., Tomarelli, R.M., Györgi, P., 1979. 1893–1976. A biographical sketch. Journal of Nutrition 109, 17–23. and from the Österreichische Nationalbibliothek ÖNB (Austrian National Library).

for infant resistance against infections. The cooperation between the two was extremely successful and led to the proof that the growth factors for *Lactobacillus bifidus* in human milk consist of oligosaccharides containing *N*-acetylglucosamine and polysaccharides (György 1954; Kuhn, 1958; György et al., 1974). In contrast, the nitrogen-free fraction in human milk did not show any bifidogenic effect.

Kuhn was interested in science at a very young age (Westphal, 1968). He did not go to elementary school but was educated by his mother before entering secondary school. Between 1910 and 1917, he attended secondary school (Döblinger Gymnasium) in Vienna together with his classmate, Wolfgang Pauli (Nobel Prize in Physics, 1945). Being 13 years old, he helped a family friend who was a professor of chemistry in Zurich to prepare the experimental classes for chemistry students. In this time, he received as a present the newest textbook of chemistry, about which Kuhn was very excited. After a short period in the Austrian army until the end of World War I, he began to study chemistry, first in Vienna and since 1919 in Munich. His PhD thesis under the supervision of Richard Willstätter (Nobel Prize in Chemistry, 1915) "The Specificity of Enzymes in Carbohydrate Metabolism" was accepted "summa cum laude" in 1922. He continued his scientific career first in Munich and between 1927 and 1929 as full professor at the Eidgenössische Technische Hochschule in Zürich. In the same year, he was appointed director of the Department of Chemistry at the newly founded "Kaiser-Wilhelm Institute for Medical Research" in Heidelberg (since 1951, Max-Planck-Institute). In 1938, Kuhn received the Nobel Prize for Chemistry for his work on carotenoids and vitamins, but due to the Nazi regime, the Prize could not be given to him until 1948.

The 1950s were a second period of enormously high research activity with Kuhn conducting investigations into immune factors and associated research on oligosaccharides in human milk and on gangliosides in the brain (Westphal, 1968). Based on studies on "bifidus factors" in milk and virus-inhibiting effects of human milk, Kuhn together with Bär, Gaue, Brossmer, and others focused on the identification and characterization of oligosaccharides in human milk (Montreuil, 1992; Kuhn, 1958; Westphal, 1968; Egge, 1992). Since 1954, numerous oligosaccharides have been purely presented and structurally elucidated by means of excellent techniques. Isolated in 1954, lacto-*N*-tetraose was identified as a key substance of HMO in human milk, and during the following years, further components were identified (Kuhn, 1958).

Kuhn had always been interested in the biological significance of isolated compounds. The observation that oligosaccharides containing lactaminic acid (nowadays: sialic acid) are cleavable by the influenza virus was of great interest. Both 3′- and 6′-lactaminyl lactose were the most easily cleavable components. Kuhn and his coworker demonstrated, for example, that the influenza virus cleaves the glycosidic linkage of lactaminic acid, and in the following years lactaminyl oligosaccharides have been identified as receptors for the influenza virus, thus explaining the virus-inhibiting effect of human milk (Kuhn, 1958; Westphal, 1968). In his lecture on resistance problems at the 100th meeting of the Society of German Natural and Medical Scientists in 1958, Kuhn explained that cells not developing such lactaminyl oligosaccharide structures on the surface had to be resistant to influenza virus (Kuhn and Brossmer, 1956; Kuhn, 1958), an observation with long-lasting influence on research even until today in the fields of chemistry, biology, and medicine.

From the beginning of their collaboration on HMOs, György in Philadelphia and Kuhn in Heidelberg found that there was a connection between the work of Tissier on bacteria and the milk fraction of Polonowski and Lespagnol, called "gynolactose." In the course of their investigations, György found an *L. bifidus* mutant solely growing in the presence of milk, which he named after its place of discovery *L. bifidus* var. *pennsilvanicus* (György et al., 1954).

György also realized that the "bifidus factor" activity is somehow related to the intestinal defense system. In 1953, he published one of his key papers, "A Hitherto Unrecognized Biochemical Difference Between Human Milk and Cow's Milk" (György, 1953). He, together with Kuhn, Rose, and Zilliken, found the highest activities in human colostrum, followed by rat colostrum, mature human milk, mature rat milk, and bovine colostrum (Table 1.7). The milk of ruminants, such as cows, ewes, and goats, showed only weak activity, if any (Table 1.8). A large number of organic compounds including known microbial growth factors, yeast extract, vitamins not present in the original *Lactobacillus* growth medium, carbohydrates, and several vegetable extracts were all ineffective in replacing the "bifidus factor." Within this close collaboration between Philadelphia and Heidelberg, many HMOs, such as lacto-*N*-tetraose, lacto-*N*-fucopentaose I, lacto-*N*-fucopentaose II, and lacto-*N*-difucohexaose, were characterized by classic methods (Montreuil, 1992; Egge, 1992).

Based on their observations that *L. bifidus* grew only in the presence of β-linked *N*-acetylglucosamine, György and Kuhn postulated that those bacteria were not able to synthesize *N*-acetylglucosamine themselves. They concluded that if an infant was fed *N*-acetylglucosamine-containing HMOs, growth of *L. bifidus* would increase and

Table 1.7 Experiments of György and Coworkers Searching for the Bifidus Factor in Human and Bovine Milk[a]

Supplement (mL/10 mL of Medium)		Acid Production in 40 h (mL of 0.1 N)
None		0.4
Human milk,	0.02	2.2
skim	0.06	7.9
	0.2	12.5
Bovine milk,	0.1	0.6
skim	0.3	0.8
	1.0	2.3

[a]*From György, P., 1953.*

Table 1.8 Experiments of György and Coworkers Searching for the Bifidus Factor in Milk From Various Species[a]

Species	Time Postpartum	Range (mL)	Unit Average (mL)	Average Dry Weight (mL)
Human colostrum[b]	1–2 days (8)[c]	0.013–0.03	0.02	2.4
	3rd day (10)	0.014–0.024	0.02	2.2
	5th day (6)	0.012–0.018	0.017	1.5
	7th day (3)	0.016–0.021	0.018	1.6
Human milk[b] (12)		0.020–0.15	0.06	5.5
Rat colostrum (3)		0.032–0.040	0.035	–
Rat milk (1)		0.13		
Cat	1st–6th days (3)	0.03–0.04	0.04	9.5
Donkey	1st–6th days (3)	0.01–0.26	0.18	18
Dog	1st–5th days (4)	0.07–0.16	0.10	21
Monkey (rhesus) colostrum	1st day (1)	–	–	25
Dog	6th–10th days (4)	0.3–>0.5	>0.4	>75
Rabbit	2nd day (1)	–	–	19
	9th day (1)	0.18	–	75
Mare (1)		–	–	50
Sow colostrum (6)		0.1–0.22	0.14	30
Sow milk (13)		0.17–0.75	0.40	60
Bovine colostrum[b] (5)		0.12–0.23	0.15	28
Bovine milk[b] (15)		1.5–4.5	2.5	250
Goat colostrum[b]	1st day (2)	0.7–0.9	0.8	85
Goat milk[b]	5th–9th days (3)	1.1–1.4	1.3	130
Ewe milk[b]	2nd–11th days (3)	1.9–2.5	2.3	250

[a]*From György, P., 1953.*
[b]*Used or calculated as skimmed milk.*
[c]*Figures in brackets indicate the number of various samples assayed.*

thus inhibit the invasion of pathogenic bacteria in two ways: (i) through the production of acetic acid and lactic acid (ratio 3:2) by which the activity of *L. bifidus* leads to a decrease in the intestinal pH, thus inhibiting the growth of various pathogenic bacteria, and (ii) by supporting the growth of *L. bifidus*, which would lead to a lack of nutrients for pathogenic microorganisms. These underlying mechanisms were already discovered in the mid-1950s but remain research topics because of the current strong interest in investigating probiotics and prebiotics and their importance for health and disease.

4. ELUCIDATION OF THE ABO AND SECRETOR/NONSECRETOR PATHWAY OF HMOs

As Kobata had a strong influence on the identification of this pathway, we refer to his contribution (see Chapter 2) for more details and summarize only briefly some important aspects.

Beginning at about 1960, the blood group ABO and the secretor system were investigated by Watkins and Morgan (Watkins, 1966) and others. Due to the large amount of HMOs in human milk, HMOs had been used already at that time as an optimal source for the elucidation of the blood group specificity. In 1967, Grollmann and Ginsburg could prove that 2′-fucosyllactose was not detectable in milk samples of women with nonsecretor status (Grollman and Ginsburg, 1967). These women express ABO blood group epitopes on their erythrocytes corresponding to their genetic AB0 background but do not express them in glycoproteins secreted by the epithelial cells of mucus-producing glands.

Kobata, first in Ginsburg's laboratory in Washington and later with his coworkers in Japan, developed a new method to determine the oligosaccharide pattern by using only a small amount of milk (reviewed in Kobata, 2000, 2003).

5. DEVELOPMENT OF NEW METHODS FOR THE ANALYSIS OF COMPLEX HMOs

Enhanced knowledge of HMOs has only been possible by establishing advanced methods for the identification and characterization of HMO within the past 60 years. The development of a new "soft ionization" method, "fast atom bombardment" (FAB), opened a completely new window into the analysis of natural compounds by using mass spectrometry (MS) (Barber et al., 1981). It became the most widely used technique in the 1980s and early 1990s and allowed ionization of nonvolatile compounds such as native or derivatized oligosaccharides, glycolipids, or peptides. The establishment of a FAB-MS instrument equipped with a newly developed high-field magnet sponsored by the Deutsche Forschungsgemeinschaft enabled the group of H. Egge in Bonn to successfully continue the structural analysis of HMOs, glycosphingolipids with blood group activity, and gangliosides. Thus, the strong history of the institute in Bonn in the search for the "bifidus factor" with Fritz Zilliken (former collaborator with Kuhn at the Max-Planck-Institute in Heidelberg and György in Philadelphia and director of the Bonn Institute between 1969 and 1986) could be continued in close collaboration with Nicolay, whose work was at that time focused on *Bifidobacteria* (György et al., 1974)

With the aid of FAB-MS, structural data could be obtained, especially of permethylated samples of oligosaccharides or glycolipids concerning molecular weight; number of sugar molecules in terms of hexoses, deoxyhexoses, and aminohexoses; sequence of sugar moieties; and in part by secondary fragment information on linkage points. In view, however, of the complexity of carbohydrate structures, a consequence of the multifunctional sugar building blocks, additional methods had to be applied for a complete structural elucidation. Here, the development of high-resolution nuclear magnetic resonance instruments operating at 500 MHz proved to be invaluable. Thanks to the cooperativity of Heinz Staab, director at the Max-Planck-Institute in Heidelberg, a close collaboration could be established with J. and U. Dabrowski, then working at the Max-Planck-Institute. This collaboration, also with P. Hanfland, resulted in a number of publications that became classics for glycosphingolipid analysis (Egge und Hanfland, 1981; Egge et al., 1982, 1983, 1984, 1985; Dabrowski et al., 1983; Hanfland et al., 1986; Egge and Katalinic, 1987). Compared with conventional methods of the determination of carbohydrate constituents, this method was highly reliable, sensitive, and specific. It allowed an exact determination of the molecular composition and the analysis of mixtures not resolved by chromatographic methods. Since the determinations could be performed with microgram quantities of substance, it was the method of choice.

6. FINAL REMARKS

This short review on the development of HMO research ends in the 1980s. However, there is a continuing strong fascination with these components, which are – together with other structures – the reason for the special character of human milk. It is impressive how clearly 50 years ago many of the HMOs could be characterized by classic analytical methods and functions like the influence of microbial composition or the effects on the immune system have been investigated. These main areas of research are still given top priority. We would like to stress that apart from the mentioned personalities who have influenced HMO research substantially, there are numerous other authors not mentioned who have also made important contributions leading to our present knowledge of HMOs.

This brief review ends with a quote from Jean Montreuil: "History demonstrates the importance of the knowledge of the primary structure to approach the metabolism, molecular biology and mechanisms of the biological activity of HMO. Only the collaboration of scientists belonging to different domains allows one to solve the problems" (Montreuil, 1992).

REFERENCES

Barber, M., Bordoli, R.S., Sedgwick, R.D., Tyler, A.N., 1981. Fast atom bombardment of solids as an ion source in mass spectrometry. Nature 293, 270–275.

Barness, L.A., Tomarelli, R.M., György, P., 1979. 1893–1976. A biographical sketch. Journal of Nutrition 109, 17–23.

Bratosin, D., Mignot, C., 2011. In memoriam Professor Emeritus Jean Montreul (1920–2010). A lifetime dedicated to the progress of science and education. Clinical Cytometry B 80, 69–70.

Dabrowski, U., Egge, H., Dabrowski, J., 1983. Proton-nuclear magnetic resonance study of peracetylated derivatives of ten oligosaccharides isolated from human milk. Archives of Biochemistry and Biophysics 224, 254–260.

Egge, H., Hanfland, P., 1981. Immunochemistry of the Lewis-blood-group system: mass spectrometric analysis of permethylated Le(a)-, Le(b)-, and H-type 1 (LedH) blood-group active and related glycosphingolipids from human plasma. Archives of Biochemistry and Biophysics 210, 396–404.

Egge, H., Peter-Katalinic, J., 1987. Fast atom bombardment mass spectrometry for the structural elucidation of glycoconjugates. Mass Spectrometry Reviews 6, 331–393.

Egge, H., Dabrowski, J., Hanfland, P., Dell, A., Dabrowski, U., 1982. High resolution 1H nuclear magnetic resonance spectroscopy and 'soft ionization' mass spectrometry of glycosphingolipids. Advances in Experimental Medicine and Biology 152, 33–34.

Egge, H., Dell, A., von Nicolai, H., 1983. Fucose containing oligosaccharides from human milk. I. Separation and identification of new constituents. Archives of Biochemistry and Biophysics 224, 235–253.

Egge, H., Dabrowski, J., Hanfland, P., 1984. Structural analysis of blood-group ABH, I, I, Lewis and related glycosphingolipids. Application of FAB mass spectrometry and high resolution proton NMR. Pure and Applied Chemistry 56, 807–8019.

Egge, H., Peter-Katalinić, J., Reuter, G., Schauer, R., Ghidoni, R., Sonnino, S., Tettamanti, G., 1985. Analysis of gangliosides using fast atom bombardment mass spectrometry. Chemistry and Physics of Lipids 37, 127–141.

Egge, H., 1992. The diversity of oligosaccharides in human milk. In: Renner, B., Sawatzki, G. (Eds.), New Perspectives in Infant Nutrition. Georg Thieme Verlag, Stuttgart, New York, pp. 12–26.

Escherich, T., 1886. Die Darmbakterien des Säuglings und ihre Beziehungen zur Physiologie der Verdauung. Enke Verlag, Stuttgart.

Grimmonprez, L., Montreuil, J., 1977. Etude des fractions glycanniques des glycosphingolipides totaux de la membrane des globules lipidiques du lait de Femme. Biochemie 59, 899–907.

Grollmann, E.F., Ginsburg, V., 1967. Correlation between secretor status and the occurrence of 2′-fucosyllactose in human milk. Biochemical and Biophysical Research Communications 28, 50–53.

György, P., Jeanloz, R.W., von Nicolay, H., Zilliken, F., 1974. Undialysable growth factors for *Lactobacillus bifidus var. pennsylvanicus*. European Journal of Biochemistry 43, 29–33.

György, P., Norris, R.F., Rose, C.S., 1954. Bifidus factor I: a variant of *Lactobacillus bifidus* requiring a special growth factor. Archives of Biochemistry and Biophysics 48, 193–201.

György, P., 1953. A hitherto unrecognized biochemical difference between human milk and cow's milk. Journal of Pediatrics 11, 98–108.

Hanfland, P., Kordowicz, M., Peter-Katalinic, J., Pfannschmidt, G., Crawford, R.J., Graham, H.A., Egge, H., 1986. Immunochemistry of the Lewis blood-group system: isolation and structures of Lewis-c active and related glycosphingolipids from the plasma of blood-group O Le(a-b-) nonsecretors. Archives of Biochemistry and Biophysics 246, 655–672.

Helmholtz, H.F., 1933. Festschrift Adalbert Czerny – an appreciation. Journal of Pediatrics 3, 5–6.

Kjeldahl, J., 1883. Neue Methode zur Bestimmung des Stickstoffs in organischen Körpern. Zeitschrift für Analytische Chemie 22, 366–382.

Kobata, A., 2000. A journey to the world of glycobiology. Glycoconj Journal 17, 443–464.

Kobata, A., 2003. Possible application of milk oligosaccharides for drug development. The Chang Gung Medical Journal 26, 620–636.

Kuhn, R., Baer, H.H., 1956. Die Konstitution der Lacto-*N*-tetraose. Chemische Berichte 89, 504–511.

Kuhn, R., Brossmer, R., 1956. Über die O-Acetyl-lactamin-säure-lactose aus Kuh-Colostrum und ihre Spaltbarkeit durch Influenza-Virus. Chemische Berichte 98, 2013–2035.

Kuhn, R., 1957. Aminozucker. Angewandte Chemie 69, 23–33.

Kuhn, R., 1958. Les oligosaccharides du lait. Bulletin de la Société de Chimie Biologique 40, 297–314.

Liebig, J., 1866. Suppe für Säuglinge. Friedrich Vieweg und Sohn, Braunschweig.

Montreuil, J., 1960. Les glucides du lait. Bulletin de la Société de Chimie Biologique 42, 1399–1440.

Montreuil, J., 1992. The saga of human milk gynolactose. In: Renner, B., Sawatzki, G. (Eds.), New Perspectives in Infant Nutrition. Georg Thieme Verlag, Stuttgart, New York, pp. 3–11.

Moro, E., 1900. Über den *Bacillus acidophilus* n. spec. Ein Beitrag zur Kenntnis der normalen Darmbakterien des Säuglings. Jahrbuch Kinderheilkunde 52, 38–55.

Nützenadel, W., 2010. Des Kindes Ernährung – Ein Rückblick in Entwicklung und Perspektiven der Kinder-und Jugendmedizin. In: Hoffmann, G.F., Eckart, W.U., Osten, P. (Eds.), 150 Jahre Pädiatrie in Heidelberg. Kirchheim Verlag, Mainz, pp. 191–209.

Polonowski, M., Lespagnol, A., 1929. Sur la nature glucidique de la substance lévogyre du lait de Femme. Bulletin de la Société de Chimie Biologique 101, 61–63.

Polonowski, M., Lespagnol, A., 1931. Sur deux nouveaux sucres du lait de femme, le gynolactose et l'allolactose. Comptes Rendu de l' Académie de Science 192, 1319.

Polonowski, M., Montreuil, J., 1954. Etude chromatographique des polyosides du lait de Femme. Comptes Rendu de l'Académie de Science 238, 2263–2264.

Rubner, M., 1889. Ein Calorimeter für physiologische und hygienische Zwecke. Zeitschrift für Biologie 25, 400–426.

Schönfeld, H., 1926. Über die Beziehungen der einzelnen Bestandteile der Frauenmilch zur Bifidusflora. Jahrbuch der Kinderheilkunde 113, 19–60.

Tissier, H., 1900. Recherches sur la flore intestinale des nourrissons (état normal et pathologique). G. Carre and C. Naud, Paris, France.

von Voit, C., 1881. Physiologie des allgemeinen Stoffwechsels und der Ernährung. Hermanns Handbuch der Physiologie. 6. Leipzig.

Watkins, W.M., 1966. Blood group specific substances. In: Gottschalk, A. (Ed.), Glycoproteins. Elsevier, Amsterdam, pp. 462–515.

Weirich, A., Hoffmann, G.F., 2005. Moro, E. (1874–1951) – a great pediatric career started at the rise of university-based pediatric research but was curtailed in the shadows of Nazi laws. European Journal of Pediatrics 164, 599–606.

Westphal, O., 1968. Richard Kuhn zum Gedächtnis. Angewandte Chemie 80, 501–540.

Wiegand, H., Egge, H., 1970. Progress in the Chemistry of Organic Natural Products XXVIII. Springer Verlag.

CHAPTER

Structures, Classification, and Biosynthesis of Human Milk Oligosaccharides

2

Akira Kobata
The Noguchi Institute, Tokyo, Japan

ABBREVIATIONS

6S 6-SO_4
A enzyme D-galactose α-3-*N*-acetylgalactosaminyltransferase
Fuc L-fucose
Gal D-galactose
GalNAc *N*-acetyl-D-galactosamine
Glc D-glucose
GlcNAc *N*-acetyl-D-glucosamine
Neu5Ac *N*-acetyl-neuraminic acid
Type I chain Galβ1-3GlcNAcβ1-
Type II chain Galβ1-4GlcNAcβ1-
β3GalT D-*N*-acetylglucosamine β-3-galactosyltransferase
β4GalT D-*N*-acetylglucosamine β-4-galactosyltransferase

Human milk contains various oligosaccharides, which are generically named human milk oligosaccharide (HMO). As described in detail in Chapter 1 of this book, many HMOs were found to serve as prebiotics, working as growth-promoting factor for *Bifidobacteria* and named Bifidus factor.

It has been known since 1900 that the feces of breast-fed babies are more acidic than those of artificially nourished babies (Tissier, 1900; Moro, 1900). This is because *Lactobacillus bifidus*, which digests lactose and produces large amounts of lactic acid and acetic acid, becomes a predominant intestinal flora of babies fed with human milk. The acidic condition in the large intestine of babies suppresses the growth of many other microorganisms and may protect babies from harmful intestinal infection (Grulee et al., 1935).

Structures of 14 HMOs were elucidated until 1965 as summarized in Table 2.1 via independent studies of Kuhn's group at the Max Planck Institute in Heidelberg, Germany, and of Montreuil's group in Lille, France.

Prebiotics and Probiotics in Human Milk. http://dx.doi.org/10.1016/B978-0-12-802725-7.00002-6

Table 2.1 Structures of Human Milk Oligosaccharides Found Up to 1965

Oligosaccharide Name	Structure	References
2'-Fucosyllactose (2'-FL)	Galβ1-4Glc 2 Fucα1	Kuhn et al. (1956a)
3-Fucosyllactose (3-FL)	Galβ1-4Glc 3 Fucα1	Montreuil (1956)
Lactodifucotetraose (LD)	Galβ1-4Glc 2 3 Fucα1 Fucα1	Kuhn and Gauhe (1958)
Lacto-*N*-tetraose (LNT)	Galβ1-3GlcNAcβ1-3Galβ1-4Glc	Kuhn and Baer (1956)
Lacto-*N*-*neo*-tetraose (LNnT)	Galβ1-4GlcNAcβ1-3Galβ1-4Glc	Kuhn and Gauhe (1962a)
Lacto-*N*-fucopentaose I (LNF-I)	Galβ1-3GlcNAcβ1-3Galβ1-4Glc 2 Fucα1	Kuhn et al. (1956b)
Lacto-*N*-fucopentaose II (LNF-II)	Galβ1-3GlcNAcβ1-3Galβ1-4Glc 4 Fucα1	Kuhn et al. (1958a)
Lacto-*N*-difucohexaose I (LND-I)	Galβ1-3GlcNAcβ1-3Galβ1-4Glc 2 4 Fucα1 Fucα1	Kuhn et al. (1958b)
Lacto-*N*-difucohexaose II (LND-II)	Galβ1-3GlcNAcβ1-3Galβ1-4Glc 4 3 Fucα1 Fucα1	Kuhn and Gauhe (1960)
3'-Sialyllactose (3'-SL)	Galβ1-4Glc 3 Neu5Acα2	Kuhn and Brossmer (1959)
6'-Sialyllactose (6'-SL)	Galβ1-4Glc 6 Neu5Acα2	Kuhn (1959)
LST-a	Galβ1-3GlcNAcβ1-3Galβ1-4Glc 3 Neu5Acα2	Kuhn and Gauhe (1965)
LST-b	Galβ1-3GlcNAcβ1-3Galβ1-4Glc 6 Neu5Acα2	Kuhn and Gauhe (1965)
LST-c	Galβ1-4GlcNAcβ1-3Galβ1-4Glc 6 Neu5Acα2	Kuhn and Gauhe (1962b)

All these oligosaccharides contain lactose at their reducing termini.

An interesting finding was that some of these oligosaccharides showed haptenic activities of human blood group determinants (Kuhn and Gauhe, 1960; Watkins, 1966): 2′-FL and LNF-I showed haptenic activity of the H determinant, LNF-II showed activity of the Le^a determinant, and LND-I showed activity of the Le^b determinant. These findings of HMOs significantly contributed to the elucidation of the structures of the H and the Lewis blood group determinants (Watkins, 1972).

1. FINDING OF THE MISSING PHENOMENA OF FUCOSYLATED OLIGOSACCHARIDES IN RELATION TO THE BLOOD TYPES OF MILK DONORS

In 1967, Grollman and Ginsburg found evidence that 2′-FL was missing in the milk samples obtained from mothers with nonsecretor blood type. The nonsecretor mothers express ABO blood group antigens on the surface of their erythrocytes according to their genetic background of the ABO locus but not on the glycoproteins, secreted from the epithelial cells of mucous glands.

Kobata et al. (1969) devised a new technique to obtain oligosaccharide patterns by using a small amount of milk samples. The method was the combination of gel filtration and paper chromatography. This method enabled them to "fingerprint" the 14 oligosaccharides in Table 2.1 by using approximately 10 mL of milk samples, as shown in Fig. 2.1A.

Interestingly, evidence revealed by the analysis of the milk samples obtained from 50 individuals was that three different oligosaccharide patterns were obtained via this analytical method. Approximately 80% of the milk samples gave the spots of all 14 oligosaccharides, as shown in Fig, 2.1A. In contrast, approximately 15% of the milk samples gave the oligosaccharide pattern shown in Fig. 2.1B. The characteristic feature of this pattern is that four oligosaccharides (2′-FL, LD, LNF-I, and LND-I) are missing as shown by the spots indicated by dotted lines in the pattern. The small gray spots, detected at the positions of the missing oligosaccharides, are minor oligosaccharides hidden under the major oligosaccharides. Written in white letters are the names assigned to the newly found minor oligosaccharides. Important evidence was that all mothers whose milk gave this oligosaccharide pattern were nonsecretors who express neither ABH blood group determinants nor Le^b determinant in their secretory glycoproteins.

The structures of the four missing oligosaccharides indicated that the missing phenomenon, found in 2′-FL by Grollman and Ginsburg, can be extended to all milk oligosaccharides containing the Fucα1-2Gal group of nonsecretor individuals. Namely, the secretory organ of nonsecretor individuals should lack the fucosyltransferase responsible for formation of the Fucα1-2Gal group.

The remaining 5% of the milk samples gave the oligosaccharide pattern as shown in Fig. 2.1C. The characteristic feature of this pattern is that the three oligosaccharides, shown by dotted lines, are missing in the pattern. Like in the case of nonsecretors, three new minor oligosaccharides were found as shown by the small gray spots in Fig. 2.1C. Examination of the blood types of the donors whose milk gave this pattern revealed that they are all Lewis negative and lacked both Le^a and Le^b antigens in their secretory glycoproteins and glycolipids on their erythrocytes.

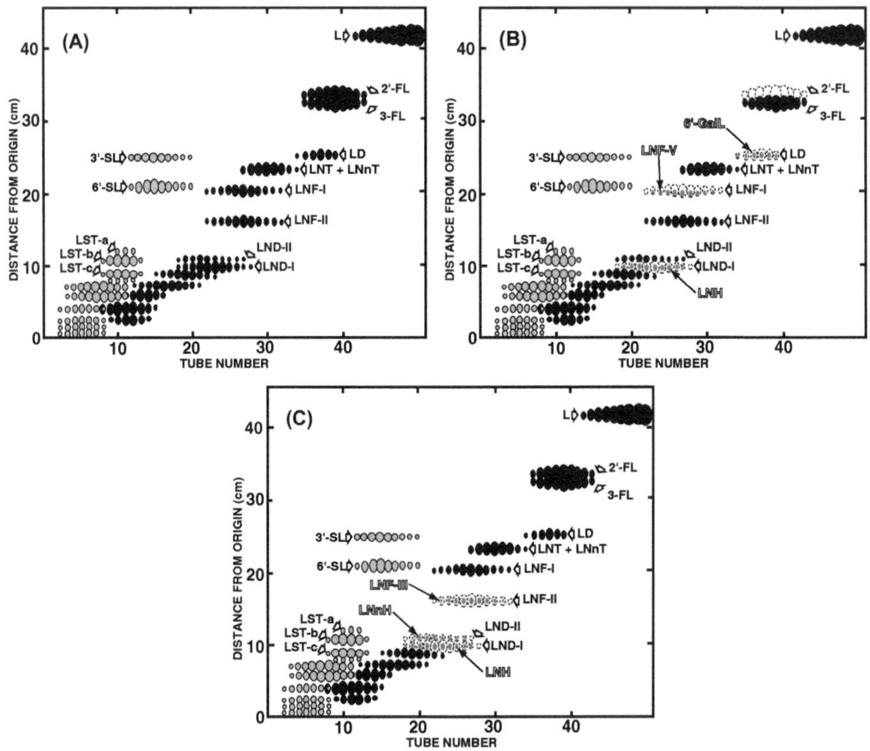

FIGURE 2.1

Three typical fingerprinting patterns obtained from the oligosaccharide fractions of human milk sample, collected from a single mother, are shown. The fraction numbers as indicated by "TUBE NUMBER" in abscissa were obtained by Sephadex G-25 column chromatography of human milk oligosaccharide fraction. Aliquot of the fractions were spotted at the origin of a sheet of a filter paper, and subjected to chromatography using ethylacetate/pyridine/acetic acid/water (5:5:1:3) as a solvent. Black spots represent oligosaccharides visualized by alkaline-$AgNO_3$ reagent, and hatched ones encircled by black lines represent those detected by both alkaline-$AgNO_3$ reagent and thiobarbituric acid reagent. Spots shown by dotted lines were missing in the pattern. Gray spots detected at the positions of missing oligosaccharides are minor oligosaccharides hidden under the major oligosaccharides. (A) the pattern obtained from milk samples of Le^{a+b+} individuals; (B) the pattern obtained from milk samples of Le^{a+b-} (nonsecretor) individuals; (C) the pattern obtained from milk samples of Le^{a-b-} individuals.

Revised from the figure in Glycoconjugate Journal 17, 443–464 (2000) with kind permission from Springer Science+Business Media.

A common feature of the three oligosaccharides missing in the milk of Lewis-negative individuals is that they all contain the Fucα1-4GlcNAc group. Based on this finding, it was concluded that another fucosyltransferase, which is responsible for formation of the Fucα1-4GlcNAc group, is not expressed in the epithelial cells of the secretory organ of the Lewis-negative individuals.

These estimations of missing phenomena of two fucosyltransferases of nonsecretor and Lewis-negative individuals were later confirmed through enzymatic studies (Shen et al., 1968; Grollman et al., 1969)

Although not confirmed at those times, it was easily estimated that six oligosaccharides—2′-FL, LD, LNF-I, LNF-II, LND-I, and LND-II—should be missing in the milk obtained from a nonsecretor and Lewis-negative mother. This estimation was confirmed by Thurl et al. (1997).

2. ENZYMES RESPONSIBLE FOR THE FORMATION OF A AND B BLOOD GROUP DETERMINANTS

Although oligosaccharides containing the blood group determinant A [GalNAcα1-3(Fucα1-2)Gal] or B [Galα1-3(Fucα1-2)Gal] were not included among the milk oligosaccharides listed in Table 2.1, the finding of the close correlation of the oligosaccharide deletion phenomena in milk and the blood type background of the donors led to an investigation of the glycosyltransferases in milk, which are related to the biosynthesis of blood group determinants. It was already reported that a large amount of the β-galactosyltransferase (D-*N*-acetylglucosamine β-4-galactosyltransferase [β4GalT]), responsible for the formation of *N*-acetyllactosamine group in the epithelial cells of the mammary gland, is secreted as a soluble form in milk (Brodbeck and Ebner, 1966). This evidence suggested that other glycosyltransferases of the epithelial cells of the mammary gland might also be excreted in soluble forms in milk. Actually, the α-fucosyltransferase responsible for formation of the Fucα1-2Gal group did exist in the milk of secretors but not in the milk of nonsecretors (Shen et al., 1968), and another α-fucosyltransferase responsible for formation of the Fucα1-4GlcNAc group did exist in the milk obtained from Lewis-positive individuals but not in the milk of Lewis-negative individuals (Grollman et al., 1969).

When UDP-[^{14}C]GalNAc was incubated with a mixture of HMOs and defatted milk obtained from a woman with blood type A, two radioactive oligosaccharides were produced in the presence of Mn^{2+}. Incubation with each purified milk oligosaccharide revealed that 2′-FL and LNF-I work as acceptors of the [^{14}C]*N*-acetylgalactosamine residue (Kobata et al., 1968a). Other milk oligosaccharides, so far known, could not accept the radioactive *N*-acetylgalactosamine. This evidence strongly suggested that the oligosaccharides containing the Fucα1-2Gal group at their nonreducing termini became acceptors of the newly found *N*-acetylgalactosaminyltransferase, which is probably responsible for formation of the blood group A determinant. Accordingly, synthesis of radioactive oligosaccharides from 2′-FL by using many milk samples obtained from individuals of different blood types were investigated. Milk samples obtained from women of blood type A or AB all showed the enzymatic activity needed to form the radioactive oligosaccharide from 2′-FL. However, none of the milk samples obtained from donors of blood type B or O showed the enzymatic activity (Kobata et al., 1968b). Important evidence is that the milk samples from nonsecretor individuals of blood type A showed the enzymatic activity at almost the same level as secretor individuals. This evidence indicated that the absence of the blood type A antigenic determinant in the glycoproteins, secreted by the epithelial cells of nonsecretor individuals, takes place not because they lack the α-*N*-acetylgalactosaminyltransferase in the epithelial cells of their secretory glands but because the cells lack the fucosyltransferase responsible for formation of the Fucα1-2Gal group, which is an essential substrate for the α-*N*-acetylgalactosaminyltransferase. The distribution of the enzyme activity, in addition to its acceptor specificity, indicated that the α-*N*-acetylgalactosaminyltransferase found in milk actually forms the blood group A determinant—GalNAcα1-3(Fucα1-2)Gal—and was named A enzyme (Kobata and Ginsburg, 1970). Because LD and LND-I cannot become the acceptor of the A enzyme, the presence of α-fucosyl residue on the adjoining monosaccharide sterically inhibits the action of A enzyme.

By using the same assay system but replacing UDP-[^{14}C]GalNAc with UDP-[^{14}C]Gal, an α-galactosyltransferase activity, which adds a galactose residue to the C-3 position of the galactose residue of the Fucα1-2Gal group of 2′-FL and LNF-I, was also detected in the milk samples obtained from blood type B and AB donors but not in milk from those from other blood types (Kobata et al., 1968b). A nonsecretor with blood type B exhibited the enzyme activity, indicating that the absence of blood type B antigenic determinant in blood type B nonsecretors is induced by the same mechanism as in the case of blood type A nonsecretors.

3. OCCURRENCE OF TWO OLIGOSACCHARIDES CONTAINING THE BLOOD GROUP A DETERMINANT IN HUMAN MILK

As described, A enzyme, purified from defatted milk obtained from blood type A individuals, adds the GalNAcα1-3 residue to the Galβ1-residue of 2′-FL and LNF-I. The structures of these enzymatic products were elucidated as P_I and P_{II} in Fig. 2.2A, respectively (Kobata and Ginsburg, 1970).

That both oligosaccharides have the haptenic activity of blood type A was confirmed in the study of Kobata and Ginsburg (1970). To 0.3 mL of anti-A antiserum, 50 μL of phosphate-buffered saline containing varying amounts of P_I or P_{II} was added. After being left for 15 min at room temperature, 5 μg of soluble blood group substance A was added, and incubation was continued for 30 min at 37°C and then left overnight at 4°C. The incubation mixtures were then centrifuged for 15 min at 10,000 rpm. The supernatant solutions were decanted, and the precipitates were washed twice with 0.3-mL aliquots of cold phosphate-buffered saline and recentrifuged. The protein contents of the precipitates were then determined colorimetrically. As shown in Fig. 2.2B, the two oligosaccharides showed almost the same haptenic activity of blood type A on a molecular basis.

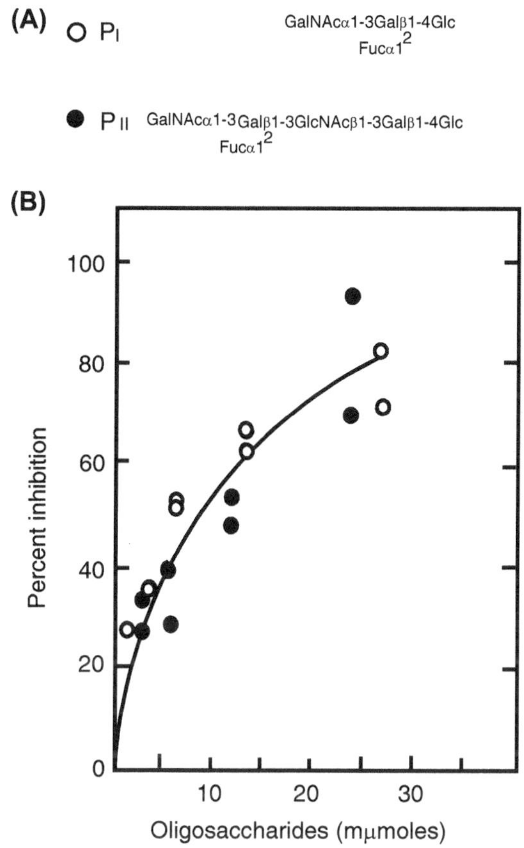

FIGURE 2.2

(A) Structures of oligosaccharides P_I and P_{II} formed by the addition of *N*-acetylgalactosamine to 2′-FL and LNF-I by A enzyme, respectively and (B) inhibition of blood group substance A, anti-A precipitin reaction by oligosaccharides P_I and P_{II}. *(Fig. B was taken from Kobata, A., Ginsburg, V., 1970).*

Whether P_I and P_{II} actually occur in human milk was investigated by measuring the haptenic activities of oligosaccharide fractions (Kobata and Ginsburg, 1970). The oligosaccharide fractions, obtained from the milk of donors with various blood types, were fingerprinted by a combination of gel-permeation and paper chromatography, and the oligosaccharides at the area of P_I and P_{II} were recovered by elution with water. The haptenic activities of the two eluates were tested by the same method described for P_I and P_{II}, and the amounts of inhibitors were estimated from the curve shown in Fig. 2.2B. It was confirmed that only the oligosaccharide fractions, obtained from individuals of blood type A or AB who were secretors, showed the presence of both P_I and P_{II}. Milk samples from a blood type A or AB nonsecretor and from those of other blood types did not contain P_I and P_{II}. The amounts of both haptenic oligosaccharides, as measured by using the data of Fig. 2.2B, varied by individual from as low as 0.2 μmol up to 13 μmol per mL of milk (Kobata and Ginsburg, 1970). These values are from one-hundredth to one-thousandth the amounts of LNT and LNF-I.

4. BIOSYNTHETIC PATHWAY OF THE ABO AND LEWIS BLOOD GROUP DETERMINANTS

Based on the oligosaccharide patterns and the enzymatic studies, the biosynthetic schema of blood group A, B, H, Le^a, and Le^b determinants were elucidated as shown in Fig. 2.3 (Grollman et al., 1970).

In the mucous epithelial cells of nonsecretor individuals, the Fucα1-2Gal group is not formed on the sugar chains of their secretory glycoproteins, because H enzyme in Fig. 2.3 is not expressed. Because the Fucα1-2Gal group, formed by the action of the fucosyltransferase, is the substrate of A and B enzymes, blood group A and B determinants could not be expressed in the sugar chains of the secretory glycoproteins of nonsecretor individuals, even if they have *A* and

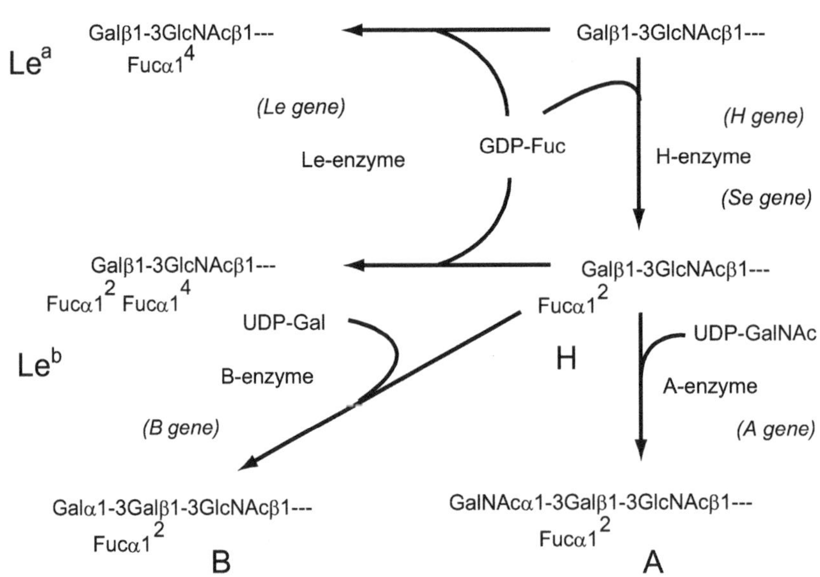

FIGURE 2.3

Biosynthetic pathway of ABO and Lewis blood group determinants.

The figure was slightly modified from that in Glycoconjugate Journal 17, 443–464 (2000) with kind permission from Springer Science+Business Media.

B genes. Expression of *H* gene, the structural gene for H enzyme, in mucous epithelial cells was originally considered to be regulated by *Se* gene (Grollman et al., 1970).

However, a gene cloning study by Ball et al. (1991) indicated that *Se* gene is also a structural gene that codes for H enzyme specifically in the secretory organs.

The *Le* gene is the structural gene of Le enzyme in Fig. 2.3. Therefore, individuals who are of *le, le* genotype lack both Le^a and Le^b antigenic determinants.

The sugar chain containing the structures of both A blood group determinant and Le^b determinant was reported to occur in the blood group substances purified from ovarian cysts by Lloyd et al. (1968). Because LND-I is not an acceptor for A enzyme as already described, Le^b determinant cannot be an acceptor for the A enzyme despite having the essential Fucα1-2Gal group. Therefore, sugar chains containing the two determinants can only be made from H determinant by the sequential action of A enzyme and then Le enzyme (Fig. 2.4).

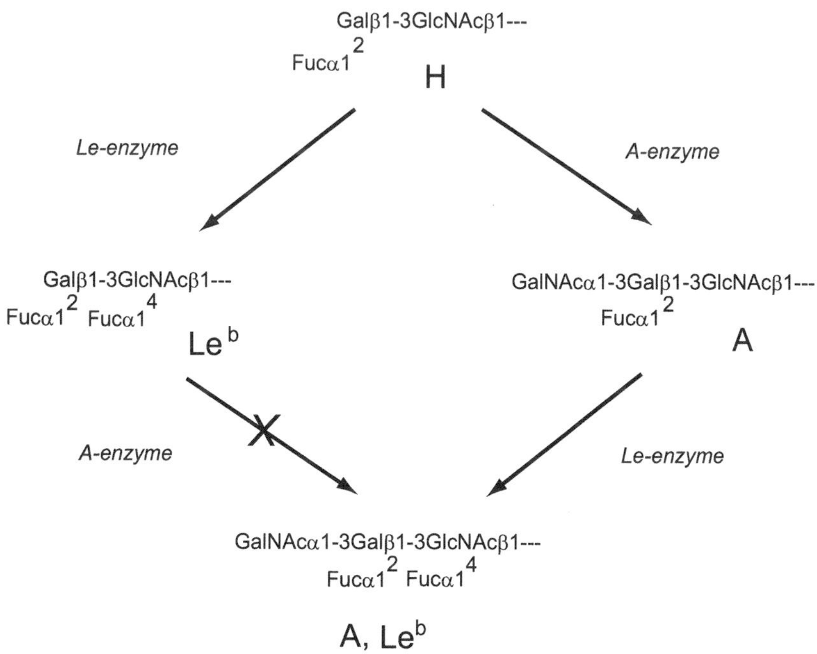

FIGURE 2.4

Biosynthetic scheme to produce A, Le^b structure.

Taken from Chang Gung Medical Journal 26: 621–635, 2003 with kind permission from Dr. Fu-Chan Wei, Editor-in-Chief.

5. STRUCTURAL CHARACTERIZATION OF NOVEL MINOR OLIGOSACCHARIDES ISOLATED FROM THE MILK OF NONSECRETOR OR LEWIS-NEGATIVE INDIVIDUALS

The structures of novel minor oligosaccharides, indicated by white letters in Fig. 2.1B and C, were subsequently elucidated as shown in Table 2.2. Among them, LNF-III has been used to clarify the role of Le^x, which is a selectin ligand, in studies on the homing of lymphocyte and migration of cancer cells through blood vessels (Fenderson et al., 1984), while LNH and LN*n*H have been useful in structural studies of branched-type ABH antigens (Yamashita et al., 1976a, 1977a).

Before the structures of these oligosaccharides had been characterized, it was thought that lactose, LNT, and LN*n*T were core units of HMO as shown in Table 2.3.

Now, LNH and LN*n*H were newly added as additional cores, and their fucosyl and sialyl derivatives were found as well (Tables 2.4 and 2.5). The structures of oligosaccharides in Table 2.4 silhouette several interesting structural rules. The Fucα1-2Gal group is not evenly distributed to the two Galβ1-GlcNAc groups of the branched arms of LNH but rather is limited to the arm extending from C-3 position of the branching Gal.

Finding of the Fucα1-3Gal group in a fucosylated LNH deserves special comment. This group is limited to the type II chain (Galβ1-4GlcNAc), in contrast to the Fucα1-2Gal group. Many fucosyltransferases have been cloned in recent years (Taniguchi et al., 2002). However, no enzyme to catalyze the formation of the Fucα1-3Gal group has been reported yet. The finding of the Fucα1-3Gal group in one of the lacto-*N*-hexaose derivatives indicates the possibility of its occurrence in the carbohydrate chains of blood group substances. It also predicts the occurrence of another novel fucosyltransferase.

Table 2.2 Novel Oligosaccharides Isolated From Milk of Nonsecretor and Lewis-Negative Individuals

Name	Structure	References
6'-Galactosyllactose (6'-GalL)	Galβ1-6Galβ1-4Glc	Yamashita and Kobata (1974)
Lacto-*N*-fucopentaose V (LNF-V)	Galβ1-3GlcNAcβ1-3Galβ1-4Glc 3 Fucα1	Ginsburg et al. (1976)
Lacto-*N*-fucopentaose III (LNF-III)	Galβ1-4GlcNAcβ1-3Galβ1-4Glc 3 Fucα1	Kobata and Ginsburg (1969)
Lacto-*N*-hexaose (LNH)	Galβ1-4GlcNAcβ1 6 Galβ1-4Glc 3 Galβ1-3GlcNAcβ1	Kobata and Ginsburg (1972a)
Lacto-*N*-*neo*-hexaose (LN*n*H)	Galβ1-4GlcNAcβ1 6 Galβ1-4Glc 3 Galβ1-4GlcNAcβ1	Kobata and Ginsburg (1972b)

Table 2.3 Human Milk Oligosaccharides With Lactose, LNT, and LNnT as Cores

Core	Name	Structure	References
Lactose			
	3'-Galactosyllactose (3'-GalL)	Galβ1-3Galβ1-4Glc	Donald and Feeney (1988)
	3-Fucosyl-3' -SL (3F-3' -SL)	Neu5Acα2-3Galβ1-4Glc 3 Fucα1	Grönberg et al. (1989)
LNT			
	Sialyl-LNF-I (S-LNF-I)	Neu5Acα2 6 Fucα1-2Galβ1-3GlcNAcβ1-3Galβ1-4Glc	Wieruszeski et al. (1985)
	Disialyl-LNT (DS-LNT)	Neu5Acα2 6 Neu5Acα2-3Galβ1-3GlcNAcβ1-3Galβ1-4Glc	Grimmonprez and Montreuil (1968)
	Disialyl-LNF-V (DS-LNF-V)	Neu5Acα2 6 Neu5Acα2-3Galβ1-3GlcNAcβ1-3Galβ1-4Glc 3 Fucα1	Grönberg et al. (1990)
LN*n*T			
	Lacto-*N*-*neo*-difucohexaose II (L*n*ND-II)	Galβ1-4GlcNAcβ1-3Galβ1-4Glc 3 3 Fucα1 Fucα1	Donald and Feeney (1988)
	3-Fucosyl-LST c (3F-LST c)	Neu5Acα2-6Galβ1-4GlcNAcβ1-3Galβ1-4Glc 3 Fucα1	Smith et al. (1987)

Table 2.4 Human Milk Oligosaccharides With LNH as a Core (References)

Galβ1-4GlcNAcβ1 6 Galβ1-4Glc Galβ1-3GlcNAcβ1 3 2 Fucα1 (Yamashita et al., 1977a)	Neu5Acα2 6 Galβ1-4GlcNAcβ1 6 Galβ1-4Glc Galβ1-3GlcNAcβ1 3 (Kobata and Ginsburg, 1972a)	Fucα1 3 Galβ1-4GlcNAcβ1 6 Galβ1-4Glc Galβ1-3GlcNAcβ1 3 6 Neu5Acα2 (Grönberg et al., 1992)	Fucα1 3 Galβ1-4GlcNAcβ1 6 Galβ1-4Glc Galβ1-3GlcNAcβ1 3 3 4 Neu5Acα2 Fucα1 (Kitagawa et al., 1989)
Fucα1 3 Galβ1-4GlcNAcβ1 6 Galβ1-4Glc Galβ1-3GlcNAcβ1 3 (Dua et al., 1985)	Neu5Acα2 6 Galβ1-4GlcNAcβ1 6 Galβ1-4Glc Galβ1-3GlcNAcβ1 3 3 Neu5Acα2 (Kitagawa et al., 1993)	Fucα1 3 Galβ1-4GlcNAcβ1 6 Galβ1-4Glc Galβ1-3GlcNAcβ1 3 3 Neu5Acα2 (Grönberg et al., 1992)	Neu5Acα2 6 Galβ1-4GlcNAcβ1 6 Galβ1-4Glc Galβ1-3GlcNAcβ1 3 2 4 Fucα1 Fucα1 (Grönberg et al., 1992)
Fucα1 3 Galβ1-4GlcNAcβ1 6 Galβ1-4Glc Galβ1-3GlcNAcβ1 3 2 Fucα1 (Yamashita et al., 1977a)	Galβ1-4GlcNAcβ1 6 Galβ1-4Glc Galβ1-3GlcNAcβ1 3 3 6 Neu5Acα2 Neu5Acα2 (Kitagawa et al., 1993)	Galβ1-4GlcNAcβ1 6 Galβ1-4Glc Galβ1-3GlcNAcβ1 3 3 4 Neu5Acα2 Fucα1 (Kitagawa et al., 1989)	Fucα1 3 Galβ1-4GlcNAcβ1 6 Galβ1-4Glc Galβ1-3GlcNAcβ1 3 3 6 Neu5Acα2 Neu5Acα2 (Yamashita et al., 1976b)
Fucα1 3 Galβ1-4GlcNAcβ1 6 Galβ1-4Glc Galβ1-3GlcNAcβ1 3 4 Fucα1 (Kobata and Ginsburg, 1972a)	Neu5Acα2 6 Galβ1-4GlcNAcβ1 6 Galβ1-4Glc Galβ1-3GlcNAcβ1 3 3 6 Neu5Acα2 Neu5Acα2 (Fievre et al., 1991)	Neu5Acα2 6 Galβ1-4GlcNAcβ1 6 Galβ1-4Glc Galβ1-3GlcNAcβ1 3 4 Fucα1 (Grönberg et al., 1992)	Fucα1 3 Galβ1-4GlcNAcβ1 6 Galβ1-4Glc Galβ1-3GlcNAcβ1 3 3 6 Neu5Acα2 Neu5Acα2 (Yamashita et al., 1976b)
Fucα1 3 Galβ1-4GlcNAcβ1 6 Galβ1-4Glc Galβ1-3GlcNAcβ1 3 2 4 Fucα1 Fucα1 (Strecker et al., 1992)		Neu5Acα2 6 Galβ1-4GlcNAcβ1 6 Galβ1-4Glc Galβ1-3GlcNAcβ1 3 2 Fucα1 (Yamashita et al., 1977a)	Neu5Acα2 6 Galβ1-4GlcNAcβ1 6 Galβ1-4Glc Galβ1-3GlcNAcβ1 3 3 4 Neu5Acα2 Fucα1 (Kitagawa et al., 1989)

Table 2.5 Human Milk Oligosaccharides With LNnH as a Core

Structure	References
Fucα1 3 Galβ1-4GlcNAcβ1 6 Galβ1-4Glc 3 Galβ1-4GlcNAcβ1 3 Fucα1	Haeuw-Fievre et al. (1993)
Neu5Acα2 6 Galβ1-4GlcNAcβ1 6 Galβ1-4Glc 3 Galβ1-4GlcNAcβ1	Kobata and Ginsburg (1972b)
Galβ1-4GlcNAcβ1 6 Galβ1-4Glc 3 Galβ1-4GlcNAcβ1 6 Neu5Acα2	Tarrago et al. (1988)
Neu5Acα2 6 Galβ1-4GlcNAcβ1 6 Galβ1-4Glc 3 Galβ1-4GlcNAcβ1 6 Neu5Acα2	Grönberg et al. (1990)
Fucα1 3 Galβ1-4GlcNAcβ1 6 Galβ1-4Glc 3 Galβ1-4GlcNAcβ1 6 Neu5Acα2	Grönberg et al. (1989)
Fucα1 2 Fucα1 3 Galβ1-4GlcNAcβ1 6 Galβ1-4Glc 3 Galβ1-4GlcNAcβ1 Neu5Acα2 6	Grönberg et al. (1989)
Neu5Acα2 6(3) Galβ1-4GlcNAcβ1 6 Galβ1-4Glc 3 Galβ1-4GlcNAcβ1 6(3) 3 Neu5Acα2 Fucα1	Yamashita et al. (1976b)

Oligosaccharides containing both Fucα1-2Gal group and sialic acid were detected. It was confirmed that these oligosaccharides could not work as the substrate of A enzyme (Kobata et al., unpublished data). Therefore, sialylation of the sugar chains may inhibit the conversion of H antigen to A antigen.

For the structural studies of these HMOs, many new sensitive analytical techniques, such as tritium labeling (Takasaki and Kobata, 1974), sequential exoglycosidase digestion (Kobata, 1979; Kobata and Takasaki, 1992), and highly sensitive methylation analysis suitable for oligosaccharides, containing amino sugars (Tai et al., 1975), were developed.

6. ADDITIONAL CORE UNITS OF HUMAN MILK OLIGOSACCHARIDES

Having been stimulated by the fact that several HMOs have been used to clarify the relationship between function and structure of sugar moieties of cell surface glycoconjugates, structural studies of higher molecular HMOs were performed.

As summarized in Table 2.6, Kobata's group found four novel core oligosaccharides: *para*-lacto-*N*-hexaose, *para*-lacto-*N*-*neo*-hexaose, lacto-*N*-octaose, and lacto-*N*-*neo*-octaose. In addition, structures of four other core oligosaccharides—*iso*-lacto-*N*-octaose, *para*-lacto-*N*-octaose, lacto-*N*-decaose, and lacto-*N*-*neo*-decaose—were characterized by other groups. The lacto-*N*-*neo*-decaose was not named in the original report but will be provisionally named as such in this review.

As such, 13 core units in total have been found for HMO to date.

All of these core oligosaccharides contain lactose at their reducing termini. Based on this evidence, all HMOs are considered to be produced by the concerted action of glycosyltransferases of epithelial cells of the mammary gland, which are responsible for elongation of the sugar chains of glycoproteins starting from the Galβ1-4GlcNAc group and of the sugar chains of glycolipids starting from the Galβ1-4Glc group in the cells. Namely, by the action of iGnT (Sasaki et al., 1997) on lactose, which is synthesized in a large amount by the action of β4GalT-I and α-lactalbumin, GlcNAcβ1-3Galβ1-4Glc is formed as shown in Fig. 2.5. All linear core oligosaccharides might be formed by the concerted actions of β4GalT (Almeida et al., 1997) and iGnT as shown in the left-hand side of Fig. 2.5. The sugar chains, produced by the concerted action of the two glycosyltransferases, are all *neo*-type, which has only the repeating structures of the Galβ1-4GlcNAcβ1-3 group. However, when the Galβ1-3GlcNAcβ1-3 group is formed by the action of β3GalT (Issiki et al., 1999) instead of β4GalT, extension of the sugar chain might stop there.

Core milk oligosaccharides with branched structures might be produced by the action of IGnT (Ropp et al., 1991) as shown in the right-hand side of Fig. 2.5.

Therefore, 13 core oligosaccharides are formed, as indicated in parentheses in Fig. 2.5.

The 13 core oligosaccharides, thus formed, are further elongated to the fucosylated and/or sialylated oligosaccharides by the actions of fucosyltransferases and/or sialyltransferases. In Table 2.7, all fucosylated *para*-lacto-*N*-hexaose and *para*-lacto-*N*-*neo*-hexaose so far reported are summarized, and in Table 2.8, all sialylated and fucosylated lacto-*N*-octaose, lacto-*N*-*neo*-octaose, and *iso*-lacto-*N*-octaose, reported so far, are summarized.

The addition of fucose and/or sialic acid to the 13 core units can produce a great variety of oligosaccharides. To date, more than 100 structures have been characterized (see Urashima et al., 2011 and Tables 2.1–2.9), and around 200 oligosaccharides

Table 2.6 Various Core Structures Found in Human Milk Oligosaccharides

Name	Structure	References
para-Lacto-*N*-hexaose (*p*LNH)	Galβ1-3GlcNAcβ1-3Galβ1-4GlcNAcβ1-3Galβ1-4Glc	Yamashita et al. (1977b)
para-Lacto-*N*-*neo*-hexaose (pLN*n*H)	Galβ1-4GlcNAcβ1-3Galβ1-4GlcNAcβ1-3Galβ1-4Glc	Yamashita et al. (1977b)
Lacto-*N*-octaose (LNO)	Galβ1-4GlcNAcβ1-3Galβ1-4GlcNAcβ1 6 Galβ1-4Glc Galβ1-3GlcNAcβ1 3	Tachibana et al. (1978)
Lacto-*N*-*neo*-octaose (LN*n*O)	Galβ1-3GlcNAcβ1-3Galβ1-4GlcNAcβ1 6 Galβ1-4Glc Galβ1-4GlcNAcβ1 3	Tachibana et al. (1978)
iso-Lacto-*N*-octaose (*i*LNO)	Galβ1-3GlcNAcβ1-3Galβ1-4GlcNAcβ1 6 Galβ1-4Glc Galβ1-3GlcNAcβ1 3	Strecker et al. (1992)
para-Lacto-*N*-octaose (*p*LNO)	Galβ1-3GlcNAcβ1-3Galβ1-4GlcNAcβ1-3Galβ1-4GlcNAcβ1-3Galβ1-4Glc	Haeuw-Fievre et al. (1993)
Lacto-*N*-decaose (LND)	Galβ1-4GlcNAcβ1 6 3 Galβ1-4GlcNAcβ1 6 Galβ1-3GlcNAcβ1 Galβ1-4Glc 3 Galβ1-3GlcNAcβ1	Bruntz et al. (1988)
Lacto-*N*-*neo*-decaose (LN*n*D)	Galβ1-4GlcNAcβ1 6 3 Galβ1-4GlcNAcβ1 6 Galβ1-4GlcNAcβ1 Galβ1-4Glc 3 Galβ1-3GlcNAcβ1	Amano et al. (2009)

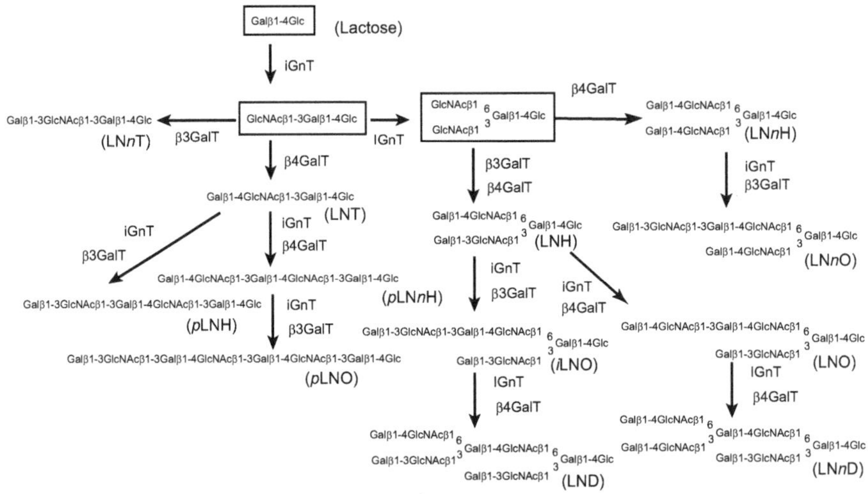

FIGURE 2.5

Biosynthetic pathways leading to various core oligosaccharides from lactose. Thirteen cores are indicated by parentheses.

have been detected by using microfluidic high-performance liquid chromatography (HPLC) chip mass spectrometry as described by Ninonuevo et al. (2006).

Structures of the derivatives of lacto-*N*-decaose and lacto-*N*-*neo*-decaose were not frequently reported. Chai et al. (2005) elucidated the structure of lacto-*N*-decaose and its monofucosylated derivative via electrospray tandem mass spectrometry and ^{1}H nuclear magnetic resonance spectrometry. Recently, Amano et al. (2009) prepared neutral oligosaccharide fraction from milk obtained from a woman with blood type A, Le^{b+} via anion-exchange chromatography. Further fractionation was performed via affinity chromatography by using an *Aleuria aurantia* lectin (AAL)-Sepharose column and reverse–phase HPLC after labeling with a pyrene derivative. This pyrene labeling allowed identification by negative-MALDI-TOFMS^{n} analysis of 22 oligosaccharides with decaose cores as listed in Table 2.9. Mono-, di-, tri-, and tetrafucosylated decaose fractions obtained via AAL-Sepharose column chromatography contained three, nine, six, and four isomers, respectively. Among the 22 oligosaccharides, the monofucosylated lacto-*N*-decaose reported by Chai et al. (2005) was included.

It can be expected that further novel oligosaccharides will be characterized using advances in mass spectrometry. Although only one tetrafucosyl derivative of *para*-lacto-*N*-octaose has been characterized so far (Haeuw-Fievre et al., 1993), additional fucosyl or sialyl derivatives of this core oligosaccharide will be characterized in the near future.

7. FUTURE PROSPECTS

Because of the mechanisms of biosynthesis so far described, HMOs print out part of the structures of the sugar chains of glycoconjugates of the epithelial cells. The sugar

Table 2.7 Human Milk Oligosaccharides Containing *para*-Lacto-*N*-hexaose (*para*-LNH) and *para*-Lacto-*N*-*neo*-hexaose (*para*-LN*n*H) as Cores

Core	Structure	References
***para*-LNH**		
	Galβ1-3GlcNAcβ1-3Galβ1-4GlcNAcβ1-3Galβ1-4Glc 3 Fucα1	Bruntz et al. (1988)
	Galβ1-3GlcNAcβ1-3Galβ1-4GlcNAcβ1-3Galβ1-4Glc 4 Fucα1	Bruntz et al. (1988)
	Galβ1-3GlcNAcβ1-3Galβ1-4GlcNAcβ1-3Galβ1-4Glc 4 Fucα1 Fucα1 3	Yamashita et al. (1977b)
	Galβ1-3GlcNAcβ1-3Galβ1-4GlcNAcβ1-3Galβ1-4Glc 2 4 3 Fucα1 Fucα1 Fucα1	Strecker et al. (1988)
	Galβ1-3GlcNAcβ1-3Galβ1-4GlcNAcβ1-3Galβ1-4Glc 4 3 3 Fucα1 Fucα1 Fucα1	Bruntz et al. (1988)
	6S I Galβ1-3GlcNAcβ1-3Galβ1-4GlcNAcβ1-3Galβ1-4Glc 2 3 Fucα1 Fucα1	Guerardel et al. (1999)
	6S I Galβ1-3GlcNAcβ1-3Galβ1-4GlcNAcβ1-3Galβ1-4Glc 4 3 Fucα1 Fucα1	Guerardel et al. (1999)
	6S I Galβ1-3GlcNAcβ1-3Galβ1-4GlcNAcβ1-3Galβ1-4Glc 2 4 3 Fucα1 Fucα1 Fucα1	Guerardel et al. (1999)
***para*-LN*n*H**		
	Galβ1-4GlcNAcβ1-3Galβ1-4GlcNAcβ1-3Galβ1-4Glc 3 3 Fucα1 Fucα1	Yamashita et al. (1977b)
	Galβ1-4GlcNAcβ1-3Galβ1-4GlcNAcβ1-3Galβ1-4Glc 3 3 3 Fucα1 Fucα1 Fucα1	Bruntz et al. (1988)

chains of epithelial glycoconjugates play roles of many recognition phenomena, so some of the HMOs may work as the decoy of these biological phenomena.

Much evidence that indicates virulent enteric bacteria and viruses start infection by binding to particular sugar chains of glycoconjugates on the surface of their target cells was presented recently (Newburg et al., 2005; Hickey, 2012). Therefore, milk oligosaccharides are expected to be useful in inhibiting infection by these bacteria and viruses.

The key to the success of this line of study is how one will be able to develop an effective method to pick up minor but useful oligosaccharides from the mixture of a large number of different milk oligosaccharides. Kitagawa et al. (1988) generated a

Table 2.8 Human Milk Oligosaccharides Containing Lacto-*N*-octaose, Lacto-*N*-*neo*-octaose, and *iso*-Lacto-*N*-octaose as Cores (References)

Lacto-*N*-octaose	***iso*-Lacto-*N*-octaose**
Fucα1 3 Galβ1-4GlcNAcβ1-3Galβ1-4GlcNAcβ1 6 Galβ1-4Glc Galβ1-3GlcNAcβ1 3 (Yamashita et al., 1976c)	Fucα1 3 Galβ1-3GlcNAcβ1-3Galβ1-4GlcNAcβ1 6 Galβ1-4Glc Galβ1-3GlcNAcβ1 3 (Kogelberg et al., 2004)
Fucα1 3 Fucα1 3 Galβ1-4G cNAcβ1-3Galβ1-4GlcNAcβ1 6 Galβ1-4Glc Galβ1-3GlcNAcβ1 3 (Tachibana et al., 1978)	Fucα1 4 Fucα1 3 Galβ1-3GlcNAcβ1-3Galβ1-4GlcNAcβ1 6 Galβ1-4Glc Galβ1-3GlcNAcβ1 3 (Strecker et al., 1989)
Fucα1 3 Galβ1-4G cNAcβ1-3Galβ1-4GlcNAcβ1 6 Galβ1-4Glc Galβ1-3GlcNAcβ1 3 4 Fucα1 (Tachibana et al., 1978)	Fucα1 3 Galβ1-3GlcNAcβ1-3Galβ1-4GlcNAcβ1 6 Galβ1-4Glc Galβ1-3GlcNAcβ1 3 2 Fucα1 (Strecker et al., 1989)
Fucα1 3 Fucα1 3 Galβ1-4G cNAcβ1-3Galβ1-4GlcNAcβ1 6 Galβ1-4Glc Galβ1-3GlcNAcβ1 3 4 Fucα1 (Tachibana et al., 1978)	Fucα1 2 Fucα1 3 Galβ1-3GlcNAcβ1-3Galβ1-4GlcNAcβ1 6 Galβ1-4Glc Galβ1-3GlcNAcβ1 3 2 Fucα1 (Strecker et al., 1992)
Fucα1 3 Galβ1-4GlcNAcβ1-3Galβ1-4GlcNAcβ1 6 Galβ1-4Glc Galβ1-3GlcNAcβ1 3 3 4 Neu5Acα2 Fucα1 (Kitagawa et al., 1991a)	Fucα1 4 Fucα1 3 Galβ1-3GlcNAcβ1-3Galβ1-4GlcNAcβ1 6 Galβ1-4Glc Galβ1-3GlcNAcβ1 3 4 Fucα1 (Kogelberg et al., 2004)

Lacto-*N*-*neo*-octaose

```
                              Fucα1 3
Galβ1-3GlcNAcβ1-3Galβ1-4GlcNAcβ1 6
                                   Galβ1-4Glc
                  Galβ1-4GlcNAcβ1 3
(Yamashita et al., 1976c)

      Fucα1 4                 Fucα1 3
Galβ1-3GlcNAcβ1-3Galβ1-4GlcNAcβ1 6
                                   Galβ1-4Glc
                  Galβ1-4GlcNAcβ1 3
(Tachibana et al., 1978)

                              Fucα1 3
Galβ1-3GlcNAcβ1-3Galβ1-4GlcNAcβ1 6
                                   Galβ1-4Glc
                  Galβ1-4GlcNAcβ1 3
                         Fucα1 3
(Tachibana et al., 1978)

    Fucα1 4                   Fucα1 3
Galβ1-3GlcNAcβ1-3Galβ1-4GlcNAcβ1 6
                                   Galβ1-4Glc
                  Galβ1-4GlcNAcβ1 3
                         Fucα1 3
(Tachibana et al., 1978)

Fucα1 2                       Fucα1 3
   Galβ1-3GlcNAcβ1-3Galβ1-4GlcNAcβ1 6
                                      Galβ1-4Glc
                  Galβ1-3GlcNAcβ1 3
                      2        4
              Fucα1      Fucα1
(Haeuw-Fievre et al., 1993)

Fucα1  2  Fucα1  4            Fucα1 3
   Galβ1-3GlcNAcβ1-3Galβ1-4GlcNAcβ1 6
                                      Galβ1-4Glc
                  Galβ1-3GlcNAcβ1 3
                      2        4
              Fucα1      Fucα1
(Haeuw-Fievre et al., 1993)

   Galβ1-3GlcNAcβ1-3Galβ1-4GlcNAcβ1 6
                                      Galβ1-4Glc
                  Galβ1-3GlcNAcβ1 3
                      3        4
         Neu5Acα2        Fucα1
(Kitagawa et al., 1991a)

                              Fucα1 3
   Galβ1-3GlcNAcβ1-3Galβ1-4GlcNAcβ1 6
                                      Galβ1-4Glc
                  Galβ1-3GlcNAcβ1 3
                      3        4
         Neu5Acα2        Fucα1
(Kitagawa et al., 1991a)

       Fucα1 4
   Galβ1-3GlcNAcβ1-3Galβ1-4GlcNAcβ1 6
                                      Galβ1-4Glc
                  Galβ1-3GlcNAcβ1 3
                      3        4
         Neu5Acα2        Fucα1
(Kitagawa et al., 1991a)

Fucα1 2                       Fucα1 3
   Galβ1-3GlcNAcβ1-3Galβ1-4GlcNAcβ1 6
                                      Galβ1-4Glc
                  Galβ1-3GlcNAcβ1 3
                      3        4
         Neu5Acα2        Fucα1
(Kitagawa et al., 1993)
```

Table 2.9 Fucosyl Derivatives of Lacto-*N*-decaose and Lacto-*N*-*neo*-decaose in HMO as Determined by Negative-Ion MALDI-QIT-TOFMS^n

Lacto-*N*-decaose

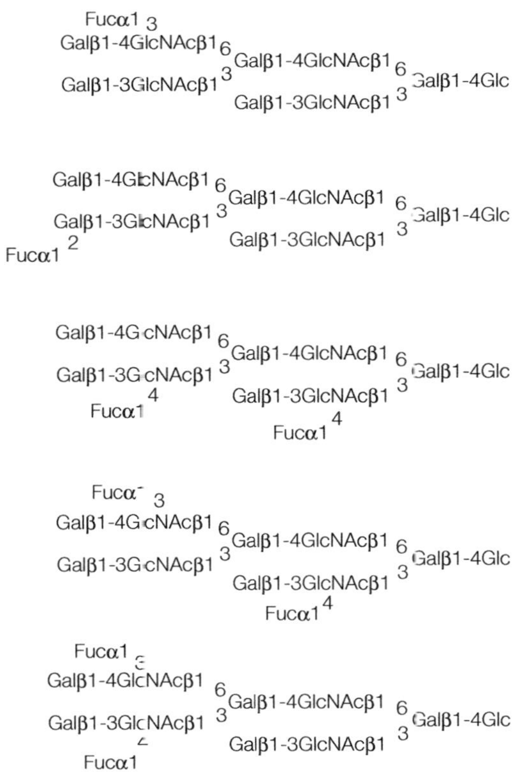

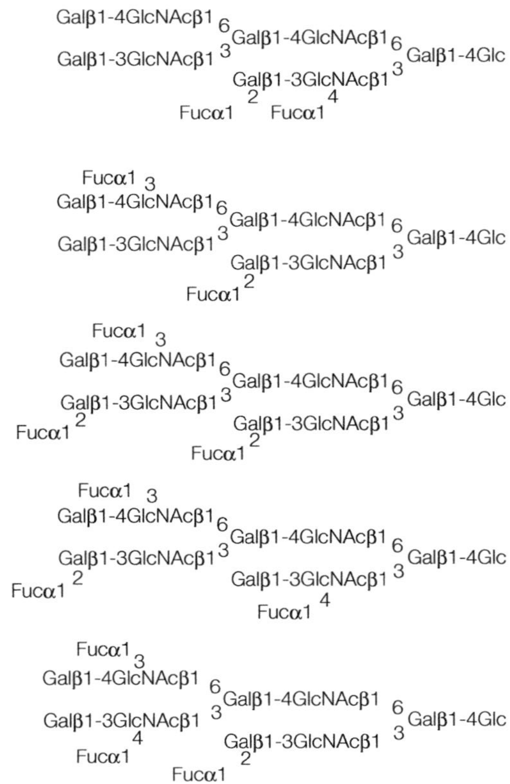

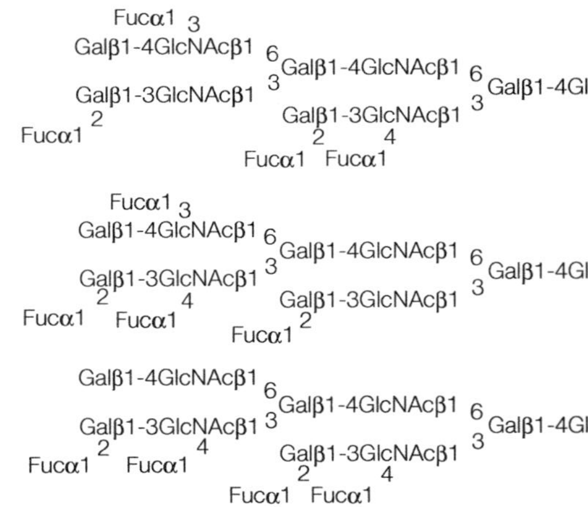

Lact-*N*-*neo*-decaose

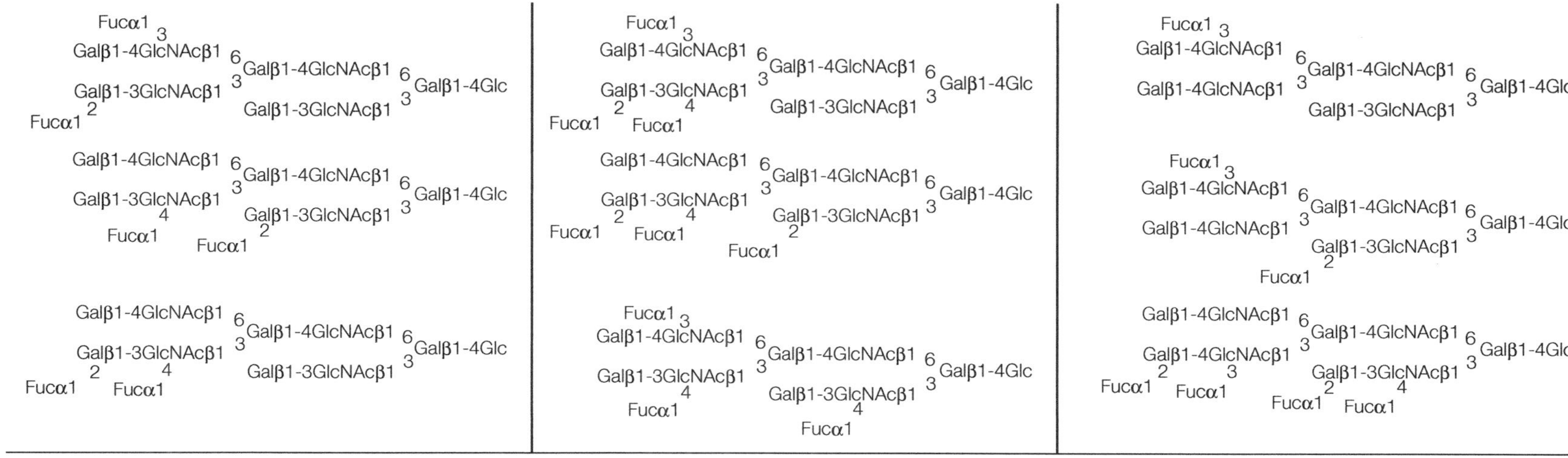

From Amano, J., Osanai, M., Orita, T., Sugahara, D., Osumi, K., 2009. *Structural determination by negative-ion MALDI-QIT-TOFMS after pyrene derivatization of variously fucosylated oligosaccharides with branched decaose cores from human milk. Glycobiology 19, 601–614.* MALDI, *Matrix assisted laser desorption/ionization;* QIT, *quadrupole ion trap;* TOF MS, *time of flight mass spectrometry.*

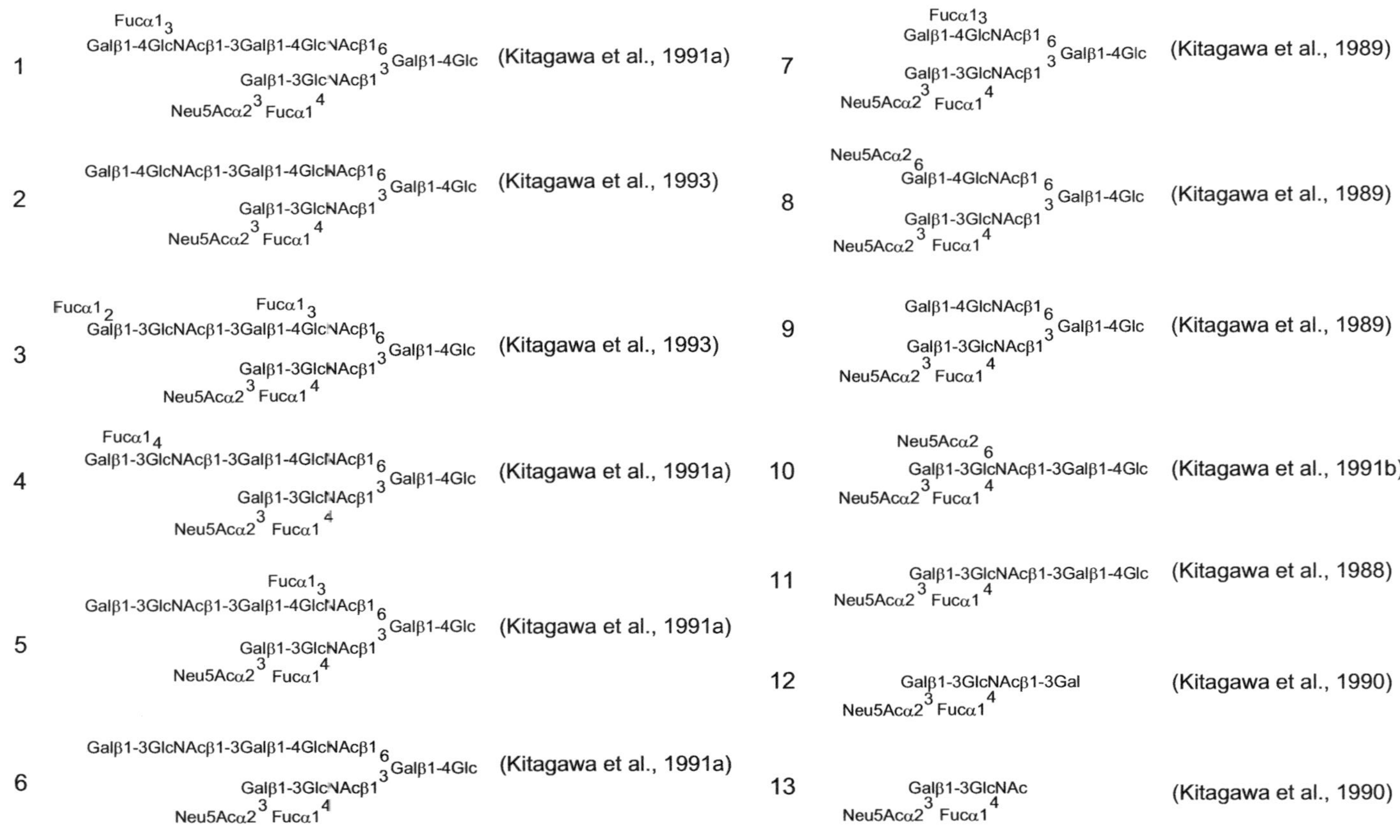

FIGURE 2.6

Structures of human milk oligosaccharides containing the sialyl-Le[a] group, collected by affinity chromatography using an immobilized monoclonal antibody, MSW 113.

monoclonal antibody named MSW 113 by using a human colonic cancer cell line, SW 1116, as the immunogen.

They reported the structures of a series of HMOs, which were retained by an immobilized column of MSW 113. As shown by 1–13 in Fig. 2.6, they are oligosaccharides of various sizes containing the sialyl-Le^a determinant in common. Among them, two oligosaccharides 12 and 13, which occur as very minor components in the oligosaccharide fraction retained by the column, have unusual features. They do not contain lactose but contain either GlcNAc or Gal residue at their reducing termini.

Therefore, the mechanism to produce oligosaccharides 12 and 13, which lack a lactose group, is totally unknown. We speculate that they might be produced from larger milk saccharides by an unknown degradation mechanism.

In any event, the report of Kitagawa et al. indicated that we would be able to pick up even a very minor unusual oligosaccharide with particular ligand specificity, if a proper affinity chromatographic method is devised by isolating receptor proteins on the surface of bacteria and viruses. Perhaps this can be performed in the near future by collaborating with the bacteriologists and virologists who are investigating virulence factors by cloning the surface lectins of bacteria and viruses.

The report of Perret et al. (2005) can be considered as a pioneering work for this line of investigation.

REFERENCES

Almeida, R., Amado, M., David, L., Levery, S.B., Holmes, E.H., Merkx, G., van Kessel, A.G., Rygaard, E., Hassan, H., Bennett, E., Clausen, H., 1997. A family of human β4-galactosyltransferases: cloning and expression of two novel UDP-galactose:β-*N*-acetylglucosamine β1,4-galactosyltransferases, β4Gal-T2 and β4Gal-T3. Journal of Biological Chemistry 272, 31979–31991.

Amano, J., Osanai, M., Orita, T., Sugahara, D., Osumi, K., 2009. Structural determination by negative-ion MALDI-QIT-TOFMS after pyrene derivatization of variously fucosylated oligosaccharides with branched decaose cores from human milk. Glycobiology 19, 601–614.

Ball, S.P., Tongue, N., Gibaud, A., Le Pendu, J., Mollicone, R., Gerald, G., Oriol, R., 1991. The human chromosome 19 linkage group FUT1 (H), FUT2 (SE), LE, LU, OEOD, C3, APOC2, D19S7 and D19S9. Annals of Human Genetics 55, 225–233.

Brodbeck, N., Ebner, K.E., 1966. Resolution of a soluble lactose synthetase into two protein components and solubilization of microsomal lactose synthetase. Journal of Biological Chemistry 241, 762–764.

Bruntz, R., Dabrowski, U., Dabrowski, J., Ebersold, A., Peter-Katalinic, J., Egge, H., 1988. Fucose-containing oligosaccharides from human milk from a donor of blood group O Le(a) nonsecretor. Biological Chemistry Hoppe-Seyler 369, 257–273.

Chai, W., Piskarev, V.E., Zhang, Y., Lawson, A.M., Kogelberg, H., 2005. Structural determination of novel lacto-*N*-decaose and its monofucosylated analogue from human milk by electrospray tandem mass spectrometry and ^{1}H NMR spectroscopy. Archives of Biochemistry and Biophysics 434, 116–127.

Donald, A.S.R., Feeney, J., 1988. Separation of human milk oligosaccharides by recycling chromatography. First isolation of lacto-N-neo-difucohexaose and 3′-galactosyllactose from this source. J. Carbohydrate Research 178, 79–91.

Dua, V.K., Goso, K., Dube, V.E., Bush, C.A., 1985. Characterization of lacto-N-hexaose and two fucosylated derivatives from human milk by high-performance liquid chromatography and proton NMR spectroscopy. Journal of Chromatography 328, 259–269.

Fenderson, B.A., Zehavi, U., Hakomori, S., 1984. A multivalent lacto-*N*-fucopentaose III-lysyllysine conjugate decompacts preimplantation mouse embryos, while the free oligosaccharide is ineffective. Journal of Experimental Medicine 160, 1591–1596.

Fievre, S., Wieruszeski, J.-M., Michalski, J.-C., Lemoine, J., Montreuil, J., Strecker, G., 1991. Primary structure of a trisialylated oligosaccharide from human milk. Biochemical and Biophysical Research Communications 177, 720–725.

Ginsburg, V., Zopf, D.A., Yamashita, K., Kobata, A., 1976. Oligosaccharides of human milk. Isolation of a new pentasaccharide, lacto-N-fucopentaose V. Archives of Biochemistry and Biophysics 175, 565–568.

Grimmonprez, L., Montreuil, J., 1968. Physico-chemical study of 6 new oligosides isolated from human milk. Bulletin de la Societe de Chimie Biologique 50, 843–855.

Grollman, E.F., Ginsburg, V., 1967. Correlation between secretor status and the occurrence of 2'-fucosyllactose in human milk. Biochemical and Biophysical Research Communications 28, 50–53.

Grollman, E.F., Kobata, A., Ginsburg, V., 1969. An enzymatic basis for Le(a^-b^-) blood type in humans. Journal of Clinical Investigation 48, 1489–1494.

Grollman, E.F., Kobata, A., Ginsburg, V., 1970. Enzymatic basis of blood types in man. Proceedings of New York Academy of Sciences of the United States of America 169, 225–233.

Grönberg, G., Lipniunas, P., Lungren, T., Erlansson, K., Lindh, F., Nilsson, B., 1989. Isolation of monosialylated oligosaccharides from human milk and structural analysis of three new compounds. Carbohydrate Research 191, 261–278.

Grönberg, G., Lipniunas, P., Lundgren, T., Lindh, F., Nilsson, B., 1990. Isolation and structural analysis of three new disialylated oligosaccharides from human milk. Archives of Biochemistry and Biophysics 278, 297–311.

Grönberg, G., Lipniunas, P., Lundgren, T., Lindh, F., Nilsson, B., 1992. Structural analysis of five new monosialylated oligosaccharides from human milk. Archives of Biochemistry and Biophysics 296, 597–610.

Grulee, C., Sanford, H., Schwartz, H., 1935. Breast and artificially fed infants; study of the age incidence in morbidity and mortality in 20,000 cases. JAMA 104, 1986–1988.

Guerardel, Y., Morelle, W., Plancke, Y., Lemoine, J., Strecker, G., 1999. Structural analysis of three sulfated oligosaccharides isolated from human milk. Carbohydrate Research 320, 230–238.

Haeuw-Fievre, S., Wieruszeski, J.–M., Plancke, Y., Michalski, J.C., Montreuil, J., Strecker, G., 1993. Primary structure of human milk octa-, dodeca-, and tridecasaccharides determined by combination of ^{1}H-NMR spectrosgopy and fast-atom-bombardment mass spectrometry. Evidence for anew core structure, the *para*-lacto-*N*-octaose. European Journal of Biochemistry 215, 361–371.

Hickey, R.M., 2012. The role of oligosaccharides from human milk and other sources in prevention of pathogen adhesion. International Dairy Journal 22, 141–146.

Issiki, S., Togayachi, A., Kudo, T., Nishihara, S., Watanabe, M., Kubota, T., Kitajima, M., Shiraishi, K., Andoh, T., Narimatsu, H., 1999. Cloning, expression, and characterization of a novel UDP-galactose:β-*N*-acetylglucosamine,β1,3-galactosyltransferase (β3GalT-V) responsible for synthesis of type-1 chain in colorectal and pancreatic epithelia and tumor cells derived therefrom. Journal of Biological Chemistry 274, 12499–12507.

Kitagawa, H., Nakada, H., Numata, Y., Kurosaka, A., Fukui, S., Funakoshi, I., Kawasaki, T., Yamashina, I., 1988. Immunoaffinity isolation of a sialyl-Le(a) oligosaccharide from human milk. Journal of Biochemistry 104, 591–594.

Kitagawa, H., Nakada, H., Kurosaka, A., Hiraiwa, N., Numata, Y., Fukui, S., Funakoshi, I., Kawasaki, T., Yamashina, I., Shimada, I., 1989. Three novel oligosaccharides with the sialyl-Lea structure in human milk: isolation by immunoaffinity chromatography. Biochemistry 28, 8891–8897.

Kitagawa, H., Nakada, H., Numata, Y., Kurosaka, A., Fukui, S., Funakoshi, I., Kawasaki, T., Shimada, I., Unagaki, F., Yamashina, I., 1990. Occurrence of tetra- and pentasaccharides with the sialyl-Le(a) structure in human milk. J. Biol. Chem. 265, 4859–4862.

Kitagawa, H., Nakada, H., Fukui, S., Funakoshi, I., Kawasaki, T., Yamashina, I., Tate, S., Inagaki, F., 1991a. Novel oligosaccharides with the sialyl-Lea structure in human milk. Biochemistry 30, 2869–2876.

Kitagawa, H., Takaoka, M., Nakada, H., Fukui, S., Funakoshi, I., Kawasaki, T., Tate, S., Inagaki, F., Yamashina, I., 1991b. Isolation and structural studies of human milk oligosaccharides that are reactive with a monoclonal antibody MSW 113. J. Biochem. 110, 598–604.

Kitagawa, H., Nakada, H., Fukui, S., Funakoshi, I., Kawasaki, T., Yamashina, I., Tate, S., Inagaki, F., 1993. Novel oligosaccharides with the sialyl-Le(a) structure in human milk. J. Biochem. 115, 504–508.

Kobata, A., 1979. Use of endo- and exoglycosidases for structural studies of glycoconjugates. Analytical Biochemistry 100, 1–14.

Kobata, A., Ginsburg, V., 1969. Oligosaccharides of human milk. II. Isolation and characterizeation of a new pentasaccharide, lacto-N-fucopentaose. J. Biol. Chem. 244, 5496–5502.

Kobata, A., Ginsburg, V., 1970. UDP-*N*-acetyl-D-galactosamine:D-Galactose α-3-*N*-acetyl-D-galactosaminyltransferase, a product of gene that determine blood type A in man. Journal of Biological Chemistry 245, 1484–1490.

Kobata, A., Ginsburg, V., 1972a. Oligosaccharides of human milk. III. Structure of a new hexasaccharide, lacto-N-hexaose. J. Biol. Chem. 1525–1529.

Kobata, A., Ginsburg, V., 1972b. Oligosaccharides of human milk. IV. Isolation and characterization of a new hexasaccharide, lacto-*N-neo*-hexaose. Arch. Biochem. Biophys. 150, 273–281.

Kobata, A., Grollman, E.F., Ginsburg, V., 1968a. An enzymatic basis of blood type A in humans. Archives of Biochemistry and Biophysics 124, 609–612.

Kobata, A., Grollman, E.F., Ginsburg, V., 1968b. An enzymatic basis of blood type B in humans. Biochemical and Biophysical Research Communications 32, 272–277.

Kobata, A., Takasaki, S., 1992. Structural characterization of oligosaccharides from glycoproteins. 4A Glycosidase treatment and other methods, including methylation analysis. In: Fukuda, M., Kobata, A. (Eds.), Glycobiology: A Practical Approach. IRL Press, Oxford, pp. 165–185.

Kobata, A., Tsuda, M., Ginsburg, V., 1969. Oligosaccharides of human milk. I. Isolation and characterization. Archives of Biochemistry and Biophysics 130, 509–513.

Kogelberg, H., Piskarev, V.E., Zhang, Y., Lawson, A.M., Chai, W., 2004. Determination by electrospray mass spectrometry and 1H-NMR spectroscopy of primary structures of variously fucosylated neutral oligosaccharides based on the iso-lacto-N-octaose core. European Journal of Biochemistry 271, 1172–1186.

Kuhn, R., 1959. Biochemie der Rezeptoren und Resistenzfaktoren. Von der Widerstandsfähigkeit der Lebewesen gegen Einwirkungen der Umwelt. Naturwissenschaften 46, 43–50.

Kuhn, R., Baer, H.H., 1956. Die Konstitutionen der Lacto-*N*-tetraose. Chemische Berichte 89, 504–511.

Kuhn, R., Baer, H.H., Gauhe, A., 1956a. Kristallisierte fucoside-lactose. Chemische Berichte 89, 2513.

Kuhn, R., Baer, H.H., Gauhe, A., 1956b. Kristallisation und Konstitutionsermittlung der Lacto-*N*-fucopentaose I. Chemische Berichte 89, 2514–2523.

Kuhn, R., Baer, H.H., Gauhe, A., 1958a. Die Konstitution der Lacto-*N*-fucopentaose II. Chemische Berichte 91, 364.

Kuhn, R., Baer, H.H., Gauhe, A., 1958b. 2-α-L-Fucopyranosyl-D-galaktose und 2-α-L-fucopyranosyl-D-talose. Justus Liebigs Annalen der Chemie 611, 242–249.

Kuhn, R., Brossmer, R., 1959. Uber das durch Viren der Influenza-Gruppe spaltbare Trisaccharid der Milch. Chemische Berichte 92, 1667–1671.

Kuhn, R., Gauhe, A., 1958. Uber die lacto-difuco-tetraose der Frauenmilch. Justus Liebigs Annalen der Chemie 611, 249–252.

Kuhn, R., Gauhe, A., 1960. Über ein kristallisiertes, Le^a-aktives Hexasaccharid aus Frauenmilch. Chemische Berichte 93, 647–651.

Kuhn, R., Gauhe, A., 1962a. Die Konstitution der Lacto-*N-neo*tetraose. Chemische Berichte 95, 518–522.

Kuhn, R., Gauhe, A., 1962b. Uber drei saure pentasaccharide aus frauenmilch. Chemische Berichte 95, 513–517.

Kuhn, R., Gauhe, A., 1965. Bestimmung der Bindungsstelle von sialinsäureresten in Oligosaccharides mit Hilfe von Periodat. Chemische Berichte 98, 395–413.

Lloyd, K.O., Kabat, E.A., Licerio, E., 1968. Immunochemical studies on blood groups XXXVIII. Structures and activities of oligosaccharides produced by alkaline degradation of blood-group A, B, H, Le^a and Le^b substances. Biochemistry 7, 2976–2990.

Montreuil, J., 1956. Structure of two triholosides isolated from human milk. Comptes Rendus de l'Académie des Sciences 242, 192–193.

Moro, E., 1900. Morphologi und bakteriologisch untersuchungen über die Darmbakterien des Säuglings: die Bakterium-flora des normalen Frauenmilchstuls. Jahrb Kinderheilkd 61, 686–734.

Newburg, D.S., Ruiz-Palacios, G.M., Morrow, A.L., 2005. Human milk glycans protect infants against enteric pathogens. Annual Review of Nutrition 25, 37–58.

Ninonuevo, M.R., Park, Y., Yin, H., Zhang, J., Ward, R.E., Clowers, B.H., German, J.B., Freeman, S.L., Kileen, K., Grim, R., Lebilla, C.B., 2006. A strategy for annotating the human milk glycome. Journal of Agricultural and Food Chemistry 54, 7471–7480.

Perret, S., Sabin, C., Dumon, C., Pokorná, M., Gautier, C., Galanina, O., Ilia, S., Bovin, N., Desmadril, M., Gilboa-Garber, N., Wimmerová, M., Michell, E.P., Imberty, A., 2005. Structural basis for the interaction between human milk oligosaccharides and the bacterial lectin PA-IIL of *Pseudomonas aeruginosa*. Biochemical Journal 389, 325–332.

Ropp, P.A., Little, M.R., Cheng, P.W., 1991. Mucin biosynthesis: purification and characterization of a mucin β6 *N*-acetylglucosaminyltransferase. Journal of Biological Chemistry 266, 23863–23871.

Sasaki, K., Kurata-Miura, K., Ujita, M., Angata, K., Kitagawa, S., Sekine, S., Nishi, T., Fukuda, M., 1997. Expression cloning of cDNA encoding a human β-1,3-*N*-acetylglucosaminyltransferase that is essential for poly-*N*-acetyllactosamine synthesis. Proceedings of National Academy of Sciences of the United States of America 94, 14294–14299.

Shen, L., Grollman, E.F., Ginsburg, V., 1968. An enzymatic basis for secretor status and blood group substance specificity in humans. Proceedings of National Academy of Sciences of the United States of America 59, 224–230.

Smith, D.F., Prieto, P.A., McCrumb, D.K., Wang, W.C., 1987. A novel sialylfucopentaose in human milk. Presence of this oligosaccharides is not dependent on expression of the secretor or Lewis fucosyltransferases. Journal of Biological Chemistry 262, 12040–12047.

Strecker, G., Fievre, S., Wieruszeski, J.M., Michalski, J.C., Montreuil, J., 1992. Primary structure of four human milk octa- nona- and undeca-saccharides established by 1H- and 13C-nuclear magnetic resonance spectroscopy. Carbohydrate Research226, 1–14.

Strecker, G., Wieruszeski, J.–M., Michalski, J.–C., Montreuil, J., 1988. Structure of a new nonasaccharide isolated from human milk; IV^2Fuc, V^4Fuc, III^3Fuc-*p*-Lacto-*N*-hexaose. Glycoconjugate Journal 5, 385–396.

Strecker, G., Wieruszeski, J.M., Michalski, J.C., Montreuil, J., 1989. Primary structure of human milk nona- and decasaccharides determined by a combination of fast atom bombardment mass spectrometry and 1H-/13C-nuclear magnetic resonance spectroscopy. Evidence for a new core structure, iso-lacto-*N*-octaose. Glycoconjugate Journal 6, 169–182.

Tachibana, Y., Yamashita, K., Kobata, A., 1978. Oigosaccharides of human milk: structural studies of di- and trifucosyl derivatives of lacto-N-octaose and lacto-N-neooctaose. Archives of Biochemistry and Biophysics 188, 83–89.

Tai, T., Yamashita, K., Kobata, A., 1975. Synthesis and mass fragmentographic analysis of partially O-methylated 2-N-methylglucosamines. Journal of Biochemistry 78, 679–686.

Takasaki, S., Kobata, A., 1974. Microdetermination of individual neutral and amino sugars and N-acetylneuraminic acid in complex saccharides. Journal of Biochemistry 76, 783–789.

Taniguchi, N., Honke, K., Fukuda, M., 2002. Handbook of Glycosyltransferases and Related Genes. Springer-Verlag, Tokyo Berlin Heidelberg New York.

Tarrago, M.T., Tucker, K.H., van Halbeek, H., Smith, D.F., 1988. A novel sialylhexasaccharide from human milk: purification by affinity chromatography on immobilized wheat germ agglutinin. Archives of Biochemistry and Biophysics 267, 353–362.

Thurl, S., Henker, J., Siegel, M., Tovar, K., Sawatzki, G., 1997. Detection of four human milk groups with respect to Lewis blood group dependent oligosaccharides. Glycoconjugate Journal 14, 795–799.

Tissier, H., 1900. Recherches sur la flore intestinale de nourissons Ph.D. thesis. Univ. Paris, Paris, France.

Urashima, T., Kitaoka, M., Terabayashi, T., Fukuda, K., Ohnishi, M., Kobata, A., 2011. Chapter 1. Milk oligosaccharides. In: Gordon, N.S. (Ed.), Oligosaccharides: Sources, Properties and Applications. Nova Science Publishers, Inc, pp. 1–58.

Watkins, W.M., 1966. Blood group specific substances. In: Gottschalk, A. (Ed.), Glycoproteins, second ed. Elsevier, Amsterdam, pp. 462–515.

Watkins, W.M., 1972. Blood group specific substances. In: Gottschalk, A. (Ed.), Glycoproteins. Elsevier, Amsterdam, pp. 830–891.

Wieruszeski, J.-M., Chekkor, A., Bouquelet, S., Montreuil, J., Stecker, G., Peter-Katalinic, J., et al., 1985. Structure of two new oligosaccharides isolated from human milk: sialylated lacto-N-focopentaoses I and II. Carbohydrate Research 137, 127–138.

Yamashita, K., Kobata, A., 1974. Oligosaccharides of human milk V. Isolation and characterization of a new trisaccharide, 6′-galactosyllactose. Archives of Biochemistry and Biophysics 161, 164–170.

Yamashita, K., Tachibana, Y., Takasaki, S., Kobata, A., 1976a. ABO blood group determinants with branched cores. Nature 262, 702–703.

Yamashita, K., Tachibana, Y., Kobata, A., 1976b. Oligosaccharides of human milk: Isolation and characterization of three new disialylfucosylhexasaccharides. Archives of Biochemistry and Biophysics 174, 582–591.

Yamashita, K., Tachibana, Y., Kobata, A., 1976c. Oligosaccharides of human milk: isolation and characterization of two new nonasaccharides, monofucosyllacto-N-octaose and monofucosyllacto-N-neooctaose. Biochemistry 15, 3950–3955.

Yamashita, K., Tachibana, Y., Kobata, A., 1977a. Oligosaccharides of human milk; Structures of three lacto-*N*-hexaose derivatives with H-haptenic structure. Archives of Biochemistry and Biophysics 182, 546–555.

Yamashita, K., Tachibana, Y., Kobata, A., 1977b. Oligosaccharides of human milk. Structural studies of two new octasaccharides, difucosyl derivatives of para-lacto-N-hexaose and para-lacto-N-neohexaose. Journal of Biological Chemistry 252, 5408–5411.

CHAPTER

Oligosaccharides in the Milk of Other Mammals

3

Tadasu Urashima[1], Michael Messer[2], Olav T. Oftedal[3]

[1]Obihiro University of Agriculture and Veterinary Medicine, Obihiro, Hokkaido, Japan; [2]The University of Sydney, Sydney, NSW, Australia; [3]Smithsonian Environmental Research Center, Edgewater, MD, United States

1. INTRODUCTION

Mammalian milk/colostrum usually contains, in addition to lactose, a mixture of many varieties of oligosaccharides (Jenness et al., 1964; Urashima et al., 2007a, 2014b). Human colostrum contains 22–24 g/L, while mature milk contains 12–13 g/L of human milk oligosaccharides (HMOs) (Newburg et al., 1995; Urashima et al., 2012a). In human milk, oligosaccharides constitute the third highest solid component after lactose and lipids, and their concentration is higher than that of protein (Newburg et al., 1995). The structures of more than 100 HMOs have been characterized to date (Urashima et al., 2011a,b; Kobata, 2010); almost all contain a lactose structure -Gal(β1-4)Glc at their reducing ends. More than 200 HMOs have been detected by analysis with microfluidic chip high-performance liquid chromatography (HPLC)–time of flight mass spectrometry (TOFMS) (Ninonuevo et al., 2006). The structures of those HMOs that have been characterized to date have been described and listed in several reviews (Urashima et al., 2007a, 2009a, 2011a,b; Kobata, 2010; see Chapter 2).

The milks/colostra of nonhuman mammals also contain oligosaccharides whose chemical structures differ among species (Urashima et al., 2001b, 2007a, 2011a, 2012b, 2014b; Messer and Urashima, 2002). In this review, we construct an updated database of milk oligosaccharide structures found in nonhuman mammals and provide some discussion of the gastrointestinal (GI) digestion and absorption, biological function, and evolutionary importance of milk oligosaccharides. Various methods have been used for structural characterization of milk oligosaccharides by different authors, and there are differences among methods in detection sensitivity. It is likely that for most studied species the most abundant milk oligosaccharides have been characterized. However, as more-sensitive methods are used and larger samples are studied, we expect that additional oligosaccharide structures will be discovered. In most cases when we consider that a given oligosaccharide structure may be absent in a particular taxon, we cannot be certain that it may not occur in trace amounts.

Prebiotics and Probiotics in Human Milk. http://dx.doi.org/10.1016/B978-0-12-802725-7.00003-8

This review concludes with a discussion of the potential industrial utilization of oligosaccharides of milk/colostrum of domestic dairy farm animals based on their characterized chemical structures and concentrations as well as on studies of their physiological functions.

2. STRUCTURES OF MILK OLIGOSACCHARIDES OF NONHUMAN MAMMALS

2.1 PLACENTAL MAMMALS (INFRACLASS EUTHERIA)

2.1.1 Nonhuman Primates (Oligosaccharides in Table 3.1)

Milk oligosaccharides have been studied in four groups of primates: (1) apes, including the chimpanzee (Urashima et al., 2009b), bonobo (Urashima et al., 2009b), gorilla (Urashima et al., 2009b), orangutan (Urashima et al., 2009b), and siamang (Urashima et al., 2009b); (2) Old World monkeys, including rhesus macaque (Goto et al., 2010), toque macaque (Goto et al., 2010), and Hamadryas baboon (Goto et al., 2010); (3) New World monkeys, including tufted capuchin (Goto et al., 2010; Urashima et al., 1999a), mantled howler (Goto et al., 2010), and Bolivian squirrel monkey (Goto et al., 2010); and (4) strepsirrhine primates, including greater galago (Taufik et al., 2012), aye-aye (Taufik et al., 2012), Coquerel's sifaka (Taufik et al., 2012), and mongoose lemur (Taufik et al., 2012). Oligosaccharides were separated by gel liquid chromatography and HPLC, and structures were determined via ^{1}H nuclear magnetic resonance (NMR) spectroscopy (Table 3.1).

We observed that there are differences in the pattern of milk oligosaccharides among primate species and that there is a characteristic difference between human and nonhuman primates. Among apes, the milk or colostrum of the chimpanzee, bonobo, and orangutan contain both type I oligosaccharides [i.e., saccharides containing the Gal(β1-3)GlcNAc (lacto-*N*-biose I, LNB) structure] and type II oligosaccharides [i.e., saccharides containing the Gal(β1-4)GlcNAc (*N*-acetyllactosamine, LacNAc) structure] (Urashima et al., 2009b). The relative predominance of type I and type II oligosaccharides can be assessed from the observed ratio of Gal(β1-3)GlcNAc(β1-3)Gal(β1-4)Glc (lacto-*N*-tetraose, LNT) to Gal(β1-4)GlcNAc(β1-3)Gal(β1-4)Glc (lacto-*N*-neotetraose, LN*n*T) and the observed ratio of Fuc(α1-2)Gal(β1-3)GlcNAc(β1-3)Gal(β1-4)Glc (lacto-*N*-fucopentaose I, LNFP-I) to Gal(β1-4)[Fuc(α1-3)]GlcNAc(β1-3)Gal(β1-4)Glc (lacto-*N*-fucopentaose III, LNFP-III). In humans, the type I oligosaccharides predominate over the type II (Urashima et al., 2012a; Asakuma et al., 2008; Chaturvedi et al., 2001; Thurl et al., 2010), whereas in the above-mentioned three species of apes, the type II predominates over the type I (Urashima et al., 2009b). Only type II oligosaccharides could be detected in the milk of gorilla and siamang (Urashima et al., 2009b). The predominance of type I oligosaccharides in human milk is a uniquely human characteristic, as we have not found this to occur in any other mammal that has been studied (Urashima et al., 2012a).

Table 3.1 Milk Oligosaccharides of Primates

No.	Oligosaccharide	Structure	References
Chimpanzee *(Pan troglodytes)* Milk			
Neutral oligosaccharides			
1	2′-FL	Fucα1-2Galβ1-4Glc	Urashima et al. (2009b)
2	3-FL	Galβ1-4Glc 3 Fucα1	Urashima et al. (2009b)
3	LNT	Galβ1-3GlcNAcβ1-3Galβ1-4Glc	Urashima et al. (2009b)
4	LNnT	Galβ1-4GlcNAcβ1-3Galβ1-4Glc	Urashima et al. (2009b)
5	LNFP III	Galβ1-4GlcNAcβ1-3Galβ1-4Glc 3 Fucα1	Urashima et al. (2009b)
Acidic oligosaccharides			
6	3′-SL	Neu5Acα2-3Galβ1-4Glc	Urashima et al. (2009b)
7	3′-Neu5GcL	Neu5Gcα2-3Galβ1-4Glc	Urashima et al. (2009b)
Bonobo *(Pan paniscus)* Milk			
Neutral oligosaccharides			
1	2′-FL	Fucα1-2Galβ1-4Glc	Urashima et al. (2009b)
2	3-FL	Galβ1-4Glc 3 Fucα1	Urashima et al. (2009b)
3	LNT	Galβ1-3GlcNAcβ1-3Galβ1-4Glc	Urashima et al. (2009b)
4	A-tetrasaccharide	GalNAcα1-3Galβ1-4Glc 2 Fucα1	Urashima et al. (2009b)
5	LNFP I	Fucα1-2Galβ1-3GlcNAcβ1-3Galβ1-4Glc	Urashima et al. (2009b)
6	LNFP III	Galβ1-4GlcNAcβ1-3Galβ1-4Glc 3 Fucα1	Urashima et al. (2009b)
Acidic oligosaccharides			
7	3′-SL	Neu5Acα2-3Galβ1-4Glc	Urashima et al. (2009b)

Continued

Table 3.1 Milk Oligosaccharides of Primates—cont'd

No.	Oligosaccharide	Structure	References
8	6′-SL	Neu5Acα2-6Galβ1-4Glc	Urashima et al. (2009b)
9	3′-Neu5GcL	Neu5Gcα2-3Galβ1-4Glc	Urashima et al. (2009b)
Gorilla *(Gorilla gorilla)* Milk or Colostrum			
Neutral oligosaccharides			
1	2′-FL	Fucα1-2Galβ1-4Glc	Urashima et al. (2009b)
2	LNnT	Galβ1-4GlcNAcβ1-3Galβ1-4Glc	Urashima et al. (2009b)
3	B-tetrasaccharice	Galα1-3Galβ1-4Glc 2 Fucα1	Urashima et al. (2009b)
Acidic oligosaccharides			
4	3′-SL	Neu5Acα2-3Galβ1-4Glc	Urashima et al. (2009b)
5	3′-Neu5GcL	Neu5Gcα2-3Galβ1-4Glc	Urashima et al. (2009b)
Orangutan *(Pongo pygmaeus)* Colostrum			
Neutral oligosaccharides			
1	3-FL	Galβ1-4Glc 3 Fucα1	Urashima et al. (2009b)
2	β 6′-GL	Galβ1-6Galβ1-4Glc	Urashima et al. (2009b)
3	LNT	Galβ1-3GlcNAcβ1-3Galβ1-4Glc	Urashima et al. (2009b)
4	LNnT	Galβ1-4GlcNAcβ1-3Galβ1-4Glc	Urashima et al. (2009b)
5	LNFP III	Galβ1-4GlcNAcβ1-3Galβ1-4Glc 3 Fucα1	Urashima et al. (2009b)
6	DF-LNnH	Fucα1 3 Galβ1-4GlcNAcβ1 6 Galβ1-4Glc 3 Galβ1-4GlcNAcβ1 3 Fucα1	Urashima et al. (2009b)

No.	Oligosaccharide	Structure	References
Acidic oligosaccharides			
7	3′-SL	Neu5Acα2-3Galβ1-4Glc	Urashima et al. (2009b)
8	6′-SL	Neu5Acα2-6Galβ1-4Glc	Urashima et al. (2009b)
9	3′-Neu5GcL	Neu5Gcα2-3Galβ1-4Glc	Urashima et al. (2009b)
10	LST b	Neu5Acα2 6 / Galβ1-3GlcNAcβ1-3Galβ1-4Glc	Urashima et al. (2009b)
11	LST c	Neu5Acα2-6Galβ1-4GlcNAcβ1-3Galβ1-4Glc	Urashima et al. (2009b)
12	MSMFLNnH	Fucα1 3 / Galβ1-4GlcNAcβ1 6 / 3 Galβ1-4Glc / Neu5Acα2-6Galβ1-4GlcNAcβ1	Urashima et al. (2009b)
Siamang *(Symphalangus syndactylus)* Milk			
Neutral oligosaccharides			
1	LNnT	Galβ1-4GlcNAcβ1-3Galβ1-4Glc	Urashima et al. (2009b)
2	LNnH	Galβ1-4GlcNAcβ1 6 / 3 Galβ1-4Glc / Galβ1-4GlcNAcβ1	Urashima et al. (2009b)
Acidic oligosaccharides			
3	3′-SL	Neu5Acα2-3Galβ1-4Glc	Urashima et al. (2009b)
4	6′-SL	Neu5Acα2-6Galβ1-4Glc	Urashima et al. (2009b)
5	LST c	Neu5Acα2-6Galβ1-4GlcNAcβ1-3Galβ1-4Glc	Urashima et al. (2009b)
6	MSLNnH	Galβ1-4GlcNAcβ1 6 / 3 Galβ1-4Glc / Neu5Acα2-6Galβ1-4GlcNAcβ1	Urashima et al. (2009b)

Continued

Table 3.1 Milk Oligosaccharides of Primates—cont'd

No.	Oligosaccharide	Structure	References
Rhesus Macaque *(Macaca mulatta)* Milk			
Neutral oligosaccharides			
1	3-FL	Galβ1-4Glc 3 Fucα1	Goto et al. (2010)
2	β6′-GL	Galβ1-6Galβ1-4Glc	Goto et al. (2010)
3	β3′-GalNAcL	GalNAcβ1-3Galβ1-4Glc	Goto et al. (2010)
4	LNnT	Galβ1-4GlcNAcβ1-3Galβ1-4Glc	Goto et al. (2010)
5	LNFP III	Galβ1-4GlcNAcβ1-3Galβ1-4Glc 3 Fucα1	Goto et al. (2010)
Acidic oligosaccharides			
1	3′-SL	Neu5Acα2-3Galβ1-4Glc	Goto et al. (2010)
2	6′-SL	Neu5Acα2-6Galβ1-4Glc	Goto et al. (2010)
3	GM_2 tetrasaccharide	GalNAcβ1 4 Galβ1-4Glc 3 Neu5Acα2	Goto et al. (2010)
4	LST c	Neu5Acα2-6Galβ1-4GlcNAcβ1-3Galβ1-4Glc	Goto et al. (2010)
Toque Macaque *(Macaca sinica)* Milk			
Neutral oligosaccharides			
1	3-FL	Galβ1-4Glc 3 Fucα1	Goto et al. (2010)
2	LNFP III	Galβ1-4GlcNAcβ1-3Galβ1-4Glc 3 Fucα1	Goto et al. (2010)

No.	Oligosaccharide	Structure	References
Acidic oligosaccharides			
1	3′-SL	Neu5Acα2-3Galβ1-4Glc	Goto et al. (2010)
Hamadryas Baboon *(Papio hamadryas)* Milk			
Neutral oligosaccharides			
1	3-FL	Galβ1-4Glc 3 Fucα1	Goto et al. (2010)
2	DFLNnH	Fucα1 3 Galβ1-4GlcNAcβ1 6 Galβ1-4Glc 3 Galβ1-4GlcNAcβ1 3 Fucα1	Goto et al. (2010)
Acidic oligosaccharides			
1	3′-L-*O*-sulphate	3-S-Gal(β1-4)Glc	Goto et al. (2010)
2	3′-SL	Neu5Acα2-3Galβ1-4Glc	Goto et al. (2010)
3	6′-SL	Neu5Acα2-6Galβ1-4Glc	Goto et al. (2010)
4	LST c	Neu5Acα2-6Galβ1-4GlcNAcβ1-3Galβ1-4Glc	Goto et al. (2010)
Tufted Capuchin *(Cebus apella)* Milk			
Neutral oligosaccharides			
1	3-FL	Galβ1-4Glc 3 Fucα1	Urashima et al. (1999a)
2	β3′-GL	Galβ1-3Galβ1-4Glc	Urashima et al. (1999a)
3	β6′-GL	Galβ1-6Galβ1-4Glc	Urashima et al. (1999a)
4	novo-LNP I	Galβ1-4GlcNAcβ1 6 Galβ1-4Glc 3 Galβ1	Goto et al. (2010) and Urashima et al. (1999a)

Continued

Table 3.1 Milk Oligosaccharides of Primates—cont'd

No.	Oligosaccharide	Structure	References
5	LNnH	Galβ1-4GlcNAcβ1-6(Galβ1-4GlcNAcβ1-3)Galβ1-4Glc	Goto et al. (2010) and Urashima et al. (1999a)
Acidic oligosaccharides			
1	3′-SL	Neu5Acα2-3Galβ1-4Glc	Goto et al. (2010) and Urashima et al. (1999a)
2	6′-SL	Neu5Acα2-6Galβ1-4Glc	Goto et al. (2010)
3	MSLNnH	Galβ1-4GlcNAcβ1-6(Neu5Acα2-6Galβ1-4GlcNAcβ1-3)Galβ1-4Glc	Goto et al. (2010)
Mantled Howler *(Alouatta paliata)* Milk			
Acidic oligosaccharides			
1	3′-SL	Neu5Acα2-3Galβ1-4Glc	Goto et al. (2010)
2	6′-SL	Neu5Acα2-6Galβ1-4Glc	Goto et al. (2010)
Bolivian Squirrel Monkey *(Saimiri boliviensis)* Milk			
Acidic oligosaccharides			
1	3′-SL	Neu5Acα2-3Galβ1-4Glc	Goto et al. (2010)
2	6′-SL	Neu5Acα2-6Galβ1-4Glc	Goto et al. (2010)
Greater Galago *(Otolemur crassicaudatus)* Milk			
Neutral oligosaccharides			
1	β6′-GL	Galβ1-6Galβ1-4Glc	Taufik et al. (2012)
2	LNnT	Galβ1-4GlcNAcβ1-3Galβ1-4Glc	Taufik et al. (2012)
Acidic oligosaccharides			
1	3′-SL	Neu5Acα2-3Galβ1-4Glc	Taufik et al. (2012)
2	3′-Neu5GcL	Neu5Gcα2-3Galβ1-4Glc	Taufik et al. (2012)

No.	Oligosaccharide	Structure	References
Aye-Aye *(Daubentonia madagascariensis)* Milk			
Neutral oligosaccharides			
1	3-FL	Galβ1-4Glc Fucα1³	Taufik et al. (2012)
2	2′-FL	Fucα1-2Galβ1-4Glc	Taufik et al. (2012)
3	LNT	Galβ1-3GlcNAcβ1-3Galβ1-4Glc	Taufik et al. (2012)
4	LNnT	Galβ1-4GlcNAcβ1-3Galβ1-4Glc	Taufik et al. (2012)
5	DFL	Fucα1-2Galβ1-4Glc Fucα1³	Taufik et al. (2012)
6	LNFP II	Galβ1-3GlcNAcβ1-3Galβ1-4Glc Fucα1⁴	Taufik et al. (2012)
7	LNFP III	Galβ1-4GlcNAcβ1-3Galβ1-4Glc Fucα1³	Taufik et al. (2012)
8	LNFP VI	Galβ1-4GlcNAcβ1-3Galβ1-4Glc Fucα1³	Taufik et al. (2012)
9	LNnH	Galβ1-4GlcNAcβ1 6 Galβ1-4Glc Galβ1-4GlcNAcβ1 3	Taufik et al. (2012)
10	FLNnH	Fucα1 3 Galβ1-4GlcNAcβ1 6 Galβ1-4Glc Galβ1-4GlcNAcβ1 3	Taufik et al. (2012)

Continued

Table 3.1 Milk Oligosaccharides of Primates—cont'd

No.	Oligosaccharide	Structure	References
		Galβ1-4GlcNAcβ1 6 Galβ1-4Glc Galβ1-4GlcNAcβ1 3 Fucα1 3	Taufik et al. (2012)
11	DFLNnH	Fucα1 3 Galβ1-4GlcNAcβ1 6 Galβ1-4Glc Galβ1-4GlcNAcβ1 3 Fucα1 3	Taufik et al. (2012)
Acidic oligosaccharides			
1	3′-SL	Neu5Acα2-3Galβ1-4Glc	Taufik et al. (2012)
2	6′-SL	Neu5Acα2-6Galβ1-4Glc	Taufik et al. (2012)
Coquerel's Sifaka *(Propithecus coquereli)* Milk			
Neutral oligosaccharides			
1	Isoglobotriose	Galα1-3Galβ1-4Glc	Taufik et al. (2012)
2	B-tetrasaccharide	Galα1-3Galβ1-4Glc Fucα1 2	Taufik et al. (2012)
3	LNnH	Galβ1-4GlcNAcβ1 6 Galβ1-4Glc Galβ1-4GlcNAcβ1 3	Taufik et al. (2012)
Acidic oligosaccharides			
1	3′-L-*O*-sulphate	3-S-Gal(β1-4)Glc	Taufik et al. (2012)
2	3′-SL	Neu5Acα2-3Galβ1-4Glc	Taufik et al. (2012)
3	6′-SL	Neu5Acα2-6Galβ1-4Glc	Taufik et al. (2012)

No.	Oligosaccharide	Structure	References
4	DSL	Neu5Acα2 6 Neu5Acα2-3Galβ1-4Glc	Taufik et al. (2012)
5	MSLNnH	Galβ1-4GlcNAcβ1 6 Galβ1-4Glc Neu5Acα2-6Galβ1-4GlcNAcβ1 3	Taufik et al. (2012)
Mongoose Lemur *(Eulemur mongoz)* Milk			
Neutral oligosaccharides			
1	3-FL	Galβ1-4Glc 3 Fucα1	Taufik et al. (2012)
2	Isoglobotriose	Galα1-3Galβ1-4Glc	Taufik et al. (2012)
3	β6′-GL	Galβ1-6Galβ1-4Glc	Taufik et al. (2012)
4	LNnT	Galβ1-4GlcNAcβ1-3Galβ1-4Glc	Taufik et al. (2012)
5	LNFP III	Galβ1-4GlcNAcβ1-3Galβ1-4Glc 3 Fucα1	Taufik et al. (2012)
6	LNnH	Galβ1-4GlcNAcβ1 6 Galβ1-4Glc Galβ1-4GlcNAcβ1 3	Taufik et al. (2012)
7	FLNnH	Fucα1 3 Galβ1-4GlcNAcβ1 6 Galβ1-4Glc Galβ1-4GlcNAcβ1 3	Taufik et al. (2012)
		Galβ1-4GlcNAcβ1 6 Galβ1-4Glc Galβ1-4GlcNAcβ1 3 3 Fucα1	Taufik et al. (2012)

Continued

Table 3.1 Milk Oligosaccharides of Primates—cont'd

No.	Oligosaccharide	Structure	References
8	DFLNnH	Fucα1 3 Galβ1-4GlcNAcβ1 6 3 Galβ1-4Glc Galβ1-4GlcNAcβ1 3 Fucα1	Taufik et al. (2012)
Acidic oligosaccharides			
1	3′-SL	Neu5Acα2-3Galβ1-4Glc	Taufik et al. (2012)
2	6′-SL	Neu5Acα2-6Galβ1-4Glc	Taufik et al. (2012)
3	LST c	Neu5Acα2-6Galβ1-4GlcNAcβ1-3Galβ1-4Glc	Taufik et al. (2012)
4	MSLNnH	Galβ1-4GlcNAcβ1 6 3 Galβ1-4Glc Neu5Acα2-6Galβ1-4GlcNAcβ1	Taufik et al. (2012)
5	MSMFLNnH	Fucα1 3 Galβ1-4GlcNAcβ1 6 3 Galβ1-4Glc Neu5Acα2-6Galβ1-4GlcNAcβ1	Taufik et al. (2012)

In human milk, the diverse array of HMOs have been classified into 13 series based on their core structures (Table 3.2). Within each series, different structures are formed from the core group by the addition of varying numbers of Fuc and Neu5Ac. Although core groups can contain up to 10 saccharide units (e.g., lacto-*N*-decaose and lacto-*N*-neodecaose), the most abundant HMOs contain two to six saccharide units within core groups, including lactose, lacto-*N*-tetraose (type I), lacto-*N*-neotetraose (type II), lacto-*N*-hexaose (type I), and lacto-*N*-neohexaose (type II) (Table 3.2). Among primates we detected oligosaccharides with lactose

Table 3.2 The 13 Core Structures of Human (*Homo sapiens*) Milk Oligosaccharides

Structures	Name
Galβ1-4Glc	Lactose
Galβ1-3GlcNAcβ1-3Galβ1-4Glc	Lacto-*N*-tetraose
Galβ1-4GlcNAcβ1-3Galβ1-4Glc	Lacto-*N*-neotetraose
Galβ1-4GlcNAcβ1 6 3 Galβ1-4Glc Galβ1-3GlcNAcβ1	Lacto-*N*-hexaose
Galβ1-4GlcNAcβ1 6 3 Galβ1-4Glc Galβ1-4GlcNAcβ1	Lacto-*N*-neohexaose
Galβ1-3GlcNAcβ1-3Galβ1-4GlcNAcβ1-3Galβ1-4Glc	*para*-Lacto-*N*-hexaose
Galβ1-4GlcNAcβ1-3Galβ1-4GlcNAcβ1-3Galβ1-4Glc	*para*-Lacto-*N*-neohexaose
Galβ1-4GlcNAcβ1-3Galβ1-4GlcNAcβ1 6 3 Galβ1-4Glc Galβ1-3GlcNAcβ1	Lacto-*N*-octaose
Galβ1-3GlcNAcβ1-3Galβ1-4GlcNAcβ1 6 3 Galβ1-4Glc Galβ1-4GlcNAcβ1	Lacto-*N*-neooctaose
Galβ1-3GlcNAcβ1-3Galβ1-4GlcNAcβ1 6 3 Galβ1-4Glc Galβ1-3GlcNAcβ1	*iso*-Lacto-*N*-octaose
Galβ1-3GlcNAcβ1-3Galβ1-4GlcNAcβ1-3Galβ1-4GlcNAcβ1-3Galβ1-4Glc	*para*-Lacto-*N*-octaose
Galβ1-4GlcNAcβ1 6 3 Galβ1-4GlcNAcβ1 Galβ1-3GlcNAcβ1 6 3 Galβ1-4Glc Galβ1-3GlcNAcβ1	Lacto-*N*-decaose
Galβ1-4GlcNAcβ1 6 3 Galβ1-4GlcNAcβ1 Galβ1-4GlcNAcβ1 6 3 Galβ1-4Glc Galβ1-3GlcNAcβ1	Lacto-*N*-neodecaose

as a core group in all species we studied; the next most prevalent core group was lacto-*N*-neotetraose (type II in chimp, bonobo, gorilla, orangutan, siamang, rhesus macaque, toque macaque, greater galago, aye-aye, and mongoose lemur). Lacto-*N*-neohexaose core group (type II) was detected in orangutan, siamang, Hamadryas baboon, tufted capuchin, aye-aye, Coquerel's sifaka, and mongoose lemur. The type I core group lacto-*N*-tetraose was only detected in the chimp, bonobo, orangutan, and aye-aye, and no milk oligosaccharides have yet been identified in nonhuman primates that contain the larger type II core group lacto-*N*-neohexaose.

With respect to sialyl oligosaccharides, milk is known to contain two types, *N*-acetyl (Neu5Ac) and *N*-glycolyl (Neu5Gc), the latter being derived from Neu5Ac through the action of CMP-Neu5Ac hydroxylase. In human milk/colostrum, Neu5Gc-containing saccharides have never been observed as a result of the absence of this enzyme from any human tissues including lactating mammary glands (Brinkman-van den Linden et al., 2000). Among apes, however, Neu5Gc(α2-3)Gal(β1-4)Glc (3′-NGc-SL) has been found in milk/colostrum of the chimpanzee, bonobo, gorilla, and orangutan (Urashima et al., 2009b) but not in milk of the siamang (Urashima et al., 2009b). 2′-FL has been found in milk/colostrum of chimpanzee, bonobo, and gorilla (Urasima et al., 2009b) but not in that of orangutan and siamang (Urashima et al., 2009b). A-tetrasaccharide (GalNAc(α1-3)[Fuc(α1-2)]Gal(β1-4)Glc), which contains human blood group A-antigen (GalNAc(α1-3)[Fuc(α1-2)]Gal), is found in the milk/colostrum of the bonobo (Urashima et al., 2009b), while B-tetrasaccharide (Gal(α1-3)[Fuc(α1-2)] Gal(β1-4)Glc, which contains B-antigen (Gal(α1-3)[Fuc(α1-2)]Gal), is found in that of the gorilla (Urashima et al., 2009b).

In the milk of Old World monkeys, only Neu5Ac-containing saccharides, not those containing Neu5Gc, have been found (Goto et al., 2010; Urashima et al., 1999a). Similarly, Neu5Gc was found to be absent in the milk of New World monkeys. In the milk of Old World monkeys, Gal(β1-4)[Fuc(α1-3)]Glc (3-fucosyllactose, 3-FL) and LNFP-Ⅲ, which contains Lewis X (Gal(β1-4)[Fuc(α1-3)]GlcNAc), have been found, while 2′-FL has not been detected in these milks (Goto et al., 2010). As noted, in some primate milk/colostrum, LN*n*T, LN*n*H [Gal(β1-4)GlcNAc(β1-3) [Gal(β1-4)GlcNAc(β1-6)]Gal(β1-4)Glc, lacto-*N*-neohexaose] and their fucosyl and sialyl derivatives have been found (Urashima et al., 1999a, 2009b; Goto et al., 2010; Taufik et al., 2012). Gal(β1-3)[Gal(β1-4)GlcNAc(β1-6)]Gal(β1-4)Glc (lacto-*N*-novopentaose I) has been found in the milk of the tufted capuchin (Goto et al., 2010; Urashima et al., 1999a), a New World monkey, but this saccharide has not been detected in the milk/colostrum of humans, apes, or Old World monkeys. Among strepsirrhine primates, aye-aye milk exceptionally contains the type I oligosaccharides including LNT and Gal(β1-3)[Fuc(α1-4)]GlcNAc(β1-3)Gal(β1-4)Glc (lacto-*N*-fucopentaose II, LNFP-II) (Taufik et al., 2012), and greater galago milk contains 3′-Neu5Gc-SL (Taufik et al., 2012). It is interesting that Gal(α1-3)Gal(β1-4)Glc (isoglobotriose) has been found in the milk of Coquerel's sifaka and mongoose lemur (Taufik et al., 2012); this is noteworthy because in tissues of Old World monkeys and apes, the α3galactosyltransferase that catalyzes the synthesis of Gal(α1-3)Gal has been evolutionarily lost due to gene inactivation (Galili, 2005). It is also noteworthy that 2′-FL was detected in milk of the aye-aye (Taufik et al., 2012); this saccharide was not found in the milks of either Old World or New World monkeys (Goto et al., 2010; Urashima et al., 1999a).

In addition, Tao et al. (2011) studied oligosaccharides in the milks of several New and Old World monkeys and apes by glycoprofiling, using porous graphitic carbon liquid chromatography–mass spectrometry. They found that in human milk 50–80% of the oligosaccharides are fucosylated depending on the secretor/Lewis group, which compared with the milk of chimpanzees at around 50% and of gorillas with only 15%. In humans, 10–30% of the milk oligosaccharides are sialylated; similar values are found in the milk/colostrum of chimpanzees, rhesus macaque, and gorillas.

Most of the studies that have been done to date on primate milk oligosaccharides are limited by small numbers of samples, precluding study of individual variation, which is known to be important in human milk. In addition, small sample volumes complicate efforts to characterize milk oligosaccharides present at trace amounts. It is likely that additional saccharides will be detected in the future, especially with the development and application of more sensitive methods and the study of additional primate species.

2.1.2 Domestic Ruminants (Cow, Goat, Sheep, Camel, Reindeer), Horse, and Pig (Oligosaccharides in Table 3.3)

Marino et al. (2011) characterized the oligosaccharides separated from bovine colostrum, after which Albrecht et al. (2014) characterized those from bovine colostrum, ovine colostrum, goat mature milk, dromedary camel mature milk, mare colostrum, and swine colostrum. The oligosaccharide in the separated fraction was isolated by hydrophilic HPLC after derivatization with 2-aminobenzaldehyde and then characterized using a combination of data from exoglycosidase or alkali phosphatase digestion, electrospray mass spectrometry, and retention time in hydrophilic HPLC. Based on the characterized structures, it was concluded that the oligosaccharide core structures are lactose, LN*n*T, lacto-*N*-novopentaose I, LN*n*H, or GlcNAc(β1-3)[Gal(β1-4)GlcNAc(β1-6)]Gal(β1-4)Glc. Oligosaccharides based on a core of GlcNAc(β1-3)[Gal(β1-4)GlcNAc(β1-6)]Gal(β1-4)Glc have not been observed in human milk or colostrum (Urashima et al., 2011b), and only one oligosaccharide with a core of lacto-*N*-novopentaose I (Neu5Ac(α2-3)Gal(β1-3){Gal(β1-4)[Fuc(α1-3)]GlcNAc(β1-6)}Gal(β1-4)Glc) occurs at trace levels in human milk (Gronberg et al., 1992). The ratio of Neu5Ac/Neu5Gc in sialyl oligosaccharides differs depending on species as follows—97:3 in the cow, 37:64 in the goat, 6:94 in sheep, 99.9:0.1 in the pig, 99:1 in the horse, and 99.7:0.3 in the dromedary camel (Albrecht et al., 2014). Thus, Neu5Ac predominates over Neu5Gc in sialyl oligosaccharides in the milk/colostrum of most species, but Neu5Gc predominates over Neu5Ac in the milk of goat and sheep (Albrecht et al., 2014). It is noteworthy that the milk/colostrum of these domestic mammals contains sialyl oligosaccharides whose core is Gal(β1-3)Gal(β1-4)Glc (3′-galactosyllactose, 3′-GL). This type of sialyl oligosaccharide has

Table 3.3 Milk Oligosaccharides of Domestic Herbivores and Pigs

No.	Oligosaccharide	Structure	References
Bovine (Bos taurus) Colostrum or Milk			
Neutral Oligosaccharides			
1	*N*-Acetylgalactosaminylglucose	GalNAcβ1-4Glc	Marino et al. (2011) and Saito et al. (1984)
2	LacNAc	Galβ1-4GlcNAc	Marino et al. (2011) and Saito et al. (1984)
3	3-FLN	Galβ1-4GlcNAc Fucα1³	Albrecht et al. (2014) and Saito et al. (1987)
4	α3′-GalNAcL	GalNAcα1-3Galβ1-4Glc	Marino et al. (2011), Albrecht et al. (2014), and Urashima et al. (1991b)
5	Isoglobotriose	Galα1-3Galβ1-4Glc	Marino et al. (2011), Albrecht et al. (2014), and Urashima et al. (1991b)
6	β3′-GL	Galβ1-3Galβ1-4Glc	Marino et al. (2011), Albrecht et al. (2014), and Saito et al. (1987)
7	β4′-GL	Galβ1-4Galβ1-4Glc	Marino et al. (2011)
8	β6′-GL	Galβ1-6Galβ1-4Glc	Marino et al. (2011), Albrecht et al. (2014), and Saito et al. (1987)
9	*novo*-LNP I	Galβ1-4GlcNAcβ1 6 3 Galβ1-4Glc Galβ1	Marino et al. (2011) and Urashima et al. (1991b)
10	β3′-GalNAcL	GalNAcβ1-3Galβ1-4Glc	Watanabe et al. (2006)

No.	Oligosaccharide	Structure	References
11	LNnT	Galβ1-4GlcNAcβ1-3Galβ1-4Glc	Marino et al. (2011) and Albrecht et al. (2014)
12	LNnH	Galβ1-4GlcNAcβ1 6 3 Galβ1-4Glc Galβ1-4GlcNAcβ1	Marino et al. (2011) and Albrecht et al. (2014)
13	LacdiNAc	GalNAcβ1-4GlcNAc	Marino et al. (2011)
14	2′-FL	Fucα1-2Galβ1-4Glc	Marino et al. (2011)
15	3-FL	Galβ1-4Glc 3 Fucα1	Albrecht et al. (2014)
16	LNTri-II	GlcNAcβ1-3Galβ1-4Glc	Marino et al. (2011) and Albrecht et al. (2014)
17	A-tetrasaccharide	Fucα1-2Galβ1-4Glc 3 GalNAcα1	Marino et al. (2011) and Albrecht et al. (2014)
18		Galβ1-4GlcNAcβ1 6 3 Galβ1-4Glc GlcNAcβ1	Marino et al. (2011) and Albrecht et al. (2014)
Acidic Oligosaccharides			
19	3′-L-*O*-phosphate	3-P-Gal(β1-4)Glc	Cumar et al. (1965)
20	3SGal	Neu5Acα2-3Gal	Kuhn and Kauhe (1965)
21	3′-SL	Neu5Acα2-3Galβ1-4Glc	Marino et al. (2011), Albrecht et al. (2014), and Schneier and Rafelson (1966)
22	6′-SL	Neu5Acα2-6Galβ1-4Glc	Marino et al. (2011), Albrecht et al. (2014), and Schneier and Rafelson (1966)

Continued

Table 3.3 Milk Oligosaccharides of Domestic Herbivores and Pigs—cont'd

No.	Oligosaccharide	Structure	References
23	3′-Neu5GcL	Neu5Gcα2-3Galβ1-4Glc	Marino et al. (2011), Albrecht et al. (2014), and Kuhn and Gauhe (1965)
24	6′-Neu5GcL	Neu5Gcα2-6Galβ1-4Glc	Marino et al. (2011), Albrecht et al. (2014), and Veh et al. (1981)
25	6′-SLacNAc	Neu5Acα2-6Galβ1-4GlcNAc	Marino et al. (2011), Albrecht et al. (2014), and Kuhn and Gauhe (1965)
26	6′-Neu5GcLacNAc	Neu5Gcα2-6Galβ1-4GlcNAc	Marino et al. (2011) and Albrecht et al. (2014)
27	3″-S-β3′-GL	Neu5Acα2-3Gal1-3Gal1-4Glc	Marino et al. (2011) and Albrecht et al. (2014)
28	DSL	Neu5Acα2-8Neu5Acα2-3Galβ1-4Glc	Kuhn and Gauhe (1965)
29	6′-SLacNAc-1-*O*-phosphate	Neu5Acα2-6Galβ1-4GlcNAc-1-P	Parkkinen and Finne (1987)
30	6′-SLacNAc-6-*O*-phosphate	Neu5Acα2-6Galβ1-4GlcNAc-6-P	Parkkinen and Finne (1987)
31	3′-SLacNAc	Neu5Acα2-3Galβ1-4GlcNAc	Albrecht et al. (2014)
32	6′-S-β3′-GL	Galβ1-3Galβ1-4Glc Neu5Acα2^{6}	Marino et al. (2011)
33	3-SLNnT	Neu5Acα2-3Galβ1-4GlcNAcβ1-3Galβ1-4Galβ1-4Glc	Marino et al. (2011)
34	LSTc	Neu5Acα2-6Galβ1-4GlcNAcβ1-3Galβ1-4Glc	Marino et al. (2011)

No.	Oligosaccharide	Structure	References
35	3-SLNP	Neu5Acα2-3[Galβ1-4GlcNAcβ1-6 / Galβ1-3]Galβ1-4Glc	Marino et al. (2011) and Albrecht et al. (2014)
36	3-SLNnH	Neu5Acα2-3[Galβ1-4GlcNAcβ1-6 / Galβ1-4GlcNAcβ1-3]Galβ1-4Glc	Marino et al. (2011) and Albrecht et al. (2014)
37	6-SLNnH	Neu5Acα2-6[Galβ1-4GlcNAcβ1-6 / Galβ1-4GlcNAcβ1-3]Galβ1-4Glc	Marino et al. (2011) and Albrecht et al. (2014)
38	6′-SLacdiNAc	Neu5Acα2-6GalNAcβ1-4GlcNAc	Marino et al. (2011)
39		Neu5Acα2-6Galβ1-4Glc GlcNAcβ1-3	Marino et al. (2011)
40		Neu5Gcα2-8Neu5Acα2-3Galβ1-4Glc	Marino et al. (2011) and Albrecht et al. (2014)
41		Neu5Acα2-8Neu5Gcα2-3Galβ1-4Glc	Marino et al. (2011)
42	DSLN	Neu5Acα2-8Neu5Acα2-3Galβ1-4GlcNAc	Marino et al. (2011) and Albrecht et al. (2014)
43		Neu5Acα2-3GlcNAcβ1-3Galβ1-4Glc	Albrecht et al. (2014)
44		Neu5Gcα2-8Neu5Gcα2-3Galβ1-4Glc	Albrecht et al. (2014)
45	DSβ3′-GL	Neu5Acα2-3Galβ1-3Galβ1-4Glc Neu5Acα2-6	Albrecht et al. (2014)
46	6-SLNP	Neu5Acα2-6[Galβ1-4GlcNAcβ1-6 / Galβ1-3]Galβ1-4Glc	Marino et al. (2011) and Albrecht et al. (2014)

Continued

Table 3.3 Milk Oligosaccharides of Domestic Herbivores and Pigs—cont'd

No.	Oligosaccharide	Structure	References
Water Buffalo *(Bubalus bubalis)* Colostrum			
Acidic Oligosaccharides			
1	DSL	Neu5Acα2-8Neu5Acα2-3Galβ1-4Glc	Aparma and Salimath (1995)
Caprine (Capra aegagrus hircus) Colostrum or Milk			
Neutral Oligosaccharides			
1	2′-FL	Fucα1-2Galβ1-4Glc	Albrecht et al. (2014) and Urashima et al. (1994a)
2	Isoglobotriose	Galα1-3Galβ1-4Glc	Albrecht et al. (2014) and Urashima et al. (1994a)
3	β3′-GL	Galβ1-3Galβ1-4Glc	Albrecht et al. (2014) and Urashima et al. (1994a)
4	β6′-GL	Galβ1-6Galβ1-4Glc	Albrecht et al. (2014) and Urashima et al. (1994a)
5	3-FL	Galβ1-4Glc Fucα1 3	Albrecht et al. (2014)
6	3-FLN	Galβ1-4GlcNAc Fucα1 3	Albrecht et al. (2014)
7	α3′-GalNAcL	GalNAcα1-3Galβ1-4Glc	Albrecht et al. (2014)
8	LNTri-II	GlcNAcβ1-3Galβ1-4Glc	Albrecht et al. (2014)
9	LNnT	Galβ1-4GlcNAcβ1-3Galβ1-4Glc	Albrecht et al. (2014)

No.	Oligosaccharide	Structure	References
10	isoLNnT	Galβ1-4GlcNAcβ1-6Galβ1-4Glc	Albrecht et al. (2014)
11		Galβ1-4GlcNAcβ1 6 Galβ1-4Glc GlcNAcβ1 3	Albrecht et al. (2014)
12	*novo*-LNP I	Galβ1-4GlcNAcβ1 6 Galβ1-4Glc Galβ1 3	Albrecht et al. (2014)
13	LNnH	Galβ1-4GlcNAcβ1 6 Galβ1-4Glc Galβ1-4GlcNAcβ1 3	Albrecht et al. (2014)
Acidic Oligosaccharides			
14	3′-SL	Neu5Acα2-3Galβ1-4Glc	Albrecht et al. (2014), Urashima et al. (1997c), and Viverge et al. (1997)
15	6′-SL	Neu5Acα2-6Galβ1-4Glc	Albrecht et al. (2014), Urashima et al. (1997c), and Viverge et al. (1997)
16	6′-Neu5GcL	Neu5Gcα2-6Galβ1-4Glc	Albrecht et al. (2014) and Urashima et al. (1997c)
17	6′-SLN	Neu5Acα2-6Galβ1-4GlcNAc	Albrecht et al. (2014) and Urashima et al. (1997c)
18	3′-S-β6′-GL	Galβ1-6Galβ1-4Glc 3 Neu5Acα2	Viverge et al. (1997)
19	6′-S-β3′-GL	Galβ1-3Galβ1-4Glc 6 Neu5Acα2	Viverge et al. (1997)
20	3′-SLN	Neu5Acα2-3Galβ1-4GlcNAc	Albrecht et al. (2014)

Continued

Table 3.3 Milk Oligosaccharides of Domestic Herbivores and Pigs—cont'd

No.	Oligosaccharide	Structure	References
21	3′-Neu5GcLN	Neu5Gcα2-3Galβ1-4GlcNAc	Albrecht et al. (2014)
22	3′-Neu5GcL	Neu5Gcα2-3Galβ1-4Glc	Albrecht et al. (2014)
23	6′-Neu5GcLN	Neu5Gcα2-6Galβ1-4GlcNAc	Albrecht et al. (2014)
24		Neu5Acα2-3GlcNAcβ1-3Galβ1-4Glc	Albrecht et al. (2014)
25	3″-S-β3′-GL	Neu5Acα2-3Galβ1-3Galβ1-4Glc	Albrecht et al. (2014)
26	3″-Neu5Gc-β3′-GL	Neu5Gcα2-3Galβ1-3Galβ1-4Glc	Albrecht et al. (2014)
27	DSL	Neu5Acα2-8Neu5Acα2-3Galβ1-4Glc	Albrecht et al. (2014)
28		Neu5Gcα2-8Neu5Acα2-3Galβ1-4Glc	Albrecht et al. (2014)
29		Neu5Gcα2-3Galβ1-3Galβ1-4Glc 6 Neu5Acα2	Albrecht et al. (2014)
30	3Neu5GcLNP	Neu5Gcα2-3-[Galβ1-4GlcNAcβ1 6 / Galβ1 3] Galβ1-4Glc	Albrecht et al. (2014)
31	6Neu5GcLNP	Neu5Gcα2-6-[Galβ1-4GlcNAcβ1 6 / Galβ1 3] Galβ1-4Glc	Albrecht et al. (2014)
32	3Neu5GcLNnH	Neu5Gcα2-3-[Galβ1-4GlcNAcβ1 6 / Galβ1-4GlcNAcβ1 3] Galβ1-4Glc	Albrecht et al. (2014)
33	6Neu5GcLNnH	Neu5Gcα2-6-[Galβ1-4GlcNAcβ1 6 / Galβ1-4GlcNAcβ1 3] Galβ1-4Glc	Albrecht et al. (2014)

No.	Oligosaccharide	Structure	References
34		Sia(α2-3(6))Gal(β1-4)GlcNAc-UDP	Jourdian et al. (1961)
35		Sia(α2-3(6))Gal(β1-6)GlcNAc-UDP	Jourdian et al. (1961)
Ovine (Ovis aries) **Colostrum**			
Neutral Oligosaccharides			
1	Isoglobotriose	Galα1-3Galβ1-4Glc	Albrecht et al. (2014) and Urashima et al. (1989a)
2	β3′-GL	Galβ1-3Galβ1-4Glc	Albrecht et al. (2014) and Urashima et al. (1989a)
3	β6′-GL	Galβ1-6Galβ1-4Glc	Albrecht et al. (2014) and Urashima et al. (1989a)
4	2′-FL	Fucα1-2Galβ1-4Glc	Albrecht et al. (2014)
5	3-FL	Galβ1-4Glc Fucα1 3	Albrecht et al. (2014)
6	3′-FLN	Galβ1-4GlcNAc Fucα1 3	Albrecht et al. (2014)
7	α3′-GalNAcL	GalNAcα1-3Galβ1-4Glc	Albrecht et al. (2014)
8	LNTri-II	GlcNAcβ1-3Galβ1-4Glc	Albrecht et al. (2014)
9	LNnT	Galβ1-4GlcNAcβ1-3Galβ1-4Glc	Albrecht et al. (2014)
10	isoLNnT	Galβ1-4GlcNAcβ1-6Galβ1-4Glc	Albrecht et al. (2014)
11		Galβ1-4GlcNAcβ1 6 Galβ1-4Glc GlcNAcβ1 3	Albrecht et al. (2014)

Continued

Table 3.3 Milk Oligosaccharides of Domestic Herbivores and Pigs—cont'd

No.	Oligosaccharide	Structure	References
12	*novo*-LNP I	Galβ1-4GlcNAcβ1-6(Galβ1-3)Galβ1-4Glc	Albrecht et al. (2014)
13	LNnH	Galβ1-4GlcNAcβ1-6(Galβ1-4GlcNAcβ1-3)Galβ1-4Glc	Albrecht et al. (2014)
Acidic Oligosaccharides			
14	3′-SL	Neu5Acα2-3Galβ1-4Glc	Albrecht et al. (2014) and Nakamura et al. (1998)
15	6′-SL	Neu5Acα2-6Galβ1-4Glc	Albrecht et al. (2014)
16	3′-Neu5GcL	Neu5Gcα2-3Galβ1-4Glc	Albrecht et al. (2014) and Nakamura et al. (1998)
17	3′-SLN	Neu5Acα2-3Galβ1-4GlcNAc	Albrecht et al. (2014)
18	3′-Neu5GcLN	Neu5Gcα2-3Galβ1-4GlcNAc	Albrecht et al. (2014)
19	6′-SLN	Neu5Acα2-6Galβ1-4GlcNAc	Albrecht et al. (2014)
20	6′-Neu5GcL	Neu5Gcα2-6Galβ1-4Glc	Albrecht et al. (2014) and Nakamura et al. (1998)
21		Neu5Acα2-3GlcNAcβ1-3Galβ1-4Glc	Albrecht et al. (2014)
22	3″-S-β3′-GL	Neu5Acα2-3Galβ1-3Galβ1-4Glc	Albrecht et al. (2014)
23	6′-Neu5Gc-β3′-GL	Galβ1-3(Neu5Gcα2-6)Galβ1-4Glc	Albrecht et al. (2014)
24	DSL	Neu5Acα2-8Neu5Acα2-3Galβ1-4Glc	Albrecht et al. (2014)
25		Neu5Gcα2-8Neu5Acα2-3Galβ1-4Glc	Albrecht et al. (2014)

No.	Oligosaccharide	Structure	References
26		Neu5Gcα2-3Galβ1-3Galβ1-4Glc (6) Neu5Acα2	Albrecht et al. (2014)
27	3Neu5GcLNP	Neu5Gcα2-3-[Galβ1-4GlcNAcβ1 (6) / Galβ1 (3)] Galβ1-4Glc	Albrecht et al. (2014)
28	6Neu5GcLNP	Neu5Gcα2-6-[Galβ1-4GlcNAcβ1 (6) / Galβ1 (3)] Galβ1-4Glc	Albrecht et al. (2014)
29	6Neu5GcLNnH	Neu5Gcα2-6-[Galβ1-4GlcNAcβ1 (6) / Galβ1-4GlcNAcβ1 (3)] Galβ1-4Glc	Albrecht et al. (2014)
30	LacNAc-PO_4	4-P-Gal(β1-4)GlcNAc	Albrecht et al. (2014)
Bactrian Camel (Camelus bactrianus) Colostrum/Milk			
Neutral Oligosaccharides			
1	3-FL	Galβ1-4Glc (3) Fucα1	Fukuda et al. (2010)
2	β3′-GL	Galβ1-3Galβ1-4Glc	Fukuda et al. (2010)
3	β6′-GL	Galβ1-6Galβ1-4Glc	Fukuda et al. (2010)
4	*novo*-LNP I	Galβ1-4GlcNAcβ1 (6) / Galβ1 (3) Galβ1-4Glc	Fukuda et al. (2010)

Continued

Table 3.3 Milk Oligosaccharides of Domestic Herbivores and Pigs—cont'd

No.	Oligosaccharide	Structure	References
Acidic Oligosaccharides			
5	3′-SL	Neu5Acα2-3Galβ1-4Glc	Fukuda et al. (2010)
6	6′-SL	Neu5Acα2-6Galβ1-4Glc	Fukuda et al. (2010)
7	3″-S-β3′-GL	Neu5Acα2-3Galβ1-3Galβ1-4Glc	Fukuda et al. (2010)
8	LSTc	Neu5Acα2-6Galβ1-4GlcNAcβ1-3Galβ1-4Glc	Fukuda et al. (2010)
9	SLNPa	Galβ1-4GlcNAcβ1 (6) Galβ1-4Glc Neu5Acα2-3Galβ1 (3)	Fukuda et al. (2010)
10	SLNPb	Neu5Acα2-6Galβ1-4GlcNAcβ1 (6) Galβ1-4Glc Galβ1 (3)	Fukuda et al. (2010)
11	MSLNnH	Galβ1-4GlcNAcβ1 (6) Galβ1-4Glc Neu5Acα2-6Galβ1-4GlcNAcβ1 (3)	Fukuda et al. (2010)
Dromedary Camel (Camelus dromedarius) Milk			
Neutral Oligosaccharides			
1	β3′-GL	Galβ1-3Galβ1-4Glc	Albrecht et al. (2014) and Alhaj et al. (2013)
2	2′-FL	Fucα1-2Galβ1-4Glc	Albrecht et al. (2014)
3	3-FL	Galβ1-4Glc Fucα1 (3)	Albrecht et al. (2014)
4	α3′-GalNAcL	GalNAcα1-3Galβ1-4Glc	Albrecht et al. (2014)
5	LNTri-II	GlcNAcβ1-3Galβ1-4Glc	Albrecht et al. (2014)

No.	Oligosaccharide	Structure	References
6	Isoglobotriose	Galα1-3Galβ1-4Glc	Albrecht et al. (2014)
7	A-tetrasaccharide	GalNAcα1-3Galβ1-4Glc Fucα1-2	Albrecht et al. (2014)
8	β6′-GL	Galβ1-6Galβ1-4Glc	Albrecht et al. (2014)
9	LNnT	Galβ1-4GlcNAcβ1-3Galβ1-4Glc	Albrecht et al. (2014)
10	isoLNnT	Galβ1-4GlcNAcβ1-6Galβ1-4Glc	Albrecht et al. (2014)
11	LNFP III	Galβ1-4GlcNAcβ1-3Galβ1-4Glc Fucα1-3	Albrecht et al. (2014)
12		Galβ1-4GlcNAcβ1-6 Galβ1-4Glc GlcNAcβ1-3	Albrecht et al. (2014)
13	LNP I	Galβ1-4GlcNAcβ1-6 Galβ1-4Glc Galβ1-3	Albrecht et al. (2014)
14	LNnH	Galβ1-4GlcNAcβ1-6 Galβ1-4Glc Galβ1-4GlcNAcβ1-3	Albrecht et al. (2014) and Alhaj et al. (2013)
Acidic Oligosaccharides			
15	3′-SL	Neu5Acα2-3Galβ1-4Glc	Albrecht et al. (2014) and Alhaj et al. (2013)
16	6′-SL	Neu5Acα2-6Galβ1-4Glc	Albrecht et al. (2014) and Alhaj et al. (2013)
17	3′-SLN	Neu5Acα2-3Galβ1-4GlcNAc	Albrecht et al. (2014)

Continued

Table 3.3 Milk Oligosaccharides of Domestic Herbivores and Pigs—cont'd

No.	Oligosaccharide	Structure	References
18	3′-Neu5GcLN	Neu5Gcα2-3Galβ1-4GlcNAc	Albrecht et al. (2014)
19	6′-SLN	Neu5Acα2-6Galβ1-4GlcNAc	Albrecht et al. (2014)
20	3′-Neu5GcL	Neu5Gcα2-3Galβ1-4Glc	Albrecht et al. (2014)
21		Neu5Acα2-3GlcNAcβ1-3Galβ1-4Glc	Albrecht et al. (2014)
22	6′-Neu5GcL	Neu5Gcα2-6Galβ1-4Glc	Albrecht et al. (2014)
23	3″-S-β3′-GL	Neu5Acα2-3Galβ1-3Galβ1-4Glc	Albrecht et al. (2014) and Alhaj et al. (2013)
24	6′-S-β3′-GL	Galβ1-3Galβ1-4Glc 6 Neu5Acα2	Albrecht et al. (2014)
25	DSL	Neu5Acα2-8Neu5Acα2-3Galβ1-4Glc	Albrecht et al. (2014)
26	DSβ3′-GL	Neu5Acα2-3Galβ1-3Galβ1-4Glc 6 Neu5Acα2	Albrecht et al. (2014)
27	SLNPa	Galβ1-4GlcNAcβ1 6 Galβ1-4Glc Neu5Acα2-3Galβ1 3	Alhaj et al. (2013)
28	3SLNP	Neu5Acα2-3-{ Galβ1-4GlcNAcβ1 6 Galβ1-4Glc Galβ1 3 }	Albrecht et al. (2014)
29		Neu5Gcα2-3Galβ1-3Galβ1-4Glc 6 Neu5Acα2	Albrecht et al. (2014)
30	3SLNnH	Neu5Acα2-3-{ Galβ1-4GlcNAcβ1 6 Galβ1-4Glc Galβ1-4GlcNAcβ1 3 }	Albrecht et al. (2014)

No.	Oligosaccharide	Structure	References
31	MSLNnH	Galβ1-4GlcNAcβ1 6 Galβ1-4Glc Neu5Acα2-6Galβ1-4GlcNAcβ1 3	Alhaj et al. (2013)
32	GSLNnH	Neu5Acα2-6-{ Galβ1-4GlcNAcβ1 6 Galβ1-4Glc Galβ1-4GlcNAcβ1 3 }	Albrecht et al. (2014)
33	LacNAc-1-*O*-phosphate	Galβ1-4GlcNAc-1-P	Albrecht et al. (2014)
Reindeer (Rangifer tarandus) Milk			
Neutral Oligosaccharides			
1	β3′-GL	Galβ1-3Galβ1-4Glc	Taufik et al. (2014)
Acidic Oligosaccharides			
2	β6′-GL	Galβ1-6Galβ1-4Glc	Taufik et al. (2014)
3	6′-SL	Neu5Acα2-6Galβ1-4Glc	Taufik et al. (2014)
4	LSTc	Neu5Acα2-6Galβ1-4GlcNAcβ1-3Galβ1-4Glc	Taufik et al. (2014)
5	UDP-LacNAc	Galβ1-4GlcNAc-UDP	Taufik et al. (2014)
Equine (Equus ferus caballus) Colostrum			
Neutral Oligosaccharides			
1	β3′-GL	Galβ1-3Galβ1-4Glc	Albrecht et al. (2014) and Urashima et al. (1989b)
2	β6′-GL	Galβ1-6Galβ1-4Glc	Albrecht et al. (2014) and Urashima et al. (1989b)
3	LNnT	Galβ1-4GlcNAcβ1-3Galβ1-4Glc	Albrecht et al. (2014) and Urashima et al. (1991a)

Continued

Table 3.3 Milk Oligosaccharides of Domestic Herbivores and Pigs—cont'd

No.	Oligosaccharide	Structure	References
4	iso-LNnT	Galβ1-4GlcNAcβ1-6Galβ1-4Glc	Albrecht et al. (2014) and Urashima et al. (1991a)
5	*novo*-LNP I	Galβ1-4GlcNAcβ1-6(Galβ1-3)Galβ1-4Glc	Albrecht et al. (2014) and Urashima et al. (1989b)
6	LNnH	Galβ1-4GlcNAcβ1-6(Galβ1-4GlcNAcβ1-3)Galβ1-4Glc	Albrecht et al. (2014) and Urashima et al. (1991a)
7	3-FL	Galβ1-4(Fucα1-3)Glc	Albrecht et al. (2014)
8	α3′-GalNAcL	GalNAcα1-3Galβ1-4Glc	Albrecht et al. (2014)
9	LNTri-II	GlcNAcβ1-3Galβ1-4Glc	Albrecht et al. (2014)
10	Isoglobotriose	Galα1-3Galβ1-4Glc	Albrecht et al. (2014)
11		Galβ1-4GlcNAcβ1-6(GlcNAcβ1-3)Galβ1-4Glc	Albrecht et al. (2014)
12	GalLNP	Galα1-3[Galβ1-4GlcNAcβ1-6(GlcNAcβ1-3)]Galβ1-4Glc	Albrecht et al. (2014)
13	GalLNnH	Galα1-3[Galβ1-4GlcNAcβ1-6(Galβ1-4GlcNAcβ1-3)]Galβ1-4Glc	Albrecht et al. (2014)
14	DGalLNnH	Galα1-3Galβ1-4GlcNAcβ1-6(Galα1-3Galβ1-4GlcNAcβ1-3)Galβ1-4Glc	Albrecht et al. (2014)

No.	Oligosaccharide	Structure	References
15	β4′-GL	Galβ1-4Galβ1-4Glc	Diffilippo et al. (2015)
16	LNH	Galβ1-4GlcNAcβ1 6 Galβ1-4Glc Galβ1-3GlcNAcβ1 3	Difilippo et al. (2015)
Acidic Oligosaccharides			
17	LacNAc-1-*O*-phosphate	Gal(β1-4)GlcNAc-1-P	Albrecht et al. (2014) and Nakamura et al. (2001)
18	3′-SL	Neu5Acα2-3Galβ1-4Glc	Albrecht et al. (2014) and Nakamura et al. (2001)
19	3′-SLN	Neu5Acα2-3Galβ1-4GlcNAc	Albrecht et al. (2014)
20	6′-SLN	Neu5Acα2-6Galβ1-4GlcNAc	Albrecht et al. (2014)
21	3′-Neu5GcL	Neu5Gcα2-3Galβ1-4Glc	Albrecht et al. (2014)
22	6′-SL	Neu5Acα2-6Galβ1-4Glc	Albrecht et al. (2014)
23	3′-S-3-FL	Neu5Acα2-3Galβ1-4Glc 3 Fucα1	Albrecht et al. (2014)
24	3″-S-β3′-GL	Neu5Acα2-3Galβ1-3Galβ1-4Glc	Albrecht et al. (2014)
25	6′-S-β3′-GL	Galβ1-3Galβ1-4Glc 6 Neu5Acα2	Albrecht et al. (2014)
26	DSLN	Neu5Acα2-8Neu5Acα2-3Galβ1-4GlcNAc	Albrecht et al. (2014)
27	DSL	Neu5Acα2-8Neu5Acα2-3Galβ1-4Glc	Albrecht et al. (2014)
28		Neu5Gcα2-8Neu5Acα2-3Galβ1-4Glc	Albrecht et al. (2014)

Continued

Table 3.3 Milk Oligosaccharides of Domestic Herbivores and Pigs—cont'd

No.	Oligosaccharide	Structure	References
29	DSβ3′-GL	Neu5Acα2-3Galβ1-3Galβ1-4Glc Neu5Acα2 6	Albrecht et al. (2014)
30	3SLNP	Neu5Acα2-3{ Galβ1-4GlcNAcβ1 6 / Galβ1 3 } Galβ1-4Glc	Albrecht et al. (2014)
31	6SLNP	Neu5Acα2-6{ Galβ1-4GlcNAcβ1 6 / Galβ1 3 } Galβ1-4Glc	Albrecht et al. (2014)
32	3SLNnH	Neu5Acα2-3{ Galβ1-4GlcNAcβ1 6 / Galβ1-4GlcNAcβ1 3 } Galβ1-4Glc	Albrecht et al. (2014)
33	6SLNnH	Neu5Acα2-6{ Galβ1-4GlcNAcβ1 6 / Galβ1-4GlcNAcβ1 3 } Galβ1-4Glc	Albrecht et al. (2014)
34	LSTa	Neu5Acα2-3Galβ1-3GlcNAcβ1-3Galβ1-4Glc	Difilippo et al. (2015)
Porcine (Sus scropha) Colostrum			
Neutral Oligosaccharides			
1	2′-FL	Fucα1-2Galβ1-4Glc	Albrecht et al. (2014)
2	3-FL	Galβ1-4Glc 3 Fucα1	Albrecht et al. (2014)
3	Isoglobotriose	Galα1-3Galβ1-4Glc	Albrecht et al. (2014)
4	β3′-GL	Galβ1-3Galβ1-4Glc	Albrecht et al. (2014)
5	β6′-GL	Galβ1-6Galβ1-4Glc	Albrecht et al. (2014)

No.	Oligosaccharide	Structure	References
6	*novo*-LNT	GlcNAcβ1 6 Galβ1-4Glc Galβ1 3	Albrecht et al. (2014)
7	LNnT	Galβ1-4GlcNAcβ1-3Galβ1-4Glc	Albrecht et al. (2014)
8	isoLNnT	Galβ1-4GlcNAcβ1-6Galβ1-4Glc	Albrecht et al. (2014)
9	LNFP III	Galβ1-4GlcNAcβ1-3Galβ1-4Glc 3 Fucα1	Albrecht et al. (2014)
10		Galβ1-4GlcNAcβ1 6 Galβ1-4Glc GlcNAcβ1 3	Albrecht et al. (2014)
11	*novo*-LNP I	Galβ1-4GlcNAcβ1 6 Galβ1-4Glc Galβ1 3	Albrecht et al. (2014)
12	LNnH	Galβ1-4GlcNAcβ1 6 Galβ1-4Glc Galβ1-4GlcNAcβ1 3	Albrecht et al. (2014)
13	GalLNP	Galα1-3{ Galβ1-4GlcNAcβ1 6 Galβ1-4Glc Galβ1 3	Albrecht et al. (2014)
14	GalLNnH	Galα1-3{ Galβ1-4GlcNAcβ1 6 Galβ1-4Glc Galβ1-4GlcNAcβ1 3	Albrecht et al. (2014)
15	DGalLNnH	Galα1-3Galβ1-4GlcNAcβ1 6 Galβ1-4Glc Galα1-3Galβ1-4GlcNAcβ1 3	Albrecht et al. (2014)

Continued

Table 3.3 Milk Oligosaccharides of Domestic Herbivores and Pigs—cont'd

No.	Oligosaccharide	Structure	References
Acidic Oligosaccharides			
16	3′-SLN	Neu5Acα2-3Galβ1-4GlcNAc	Albrecht et al. (2014)
17	3′-SL	Neu5Acα2-3Galβ1-4Glc	Albrecht et al. (2014)
18	6′-SLN	Neu5Acα2-6Galβ1-4GlcNAc	Albrecht et al. (2014)
19	3′-Neu5GcL	Neu5Gcα2-3Galβ1-4Glc	Albrecht et al. (2014)
20		Neu5Acα2-6GlcNAcβ1-6Galβ1-4Glc	Albrecht et al. (2014)
21	6′-SL	Neu5Acα2-6Galβ1-4Glc	Albrecht et al. (2014)
22	3″-S-β3′-GL	Neu5Acα2-3Galβ1-3Galβ1-4Glc	Albrecht et al. (2014)
23	DSLN	Neu5Acα2-8Neu5Acα2-3Galβ1-4GlcNAc	Albrecht et al. (2014)
24	3-SLNnT	Neu5Acα2-3Galβ1-4GlcNAcβ1-3Galβ1-4Galβ1-4Glc	Albrecht et al. (2014)
25	LSTc	Neu5Acα2-6Galβ1-4GlcNAcβ1-3Galβ1-4Glc	Albrecht et al. (2014)
26		Neu5Acα2-3Galβ1-4GlcNAcβ1 6 Galβ1-4Glc 3 GlcNAcβ1	Albrecht et al. (2014)
27	DS-β3′-GL	Neu5Acα2-3Galβ1-3Galβ1-4Glc 6 Neu5Acα2	Albrecht et al. (2014)

No.	Oligosaccharide	Structure	References
28	3-SLNP	Neu5Acα2-3-[Galβ1-4GlcNAcβ1-6 Galβ1-3]Galβ1-4Glc	Albrecht et al. (2014)
29	6-SLNP	Neu5Acα2-6-[Galβ1-4GlcNAcβ1-6 Galβ1-3]Galβ1-4Glc	Albrecht et al. (2014)
30	3-SLNnH	Neu5Acα2-3-[Galβ1-4GlcNAcβ1-6 Galβ1-4GlcNAcβ1-3]Galβ1-4Glc	Albrecht et al. (2014)
31	6-SLNnH	Neu5Acα2-6-[Galβ1-4GlcNAcβ1-6 Galβ1-4GlcNAcβ1-3]Galβ1-4Glc	Albrecht et al. (2014)

not been detected in human milk. All the oligosaccharides characterized by Marino et al. (2011), Albrecht et al. (2014), and others (Urashima et al., 1989a,b, 1991a,b, 1994a, 1997c; Nakamura et al., 1998, 2001; Kuhn and Gauhe, 1965; Cumar et al., 1965; Scheneier and Rafelson, 1966; Veh et al., 1981; Parkkinen and Finne, 1987; Saito et al., 1984, 1987; Viverge et al., 1997; Fukuda et al., 2010; Alhaj et al., 2013; Taufik et al., 2014), other than those whose core is lactose, are type II saccharides. As these characterizations were performed using a highly sensitive method, albeit with small numbers of samples (Marino et al., 2011; Albrecht et al., 2014), it can be concluded that the type I saccharides are absent from the milk/colostrum of these species or are present at only very low concentrations. However, Difilippo et al. (2015) found Gal(β1-3)GlcNAc(β1-3)[Gal(β1-4)GlcNAc(β1-6)Gal(β1-4)Glc (lacto-*N*-hexaose, LNH) and Neu5Ac(α2-3)Gal(β1-3)GlcNAc(β1-3)Gal(β1-4)Glc (sialyl lacto-*N*-tetraose a, LST a), which are type I, in mare colostrum. These milks are reported to contain free LacNAc or sialyl LacNAc (Albrecht et al., 2014), neither of which have been detected in human milk (Urashima et al., 2011b). Further study is needed to determine if such saccharides might derive from partial hydrolysis of oligosaccharide chains on milk glycoproteins or glycolipids. Isoglobotriose and GalNAc(α1-3)Gal(β1-4)Glc (α3′-GalNAcLac), which occur in the milk/colostrum of most of these herbivores, have not been found in human milk (Urashima et al., 2011b). GalNAc(β1-4)GlcNAc (LacdiNAc) and GalNAc(β1-4)Glc, which are present in bovine colostrum (Marino et al., 2011; Saito et al., 1984), are thought to be related to nonreducing LacdiNAc in the *N*-glycan of butyrophilin, one of the milk fat globule membrane glycoproteins (Urashima et al., 2011b).

Although fucosyl oligosaccharides such as 2′-FL, 3-FL, Gal(β1-4)[Fuc(α1-3)] GlcNAc (3-fucosyllactosamine, 3-FLN), and A-tetrasaccharide have been detected in bovine colostrum (Marino et al., 2011; Albrecht et al., 2014), they are present at no more than trace concentrations, unlike the situation in human milk/colostrum. Aldredge et al. (2013) found some large fucosyl oligosaccharides in bovine colostrum, but their concentrations were very low.

The method used by Marino et al. (2011) and Albrecht et al. (2014) is highly sensitive, enabling characterizations using very small milk/colostrum samples, but does not permit determination of the linkage positions of Neu5Ac or Neu5Gc to LN*n*H or lacto-*N*-novopentaose I. In our method with ^{1}H-NMR, we were able to determine the linkage position of Neu5Ac to Gal to differentiate between Gal(β1-4) GlcNAc(β1-3) and Gal(β1-4)GlcNAc(β1-6) of LN*n*H, and between Gal(β1-3) and Gal(β1-4)GlcNAc(β1-6) of lacto-*N*-novopentaose I (Fukuda et al., 2010; Alhaj et al., 2013). However, the NMR method requires considerably larger amounts of the purified components than the MS-based method. We note that our previous characterizations of isoglobotriose (Urashima et al., 1989a, 1991b, 1994a), α3′-GalNAcLac (Urashima et al., 1991b), lacto-*N*-novopentaose I (Urashima et al., 1989b, 1991b), Gal(β1-4)GlcNAc(β1-6)Gal(β1-4)Glc (isolacto-*N*-neotetraose) (Urashima et al., 1991a), etc. were probably of assistance in the characterizations performed by Marino et al. (2011) and Albrecht et al. (2014).

2.1.2.1 UDP-Oligosaccharides

Gal(β1-4)GlcNAc-UDP has been found in reindeer milk (Taufik et al., 2014), while Sia(α2-3(6))Gal(β1-4)GlcNAc-UDP and Sia(α2-3(6))Gal(β1-6)GlcNAc-UDP have been detected in caprine colostrum (Jourdian et al., 1961). Human milk, in addition, contains Gal(β1-4)GlcNAc-UDP and Fuc(α1-2)Gal(β1-4)GlcNAc-UDP (Kobota, 1963, 1966). Neu5Gc(α2-3)Gal(β1-4)GlcNAc-UDP and Neu5Gc(α2-6)Gal(β1-4) GlcNAc-UDP have been found in ovine colostrum (Sasaki et al., 2016). It can be hypothesized that these oligosaccharides are synthesized by the activity of β4-galactosyltransferase, whose acceptor is UDP-GlcNAc, and the activities of fucosyltransferase and/or sialyltransferase. The possible physiological significance of these UDP-oligosaccharides has not been clarified.

2.1.2.2 Phosphorylated Oligosaccharides

Gal(β1-4)GlcNAc-α1-PO_4 has been found in mare colostrum (Nakamura et al., 2001), while Gal(β1-4)Glc-3-PO_4 (Cumar et al., 1965), Neu5Ac(α2-6)Gal(β1-4) GlcNAc-1-PO_4, and Neu5Ac(α2-6)Gal(β1-4)GlcNAc-6-PO_4 (Parkkinen and Finne, 1987) have been detected in bovine colostrum. In addition, phosphorylated oligosaccharides have been found by Albrecht et al. (2014) in the milk/colostrum of goat, sheep, horse, and dromedary camel. Phosphorylated oligosaccharides have so far been found only in the milk/colostrum of herbivorous mammals.

2.1.3 Carnivorous Mammals (Bear, Dog, Skunk, Mink, Coati, Seal, Hyena, Lion, and Clouded Leopard) (Oligosaccharides in Table 3.4)

In most eutherian mammals, lactose predominates over milk oligosaccharides in milk/colostrum. However, in the milk of Ursidae including Ezo brown bear, Japanese black bear, polar bear, and giant panda, milk oligosaccharides predominate over lactose (Urashima et al., 1997b, 1999b, 2000, 2003a, 2004b; Nakamura et al., 2003b). In the milks of these bears, oligosaccharides containing human blood group A antigen (GalNAc(α1-3)[Fuc(α1-2)]Gal), B antigen (Gal(α1-3) [Fuc(α1-2)]Gal, or H antigen (Fuc(α1-2)Gal) at their nonreducing ends, including A-tetrasaccharide and B-tetrasaccharide, are characteristically prominent constituents. On the other hand, the presence/absence of A or B antigen in milk oligosaccharides depends on the species of bear. Thus, A antigen– and/or B antigen–containing oligosaccharides have been detected in polar bear milk (Urashima et al., 2000, 2003a) and B antigen containing oligosaccharides have been found in Japanese black bear milk (Urashima et al., 1999b, 2004b), but only H antigen–containing oligosaccharides have been detected in Ezo brown bear milk (Urashima et al., 1997b). Although A-tetrasaccharide has been found in the milk of blood A group human donors, its concentration in the milk is very low (Sabharwal et al., 1991) and oligosaccharides containing B antigen have never been found in human milk. Oligosaccharides containing the α-Gal epitope, including isoglobotriose, are prominent in the milk of these bears and in giant panda milk (Urashima et al., 1997b, 1999b, 2000, 2003a, 2004b; Nakamura

Table 3.4 Milk Oligosaccharides of Carnivores

No.	Oligosaccharide	Structure	References
Dog *(Canis lupus familiaris)* Milk			
Neutral oligosaccharides			
1	2′-FL	Fucα1-2Galβ1-4Glc	Rostami et al. (2014) and Bubb et al. (1999)
2	A-tetrasaccharide	Fucα1-2Galβ1-4Glc 3 GalNAcα1	Rostami et al. (2014)
Acidic oligosaccharides			
3	3′-L-*O*-sulphate	3-S-Galβ1-4Glc	Rostami et al. (2014) and Bubb et al. (1999)
4	3′-SL	Neu5Acα2-3Galβ1-4Glc	Rostami et al. (2014)
5	6′-SL	Neu5Acα2-6Galβ1-4Glc	Rostami et al. (2014)
Ezo Brown Bear *(Ursus arctos yesoensis)* Milk			
Neutral oligosaccharides			
1	2′-FL	Fucα1-2Galβ1-4Glc	Urashima et al. (1997b)
2	Isoglobotriose	Galα1-3Galβ1-4Glc	Urashima et al. (1997b)
3	DF-LNnT	Fucα1-2Galβ1-4GlcNAcβ1-3Galβ1-4Glc 3 Fucα1	Urashima et al. (1997b)
4	Gal-LNFP III	Galα1-3Galβ1-4GlcNAcβ1-3Galβ1-4Glc 3 Fucα1	Urashima et al. (1997b)
5	Tetra-F-LNnH	Fucα1 3 Fucα1-2Galβ1-4GlcNAcβ1 6 Galβ1-4Glc 3 Fucα1-2Galβ1-4GlcNAcβ1 3 Fucα1	Urashima et al. (1997b)

No.	Oligosaccharide	Structure	References
6	DF D Gal-LNnH	Fucα1 3 Galα1-3Galβ1-4GlcNAcβ1 6 3 Galβ1-4Glc Galα1-3Galβ1-4GlcNAcβ1 3 Fucα1	Urashima et al. (1997b)
Japanese Black Bear *(Ursus thibetanus japonicus)* Milk			
Neutral oligosaccharides			
1	2′-FL	Fucα1-2Galβ1-4Glc	Urashima et al. (1999b)
2	Isoglobotriose	Galα1-3Galβ1-4Glc	Urashima et al. (1999b)
3	3-F-isoglobotriose	Galα1-3Galβ1-4Glc Fucα1 3	Urashima et al. (1999b)
4	B-tetrasaccharide	Galα1-3Galβ1-4Glc Fucα1 2	Urashima et al. (1999b)
5	B-pentasaccharide	Galα1-3Galβ1-4Glc Fucα1 2 Fucα1 3	Urashima et al. (1999b)
6	Gal-LNFP III	Galα1-3Galβ1-4GlcNAcβ1-3Galβ1-4Glc Fucα1 3	Urashima et al. (1999b)
7	B-heptasaccharide type II chain	Galα1-3Galβ1-4GlcNAcβ1-3Galβ1-4Glc Fucα1 2 Fucα1 3	Urashima et al. (1999b)
8	DF DGal-LNnT	Galα1-3Galβ1-4GlcNAcβ1-3Galβ1-4Glc 3 3 Fucα1 Fucα1	Urashima et al. (1999b)

Continued

Table 3.4 Milk Oligosaccharides of Carnivores—cont'd

No.	Oligosaccharide	Structure	References
9	DF DGal-LNnH	Fucα1 3 Galα1-3Galβ1-4GlcNAcβ1 6 3 Galβ1-4Glc Galα1-3Galβ1-4GlcNAcβ1 3 Fucα1	Urashima et al. (1999b)
10	TF DGal-LNnH a	Fucα1 Fucα1 2 3 Galα1-3Galβ1-4GlcNAcβ1 6 3 Galβ1-4Glc Galα1-3Galβ1-4GlcNAcβ1 3 Fucα1	Urashima et al. (1999b)
11	TF DGal-LNnH b	Fucα1 3 Galα1-3Galβ1-4GlcNAcβ1 6 3 Galβ1-4Glc Galα1-3Galβ1-4GlcNAcβ1 2 3 Fucα1 Fucα1	Urashima et al. (1999b)
Acidic oligosaccharides			
12	3′-SL	Neu5Acα2-3Galβ1-4Glc	Urashima et al. (2004b)
13	FS Gal-LNnH	Fucα1 3 Galα1-3Galβ1-4GlcNAcβ1 6 3 Galβ1-4Glc Neu5Acα2-6Galβ1-4GlcNAcβ1	Urashima et al. (2004b)
14	DFSGal-LNnH	Fucα1 Fucα1 2 3 Galα1-3Galβ1-4GlcNAcβ1 6 3 Galβ1-4Glc Neu5Acα2-6Galβ1-4GlcNAcβ1	Urashima et al. (2004b)

No.	Oligosaccharide	Structure	References
15	DS-LNnH	Neu5Acα2-6Galβ1-4GlcNAcβ1 6 Galβ1-4Glc Neu5Acα2-6Galβ1-4GlcNAcβ1 3	Urashima et al. (2004b)
Polar bear *(Ursus maritimus)* Milk			
Neutral oligosaccharides			
1	Isoglobotriose	Galα1-3Galβ1-4Glc	Urashima et al. (2000)
2	2′-FL	Fucα1-2Galβ1-4Glc	Urashima et al. (2000)
3	B-tetrasaccharide	Galα1-3Galβ1-4Glc Fucα1 2	Urashima et al. (2000)
4	3-F-isoglobotriose	Galα1-3Galβ1-4Glc Fucα1 3	Urashima et al. (2000)
5	A-tetrasaccharide	GalNAcα1-3Galβ1-4Glc Fucα1 2	Urashima et al. (2000)
6	A-pentasaccharide	GalNAcα1-3Galβ1-4Glc Fucα1 2 Fucα1 3	Urashima et al. (2000)
7	Galilipentasaccharide	Galα1-3Galβ1-4GlcNAcβ1-3Galβ1-4Glc	Urashima et al. (2000)
8	B-hexasaccharide type II chain	Galα1-3Galβ1-4GlcNAcβ1-3Galβ1-4Glc Fucα1 2	Urashima et al. (2000)
9	Gal-LNFP III	Galα1-3Galβ1-4GlcNAcβ1-3Galβ1-4Glc Fucα1 3	Urashima et al. (2000)
10	DF Gal-LNnT	Galα1-3Galβ1-4GlcNAcβ1-3Galβ1-4Glc Fucα1 3 Fucα1 3	Urashima et al. (2000)

Continued

Table 3.4 Milk Oligosaccharides of Carnivores—cont'd

No.	Oligosaccharide	Structure	References
11	DGal-LNnH	Galα1-3Galβ1-4GlcNAcβ1 6 Galβ1-4Glc 3 Galα1-3Galβ1-4GlcNAcβ1	Urashima et al. (2000)
12	DF DGal-LNnH	Fucα1 3 Galα1-3Galβ1-4GlcNAcβ1 6 Galβ1-4Glc 3 Galα1-3Galβ1-4GlcNAcβ1 3 Fucα1	Urashima et al. (2000)
Giant Panda (*Ailuropoda melanoleuca*) Milk			
Neutral oligosaccharides			
1	Isoglobotriose	Galα1-3Galβ1-4Glc	Nakamura et al. (2003b)
2	3-F-isoglobotriose	Galα1-3Galβ1-4Glc 3 Fucα1	Nakamura et al. (2003b)
Acidic oligosaccharides			
3	3′-SL	Neu5Acα2-3Galβ1-4Glc	Nakamura et al. (2003b)
4	6′-SL	Neu5Acα2-6Galβ1-4Glc	Nakamura et al. (2003b)
5	3′-S-3-FL	Neu5Acα2-3Galβ1-4Glc 3 Fucα1	Nakamura et al. (2003b)
White-Nosed Coati (*Nasua narica*) Milk			
Neutral oligosaccharides			
1	2′-FL	Fucα1-2Galβ1-4Glc	Urashima et al. (1999c)
2	Isoglobotriose	Galα1-3Galβ1-4Glc	Urashima et al. (1999c)

No.	Oligosaccharide	Structure	References
3	LNnT	Galβ1-4GlcNAcβ1-3Galβ1-4Glc	Urashima et al. (1999c)
4	LNFP IV	Fucα1-2Galβ1-4GlcNAcβ1-3Galβ1-4Glc	Urashima et al. (1999c)
5	Galilipentasaccharide	Galα1-3Galβ1-4GlcNAcβ1-3Galβ1-4Glc	Urashima et al. (1999c)
6	F Gal-LNnH	Fucα1-2 { Galβ1-4GlcNAcβ1 6 Galα1-3 { Galβ1-4GlcNAcβ1 3 Galβ1-4Glc	Urashima et al. (1999c)
American Mink *(Neovison vison)* Milk			
Neutral oligosaccharides			
1	2′FL	Fucα1-2Galβ1-4Glc	Urashima et al. (2005)
2	Isoglobotriose	Galα1-3Galβ1-4Glc	Urashima et al. (2005)
3	LNnT	Galβ1-4GlcNAcβ1-3Galβ1-4Glc	Urashima et al. (2005)
4	LNFP IV	Fucα1-2Galβ1-4GlcNAcβ1-3Galβ1-4Glc	Urashima et al. (2005)
5	Galilipentasaccharide	Galα1-3Galβ1-4GlcNAcβ1-3Galβ1-4Glc	Urashima et al. (2005)
6	LNnH	Galβ1-4GlcNAcβ1 6 Galβ1-4GlcNAcβ1 3 Galβ1-4Glc	Urashima et al. (2005)
7	F-LNnH	Fucα1-2{ Galβ1-4GlcNAcβ1 6 Galβ1-4GlcNAcβ1 3 Galβ1-4Glc	Urashima et al. (2005)
8	FS-LNnH	Fucα1-2Galβ1-4GlcNAcβ1 6 Neu5Acα2-6Galβ1-4GlcNAcβ1 3 Galβ1-4Glc	Urashima et al. (2005)

Continued

Table 3.4 Milk Oligosaccharides of Carnivores—cont'd

No.	Oligosaccharide	Structure	References
9	FGal-LNnH	Galα1-3Galβ1-4GlcNAcβ1 6 3 Galβ1-4Glc Neu5Acα2-6Galβ1-4GlcNAcβ1	Urashima et al. (2005)
Striped Skunk *(Mephitis mephitis)* Milk			
Neutral oligosaccharides			
1	2′-FL	Fucα1-2Galβ1-4Glc	Taufik et al. (2013)
2	Isoglobotriose	Galα1-3Galβ1-4Glc	Taufik et al. (2013)
3	A-tetrasaccharide	GalNAcα1-3Galβ1-4Glc Fucα1 2	Taufik et al. (2013)
4	Galilipentasaccharide	Galα1-3Galβ1-4GlcNAcβ1-3Galβ1-4Glc	Taufik et al. (2013)
Acidic oligosaccharides			
5	3′-SL	Neu5Acα2-3Galβ1-4Glc	Taufik et al. (2013)
6	GalMSLNnH	Galα1-3Galβ1-4GlcNAcβ1 6 3 Galβ1-4Glc Neu5Acα2-6Galβ1-4GlcNAcβ1	Taufik et al. (2013)
Crabeater Seal *(Lobodon carcinophagus)* Milk			
Neutral oligosaccharides			
1	2′FL	Fucα1-2Galβ1-4Glc	Urashima et al. (1997a)
Hooded Seal *(Cystophora cristata)* Milk			
Neutral oligosaccharides			
1	2′FL	Fucα1-2Galβ1-4Glc	Urashima et al. (2001a)
2	LNnT	Galβ1-4GlcNAcβ1-3Galβ1-4Glc	Urashima et al. (2001a)

No.	Oligosaccharide	Structure	References
3	LNFP IV	Fucα1-2Galβ1-4GlcNAcβ1-3Galβ1-4Glc	Urashima et al. (2001a)
4	LNnH	Galβ1-4GlcNAcβ1 6 Galβ1-4Glc Galβ1-4GlcNAcβ1 3	Urashima et al. (2001a)
5	F-LNnH a	Fucα1-2Galβ1-4GlcNAcβ1 6 Galβ1-4Glc Galβ1-4GlcNAcβ1 3	Urashima et al. (2001a)
6	F-LNnH b	Galβ1-4GlcNAcβ1 6 Galβ1-4Glc Fucα1-2Galβ1-4GlcNAcβ1 3	Urashima et al. (2001a)
7	DF-LNnH II	Fucα1-2Galβ1-4GlcNAcβ1 6 Galβ1-4Glc Fucα1-2Galβ1-4GlcNAcβ1 3	Urashima et al. (2001a)
8	*para*-LNnH	Galβ1-4GlcNAcβ1-3Galβ1-4GlcNAcβ1-3Galβ1-4Glc	Urashima et al. (2001a)
9	F-*para*-LNnH	Fucα1-2Galβ1-4GlcNAcβ1-3Galβ1-4GlcNAcβ1-3Galβ1-4Glc	Urashima et al. (2001a)
Bearded Seal *(Erignathus barbatus)* Milk			
Neutral oligosaccharides			
1	2′FL	Fucα1-2Galβ1-4Glc	Urashima et al. (2004a)
2	LNFP IV	Fucα1-2Galβ1-4GlcNAcβ1-3Galβ1-4Glc	Urashima et al. (2004a)
3	DF-LNnH II	Fucα1-2Galβ1-4GlcNAcβ1 6 Galβ1-4Glc Fucα1-2Galβ1-4GlcNAcβ1 3	Urashima et al. (2004a)

Continued

Table 3.4 Milk Oligosaccharides of Carnivores—cont'd

No.	Oligosaccharide	Structure	References
Arctic Harbour Seal *(Phoca vitulina)* Milk			
Neutral oligosaccharides			
1	2′FL	Fucα1-2Galβ1-4Glc	Urashima et al. (2003b)
2	LNnT	Galβ1-4GlcNAcβ1-3Galβ1-4Glc	Urashima et al. (2003b)
3	LNnH	Galβ1-4GlcNAcβ1 6 Galβ1-4Glc Galβ1-4GlcNAcβ1 3	Urashima et al. (2003b)
4	F-LNnH a	Fucα1-2Galβ1-4GlcNAcβ1 6 Galβ1-4Glc Galβ1-4GlcNAcβ1 3	Urashima et al. (2003b)
5	F-LNnH b	Galβ1-4GlcNAcβ1 6 Galβ1-4Glc Fucα1-2Galβ1-4GlcNAcβ1 3	Urashima et al. (2003b)
6	DF-LNnH II	Fucα1-2Galβ1-4GlcNAcβ1 6 Galβ1-4Glc Fucα1-2Galβ1-4GlcNAcβ1 3	Urashima et al. (2003b)
Acidic oligosaccharides			
7	S-LNnH	Galβ1-4GlcNAcβ1 6 Galβ1-4Glc Neu5Acα2-6Galβ1-4GlcNAcβ1 3	Urashima et al. (2003b)
8	FS-LNnH	Fucα1-2Galβ1-4GlcNAcβ1 6 Galβ1-4Glc Neu5Acα2-6Galβ1-4GlcNAcβ1 3	Urashima et al. (2003b)
9	DS-LNnH	Neu5Acα2-6Galβ1-4GlcNAcβ1 6 Galβ1-4Glc Neu5Acα2-6Galβ1-4GlcNAcβ1 3	Urashima et al. (2003b)

No.	Oligosaccharide	Structure	References
Spotted Hyena *(Crocuta crocuta)* Colostrum			
Neutral oligosaccharides			
1	2′-FL	Fucα1-2Galβ1-4Glc	Uemura et al. (2009)
2	Isoglobotriose	Galα1-3Galβ1-4Glc	Uemura et al. (2009)
3	B-tetrasaccharide	Galα1-3Galβ1-4Glc Fucα1 2	Uemura et al. (2009)
Acidic oligosaccharides			
4	3′-SL	Neu5Acα2-3Galβ1-4Glc	Uemura et al. (2009)
African Lion *(Panthera leo)* Milk			
Neutral oligosaccharides			
1	2′-FL	Fucα1-2Galβ1-4Glc	Senda et al. (2010)
2	A-tetrasaccharide	GalNAcα1-3Galβ1-4Glc Fucα1 2	Senda et al. (2010)
Acidic oligosaccharides			
3	3′-Neu5GcL	Neu5Gcα2-3Galβ1-4Glc	Senda et al. (2010)
Clouded Leopard *(Neofelis nebulosa)* Milk			
Neutral oligosaccharides			
1	Isoglobotriose	Galα1-3Galβ1-4Glc	Senda et al. (2010)
2	A-tetrasaccharide	GalNAcα1-3Galβ1-4Glc Fucα1 2	Senda et al. (2010)
Acidic oligosaccharides			
3	3′-Neu5GcL	Neu5Gcα2-3Galβ1-4Glc	Senda et al. (2010)

et al., 2003b) but have not been found in human milk. Thus there are characteristic differences between the milk oligosaccharides of bears and those of humans.

Among Carnivora other than Ursidae, A-tetrasaccharide has been found in milks of the dog (Rostami et al., 2014), striped skunk (Taufik et al., 2013), African lion (Senda et al., 2010), and clouded leopard (Senda et al., 2010), while B-tetrasaccharide has been detected in colostrum of spotted hyena (Uemura et al., 2009). Oligosaccharides containing H antigen have been detected in the milk of dog (Rostami et al., 2014; Bubb et al., 1999), mink (Urashima et al., 2005), white nose coati (Urashima et al., 1999c), and three species of seals, including hooded seal, bearded seal, and harbor seal (Urashima et al., 2001a, 2003b, 2004a; Kinoshita et al., 2009). Isoglobotriose- and α-Gal epitope–containing oligosaccharides have been found in milk/colostrum of the striped skunk (Taufik et al., 2013), mink (Urashima et al., 2005), white nose coati (Urashima et al., 1999c), spotted hyena (Uemura et al., 2009). and clouded leopard (Senda et al., 2010) but not in the milk of true seals (Urashima et al., 2001a, 2003b, 2004a; Kinoshita et al., 2009). It is worth noting that sea lions and fur seals (family Otariidae) and the walrus (family Odobenidae) lack α-lactalbumin and thus are unable to synthesize lactose or oligosaccharides containing lactose at the reducing end. Thus, such milks have only traces of carbohydrates and are devoid of lactose and oligosaccharides (Oftedal, 2011).

The core units of the milk oligosaccharides among Carnivora species are lactose, lacto-*N*-neotetraose and lacto-*N*-neohexaose. Only type II, not type I, oligosaccharides have been found. It is noteworthy that some milk oligosaccharides of the Ursidae contain Lewis X (Gal(β1-4)[Fuc(α1-3)]GlcNAc (Urashima et al., 1997b, 1999b, 2000, 2003a, 2004b; Nakamura et al., 2003b).

With respect to sialic acids of the sialyl milk oligosaccharides, Neu5Ac (but not Neu5Gc) has been detected in milk oligosaccharides of the Japanese black bear (Urashima et al., 2004b), giant panda (Nakamura et al., 2003b), dog (Rostami et al., 2014), mink (Urashima et al., 2005), stripped skunk (Taufik et al., 2013), seals (Urashima et al., 2003b, 2004a), and spotted hyena (Uemura et al., 2009). Remarkably, Neu5Gc (but not Neu5Ac) has been found in the African lion (Senda et al., 2010) and clouded leopard (Senda et al., 2010).

Concerning the ratio of milk oligosaccharides to lactose, oligosaccharides predominate over lactose in the milk of seals (Urashima et al., 2001a, 2003b, 2004a; Kinoshita et al., 2009), striped skunk (Taufik et al., 2013), mink (Urashima et al., 2005), and white nose coati (Urashima et al., 1999c), while lactose predominates over oligosaccharides in milk of the dog (Rostami et al., 2014; Bubb et al., 1999), spotted hyena (Uemura et al., 2009), African lion (Senda et al., 2010), and clouded leopard (Senda et al., 2010).

2.1.4 Elephants (Asian Elephant and African Elephant) (Oligosaccharides in Table 3.5)

Elephant milks contain a diverse array of oligosaccharides. The core units of milk oligosaccharides of Asian and African elephants are lacto-*N*-neotetraose, lacto-*N*-neohexaose, and *para*-lacto-*N*-neohexaose (Gal(β1-4)GlcNAc(β1-3)Gal(β1-4)GlcNAc(β1-3)Gal(β1-4)Glc), all of which are of type II (Uemura et al., 2006; Osthoff et al., 2008). Lacto-*N*-novopentaose I and its derivatives, which have been found in milk/colostrum of

Table 3.5 Milk Oligosaccharides of Miscellaneous Eutherians, Including Elephants and Cetaceans

No.	Oligosaccharide	Structure	References
Asian Elephant *(Elephas maximus)* Milk			
Neutral oligosaccharides			
1	Isoglobotriose	Galα1-3Galβ1-4Glc	Uemura et al. (2006)
Acidic oligosaccharides			
2	3′-SL	Neu5Acα2-3Galβ1-4Glc	Uemura et al. (2006)
3	6′-SL	Neu5Acα2-6Galβ1-4Glc	Uemura et al. (2006)
4	3′-S-3-FL	Neu5Acα2-3Galβ1-4Glc Fucα1 3	Uemura et al. (2006)
5	LST c	Neu5Acα2-6Galβ1-4GlcNAcβ1-3Galβ1-4Glc	Uemura et al. (2006)
6	MSGalLNnH	Galα1-3Galβ1-4GlcNAcβ1 6 Galβ1-4Glc Neu5Acα2-6Galβ1-4GlcNAcβ1 3	Uemura et al. (2006)
7	MSMFGalLNnH	Fucα1 3 Galα1-3Galβ1-4GlcNAcβ1 6 Galβ1-4Glc Neu5Acα2-6Galβ1-4GlcNAcβ1 3	Uemura et al. (2006)
8	MSMFLNnT I	Neu5Acα2-3Galβ1-4GlcNAcβ1-3Galβ1-4Glc Fucα1 3	Uemura et al. (2006)
9	MS-*para*-LNnH	Neu5Acα2-6Galβ1-4GlcNAcβ1-3Galβ1-4GlcNAcβ1-3Galβ1-4Glc	Uemura et al. (2006)
10	MSMF-*para*-LNnH	Neu5Acα2-3Galβ1-4GlcNAcβ1-3Galβ1-4GlcNAcβ1-3Galβ1-4Glc Fucα1 3 Fucα1 3	Uemura et al. (2006)

Continued

Table 3.5 Milk Oligosaccharides of Miscellaneous Eutherians, Including Elephants and Cetaceans—cont'd

No.	Oligosaccharide	Structure	References
African Elephant *(Loxodonta africana)* Milk			
Neutral oligosaccharides			
1	Isoglobotriose	Galα1-3Galβ1-4Glc	Osthoff et al. (2008)
2	LNFP III	Galβ1-4GlcNAcβ1-3Galβ1-4Glc Fucα1^{3}	Osthoff et al. (2008)
3	GalLNFP III	Galα1-3Galβ1-4GlcNAcβ1-3Galβ1-4Glc Fucα1^{3}	Osthoff et al. (2008)
4	DF-*para*-LNnH	Galβ1-4GlcNAcβ1-3Galβ1-4GlcNAcβ1-3Galβ1-4Glc Fucα1^{3} Fucα1^{3}	Osthoff et al. (2008)
5	DFGal-*para*-LNnH	Galα1-3Galβ1-4GlcNAcβ1-3Galβ1-4GlcNAcβ1-3Galβ1-4Glc Fucα1^{3} Fucα1^{3}	Osthoff et al. (2008)
Acidic oligosaccharides			
6	3′-SL	Neu5Acα2-3Galβ1-4Glc	Osthoff et al. (2008)
7	3′-Neu5GcL	Neu5Gcα2-3Galβ1-4Glc	Osthoff et al. (2008)
8	6′-SL	Neu5Acα2-6Galβ1-4Glc	Osthoff et al. (2008)
9	3′-S-3-FL	Neu5Acα2-3Galβ1-4Glc Fucα1^{3}	Osthoff et al. (2008)
10	LST c	Neu5Acα2-6Galβ1-4GlcNAcβ1-3Galβ1-4Glc	Osthoff et al. (2008)
11	MSMFLNnT I	Neu5Acα2-3Galβ1-4GlcNAcβ1-3Galβ1-4Glc Fucα1^{3}	Osthoff et al. (2008)

No.	Oligosaccharide	Structure	References
12	MSMFLNnT II	Neu5Acα2-6Galβ1-4GlcNAcβ1-3Galβ1-4Glc Fucα1 (3)	Osthoff et al. (2008)
13	MSLNnH	Galβ1-4GlcNAcβ1 (6) Galβ1-4Glc Neu5Acα2-6Galβ1-4GlcNAcβ1 (3)	Osthoff et al. (2008)
14	MSMFLNnH	Fucα1 (3) Galβ1-4GlcNAcβ1 (6) Galβ1-4Glc Neu5Acα2-6Galβ1-4GlcNAcβ1 (3)	Osthoff et al. (2008)
15	MSMF-*para*-LNnH II	Neu5Acα2-6Galβ1-4GlcNAcβ1-3Galβ1-4GlcNAcβ1-3Galβ1-4Glc Fucα1 (3)	Osthoff et al. (2008)
16	MSMFGalLNnH	Fucα1 (3) Galα1-3Galβ1-4GlcNAcβ1 (6) Galβ1-4Glc Neu5Acα2-6Galβ1-4GlcNAcβ1 (3)	Osthoff et al. (2008)
Laboratory Rat *(Rattus norvegicus)* Milk			
Acidic oligosaccharides			
1	3′-SL	Neu5Acα2-3Galβ1-4Glc	Kuhn (1972)
2	3′-SL-6′-*O*-sulphate	6-S-Neu5Acα2-3Galβ1-4Glc	Sturman et al. (1985) and Choi and Carubelli (1968)
3	6′-L-*O*-sulphate	6-S-Galβ1-4Glc	Choi and Carubelli (1968) and Barra and Caputto (1965)
4	β 6′galactosyl-*myo*-inositol	Galβ1-6-*myo*-inositol	Naccrato et al. (1975)

Continued

Table 3.5 Milk Oligosaccharides of Miscellaneous Eutherians, Including Elephants and Cetaceans—cont'd

No.	Oligosaccharide	Structure	References
Giant Anteater *(Myrmecophaga tridactyla)* Milk			
Neutral oligosaccharides			
1	Isoglobotriose	Galα1-3Galβ1-4Glc	Urashima et al. (2008)
Acidic oligosaccharides			
2	6′-SL	Neu5Acα2-6Galβ1-4Glc	Urashima et al. (2008)
3	6′- Neu5GcL	Neu5Gcα2-6Galβ1-4Glc	Urashima et al. (2008)
4	LST c	Neu5Acα2-6Galβ1-4GlcNAcβ1-3Galβ1-4Glc	Urashima et al. (2008)
5	Neu5GcLNnT	Neu5Gcα2-6Galβ1-4GlcNAcβ1-3Galβ1-4Glc	Urashima et al. (2008)
Island Flying Fox *(Pteropus hypomelanus)* Milk			
Neutral oligosaccharides			
1	Isoglobotriose	Galα1-3Galβ1-4Glc	Senda et al. (2011)
2	LNnT	Galβ1-4GlcNAcβ1-3Galβ1-4Glc	Senda et al. (2011)
3	LNnH	Galβ1-4GlcNAcβ1 6 Galβ1-4Glc Galβ1-4GlcNAcβ1 3	Senda et al. (2011)
Acidic oligosaccharides			
4	3′-Neu5GcL	Neu5Gcα2-3Galβ1-4Glc	Senda et al. (2011)
Beluga Whale *(Delphinapterus leucas)* Milk			
Acidic oligosaccharides			
1	3′-SL	Neu5Acα2-3Galβ1-4Glc	Urashima et al. (2002)

No.	Oligosaccharide	Structure	References
Common Bottlenose Dolphin *(Tursiops truncatus)* Milk			
Neutral oligosaccharides			
1	Globotriose	Galα1-4Galβ1-4Glc	Uemura et al. (2005)
Acidic oligosaccharides			
2	3′-SL	Neu5Acα2-3Galβ1-4Glc	Uemura et al. (2005)
3	6′-SL	Neu5Acα2-6Galβ1-4Glc	Uemura et al. (2005)
4	GM_2 tetrasaccharide	GalNAcβ1 4 Galβ1-4Glc 3 Neu5Acα2	Uemura et al. (2005)
Northern Minke Whale *(Balaenoptera acutorostrata)* Milk			
Neutral oligosaccharides			
1	2′-FL	Fucα1-2Galβ1-4Glc	Urashima et al. (2002)
2	LNnT	Galβ1-4GlcNAcβ1-3Galβ1-4Glc	Urashima et al. (2002)
3	A-tetrasaccharide	GalNAcα1-3Galβ1-4Glc 2 Fucα1	Urashima et al. (2002)
4	*para*-LNnH	Galβ1-4GlcNAcβ1-3Galβ1-4GlcNAcβ1-3Galβ1-4Glc	Urashima et al. (2002)
Acidic oligosaccharides			
5	3‴-S-LNnT	Neu5Acα2-3Galβ1-4GlcNAcβ1-3Galβ1-4Glc	Urashima et al. (2002)
6	LST c	Neu5Acα2-6Galβ1-4GlcNAcβ1-3Galβ1-4Glc	Urashima et al. (2002)
7	S-*para*-LNnH	Neu5Acα2-3Galβ1-4GlcNAcβ1-3Galβ1-4GlcNAcβ1-3Galβ1-4Glc	Urashima et al. (2002)

Continued

Table 3.5 Milk Oligosaccharides of Miscellaneous Eutherians, Including Elephants and Cetaceans—cont'd

No.	Oligosaccharide	Structure	References
Bryde's Whale *(Balaenoptera edeni)* Milk			
Acidic oligosaccharides			
1	3′-SL	Neu5Acα2-3Galβ1-4Glc	Urashima et al. (2007b)
2	6′-SL	Neu5Acα2-6Galβ1-4Glc	Urashima et al. (2007b)
3	LST c	Neu5Acα2-6Galβ1-4GlcNAcβ1-3Galβ1-4Glc	Urashima et al. (2007b)
Sei Whale *(Balaenoptera borealis)* Milk			
Acidic oligosaccharides			
1	3′-SL	Neu5Acα2-3Galβ1-4Glc	Urashima et al. (2007b)
2	6′-SL	Neu5Acα2-6Galβ1-4Glc	Urashima et al. (2007b)
3	LST c	Neu5Acα2-6Galβ1-4GlcNAcβ1-3Galβ1-4Glc	Urashima et al. (2007b)

cows (Marino et al., 2011; Albrecht et al., 2014; Urashima et al., 1991b), goats (Albrecht et al., 2014), sheep (Albrecht et al., 2014), camels (Albrecht et al., 2014; Fukuda et al., 2010; Alhaj et al., 2013), horses (Albrecht et al., 2014; Urashima et al., 1989b), pigs (Albrecht et al., 2014), and capuchin (Goto et al., 2010; Urashima et al., 1999a), have not been detected in the milk of either elephant species. Some elephant oligosaccharides contain Lewis X and/or α-Gal epitope, but those containing ABH antigens have not been found. It is also noteworthy that oligosaccharides containing sialyl Lewis X (Neu5Ac(α2-3)Gal(β1-4)[Fuc(α1-3)]GlcNAc) have been found in elephant milks. Neu5Ac predominates over Neu5Gc in elephant milk sialyl oligosaccharides, but 3′-NGc-SL has been detected in milk of the African elephant (Osthoff et al., 2008).

2.1.5 Cetaceans (Oligosaccharides in Table 3.5)

The core units of minke whale milk oligosaccharides are lacto-*N*-neotetraose and para-lacto-*N*-neohexaose, both of which are of type II (Urashima et al., 2002). This milk also contained A-tetrasaccharide (Urashima et al., 2002). It is noteworthy that bottlenose dolphin milk contained Neu5Ac(α2-3)[GalNAc(β1-4)]Gal(β1-4)Glc (GM2 tetrasaccharide) and Gal(α1-4)Gal(β1-4)Glc (globotriose) (Uemura et al., 2005), which is yet to be found in the milk/colostrum of other species. The sialyl oligosaccharides of minke whale, bottlenose dolphin, beluga, Brydes whale, and sei whale contained Neu5Ac but not Neu5Gc (Urashima et al., 2002, 2007b; Uemura et al., 2005).

2.1.6 Other Eutherians (Oligosaccharides in Table 3.5)

Among other eutherian mammals, milk oligosaccharides have been studied in the Norway rat (Sturman et al., 1985; Choi et al., 1968; Barra et al., 1965; Kuhn, 1972; Naccrato et al., 1975), giant anteater (Urashima et al., 2008), and island flying fox (Senda et al., 2011). It is noteworthy that rat milk contains Neu5Ac(α2-3)Gal(β1-4)Glc-6′-SO_3 (Sturman et al., 1985), Gal(β1-4)Glc-6′-SO_3 (Choi et al., 1968) and Gal(β1-6)-myo-inositol (Naccrato et al., 1975). Isoglobotriose has been found in milk of the giant anteater (Urashima et al., 2008) and island flying fox (Senda et al., 2011). The sialic acids of milk oligosaccharides are Neu5Ac in the rat (Sturman et al., 1985; Naccrato et al., 1975), Neu5Gc in the flying fox (Senda et al., 2011), and both Neu5Ac and Neu5Gc in the giant anteater (Urashima et al., 2008).

2.2 MARSUPIALS (INFRACLASS METATHERIA) (OLIGOSACCHARIDES IN TABLE 3.6)

Among marsupials, milk oligosaccharides have been characterized in the tammar wallaby (Messer et al., 1980, 1982; Collins et al., 1981; Bradbury et al., 1983; Urashima et al., 1994b), red kangaroo (Anraku et al., 2012), koala (Urashima et al., 2013b), common brushtail possum (Urashima et al., 2014a), and eastern quoll (Urashima et al., 2015b). In addition, milk oligosaccharides of other marsupials, including Eastern gray kangaroo (Messer and Mossop, 1977), eastern quoll (Messer et al., 1987), mouse opossum, *Monodelphis domestica* (Crisp et al., 1989b), and ringtail possum (Munks et al., 1991) have been studied by thin layer chromatography; the results

Table 3.6 Milk Oligosaccharides of Marsupials

No.	Oligosaccharide	Structure	References
Tammar wallaby *(Macropus eugenii)* Milk			
Neutral oligosaccharides			
1	β 3′-GL	Galβ1-3Galβ1-4Glc	Messer et al. (1980)
2	Di-GalL	Galβ1-3Galβ1-3Galβ1-4Glc	Collins et al. (1981)
3	Tri-GalL	Galβ1-3Galβ1-3Galβ1-3Galβ1-4Glc	Collins et al. (1981)
4	Tetra-GalL	Galβ1-3Galβ1-3Galβ1-3Galβ1-3Galβ1-4Glc	Collins et al. (1981)
5	Penta-GalL	Galβ1-3Galβ1-3Galβ1-3Galβ1-3Galβ1-3Galβ1-4Glc	Collins et al. (1981)
6	*novo*-LNT	GlcNAcβ1 6 Galβ1-4Glc Galβ1 3	Messer et al. (1980)
7	*novo*-LNP I	Galβ1-4GlcNAcβ1 6 Galβ1-4Glc Galβ1 3	Bradbury et al. (1983)
8	Gal-*novo*-LNP I	Galβ1-4GlcNAcβ1 6 Galβ1-4Glc Galβ1-3Galβ1 3	Bradbury et al. (1983)
Red Kangaroo *(Macropus rufus)* Milk			
Acidic oligosaccharides			
1	3′-SL	Neu5Acα2-3Galβ1-4Glc	Anraku et al. (2012)
2	3″-S- β3′-GL	Neu5Acα2-3Galβ1-3Galβ1-4Glc	Anraku et al. (2012)
3		Neu5Acα2-3Galβ1-3Galβ1-3Galβ1-4Glc	Anraku et al. (2012)
4	SLNPa	Galβ1-4GlcNAcβ1 6 Galβ1-4Glc Neu5Acα2-3Galβ1 3	Anraku et al. (2012)

No.	Oligosaccharide	Structure	References
5	SLNPb	Neu5Acα2-6Galβ1-4GlcNAcβ1 6 Galβ1-4Glc Galβ1 3	Anraku et al. (2012)
6	SLNPc	Neu5Acα2-3Galβ1-4GlcNAcβ1 6 Galβ1-4Glc Galβ1 3	Anraku et al. (2012)
7		Neu5Acα2-3Galβ1-3Galβ1-3Galβ1-3Galβ1-4Glc	Anraku et al. (2012)
8		Galβ1-4GlcNAcβ1 6 Galβ1-4Glc Neu5Acα2-3Galβ1-3Galβ1 3	Anraku et al. (2012)
9		Neu5Acα2-3Galβ1-4GlcNAcβ1 6 Galβ1-4Glc Galβ1-3Galβ1 3	Anraku et al. (2012)
10		3-S-Galβ1-3Galβ1-3Galβ1-4Glc	Anraku et al. (2012)
11		3-S-Galβ1-3Galβ1-3Galβ1-3Galβ1-4Glc	Anraku et al. (2012)
12		Galβ1-4GlcNAcβ1 6 Galβ1-4Glc 3-S-Galβ1-3Galβ1 3	Anraku et al. (2012)
13		3-S-Galβ1-4GlcNAcβ1 6 Galβ1-4Glc Galβ1-3Galβ1 3	Anraku et al. (2012)
14		3-S-Galβ1-3Galβ1-3Galβ1-3Galβ1-3Galβ1-4Glc	Anraku et al. (2012)

Continued

Table 3.6 Milk Oligosaccharides of Marsupials—cont'd

No.	Oligosaccharide	Structure	References
15		Galβ1-4GlcNAcβ1 6 Galβ1-4Glc 3-S-Galβ1-3Galβ1-3Galβ1 3	Anraku et al. (2012)
16		3-S-Galβ1-4GlcNAcβ1 6 Galβ1-4Glc Galβ1-3Galβ1-3Galβ1 3	Anraku et al. (2012)
Common Brushtail Possum *(Trichosurus vulpecula)* Milk			
Neutral oligosaccharides			
1	β 3′-GL	Galβ1-3Galβ1-4Glc	Urashima et al. (2014a)
2	Di-GalL	Galβ1-3Galβ1-3Galβ1-4Glc	Urashima et al. (2014a)
3	Tri-GalL	Galβ1-3Galβ1-3Galβ1-3Galβ1-4Glc	Urashima et al. (2014a)
4	Tetra-GalL	Galβ1-3Galβ1-3Galβ1-3Galβ1-3Galβ1-4Glc	Urashima et al. (2014a)
5	*novo*-LNP I	Galβ1-4GlcNAcβ1 6 Galβ1-4Glc Galβ1 3	Urashima et al. (2014a)
6	Gal-*novo*-LNP I	Galβ1-4GlcNAcβ1 6 Galβ1-4Glc Galβ1-3Galβ1 3	Urashima et al. (2014a)
7	Gal-*novo*-LNP II	Galβ1-4GlcNAcβ1 6 Galβ1-3Galβ1-4Glc Galβ1 3	Urashima et al. (2014a)

No.	Oligosaccharide	Structure	References
Acidic oligosaccharides			
8	3″-S- β3′-GL	Neu5Acα2-3Galβ1-3Galβ1-4Glc	Urashima et al. (2014a)
9		Galβ1-4GlcNAcβ1-6 Galβ1-4Glc 3-S-Galβ1-3	Urashima et al. (2014a)
10		3-S-Galβ1-4GlcNAcβ1-6 Galβ1-4Glc Galβ1-3	Urashima et al. (2014a)
11		Neu5Acα2-3Galβ1-3Galβ1-3Galβ1-4Glc	Urashima et al. (2014a)
12	SLNPa	Galβ1-4GlcNAcβ1-6 Galβ1-4Glc Neu5Acα2-3Galβ1-3	Urashima et al. (2014a)
13		Galβ1-4GlcNAcβ1-6 Galβ1-4Glc 3-S-Galβ1-3Galβ1-3	Urashima et al. (2014a)
14		3-S-Galβ1-4GlcNAcβ1-6 Galβ1-4Glc Galβ1-3Galβ1-3	Urashima et al. (2014a)
15	SLNPb	Neu5Acα2-6Galβ1-4GlcNAcβ1-6 Galβ1-4Glc Galβ1-3	Urashima et al. (2014a)
16		Neu5Acα2-3Galβ1-3Galβ1-3Galβ1-3Galβ1-4Glc	Urashima et al. (2014a)

Continued

Table 3.6 Milk Oligosaccharides of Marsupials—cont'd

No.	Oligosaccharide	Structure	References
17		3-S-Galβ1-3Galβ1-3Galβ1-3Galβ1-3Galβ1-4Glc	Urashima et al. (2014a)
18		Galβ1-4GlcNAcβ1 6 Galβ1-4Glc 3 Neu5Acα2-3Galβ1-3GlcNAcβ1	Urashima et al. (2014a)
19		Galβ1-4GlcNAcβ1 6 Galβ1-4Glc 3 3-S-Galβ1-3Galβ1-3Galβ1	Urashima et al. (2014a)
20		3-S-Galβ1-4GlcNAcβ1 6 Galβ1-4Glc 3 Galβ1-3Galβ1-3Galβ1	Urashima et al. (2014a)
21		Neu5Acα2-6Galβ1-4GlcNAcβ1 6 Galβ1-4Glc 3 Galβ1-3Galβ1	Urashima et al. (2014a)
Koala *(Phascolarctos cinereus)* Milk			
Neutral oligosaccharides			
1	β3′-GL	Galβ1-3Galβ1-4Glc	Urashima et al. (2013b)
2	3″,3′-DGL	Galβ1-3Galβ1-3Galβ1-4Glc	Urashima et al. (2013b)
3	novo-LNP I	Galβ1-4GlcNAcβ1 6 Galβ1-4Glc 3 Galβ1	Urashima et al. (2013b)
4	FLNP	Fucα1 3 Galβ1-4GlcNAcβ1 6 Galβ1-4Glc 3 Galβ1	Urashima et al. (2013b)

No.	Oligosaccharide	Structure	References
Acidic oligosaccharides			
5	3′-SL	Neu5Acα2-3Galβ1-4Glc	Urashima et al. (2013b)
6	3″-S-3′-GL	Neu5Acα2-3Galβ1-3Galβ1-4Glc	Urashima et al. (2013b)
7	SLNPa	Galβ1-4GlcNAcβ1 6 Galβ1-4Glc Neu5Acα2-3Galβ1 3	Urashima et al. (2013b)
8	SLNPb	Neu5Acα2-6Galβ1-4GlcNAcβ1 6 Galβ1-4Glc Galβ1 3	Urashima et al. (2013b)
9	SLNPc	Neu5Acα2-3Galβ1-4GlcNAcβ1 6 Galβ1-4Glc Galβ1 3	Urashima et al. (2013b)
10	FSLNP	Fucα1 3 Galβ1-4GlcNAcβ1 6 Galβ1-4Glc Neu5Acα2-3Galβ1 3	Urashima et al. (2013b)
Eastern quoll *(Dasyurus viverrinus)* Milk			
Neutral oligosaccharides			
1	β 3′-GL	Galβ1-3Galβ1-4Glc	Urashima et al. (2015b)
2	3″,3′-DGL	Galβ1-3Galβ1-3Galβ1-4Glc	Urashima et al. (2015b)
3	*novo*-LNP I	Galβ1-4GlcNAcβ1 6 Galβ1-4Glc Galβ1 3	Urashima et al. (2015b)

Continued

Table 3.6 Milk Oligosaccharides of Marsupials—cont'd

No.	Oligosaccharide	Structure	References
4	Gal-*novo*-LNF II	Galβ1-4GlcNAcβ1 6 Galβ1-3Galβ1-4Glc Galβ1 3	Urashima et al. (2015b)
5	Gal-*novo*-LNF I	Galβ1-4GlcNAcβ1 6 Galβ1-4Glc Galβ1-3Galβ1 3	Urashima et al. (2015b)
6	Gal-*novo*-LNF III	Galβ1-3Galβ1-4GlcNAcβ1 6 Galβ1-4Glc Galβ1 3	Urashima et al. (2015b)
7	*novo*-LNO	Galβ1-4GlcNAcβ1 Galβ1-4GlcNAcβ1 6 6 Galβ1-3Galβ1-3Galβ1-4Glc	Urashima et al. (2015b)
Acidic oligosaccharides			
8	3′-SL	Neu5Acα2-3Galβ1-4Glc	Urashima et al. (2015b)
9		Galβ1-4GlcNAcβ1 6 Galβ1-4Glc 3-S-Galβ1 3	Urashima et al. (2015b)
10		3-S-Galβ1-4GlcNAcβ1 6 Galβ1-4Glc Galβ1 3	Urashima et al. (2015b)
11	SLNPa	Galβ1-4GlcNAcβ1 6 Galβ1-4Glc Neu5Acα2-3Galβ1 3	Urashima et al. (2015b)
12	SLNPc	Neu5Acα2-3Galβ1-4GlcNAcβ1 6 Galβ1-4Glc Galβ1 3	Urashima et al. (2015b)

No.	Oligosaccharide	Structure	References
13	SLNOa	Galβ1-4GlcNAcβ1 Galβ1-4GlcNAcβ1 6 6 Neu5Acα2-3Galβ1-3Galβ1-3Galβ1-4Glc	Urashima et al. (2015b)
14	SLNOb	Neu5Acα2-3 Galβ1-4GlcNAcβ1 Galβ1-4GlcNAcβ1 6 6 Galβ1-3Galβ1-3Galβ1-4Glc	Urashima et al. (2015b)

suggest that milk oligosaccharides are similar to those of the tammar wallaby across all marsupial species, even including, remarkably, a South American species.

The neutral oligosaccharides of the tammar wallaby can be classified into an unbranched major series, expressed as [Gal(β1-3)]$_{n=1-5}$Gal(β1-4)Glc (Messer et al., 1980; Collins et al., 1981), and a branched minor series, including lacto-*N*-novopentaose I and Gal(β1-3)Gal(β1-3)[Gal(β1-4)GlcNAc(β1-6)]Gal(β1-4)Glc (Messer et al., 1982; Bradbury et al., 1983). Lactating tammar wallaby mammary glands have been shown to contain β4-galactosyltransferase, β3-galactosyltransferase, and β6-*N*-acetylglucosaminyltransferase activities (Messer et al., 1991; Urashima et al., 1992); these are most likely involved in the biosynthesis of the major and minor series of milk oligosaccharides. The β3-galactosyltransferase is a novel enzyme that transfers Gal from UDP-Gal to Lac to synthesize Gal(β1-3)Gal(β1-4)Glc (3′-GL) and to 3′-GL to synthesize Gal(β1-3)Gal(β1-3)Gal(β1-4)Glc (digalactosyllactose), while the β6-*N*-acetylglucosaminyltransferase transfers GlcNAc from UDP-GlcNAc to 3′-GL to synthesize Gal(β1-3)[GlcNAc(β1-6)]Gal(β1-4)Glc (lacto-*N*-novotetraose).

The acidic milk oligosaccharides of the red kangaroo have been shown to be sialylated or sulfated derivatives of neutral oligosaccharides, both unbranched and branched, that are similar or identical to those found in tammar wallaby milk. They contained nonreducing α(2-3) linked Neu5Ac or *O*-3 sulfated Gal linked to a penultimate Gal(β1-3) residue and α(2-3/6) linked Neu5Ac linked to a Gal(β1-4) residue of *N*-acetyllactosamine of a branched unit (Anraku et al., 2012).

The neutral and acidic milk oligosaccharides of the common brushtail possum are similar to tammar wallaby neutral and red kangaroo acidic oligosaccharides, respectively (Urashima et al., 2014a). It is noteworthy, however, that this milk contains a novel hexasaccharide. Gal(β1-3)[Gal(β1-4)GlcNAc(β1-6)]Gal(β1-3)Gal(β1-4)Glc, in which the GlcNAc(β1-6) residue is linked to a penultimate β(1-3) linked Gal but not to a β(1-4) linked Gal. This is consistent with the presence of a β6-*N*-acetylglucosaminyltransferase in lactating tammar mammary glands, which transfers GlcNAc to the penultimate Gal of Gal(β1-3)Gal(β1-3)Gal(β1-4)Glc as well as of 3′-GL (Urashima et al., 1992). The presence of this hexasaccharide suggests that lactating mammary glands of the common brushtail possum contain a β6-*N*-acetylglucosaminyltransferase with the same substrate specificity as that of the tammar wallaby.

Eastern quoll milk contains Gal(β1-3)[Gal(β1-4)GlcNAc(β1-6)]Gal(β1-3)[Gal(β1-4)GlcNAc(β1-6)]Gal(β1-4)Glc (lacto-*N*-novooctaose) and its sialyl derivatives as well as lacto-*N*-novopentaose I and its sialyl derivatives (Urashima et al., 2015b). It is noteworthy that, in contrast to the milk oligosaccharides of other marsupials, branched oligosaccharides predominate over linear ones. This suggests that in the lactating mammary glands of the eastern quoll, the activity of the above-mentioned β6-*N*-acetylglucosaminyltransferase is greater than in that of the tammar wallaby or brushtail possum.

Some of the neutral as well as acidic oligosaccharides of the koala have been found to contain a Fuc residue (Urashima et al., 2013b). This is noteworthy because fucosyl oligosaccharides have not so far been detected in any other marsupial milks. One can hypothesize that the milk of the common ancestor of living marsupials had contained fucosyl oligosaccharides that had been lost in marsupials other than the koala. Sulfated milk oligosaccharides have not been found in the koala (Urashima et al., 2013b).

It is apparent that there is relatively little heterogeneity of milk oligosaccharides among marsupial species compared with that among eutherians. Furthermore, lactose is no more than a minor milk saccharide in all those marsupials whose milk carbohydrates have been studied, which include a South American species in addition to at least five Australian marsupials (Munk et al., 1991).

2.3 MONOTREMES (INFRACLASS PROTOTHERIA) (OLIGOSACCHARIDES IN TABLE 3.7)

The neutral and acidic milk oligosaccharides of both the echidna and the platypus have been characterized (Messer and Kerry, 1973; Messer, 1974; Kamerling et al., 1982; Jenkins et al., 1984; Amano et al., 1985; Oftedal et al., 2014; Urashima et al., 2015a). Lactose is only a minor saccharide in the milk of both monotremes (Messer and Kerry, 1973; Amano et al., 1985; Oftedal et al., 2014; Urashima et al., 2015a), as in marsupials and some eutherians. Unlike marsupials and eutherians, however, the main sialyl milk oligosaccharides of Tasmanian, Kangaroo Island, and New South Wales echidnas and of the platypus all contain a 4-*O*-acetyl group attached to the Neu5Ac residue (Messer and Kerry, 1973; Messer, 1974; Kamerling et al., 1982; Oftedal et al., 2014; Urashima et al., 2015a). Thus, the major milk oligosaccharide of the Kangaroo Island echidna and of the Tasmanian echidna early in lactation was found to be Neu4,5Ac_2(α2-3)Gal(β1-4)Glc, and it has been hypothesized that this reflects the status of milk carbohydrates in the common ancestor of mammals (Oftedal et al., 2014). In late lactation milk of the Tasmanian echidna, the concentrations of the neutral oligosaccharides Gal(α1-3)[Fuc(α1-2)]Gal(β1-4)[Fuc(α1-3)]Glc (B-pentasaccharide) and B-tetrasaccharide both increased (Oftedal et al., 2014), but B-penta and -tetrasaccharides have not been found in the milk of either Kangaroo Island or New South Wales echidnas, in which Fuc(α1-2)Gal(β1-4)Glc is the predominant neutral oligosaccharide (Messer and Kerry, 1973; Jenkins et al., 1984). The presence/absence of B antigen in milk oligosaccharides among the Tasmanian subspecies of the echidna may be similar to that among Ursidae species (Japanese black bear, polar bear, Ezo brown bear) (Urashima et al., 1997b, 1999b, 2000, 2004b). Lacto-*N*-fucopentaose III, a minor saccharide in the Tasmanian echidna milk, is the only milk oligosaccharide whose core is lacto-*N*-neotetraose but not lactose.

The predominant neutral oligosaccharide in milk of the platypus is Fuc(α1-2)Gal(β1-4)[Fuc(α1-3)]Glc (Messer and Kerry, 1973; Jenkins et al., 1984). The core structures of platypus neutral milk oligosaccharides are lactose, lacto-*N*-neotetraose, lacto-*N*-tetraose, or lacto-*N*-neohexaose, and many oligosaccharides contain Lewis X or Lewis Y (Fuc(α1-2)Gal(β1-4)[Fuc(α1-3)]GlcNAc) (Amano et al., 1985). Most of the acidic oligosaccharides in platypus milk contain Neu4,5Ac_2 and the core structures are lactose, lacto-*N*-neotetraose, or lacto-*N*-neohexaose (Urashima et al., 2015a). The presence of lacto-*N*-neotetraose or lacto-*N*-neohexaose as core units in major milk oligosaccharides represents a significant difference between platypus and echidna.

Table 3.7 Milk Oligosaccharides of Monotremes

No.	Oligosaccharide	Structure	References
Platypus (*Ornithorhynchus anatinus*) Milk			
Neutral oligosaccharides			
1	LDFT	Fucα1-2Galβ1-4Glc Fucα1 3	Messer and Kerry (1973) and Jenkins et al. (1984)
2	LNFP III	Galβ1-4GlcNAcβ1-3Galβ1-4Glc 3 Fucα1	Amano et al. (1985)
3	LNDFH III	Fucα1-2Galβ1-4GlcNAcβ1-3Galβ1-4Glc Fucα1 3	Amano et al. (1985)
4	DF-LNnT	Galβ1-4GlcNAcβ1-3Galβ1-4Glc Fucα1 3 Fucα1 3	Amano et al. (1985)
5	LNDFH I	Fucα1-2Galβ1-3GlcNAcβ1-3Galβ1-4Glc Fucα1 4	Amano et al. (1985)
6	DF-LNnH I	Fucα1 3 Galβ1-4GlcNAcβ1 6 Galβ1-4Glc Galβ1-4GlcNAcβ1 3 Fucα1 3	Amano et al. (1985)
7	TF-LNnH a	Fucα1 3 Fucα1-2Galβ1-4GlcNAcβ1 6 Galβ1-4Glc Galβ1-4GlcNAcβ1 3 Fucα1 3	Amano et al. (1985)

No.	Oligosaccharide	Structure	References
8	TF-LNnH b	Fucα1 3 Galβ1-4GlcNAcβ1 6 3 Galβ1-4Glc Fucα1-2Galβ1-4GlcNAcβ1 3 Fucα1	Amano et al. (1985)
Acidic oligosaccharides			
9		4-O-Ac-Neu5Acα2-3Galβ1-4Glc	Urashima et al. (2015a)
10		Neu5Acα2-3Galβ1-4Glc	Urashima et al. (2015a)
11		Fucα1 3 4-O-Ac-Neu5Acα2-3Galβ1-4GlcNAcβ1 6 3 Galβ1-4Glc 4-O-Ac-Neu5Acα2-3Galβ1-4GlcNAcβ1 and /or 4-O-Ac-Neu5Acα2-3Galβ1-4GlcNAcβ1 6 3 Galβ1-4Glc 4-O-Ac-Neu5Acα2-3Galβ1-4GlcNAcβ1 3 Fucα1	Urashima et al. (2015a) Urashima et al. (2015a)
12		Fucα1 3 4-O-Ac-Neu5Acα2-3Galβ1-4GlcNAcβ1 6 3 Galβ1-4Glc Galβ1-4GlcNAcβ1 and /or Fucα1 3 Galβ1-4GlcNAcβ1 6 3 Galβ1-4Glc 4-O-Ac-Neu5Acα2-3Galβ1-4GlcNAcβ1	Urashima et al. (2015a) Urashima et al. (2015a)

Continued

Table 3.7 Milk Oligosaccharides of Monotremes—cont'd

No.	Oligosaccharide	Structure	References
13		4-O-Ac-Neu5Acα2-3Galβ1-4GlcNAcβ1 6 Galβ1-4Glc Galβ1-4GlcNAcβ1 3 Fucα1 3 and /or	Urashima et al. (2015a)
		Galβ1-4GlcNAcβ1 6 Galβ1-4Glc 4-O-Ac-Neu5Acα2-3Galβ1-4GlcNAcβ1 3 Fucα1 3	Urashima et al. (2015a)
14		4-O-Ac-Neu5Acα2-3Galβ1-4GlcNAcβ1-3Galβ1-4Glc Fucα1 3	Urashima et al. (2015a)
15		4-O-Ac-Neu5Acα2-3Galβ1-4GlcNAcβ1-3Galβ1-4Glc	Urashima et al. (2015a)
16		Fucα1 3 Galβ1-4GlcNAcβ1 6 Galβ1-4Glc 4-O-Ac-Neu5Acα2-3Galβ1-4GlcNAcβ1 3 Fucα1 3 and /or	Urashima et al. (2015a)
		Fucα1 3 4-O-Ac-Neu5Acα2-3Galβ1-4GlcNAcβ1 6 Galβ1-4Glc Galβ1-4GlcNAcβ1 3 Fucα1 3	Urashima et al. (2015a)

No.	Oligosaccharide	Structure	References
17		Fucα1 3 Gapβ1-4GlcNAcβ1 6 Galβ1-4Glc 4-O-Ac-Neu5Acα2-6Galβ1-4GlcNAcβ1 3 and /or 4-O-Ac-Neu5Acα2-6Galβ1-4GlcNAcβ1 6 Galβ1-4Glc Galβ1-4GlcNAcβ1 3 3 Fucα1	Urashima et al. (2015a) Urashima et al. (2015a)
18		Fucα1 3 Fucα1-2Galβ1-4GlcNAcβ1 6 Galβ1-4Glc 4-O-Ac-Neu5Acα2-3Galβ1-4GlcNAcβ1 3 3 Fucα1 and /or Fucα1 3 4-O-Ac-Neu5Acα2-3Galβ1-4GlcNAcβ1 6 Galβ1-4Glc Fucα1-2Galβ1-4GlcNAcβ1 3 3 Fucα1	Urashima et al. (2015a) Urashima et al. (2015a)
19		Fucα1 3 Fucα1-2Galβ1-4GlcNAcβ1 6 Galβ1-4Glc 4-O-Ac-Neu5Acα2-6Galβ1-4GlcNAcβ1 3 and /or 4-O-Ac-Neu5Acα2-6Galβ1-4GlcNAcβ1 6 Galβ1-4Glc Fucα1-2Galβ1-4GlcNAcβ1 3 3 Fucα1	Urashima et al. (2015a) Urashima et al. (2015a)

Continued

Table 3.7 Milk Oligosaccharides of Monotremes—cont'd

No.	Oligosaccharide	Structure	References
20		Fucα1 (3) Fucα1-2Galβ1-4GlcNAcβ1 (6) Galβ1-4Glc 4-O-Ac-Neu5Acα2-3Galβ1-4GlcNAcβ1 (3) and /or	Urashima et al. (2015a)
		4-O-Ac-Neu5Acα2-3Galβ1-4GlcNAcβ1 (6) Galβ1-4Glc Fucα1-2Galβ1-4GlcNAcβ1 (3) Fucα1 (3)	Urashima et al. (2015a)
Short-Beaked Echidna *(Tachyglossus aculeatus)* Milk			
Neutral oligosaccharides			
-	2′-FL	Fucα1-2Galβ1-4Glc	Messer and Kerry (1973), Jenkins et al. (1984), and Oftedal et al. (2014)
2	LDFT	Fucα1-2Galβ1-4Glc Fucα1 (3)	Messer and Kerry (1973), Jenkins et al. (1984), and Oftedal et al. (2014)
3	B-tetrasaccharide	Galα1-3Galβ1-4Glc Fucα1 (2)	Oftedal et al. (2014)
4	B-pentasaccharide	Galα1-3Galβ1-4Glc Fucα1 (2) Fucα1 (3)	Oftedal et al. (2014)
5	LNFP III	Galβ1-4GlcNAcβ1-3Galβ1-4Glc Fucα1 (3)	Oftedal et al. (2014)
Acidic oligosaccharides			
6	3′-SL	Neu5Acα2-3Galβ1-4Glc	Messer and Kerry (1973), Messer (1974), and Oftedal et al. (2014)

No.	Oligosaccharide	Structure	References
7	4-*O*-Ac-3′-SL	4-O-Ac-Neu5Acα2-3Galβ1-4Glc	Messer and Kerry (1973), Messer (1974), Kamerling et al. (1982), and Oftedal et al. (2014)
8	di-*O*-Ac-3′-SL	4-O-Ac-U-O-AcNeu5Acα2-3Galβ1-4Glc where U = 7 , 8 or 9	Oftedal et al. (2014)
9	4-*O*-Ac-3′-SL-*O*-sulfate	4-O-Ac-Neu5Acα2-3Galβ1-4Glc-S S=sulfate	Oftedal et al. (2014)

F, Fucose; *L*, lactose; *S*, sialyl; *DF*, difucosyl; *TF*, trifucosyl; *DS*, disialyl; *TS*, trisialyl; *FS*, fucosyl sialyl; *DFS*, difucosyl sialyl; *TFS*, trifucosyl sialyl; *FDS*, fucosyl disialyl; *DGal*, digalactosyl; *FL*, fucosyllactose; *GL*, galactosyllactose; *LDFT*, lacto difucotetraose; *LNT*, lacto-N-tetraose; *LNnT*, lacto-N-neotetraose; *LNFP*, lacto-N-fucopentaose; *LNP*, lacto-N-pentaose; *LNDFH*, lacto-N-difucohexaose; *LNH*, lacto-N-hexaose; *LNnH*, lacto-N-neohexaose; *LNO*, lacto-N-octaose; *LND*, lacto-N-decaose.

The presence of 4-*O*-acetyl Neu5Ac (Neu4,5Ac$_2$) in the acidic milk oligosaccharides is the major unique and significant feature of monotreme milk. The 4-*O*-acetyl group in sialic acids is known to inhibit the actions of bacterial sialidases, and we have suggested that this inhibition would prevent or reduce bacterial growth in milk that may collect on or around the monotreme mammary patch (in the absence of a nipple) during suckling. This would tend to protect the neonatal monotreme against pathogens and could be of significance in relation to the evolution of mammals (Oftedal et al., 2014).

2.4 COMPARISON OF STRUCTURES OF MILK OLIGOSACCHARIDES AMONG MAMMALIAN SPECIES

Some milk oligosaccharides of the platypus, a monotreme, and of diverse eutherians including humans, many other primates, bears and some other carnivores, ruminants, horses, pigs, and elephants, contain core units of lacto-*N*-neotetraose and lacto-*N*-neohexaose (Urashima et al., 2011b, 1997b, 1999b, 2004b, 2015a; Uemura et al., 2006; Osthoff et al., 2008; Amano et al., 1985). Thus, these, along with lactose, must be considered the most universal core structures in milk oligosaccharides. However, the milk oligosaccharides of all marsupials as far studied, including the tammar wallaby, red kangaroo, koala, brushtail possum, and eastern quoll, do not have core units of lacto-*N*-neotetraose or lacto-*N*-neohexaose but rather have in common a core unit that can be expressed as [Gal(β1-3)]nGal(β1-4)Glc (Messer et al., 1980; Collins et al., 1981; Anraku et al., 2012; Urashima et al., 2013b, 2014a, 2015b). Such Gal(β1-3)Gal–based types of oligosaccharides have not been found in the milk of monotremes and, other than Gal(β1-3)Gal(β1-4)Glc (β3′-GL) and its sialyl derivative Neu5Ac(α2-3)Gal(β1-3)Gal(β1-4)Glc (3″-S-β3′-GL), have not been detected in the milk of eutherians. Thus, Messer and Urashima (2002) suggested that with respect to milk oligosaccharides, eutherians resemble monotremes more than they do marsupials.

However, a somewhat different picture emerges from the distribution of lacto-*N*-novopentaose I and/or its sialyl derivatives. They have been detected in the milk/colostrum of marsupials (Urashima et al., 1994b, 2013b, 2014a, 2015b; Anraku et al., 2012) as well as some eutherians including cows (Marino et al., 2011; Albrecht et al., 2014; Urashima et al., 1991b), goats (Albrecht et al., 2014), sheep (Albrecht et al., 2014), camels (Albrecht et al., 2014; Fukuda et al., 2010; Alhaj et al., 2013), horses (Albrecht et al., 2014; Urashima et al., 1989b), pigs (Albrecht et al., 2014), and capuchins (Goto et al., 2010; Urashima et al., 1999a). In addition, fucosyl sialyl lacto-*N*-novopentaose I has been found in the milk of the koala (Urashima et al., 2013b) and as a very minor saccharide in human milk (Gronberg et al., 1992). By contrast, the core unit lacto-*N*-novopentaose I has yet to be found in the milk of monotremes, suggesting that this oligosaccharide core unit is common to marsupials and some eutherians but missing (or at very low levels) in the two extant monotremes. Its presence or absence is presumably related to the presence or absence of one or more *N*-acetylglucosaminyltransferase activities in the lactating mammary glands of these species or else depends on the presence or absence of Gal(β1-3)Gal(β1-4)Glc, the substrate for β6*N*-acetylglycosaminyltransferase in the synthesis of lacto-*N*-novotetraose [refer to Fig. 1.14 of Urashima et al. (2014b)]. In marsupials, the presence of [Gal(β1-3)]nGal(β1-4)Glc oligosaccharides larger than a tetrasaccharide is probably due to high activity of the β3-galactosyltransferase, which is specifically found in marsupial lactating mammary glands (Messer et al., 1991) but appears to be absent in monotremes.

The presence/absence of the nonreducing units of ABH antigen, α-Gal epitope, Lewis X, and Lewis Y varies depending on mammalian species. Oligosaccharides that contain A antigen have been found in the milk/colostrum of the bonobo (Urasima et al., 2009b), dog (Rostami et al., 2014), striped skunk (Taufik et al., 2013), polar bear (Urashima et al., 2000, 2003a), African lion (Senda et al., 2010), clouded leopard (Senda et al., 2010), cow (Marino et al., 2011; Albrecht et al., 2014), dromedary camel (Albrecht et al., 2014), and minke whale (Urashima et al., 2002), while B antigen–containing oligosaccharides have been detected in the milk/colostrum of the gorilla (Urashima et al., 2009b), Coquerel's sifaka (Taufik et al., 2012), Japanese black bear (Urashima et al., 1999b, 2004b), polar bear (Urashima et al., 2000), spotted hyena (Uemura et al., 2009), and Tasmanian echidna (Oftedal et al., 2014). Oligosaccharides that contain H antigen have been found in the milk/colostrum of humans (Urashima et al., 2011b), the chimpanzee (Urashima et al., 2009b), bonobo (Urashima et al., 2009b), gorilla (Urashima et al., 2009b), aye-aye (Taufik et al., 2012), cow (Marino et al., 2011; Albrecht et al., 2014), goat (Albrecht et al., 2014), sheep (Albrecht et al., 2014), dromedary camel (Albrecht et al., 2014), pig (Albrecht et al., 2014), dog (Rostami et al., 2014; Bubb et al., 1999), brown bear (Urashima et al., 1997b), Japanese black bear (Urashima et al., 1999b), polar bear (Urashima et al., 2000), mink (Urashima et al., 2005), white-nosed coati (Urashima et al., 1999c), several seals (Urashima et al., 2001a, 2003b, 2004a; Kinoshita et al., 2009), and minke whale (Urashima et al., 2002), and small amounts of this type of oligosaccharide also occur in species whose milk/colostrum contains oligosaccharides that contain A or B antigens. α-Gal epitope–containing oligosaccharides have been detected in the milk/colostrum of the sifaka (Taufik et al., 2012), mongoose lemur (Taufik et al., 2012), cow (Marino et al., 2011; Albrecht et al., 2014; Urashima et al., 1991b), goat (Albrecht et al., 2014; Urashima et al., 1994a), sheep (Albrecht et al., 2014; Urashima et al., 1989a), dromedary camel (Albrecht et al., 2014), horse (Albrecht et al., 2014), pig (Albrecht et al., 2014), skunk (Taufik et al., 2013), mink (Urashima et al., 2005), coati (Urashima et al., 1999c), bears (Urashima et al., 1997b, 1999b, 2000, 2003a, 2004b), giant panda (Nakamura et al., 2003b), leopard (Senda et al., 2010), hyena (Uemura et al., 2009), elephants (Uemura et al., 2006; Osthoff et al., 2008), giant anteater (Urashima et al., 2008), and flying fox (Senda et al., 2011). Oligosaccharides containing Lewis X have been found in the milk/colostrum of humans (Urashima et al., 2011b), chimpanzee (Urashima et al., 2009b), bonobo (Urashima et al., 2009b), orangutan (Urashima et al., 2009b), rhesus macaque (Goto et al., 2010), capuchin (Urashima et al., 1999a), toque macaque (Goto et al., 2010), baboon (Goto et al., 2010), aye-aye (Taufik et al., 2012), mongoose lemur (Taufik et al., 2012), cow (Marino et al., 2011; Albrecht et al., 2014), goat (Albrecht et al., 2014), sheep (Albrecht et al., 2014), camel (Albrecht et al., 2014; Fukuda et al., 2010), horse (Albrecht et al., 2014), pig (Albrecht et al., 2014), bears (Urashima et al., 1997b, 1999b, 2000, 2003a, 2004b), giant panda (Nakamura et al., 2003b), elephants (Uemura et al., 2006; Osthoff et al., 2008), koala (Urashima et al., 2013b), echidna (Messer and Kerry, 1973; Jenkins et al., 1984; Oftedal et al., 2014), and platypus (Messer and Kerry, 1973; Jenkins et al., 1984; Amano et al., 1985; Urashima et al., 2015a).

Neu5Ac is the sole or predominant molecular unit of sialic acid of sialyl milk oligosaccharides in most mammalian species, while Neu5Gc is the predominant or only unit of sialic acid in the milk/colostrum of sheep (Albrecht et al., 2014), goat (Albrecht et al., 2014), lion (Senda et al., 2010), clouded leopard (Senda et al., 2010), and flying fox (Senda et al., 2011). As noted, milk of the monotremes echidna and platypus contains 4-*O*-acetylated Neu5Ac in the dominant sialyl oligosaccharides (Messer and Kerry, 1973; Messer, 1974; Kamerling et al., 1982; Oftedal et al., 2014; Urashima et al., 2015a). Trace levels of an unspecified *O*-acetyl-Neu5Ac-Gal(β1-4) Glc have been found in the milk/colostrum of the cow, goat, and horse (Albrecht et al., 2014).

Sulfate-containing oligosaccharides have been found in the milk/colostrum of humans (Urashima et al., 2011b), the baboon (Goto et al., 2010), sifaca (Taufik et al., 2012), dog (Rostami et al., 2014; Bubb et al., 1999), bearded seal (Urashima et al., 2004a; Kinoshita et al., 2009), rat (Sturman et al., 1985; Choi et al., 1968; Barra et al., 1965), red kangaroo (Anraku et al., 2012), brushtail possum (Urashima et al., 2014a), eastern quoll (Urashima et al., 2015b), and Tasmanian echidna (Oftedal et al., 2014), while phosphate-containing saccharides have been detected in the milk/colostrum of cow (Albrecht et al., 2014; Cumar et al., 1965; Parkkinen and Finne, 1987), goat (Albrecht et al., 2014), sheep (Albrecht et al., 2014), horse (Albrecht et al., 2014; Nakamura et al., 2001) and dromedary camel (Albrecht et al., 2014).

Thus, the presence/absence of these nonreducing units (i.e., sialic acid species and sulfate/phosphate) shows considerable variation among mammalian species.

2.5 BIOSYNTHESIS OF LACTOSE AND MILK OLIGOSACCHARIDES: IMPORTANCE OF α-LACTALBUMIN

Lactose is synthesized within the Golgi apparatus in secretory cells in lactating mammary glands from UDP-Gal (donor) and glucose (acceptor) via transgalactosylation catalyzed by lactose synthase, whereas milk oligosaccharides are synthesized via various specific glycosyltransferases that transfer monosaccharide residues to lactose and/or small lactose-based oligosaccharides as acceptors. Lactose synthase is a complex formed by membrane-bound β4-galactosyltransferase I (β4Gal-T1) and α-lactalbumin, which is one of the whey proteins. Tissues other than lactating mammary glands and milk do not contain α-lactalbumin but do contain β4Gal-T1, which transfers galactose from UDP-Gal to nonreducing GlcNAc residues in glycoconjugates, producing *N*-acetyllactosamine [Gal(β1-4)GlcNAc] units. In lactating mammary glands, the binding of α-lactalbumin to β4Gal-T1 changes its preferred acceptor from GlcNAc to free glucose. Thus, the expression of α-lactalbumin within the mammary gland is the key to the secretion of lactose in milk.

It has been suggested that the ratio of milk oligosaccharides to lactose is determined mainly by the rate of lactose synthesis (Messer and Urashima, 2002). When the lactose synthesis rate is low, most of the lactose produced within the Golgi apparatus would serve as an acceptor for the glycosyltransferases that generate milk oligosaccharides, and thus the ratio of milk oligosaccharides to lactose in secreted milk would be relatively high. When, however, the rate of lactose production is high, only a small proportion of the nascent lactose would function as an acceptor, and the ratio of oligosaccharides to lactose in secreted milk would consequently be relatively low.

Interestingly, the rate at which lactose is synthesized is primarily controlled by the expression level of α-lactalbumin within the mammary gland, although upregulation of β4Gal-T1 by a mammary specific mechanism is also important (Shaper et al., 1998). It follows that in most eutherian species, in whose milk lactose is the predominant saccharide, the level of expression of α-lactalbumin within the mammary glands is likely to be higher, relative to the expression and activity of glycosyltransferases, than in monotremes, marsupials, and those species of Carnivora in which milk oligosaccharides predominate over lactose (Messer and Urashima, 2002). The hypothesis that the high ratio of milk oligosaccharides to lactose in monotremes is due to low expression of α-lactalbumin within the mammary gland is supported by the finding that the α-lactalbumin concentration is low in the milks of the platypus (Shaw et al., 1993) and echidna (Messer et al., 1997), when compared with other milks.

2.6 THE EVOLUTION OF MILK OLIGOSACCHARIDES IN A BIOLOGICAL CONTEXT

Given that almost all milk oligosaccharides contain the lactose structure at the reducing end and are synthesized via addition of monosaccharide moieties to lactose, it is apparent that milk oligosaccharides could not evolve until α-lactalbumin-mediated synthesis of lactose had been achieved. α-Lactalbumin has been found only in milk or lactating mammary glands. Lysozymes, which cleave the bond in peptidoglycans of bacterial cell walls, are found in many tissues of other vertebrates and in insects. Since the discovery that the amino acid sequence of α-lactalbumin is similar to that of c-type lysozyme, this similarity was found to extend to their secondary and tertiary structures and the arrangement of their genes (McKenzie and White, 1991). As the gene for c-lysozyme is more broadly distributed and phylogenetically older than that for α-lactalbumin, it appears that α-lactalbumin derived from c-lysozyme via gene duplication and subsequent base pair substitutions. The amino acid substitutions that occurred resulted in loss of bacteriolytic activity and the gain of a novel ability to bind to β4Gal-T1. Based on molecular clock estimates, the divergence of c-lysozyme and α-lactalbumin occurred about 300 million years ago (Prager and Wilson, 1988), or about 110 million years before the advent of the earliest mammals in the Jurassic (Luo et al., 2011). This is consistent with other evidence indicating an ancient origin of lactation among the Synapsida (ancestral group from which mammals evolved) during the Carboniferous (Oftedal, 2002a, 2012, 2013).

However, the earliest form of lactation ("protolactation") may have been quite different from milk production. First, the earliest mammary glands were likely tubular apocrine-like glands that secreted onto a hairy integument, as nipples did not evolve until much later (Oftedal and Dhouailly, 2013). Second, the earliest function of protolactation may have been provision of water, some nutrients, and protective (antibacterial) compounds to the surface of incubated eggs (Oftedal, 2002b). Third, some constituents, such as large casein micelles and milk fat globules, would have taken time to evolve from their precursor secretory calcium-binding phosphoproteins and apical blebs (Oftedal, 2013). Thus the initial secretion was likely dilute, produced in small quantities, and applied to incubated eggs.

So how early in synapsid evolution did milk oligosaccharides appear? Since milk oligosaccharides are found in monotremes, marsupials, and eutherians, albeit with some differences in structure, we conclude that milk oligosaccharides preceded the divergence of these lineages; that is, were already present in the ancestors of early mammals (i.e., mammaliaforms) more than 190 million years ago. This assumes that milk oligosaccharide synthesis evolved once rather than separately via parallel evolution in each mammalian lineage, and the general overlap, and similarities in oligosaccharide structures among monotremes, marsupials, and eutherians (see earlier) support this assumption. On the other hand, there are aspects of monotreme acidic oligosaccharides (4-*O*-acetylation of sialic acid) and marsupial long-chain oligosaccharides [linear and branched Gal(β1-3)nGal] that appear to be unique to these lineages.

However, another alternative is that milk oligosaccharides evolved concurrent with lactose, that is, about 300 million years ago. It has been suggested that once α-lactalbumin evolved the ability to modify the acceptor preference of β4Gal-T1, leading to lactose production, that glycosyltransferases—otherwise employed in chain elongation and epitope decoration of glycoconjugates—could have added other monosaccharide moieties to the newly formed lactose, producing oligosaccharides (Messer and Urashima, 2002). This would presumably have been favored by the low lactose secretion rate in proto-mammary glands. Given that one of the earliest functions of proto-lactation in early synapsids may have been provision of moisture and protective compounds to the surface of incubated eggs (Oftedal, 2002b), it is possible that the selective forces favoring oligosaccharides included potential antimicrobial or prebiotic effects. Of course, such beneficial effects might also protect the surface of maternal skin, onto which proto-milk was secreted, and, after ingestion by hatchlings, their oral cavity and digestive tract.

This scenario is supported by recent evidence on the acidic oligosaccharides of monotremes: the short-beaked echidna (Oftedal et al., 2014) and platypus (Urashima et al., 2015a). Monotremes retain what is believed to be the ancestral form of reproduction: (1) Eggs are laid and incubated in a pouch or incubatorium. (2) The young are immature (altricial) at hatching. (3) The young feed posthatching via suckling on initially dilute milk secreted onto the skin in a mammary patch (there are no nipples). (4) Lactation entails a prolonged period of dependence. Although it has not been studied directly, it is reasonable to assume that the immune system is poorly developed at birth (as in altricial marsupials; Bisana et al., 2013) and the moist pouch/incubatorium provides a potential site for microbial proliferation. The unique feature of milk oligosaccharides—which include a variety of core structures and both fucosyl and sialyl derivatives—is that the sialyl oligosaccharides contain predominantly 4-*O*-acetyl-sialic acid (Neu4,5Ac_2) rather than sialic acid (Neu5Ac). 4-*O*-Acetylation of sialic acid appears to be a lockup mechanism that prevents microbial sialidases from catabolizing sialic acid, likely due to steric hindrance of binding by these enzymes (Schauer et al., 2011; Oftedal et al., 2014). It is thought that these species resemble ancestral synapsids in having oligosaccharides evolutionarily molded to confront potential microbial assaults on the skin as well as in the oral cavity and digestive tract of the hatchlings.

Regardless of when oligosaccharides first appeared during synapsid evolution, they subsequently diversified into an immense array of structures, as described earlier. Some may represent evolutionary responses to specific microbial challenges, others may be generic protective compounds, and still others may provide for specific needs in offspring. Unfortunately, little is known about the biological effects or benefits of the vast array of milk oligosaccharides in nonhuman milks. Moreover, lactose has come to predominate in the milks of most eutherian taxa. If the expression of α-lactalbumin was low within the mammary glands of the synapsid ancestors of mammals, subsequent evolutionary increase in α-lactalbumin expression must have occurred in mammary glands in the eutherian lineage, since most extant eutherian species secrete lactose as the predominant milk saccharide (Messer and Urashima, 2002).

Another intriguing question is when an enzyme system to digest lactose evolved in the offspring. If the hypotheses about protolactation are correct—that the initial protomilk was dilute and applied to eggs, rather than ingested by young, and oligosaccharides rather than lactose predominated—there may have been little selective benefit for a digestive process. Even now, it is not certain if and how species with a predominance of oligosaccharides in milk are able to use them as sources of energy and organic substrates. In rats, it is believed that milk oligosaccharides are taken up by endocytosis and digested by intracellular lysosomal enzymes (Duncan et al., 2009), and the same may be true of monotremes (Oftedal et al., 2014) and marsupials (Messer et al., 1989). It is likely that small intestinal brush border lactase activity evolved and became upregulated as lactose synthesis increased, as it is required for digestion of the higher lactose milks of most eutherians (Messer and Urashima, 2002; Oftedal, 2013). In extant mammals, lactase activity in the brush border of the small intestine is found in most suckling eutherians (except species devoid of milk lactose, such as sea lions) but not in suckling macropods (Messer et al., 1989) or in other examined suckling marsupials (except for the late lactation stage of the brush-tailed possum) (Crisp et al., 1989a) or in suckling short-beaked echidna, a monotreme (Stewart et al., 1983).

3. DAIRY FARM ANIMALS AS POTENTIAL SOURCES FOR HUMAN MILK OLIGOSACCHARIDES REPLACER

Human mature milk and colostrum contain 12–13 g/L and 22–24 g/L of milk oligosaccharides, respectively, and the structures of more than 100 HMOs have been characterized to date (Newburg et al., 1995; Urashima et al., 2011b, 2012a). By way of comparison, bovine colostrum collected immediately postpartum contains only around 1 g/L of oligosaccharides, and this concentration rapidly decreases after 48 h (Nakamura et al., 2003a). It has been recognized that HMOs have several biological functions (Urashima et al., 2007a, 2009a, 2011a,b; Newburg et al., 1995; Kobata, 2010). They stimulate the growth of beneficial microorganisms in the infant colon, they act as receptor analogs that inhibit the attachment of pathogenic microorganisms to the colonic mucosa, and small amounts are absorbed into the circulation, where they modulate immunoreactivity.

Human infant formulas are produced from mature bovine milk. Since HMOs have several important biological functions, other materials whose functions are similar to those of HMOs might profitably be incorporated into milk replacers, because mature bovine milk contains only trace amounts of oligosaccharides. Prebiotics such as galacto- and fructo-oligosaccharides and lactulose have been incorporated into infant formulas, but these are not present or are present at only trace levels in human milk. Similarly, galacto-oligosaccharides have been incorporated into some milk replacers for marsupials. It is to be expected that oligosaccharides separated from bovine colostrum, from cheese whey, or from the milk/colostrum of other domestic farm animals can be used as additives to infant formulas and functional foods. The following section discusses the possibility, in the near future, of the industrial utilization of the milk oligosaccharides of dairy farm animals, based on their chemical structures and their concentrations, as well as on their known biological functions.

3.1 DIFFERENCES BETWEEN HUMAN MILK OLIGOSACCHARIDES AND BOVINE MILK OLIGOSACCHARIDES

Discussion of the possible utilization of bovine milk oligosaccharides (BMOs) requires knowledge of the differences between milk oligosaccharide structures produced by women and cows. Table 3.3 shows the chemical structures of the oligosaccharides in milk/colostrum of dairy domestic farm animals including cows, goats, sheep, camels, and horses; they are described in Section 2.1.2 of this chapter.

In HMOs, 2'-fucosyllactose and oligosaccharides whose core is lacto-*N*-tetraose are predominant, and type I oligosaccharides predominate over type II (Urashima et al., 2012a). In BMOs, type II oligosaccharides whose core units are LN*n*T, lacto-*N*-novopentaose I, or LN*n*H have been detected, but the type I have not. The only oligosaccharide whose core is lacto-*N*-novopentaose I, (Neu5Ac(α2-3){Gal(β1-4)[Fuc(α1-3)]GlcNAc(β1-6)}Gal(β1-4)Glc), was found in human milk (Gronberg et al., 1992), but its concentration was very low. The ratio of lacto-*N*-novopentaose I–containing oligosaccharides to other oligosaccharides is very different in bovine compared with human milk. In BMOs, a few sialyl oligosaccharides contain galactosyllactose (Marino et al., 2011; Albrecht et al., 2014), but this type of oligosaccharide has not been found in HMOs. In human milk, neutral oligosaccharides predominate over acidic ones and the ratio of fucosyl oligosaccharides to total HMOs is relatively high, whereas in bovine milk/colostrum acidic predominate over neutral oligosaccharides, and the concentration of fucosyl oligosaccharides is very low. LacNAc, LacdiNAc, and GalNAc(β1-4)Glc, found in bovine colostrum, have not been detected in human milk or colostrum. Bovine colostrum contains isoglobotriose and GalNAc(α1-3)Gal(β1-4)Glc, which have α-Gal or α-GalNAc in their structures, but these have not been found in human milk.

Such differences in milk oligosaccharides between human and bovine milk must be considered in relation to the potential utilization of BMOs as additives in the food industry.

3.2 QUANTITATIVE ASPECTS OF BOVINE MILK OLIGOSACCHARIDES

The concentration of predominant BMOs (3′-SL, 6′-SL, 6′-SLN, and DSL) in milk has been estimated to be considerably lower than that of HMOs. Table 3.8 [from reference Fong et al. (2011)] shows the concentrations of several BMOs in colostrum, mature milk, defatted mature milk, and infant formula produced from bovine mature milk. The data were obtained by quantitation of BMOs with reverse-phase HPLC after derivatization with 2-aminopyridine, etc., or a combination of high pH anion exchange HPLC and detection with pulse amperometry (HPEAC-PAD) of the underivatized BMO fraction (Nakamura et al., 2003a; Martin-Sosa et al., 2003; McJarrow et al., 2004).

Fig. 3.1 [from Nakamura et al. (2003a)] shows the changes in the concentrations of 3′-SL, 6′-SL, and 6′-SLN in bovine colostrum/transition milk from immediately after parturition to 168 h postpartum. The concentrations rapidly decreased up to 48 h postpartum, after which they declined more slowly. In humans, the concentration of HMOs in mature milk is lower than it is in the colostrum but is still much higher than in mature bovine milk.

Fong et al. (2011) developed a method for the quantitation of different BMOs using hydrophilic interaction chromatography HPLC with high-resolution selected reaction monitoring–MS (HILIC HPLC-HRSRM-MS). They determined the concentrations of five BMOs [3′-SL, 6′-SL, 6′-SLN, DSL, and *N*-acetylgalactosaminyllactose (GNL)] in bovine mature defatted milk, homogenized mature milk, nonpasteurized mature milk, bovine colostrum, and infant formula. They extracted the BMO fraction with chloroform/methanol and acetonitrile, separated the BMOs by hydrophilic interaction HPLC with a Kintex HILIC column using 50 mmol/L ammonium acetate (pH 4.5) and 100% acetonitrile as elution solvent, and performed thermoelectrospray ionization–MS for each component. The concentration dependence and recovery of the peak areas of ion monitor of MS were determined for five BMOs with oligosaccharide standards.

Table 3.8 Concentrations of Oligosaccharides in Samples of Bovine Milk, Bovine Colostrum, and Infant Formula (Number of Samples and Coefficient of Variation in Parentheses)

	3′SL (μg/mL)	6′SL (μg/mL)	6′SLN (μg/mL)	DSL (μg/mL)	GNL (μg/mL)
Skim milk 1	51 ± 4 (30, 9%)	6.3 ± 0.4 (8, 6%)	0.13 ± 0.02 (2, 14%)	1.5 ± 0.1 (2, 6%)	2.6 ± 0.3 (2, 10%)
Skim milk 2	55 ± 4 (2, 6%)	9 ± 0.2 (2, 2%)	0.10 ± 0.02 (2, 17%)	2.1 ± 0.3 (2, 14%)	3.4 ± 0.4 (2, 13%)
Homogenized milk	48 ± 4 (6, 8%)	9.6 ± 0.8 (3, 8%)	0.1 ± 0.03 (3, 14%)	3.1 ± 0.2 (3, 6%)	2.4 ± 0.1 (3, 2%)
Unpasteurized milk	47 ± 4 (6, 9%)	3.6 ± 0.3 (2, 9%)	<LOD	0.54 ± 0.01 (2, 14%)	<LOD (2%)
Mature milk (Martin-Sosa et al.)	94–119	67–88	145–176	41–77	
Mature milk (μg/mL, McJarrow and van Amelsfort-Schoonbeek)	35–50	14–25	9–12	2–7	3–4
Mature milk (7 d postpartum, Nakamura et al.)	30	25	12	ND	
Colostrum (second milking)	1245 ± 82 (7, 7%)	85 ± 6 (7, 7%)	119 ± 7 (7, 6%)	126 ± 8 (2, 8%)	1 ± 0.1 (2, 12%)
Colostrum (fourth milking)	739 ± 53 (5, 7%)	73 ± 2 (5, 2%)	117 ± 10 (5, 8%)	80 ± 7 (2, 9%)	1 ± 0.1 (2, 10%)
Colostrum (Martin-Sosa et al.)	354	147	210	135	
Colostrum (μg/mL, McJarrow and van Amelsfort-Schoonbeek)	261–867	92–243	97–239	166–283	20–65
Colostrum (Nakamura et al.)	850	141	117	ND	
Infant formula 1	17 ± 4 (2, 8%)	3.8 ± 0.2 (2, 10%)	<LOD	0.8 ± 0.1 (2, 13%)	<LOD
Infant formula 2	19 ± 1 (2, 6%)	4.6 ± 0.5 (2, 10%)	<LOD	0.5 ± 0.02 (2, 5%)	<LOD

Adapted from reference Fong, B., Ma, K., McJarrow, P., 2011. Quantification of bovine milk oligosaccharides using liquid chromatography-selected reaction monitoring-mass spectrometry. Journal of Agricultural and Food Chemistry 59, 9788–9795.

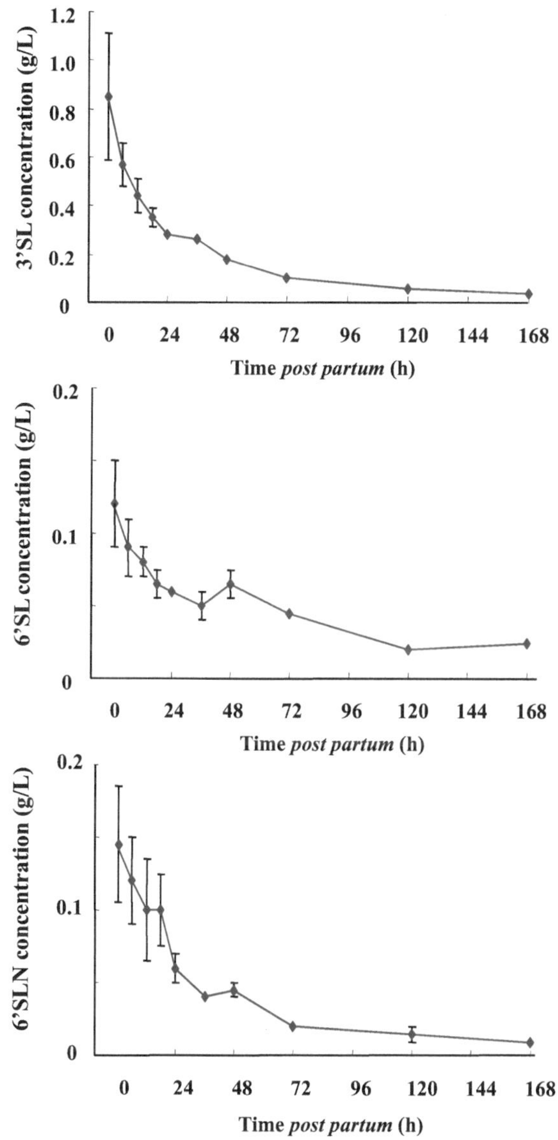

FIGURE 3.1

Changes in the concentrations of 3′-SL, 6′-SL, and 6′-SLN in Holstein bovine colostrum during early lactation. Values are indicated as means ± SD ($n = 4$).

Reproduced from a figure in reference Nakamura, T., Kawase, H., Kimura, K., Watanabe, Y., Ohtani, M., Arai, I., Urashima, T. 2003a. Concentration of sialyloligosaccharides in bovine colostrum and milk during the prepartum and early lactation. Journal of Dairy Science 86, 1315-1320.

They first attempted to use a hydrocarb graphited carbon column to separate BMOs and found that their BMO standards achieved very poor chromatographic separation, with line broadening and significant tailing of peaks. These problems disappeared, however, when they used hydrophilic interaction HPLC with a Kintex HILIC column. In samples of mature bovine milk (defatted milk, homogenized milk, and nonpasteurized milk), the values they determined were 47–55 mg/L for 3′-SL, 3.6–9.6 mg/L for 6′-SL, less than 0.13 mg/L for 6′-SLN, 0.54–3.1 mg/L for DSL, and 3.4 mg/L for GNL (Table 3.8). In colostrum, collected at the second or fourth milking from the same cow, the concentrations of 3′-SL, 6′-SL, 6′-SLN, and DSL were much higher than those in the mature milk, while that of GNL was lower (Table 3.8). The concentration of 3′-SL was twice as high in the sample collected at the second milking than in that collected at the fourth milking, but no significant differences in the concentrations of 6′-SL and 6′-SLN were observed between the two milking samples. In infant formula, the concentration of each oligosaccharide was 30–50% lower than that in the mature milk samples. As this quantitation method does not require any derivatization of oligosaccharides, it might in the future be used more frequently in view of its convenience.

Liu et al. (2014) subsequently improved the quantitative analysis of 3′-SL, 6′-SL, and 6′-SLN in bovine mature milk using a method based on the use of hydrophilic interaction liquid chromatography with a Luna HILIC column coupled to MS in negative ion mode. The concentrations of 3′-SL, 6′-SL, and 6′-SLN were determined to be 116–199 mg/L, 6–32 mg/L, and 0.27–1.2 mg/L, respectively.

3.3 FUTURE INDUSTRIAL USE OF MILK OLIGOSACCHARIDES OF DOMESTIC FARM ANIMALS

As described, the concentration of milk oligosaccharides is much lower in bovine milk than in human milk. This is a limitation to the utilization of BMOs as food additives in industry, but since bovine colostrum contains larger amounts of oligosaccharides than bovine milk, it is possible that it will be used in the near future.

These data suggest several biological functions for BMOs, as follows. It is thought that the adhesion of *Neisseria meningitidis*, which causes meningitis and septicemia, is mediated via type IV pili. A microtiter pili-binding assay was used to investigate the binding of type IV pili isolated from *N. meningitidis* to various glycoproteins. Inhibition of pili binding to bovine thyroglobulin by fractionated BMOs was demonstrated (Hakkarainen et al., 2005). The binding of *Neisseria* pili to bovine thyroglobulin was most effective and was clearly inhibited by neutral and acidic BMOs at concentrations of 1–2 g/L.

The bovine acidic oligosaccharide fraction, in which 3′-SL is dominant, can possibly be used as an antiadhesion agent against enteropathogenic *Escherichia coli* (EPEC). Angeloni et al. (2005) found that on exposure to 3′-SL, EPEC adhesion to Caco-2 cells was reduced by 50% compared with control cells. They found that on exposure to 3′-SL, Caco-2 cells changed their cell surface glycan profile in that the expression of α(2-3) and α(2-6) linked sialic acid residues was significantly reduced, while that of fucose and galactose residues was also diminished. These results suggest a novel mechanism by which milk oligosaccharides, such as 3′-SL, regulate bacteria–host interactions.

Fractions containing milk oligosaccharides, in the form of the supernatant separated from colostrum and from transitional, mature, and late lactation milk of Spanish brown cows following ethanol precipitation and subsequent centrifugation, were used to investigate inhibition of hemagglutination by seven enterotoxigenic *E. coli* strains (K99, FK, F41, F17, B16, B23, and B64) (Martin et al., 2002) that had been isolated from diarrheal calves. The fractions from the transitional and mature milk inhibited hemagglutination by all of these strains, whereas those from the colostrum and late lactation milk produced weaker inhibition. These data suggest that BMO can be used as antiinfectional agents for humans and for cows.

Terabayashi et al. have been attempting to enhance the possible biological function of bovine colostrum sialyl oligosaccharides via chemical modification (Terabayashi et al., 2006). The OH-1 at the reducing end of the oligosaccharides was substituted by an amino group, using an amination reaction with saturated ammonium hydrogen carbonate. These amino derivatives were then condensed with lauric acid using a reagent for amidation, DMT-MM (4-(4,6-dimethoxy-1,3,5-triazin)-2-yl)-4-methylmorpholinium chloride. It was observed that the sialyl glycosides, synthesized by the condensation of 3′-SL with this long chain fatty acid, inhibited the infection of MDCK cells by human type influenza virus A/PR/8 (H1N1).

Campylobacter jejuni is the leading cause of acute bacterial infectious diarrhea in humans. It has been suggested that 2′-FL, a predominant HMO in secretor donor human milk, inhibits the adherence of this organism to the infant colonic mucosa. Lane et al. (2012b) observed inhibition of invasion and translocation of *C. jejuni* to HT-29 epithelial cells by colostral BMOs, in an experiment involving coculture of bacteria and HT-29 cells in the presence of BMOs and the authentic oligosaccharides. The addition of BMOs reduced the invasion of HT-29 cells by *C. jejuni* by 50% compared with the control, and this antiinvasion effect was dose-dependent at concentrations of 0.25, 0.5, 1.0, and 5.0 mg/mL. However, when BMOs were pretreated with periodate, no such inhibition was observed. The addition of 5 mg/mL BMOs or 1 mg/mL of 3′-SL reduced the translocation of *C. jejuni* into HT-29 cells by 80% and 50%, respectively, 5 h after infection of the cells by this organism. Although it has been suggested that 2′-FL inhibits infection of the epithelial cells by *C. jejuni* by an anti-adhesion mechanism, the data suggest that BMOs, including 3′-SL, inhibit infection by a different mechanism, because 2′-FL has not been found in BMOs or is present at only very low concentrations.

Lane et al. (2012a) confirmed inhibition by BMOs of the translocation of *E. coli* P1422 into HT-29 cells in a coculture experiment, and analyzed the attachment of BMOs to these bacteria by their original methods. 3′-SL (20 μg/mL), or BMOs at a concentration that corresponded to 20 μg/mL of 3′-SL, was suspended in 1×10^9 CFU/mL of bacteria in saline, and the bacterial cells were removed via centrifugation. This exposure of the oligosaccharides to the bacteria was performed once, 5 times, or 10 times. The concentration of each oligosaccharide in the supernatant was determined by HPEAC-PAD without derivatization or by hydrophilic interaction HPLC after derivatization with 2-aminobenzaldehyde. The results indicated that the concentration of 3′-SL (20 μg/mL) in the supernatant was reduced by 4% and 11% when exposed to the bacteria 5 times and 10 times, respectively. The concentrations of 6′-SLN (4 μg/mL) and of DSL (2.2 μg/mL) decreased by 11% and by 15% after five exposures, and by 13% and 18% after 10 exposures, whereas the peak area of 6′-SL (i.e., its concentration) was not significantly reduced by exposure to the bacteria. The authors emphasized that this represents a simple method for the detection of specific oligosaccharides among milk oligosaccharides that inhibit the attachment of certain pathogenic microorganisms to cells, but further experiments with several bacterial strains and milk oligosaccharides are required to confirm the reliability of this method.

Hester et al. (2013) tested the antirotavirus (RV) activity of 3′-SL and 6′-SL, which are predominant oligosaccharides in bovine colostrum, in an established *in vitro* system for assessing cellular binding and viral infectivity/replication to uroepithelial MA-104 cells. 3′-SL and 6′-SL were tested against the sialidase-sensitive porcine OSU strain and the nonsensitive human RV Wa strain. The RV Wa strain was not inhibited by these oligosaccharides, but RV OSU strain infectivity was dose-dependently inhibited. 3′-SL and 6′-SL concordantly inhibited ^{125}I-radiolabeled RV cellular binding and infectivity/replication at a 1–3 mg/mL concentration. In the immunohistochemical study with peroxidase, the inhibition of infection of the cells was dose-dependently observed for 2–6 mg/mL of 3′-SL and 6′-SL by 20–74% and by 61–83%, respectively. The data suggest that, in future, BMO may be used as an anti-RV infection reagent.

It is expected that BMOs would potentially be an excellent source for utilization as immunomodulating agents, as suggested by the following. Lane et al. (2013) compared the transcriptional response of colonic epithelial cells (HT-29) to the entire pool of HMOs and bovine colostrum oligosaccharides (BCOs), to determine whether BMOs had effects on gene expression that were similar to those of HMOs. They observed changes in the expression profiles of immune system–associated glycogenes, after 24-h exposure of HT-29 cells that had been grown in McCoy 5A broth to BCOs, HMOs, or 3′-SL for 24 h. Reverse transcriptase–polymerase chain reaction (RT-PCR) analysis revealed that HMOs and BCOs influenced the expression of cytokines [interleukin (IL)-1β, IL-8, colony-stimulating factor 2 granulocyte-macrophage (GM-CSF2), IL-17C, and platelet factor 4 (PF4)], chemokines [chemokine (C-X-C motif) ligand 1 (CXCL1), chemokine (C-X-C motif) ligand 3 (CXCL3), chemokine (C–C motif) ligand 20 (CCL20), chemokine (C-X-C motif) ligand 2 (CXCL2), chemokine (C-X-C motif) ligand 6 (CXCL6), chemokine (C–C motif) ligand 5 (CCL5), and chemokine (C-X3-C motif) ligand 1 (CXCL1)], and cell surface receptors [interferon γ receptor 1 (IFNGR1), intercellular adhesion molecule-1 (ICAM-1), intercellular adhesion molecule-2 (ICAM-2), and IL-10 receptor α (IL10RA)]. These data suggest that milk oligosaccharides contribute to the development and maturation of the intestinal immune response and that bovine milk may be an attractive commercially viable source of oligosaccharides for such application.

Mature human milk contains 0.7 g/L, on average, of sialic acid, a concentration that is significantly greater than that (0–0.2 g/L) in milk replacers, which are based on mature bovine milk. It has been reported that the levels of gangliosides and of sialylglycoproteins in the brains of breastfed infants are higher than those in bottle-fed infants (Wang et al., 2003), raising the question as to whether sialyl oligosaccharides or sialyl glycoconjugates should be added to infant formulas. In a study using piglets, feeding of caseinoglycopeptide separated from cheese whey elevated the level of sialic acid in brain glycoproteins and glycolipids and the levels of the mRNAs for polysialyltransferase IV (ST8SIA4) and UDP-*N*-acetylglucosamine-2-epimerase (GNA). ST8SIA4 is a key enzyme for sialyl glycoconjugate biosynthesis, while GNA is a rate-controlling enzyme in the de novo synthesis of sialic acid (Wang et al., 2007). In addition, the learning performance and memory of the piglets were found to have improved after feeding of these glycoconjugates. Significant dose–response relations were observed in the hippocampus between the degree of sialic acid supplementation and the mRNA levels of ST8SIA4 and GNE, corresponding to proportionate increases in *protein-bound* sialic acid concentrations in the frontal cortex. These results suggest that the sialic acid of the caseinoglycopeptide supplement was absorbed and then used to form brain sialyl glycopeptides and gangliosides, which may have enhanced learning abilities in this model animal.

Furthermore, it has been found that when adult rats were fed sialyllactose, there was an increase in their brain ganglioside contents, including GM_3 [Neu5Ac(α2-3)Gal(β1-4)Glc-Cer], and an improvement in their ability to learn to swim (Sakai et al., 2006). These data suggest that sialyl oligosaccharides or sialyl glycoconjugates, isolated from bovine colostrum or cheese whey, can be used as potential brain-activating factors and be incorporated into infant formula and the other functional foods.

It has been reported that the milk of grazing cows contains higher concentrations of sialic acid than that of nongrazing cows (Asakuma et al., 2010); the former would therefore be a more suitable source of sialyl glycoconjugates.

4. CONCLUDING REMARKS

It can be expected that, in the near future, the oligosaccharides separated from the milk/colostrum of cows and other domestic farm animals, and from cheese whey freed from lactose, can probably be used as antiinfection and/or immunomodulating agents in bio-functional foods, including infant formulas. In this connection, it is worth noting that Mehra et al. (2014) characterized the structures of oligosaccharides in the mother liquor prepared from cheese whey by membrane technology and lactose crystallization. Data on the chemical structures as well as the concentrations of milk oligosaccharides constitute basic information that is likely to have increasing importance in the food industry.

The growth of and safety for infants fed formula supplemented with a mixture of BMOs were recently evaluated by Meli et al. (2014). This mixture, which was generated from whey permeate, contains galacto-oligosaccharides and other oligosaccharides from bovine milk, such as 3′- and 6′-SL. Healthy term infants 14 days old or older were randomly assigned to receive standard formula (control, $n=84$), standard formula with BMOs (IF-BMO; $n=99$), or standard formula with BMOs and probiotics (*Bifidobacterium longum, Lactobacillus rhamnosus*) (IF-BMO+Pro; $n=98$). A breastfed reference group was also enrolled ($n=30$). The primary outcome was mean weight gain/day from enrollment to age 4 months (noninferiority margin: −3.0 g/day). Mean differences in weight gain between the control and IF-BMO and IF-BMO+Pro group were <1 g/day, with 97.5% confidence intervals above −3.0 g/day, indicating noninferior weight gain in the BMO formula groups. Compared with control, infants in the BMO groups had more frequent ($p<.0001$) and softer ($p=.0003$) stools. Stool bifidobacteria and lactobacilli counts were higher with IF-BMO+Pro compared with control ($p<.05$), whereas *Clostridia* counts were lower ($p<.05$) in both BMO groups compared with the control. These data suggest that BMO-containing infant formulas of benefit to bottle-fed infants will be developed in the near future.

With the methodical development of chemical characterization using small scale samples, structural information on milk oligosaccharides of domestic farm animals has increasingly been accumulating, especially during the last 10 years. This progress enables us to discuss, in detail, evolutionary aspect of milk oligosaccharides among mammalian species (Urashima et al., 2001b, 2007a, 2012b, 2014b; Messer and Urashima, 2002). In addition, physiological studies on bovine milk/colostrum oligosaccharides as well as HMOs have recently increased (Urashima et al., 2011b, 2013a). It is to be hoped that not only basic studies in this area but also applied studies on oligosaccharides of milk/colostrum of domestic farm animals, or relevant artificial saccharides, will increasingly be used in the food and/or pharmaceutical industries.

REFERENCES

Albrecht, S., Lane, J.A., Marino, K., Al Busadah, K.A., Carrington, S.D., Hickey, R.M., Rudd, P.M., 2014. A comparative study of free oligosaccharides in the milk of domestic animals. British Journal of Nutrition 111, 1313–1328.

Aldredge, D.L., Geronimo, M.R., Hua, S., Nwosu, C.C., Lebrilla, C.B., Barile, D., 2013. Annotation and structural elucidation of bovine milk oligosaccharides and determination of novel fucosylated structures. Glycobiology 23, 664–676.

Alhaj, O.A., Taufik, E., Handa, Y., Fukuda, K., Saito, T., Urashima, T., 2013. Chemical characterization of oligosaccharides in commercially pasteurized dromedary camel (*Camelus dromedaries*) milk. International Dairy Journal 28, 70–75.

Amano, J., Messer, M., Kobata, A., 1985. Structures of the oligosaccharides isolated from milk of the platypus. Glycoconjugate Journal 2, 121–135.

Angeloni, S., Ridet, J.L., Kusy, N., Gao, H., Crevoisier, F., Guinchard, D., Kochhar, S., Sigrist, H., Sprenger, N., 2005. Glycoprofiling with micro-arrays of glycoconjugates and lectins. Glycobiology 15, 31–45.

Anraku, T., Fukuda, K., Saito, T., Messer, M., Urashima, T., 2012. Chemical characterization of acidic oligosaccharides in milk of the red kangaroo (*Macropus rufus*). Glycoconjugate Journal 29, 147–156.

Aparna, H.S., Salimath, P.V., 1995. Disialyl lactose from buffalo colostrum: isolation and characterization. Carbohydrate Research 268, 313–318.

Asakuma, S., Urashima, T., Akahori, M., Ohbayashi, H., Nakamura, T., Kimura, K., Watanabe, Y., Arai, I., Sanai, Y., 2008. Variation of major neutral oligosaccharides levels in human colostrum. European Journal of Clinical Nutrition 62, 488–494.

Asakuma, S., Ueda, Y., Akiyama, F., Uemura, Y., Miyagi, M., Nakamura, M., Murai, M., Urashima, T., 2010. Effect of grazing on the concentrations of total sialic acid and hexose in bovine milk. Journal of Dairy Science 93, 4850–4854.

Barra, W.C., Caputto, R., 1965. Isolation and identification of a lactose sulfate ester from rat mammary gland. Biochimica et Biophysica Acta 101, 367–369.

Bisana, S., Kumar, S., Rismiller, P., Nicol, S.C., Lefèvre, C., Nicholas, K.R., Sharp, J.A., 2013. Identification and functional characterization of a novel monotreme-specific antibacterial protein expressed during lactation. PLoS One 8 (1), e53686.

Bradbury, J.H., Collins, J.G., Jenkins, G.A., Trifonoff, E., Messer, M., 1983. ^{13}C-NMR study of the structures of two branched oligosaccharides from marsupial milk. Carbohydrate Research 122, 327–331.

Brinkman-van den Linden, E.C., Sjoberg, E.R., Raj Juneja, L., Crocker, P.R., Varki, N., Varki, A.J., 2000. Loss of N-glycolylneuraminic acid in human evolution, implication for sialic acid recognition by siglecs. Journal of Biological Chemistry 275, 8633–8640.

Bubb, W.A., Urashima, T., Kohso, K., Nakamura, T., Arai, I., Saito, T., 1999. Occurrence of an unusual lactose sulfate in dog milk. Carbohydrate Research 318, 123–128.

Chaturvedi, P., Warren, C.D., Altaya, M., Morro, A.L., Ruiz-Palacios, G., Pickerling, L.K., Newburg, D.S., 2001. Fucosylated human milk oligosaccharides vary between individuals and over the course of lactation. Glycobiology 11, 365–372.

Choi, H.U., Carubelli, R., 1968. Neuramin-lactose, neuramin-lactose sulfate, and lactose sulfate from rat mammary glands. Isolation, purification, and permethylation studies. Biochemistry 7, 4423–4430.

Collins, J.G., Bradbury, J.H., Trifonoff, E., Messer, M., 1981. Structures of four new oligosaccharides from marsupial milk, determined mainly by ^{13}C-NMR spectroscopy. Carbohydrate Research 92, 136–140.

Crisp, E.A., Messer, M., Cowan, P.E., 1989a. Intestinal lactase (β-galactosidase) and other disaccharidase activities of suckling and adult common brushtail possums, *Trichosurus valpercula* (Marsupialia: Phalangeridae). Reproduction, Fertility and Development 1, 315–324.

Crisp, E.A., Messer, M., Vandeberg, J.L., 1989b. Changes in milk carbohydrates during lactation in a didelphid marsupial, *Monodelphis domestica*. Physiology and Zoology 62, 1117–1125.

Cumar, F.A., Ferchmin, P.A., Caputto, R., 1965. Isolation and identification of a lactose phosphate ester from cow colostrum. Biochemical and Biophysical Research Communications 20, 60–62.

Difilippo, E., Willems, H.A.M., Vendrig, J.C., Fink-Gremmels, J., Gruppen, H., Schols, H.A., 2015. Comparison of milk oligosaccharides pattern in colostrum of different horse breeds. Journal of Agricultural and Food Chemistry 53, 4805–4814.

Duncan, P.I., Raymond, F., Fuerholz, A., Sprenger, N., 2009. Sialic acid utilisation and synthesis in the neonatal rat revisited. PLoS One 4 (12), e8241.

Fong, B., Ma, K., McJarrow, P., 2011. Quantification of bovine milk oligosaccharides using liquid chromatography-selected reaction monitoring-mass spectrometry. Journal of Agricultural and Food Chemistry 59, 9788–9795.

Fukuda, K., Yamamoto, Y., Ganrorig, K., Khuukhenbaatar, J., Senda, A., Saito, T., Urashima, T., 2010. Chemical characterization of the oligosaccharides in Bactrian camel (*Camelus bactrianus*) milk and colostrum. Journal of Dairy Science 93, 5572–5587.

Galili, U., 2005. The α-gal epitope and the anti-gal antibody in xenotransplantation and in cancer immunotherapy. Immunology and Cell Biology 83, 674–686.

Goto, K., Fukuda, K., Senda, A., Saito, T., Kimura, K., Glander, K.E., Hinde, K., Dittus, W., Milligan, L.A., Power, M.L., Oftedal, O.T., Urashima, T., 2010. Chemical characterization of oligosaccharides in the milk of six species of new and old world monkeys. Glycoconjugate Journal 27, 703–715.

Gronberg, G., Lipniunas, P., Lundgren, T., Lindh, F., Nilsson, B., 1992. Structural analysis of five new monosialylated oligosaccharides from human milk. Archives of Biochemistry and Biophysics 296, 597–610.

Hakkarainen, J., Toivanen, M., Leinonen, A., Frangsmyr, L., Stronberg, N., Lapinjoki, S., Nassif, X., Tikkanen-Kaukanen, C., 2005. Human and bovine milk oligosaccharides inhibit *Neisseria meningitidis* pili attachment *in vitro*. Journal of Nutrition 135, 2445–2448.

Hester, S.N., Chen, X., Li, M., Monaco, M.H., Comstock, S.S., Kuhlenschmidt, T.B., Kuhlenschmidt, M.S., Donovan, S.M., 2013. Human milk oligosaccharides inhibit rotavirus infectivity *in vitro* and in acutely infected piglets. British Journal of Nutrition 110, 1233–1242.

Jenkins, G.A., Bradbury, J.H., Messer, M., Trifonoff, E., 1984. Determination of the structures of fucosyl-lactose and difucosyl-lactose from the milk of monotremes, using ^{13}C-n.m.r. spectroscopy. Carbohydrate Research 126, 157–161.

Jenness, R.E., Regehr, E.A., Sloan, R.E., 1964. Comprehensive studies of milks. Ⅱ. Dialyzable carbohydrates. Comparative Biochemistry and Physiology 13, 339–352.

Jourdian, G.W., Shimizu, F., Roseman, S., 1961. Isolation of nucleotide – oligosaccharides containing sialic acid. Federation Proceedings 20, 161.

Kamerling, J.P., Dorland, L., van Halbeek, H., Vliegenthart, J.F.G., Messer, M., Schauer, R., 1982. Structural studies of 4-O-acetyl-α-N-acetylneuraminyl-(2,3)-lactose, the main oligosaccharide in echidna milk. Carbohydrate Research 100, 331–340.

Kinoshita, M., Ohta, H., Higaki, K., Kojima, Y., Urashima, T., Nakajima, K., Suzuki, M., Kovacs, K.M., Lydersen, C., Hayakawa, T., Kakehi, K., 2009. Structural characterization of multi-branched oligosaccharides from seal milk by combination of off-line HPLC-MALDI-TOF MS and sequential exoglycosidase digestion. Analytical Biochemistry 388, 242–253.

Kobata, A., 1963. The acid soluble nucleotides of milk. Ⅱ. Isolation and identification of two novel uridine nucleotides of oligosaccharide conjugates from human milk and colostrum. Journal of Biochemistry Tokyo 53, 167–175.

Kobata, A., 1966. The acid soluble nucleotides of milk. Ⅳ. The chemical structure of UDP-X3. Journal of Biochemistry Tokyo 59, 63–66.

Kobata, A., 2010. Structures and application of oligosaccharides in human milk. Proceedings of Japan Academy, Series B, Physical and Biological Sciences 86, 1–17.

Kuhn, N.J., 1972. The lactose and neuraminyllactose content of rat milk and mammary tissue. Biochemical Journal 130, 177–180.

Kuhn, R., Gauhe, A., 1965. Bestimmung der Bindungsstelle von Sialinsäureresten in Oligosaccharides mit Hilfe von Perjodat. Chemische Berichte 98, 395–413.

Lane, J.A., Marino, K., Rudd, P.M., Carrington, S.D., Slattery, H., Hickey, R.M., 2012a. Methodologies for screening of bacteria-carbohydrate interactions: anti-adhesive milk oligosaccharides as a case study. Journal of Microbiological Methods 90, 53–59.

Lane, J.A., Marino, K., Naughton, J., Kavanaugh, D., Clyne, M., Carrington, S.D., Hickey, R.M., 2012b. Anti-infective bovine colostrum oligosaccharides: *Campylobacter jejuni* as a case study. International Journal of Food Microbiology 157, 182–188.

Lane, J.A., O'Callaghan, J., Carrington, S.T., Hickey, R.M., 2013. Transcriptional response of HT-29 intestinal epithelial cells in human and bovine milk oligosaccharides. British Journal of Nutrition 110, 2127–2137.

Liu, Z., Moate, P., Cocks, B., Rochfort, S., 2014. A simple LC-MS method for quantification of major free oligosaccharides in bovine milk. Journal of Agricultural and Food Chemistry 62, 11568–11574.

Luo, Z.X., Yuan, C.X., Meng, Q.J., Ji, Q., 2011. A Jurassic eutherian mammal and divergence of marsupials and placentals.. Nature 476, 442–455.

Marino, K., Lane, J.A., Abrahams, J.L., Struwe, W.B., Harvey, D.J., Marotta, M., Hickey, R.M., Rudd, P.M., 2011. Method for milk oligosaccharide profiling by 2-aminobenzamide labeling and hydrophilic interaction chromatography. Glycobiology 21, 1317–1330.

Martin, M.J., Martin-Sosa, S., Hueso, P., 2002. Binding of milk oligosaccharides by several enterotoxigenic *Escherichia coli* strains isolated from calves. Glycoconjugate Journal 19, 5–11.

Martin-Sosa, S., Martin, M.J., Garcia-Pardo, L.A., Hueso, P., 2003. Sialyloligosaccharides in human and bovine milk and in infant formulas: variations with the progression of lactation. Journal of Dairy Science 86, 52–59.

McJarrow, P., van Amelsfort-Schoonbeek, J., 2004. Bovine sialyl oligosaccharides: seasonal variations in their concentrations in milk, and a comparison of the colostrum of Jersey and Fiesian cows. International Dairy Journal 14, 571–579.

McKenzie, H.A., White Jr., F.H., 1991. Lysozyme and α-lactalbumin, structure, function, and interrelationships. Advances in Protein Chemistry 41, 174–315.

Mehra, R., Barille, D., Marotta, M., Lebrilla, C.B., Chu, C., German, J.B., 2014. Novel high-molecular weight fucosylated milk oligosaccharides identified in dairy streams. PLoS One 9, e96040.

Meli, F., Puccio, G., Cajozzo, C., Ricottone, G.L., Pecquet, S., Sprenger, N., Steenhout, P., 2014. Growth and safety evaluation of infant formulae containing oligosaccharides derived from bovine milk: a randomized, double-blind, noninferiority trial. BMC Pediatrics 14, 306–316.

Messer, M., Kerry, K.R., 1973. Milk carbohydrates of the echidna and the platypus. Science 180, 201–203.

Messer, M., 1974. Identification of N-acetyl-4-O-acetylneuraminyl-lactose in echidna milk. Biochemical Journal 139, 415–420.

Messer, M., Mossop, G.S., 1977. Milk carbohydrates of marsupials. 1. Partial separation and characterization of neutral milk oligosaccharides of the eastern grey kangaroo. Australian Journal of Biological Science 30, 379–388.

Messer, M., Trifonoff, E., Stern, W., Collins, J.G., Bradbury, J.H., 1980. Structure of a marsupial milk trisaccharide. Carbohydrate Research 83, 327–334.

Messer, M., Trifonoff, E., Collins, J.G., Bradbury, J.H., 1982. Structure of a branched tetrasaccharide from marsupial milk. Carbohydrate Research 102, 316–320.

Messer, M., FitzGerald, P.A., Merchant, J.C., Green, B., 1987. Changes in milk carbohydrates during lactation in the eastern quoll, *Dasyurus viverrinus* (Marsupialia). Comparative Biochemistry and Physiology 88B, 1083–1086.

Messer, M., Crisp, E.A., Czolij, R., 1989. Lactose digestion in suckling macropods. In: Grigg, G., Jarman, P., Hume, I. (Eds.), Kangaroos, Wallabies and Rat Kangaroos. Surry Beaty & Sons Pty Ltd., Australia, pp. 217–221.

Messer, M., Nicholas, K.R., 1991. Biosynthesis of marsupial milk oligosaccharides: characterization and developmental changes of two galactosyltransferases in lactating mammary glands of the tammar wallaby, *Macropus eugenii*. Biochimica et Biophysica Acta 1077, 79–85.

Messer, M., Griffiths, M., Rismiller, P.D., Shaw, B.C., 1997. Lactose synthesis in a monotremes, the echidnas (*Tachyglossus aculeatus*): isolation and amino acid sequence of echidna α-lactalbumin. Comparative Biochemistry and Physiology B118, 403–410.

Messer, M., Urashima, T., 2002. Evolution of milk oligosaccharides and lactose. Trends in Glycoscience and Glycotechnology 14, 153–176.

Munks, S.A., Green, B., Newgrain, K., Messer, M., 1991. Milk composition in the common ringtail possum, *Pseudocheirus peregrinus* (Petauridae: Marsupialia). Australian Journal of Zoology 39, 403–416.

Naccrato, W.F., Ray, R.E., Wells, W.W., 1975. Characterization and tissue distribution of 6-O-β-D-galactopyranosyl myo-inositol in the rat. Journal of Biological Chemistry 250, 1872–1876.

Nakamura, T., Urashima, T., Nakagawa, M., Saito, T., 1998. Sialyllactose occurs as free lactones in ovine colostrum. Biochimica et Biophysica Acta 1381, 286–292.

Nakamura, T., Amikawa, S., Harada, T., Saito, T., Arai, I., Urashima, T., 2001. Occurrence of an unusual phosphorylated N-acetyllactosamine in horse colostrum. Biochimica et Biophysica Acta 1525, 13–18.

Nakamura, T., Kawase, H., Kimura, K., Watanabe, Y., Ohtani, M., Arai, I., Urashima, T., 2003a. Concentrations of sialyloligosaccharides in bovine colostrum and milk during the prepartum and early lactation. Journal of Dairy Science 86, 1315–1320.

Nakamura, T., Urashima, T., Mizukami, T., Fukushima, M., Arai, I., Senshu, T., Imazu, K., Nakao, T., Saito, T., Ye, Z., Zuo, H., Wu, K., 2003b. Composition and oligosaccharides of a milk sample of the giant panda, *Ailuropoda melanoleuca*. Comparative Biochemistry and Physiology B135, 439–448.

Newburg, D.S., Naubauer, S.H., 1995. Carbohydrates in milks: analysis, quantities and significance. In: Jensen, R.G. (Ed.), Handbook of Milk Composition. Academic Press, San Diego, pp. 273–349.

Ninonuevo, M.R., Park, Y., Yin, H., Zhang, J., Ward, R.E., Clowers, B.H., German, J.B., Freeman, S.L., Killeen, K., Grimm, R., Lebrilla, C.B., 2006. A strategy for annotating the human milk glycome. Journal of Agricultural and Food Chemistry 54, 7471–7480.

Oftedal, O.T., 2002a. The mammary gland and its origin during synapsid evolution. Journal of Mammary Gland Biology and Neoplasia 7, 225–252.

Oftedal, O.T., 2002b. The origin of lactation as a water source for parchment-shelled eggs. Journal of Mammary Gland Biology and Neoplasia 7, 253–266.

Oftedal, O.T., 2011. Milk of marine mammals. In: Fuquay, J.W., Fox, P.F., McSweeney, P.H.L. (Eds.), Encyclopedia of Dairy Science, vol. 3. second ed. Academic Press, San Diego, pp. 563–580.

Oftedal, O.T., 2012. The evolution of milk secretion and its ancient origins. Animal 6, 355–368.

Oftedal, O.T., 2013. Origin and evolution of the major constituents of milk. In: McSweeney, P.H.L., Fox, P.F. (Eds.), Advanced Dairy Chemistry, vol. 1A. fourth ed. Springer Science + Buisiness Media, New York, pp. 1–42.

Oftedal, O.T., Dhouailly, D., 2013. Evo-Devo of the mammary gland. Journal of Mammary Gland Biology and Neoplasia 18 (2), 105–120.

Oftedal, O.T., Nicol, S.C., Davies, N.W., Sekii, N., Taifik, E., Fukuda, K., Saito, T., Urashima, T., 2014. Can an ancestral condition for milk oligosaccharides be determined? Evidence from the Tasmanian echidna (*Tachyglossus aculeatus setosus*). Glycobiology 24, 826–839.

Osthoff, G., Dickens, L., Urashima, T., Bonnet, S.L., Uemura, Y., van der Westhuizen, J.H., 2008. Structural characterization of oligosaccharides in the milk of an African elephant (*Loxodonta africana africana*). Comparative Biochemistry and Physiology B150, 74–84.

Parkkinen, J., Finne, J., 1987. Isolation of sialyl oligosaccharides and sialyl oligosaccharides phosphates from bovine colostrum and human urine. Methods in Enzymology 138, 289–300.

Prager, E.M., Wilson, A.C., 1988. Ancient origin of lactalbumin from lysozyme: analysis of DNA and amino acid sequence. Journal of Molecular Evolution 27, 326–335.

Rostami, S.M., Benet, T., Spears, J., Reynolds, A., Satyaraj, E., Sprenger, N., Austin, S., 2014. Milk oligosaccharides over time of lactation from different dog breeds. PLoS One 9, e99824.

Sabharwal, H., Sjoblad, S., Lundblad, A., 1991. Affinity chromatographic identification and quantitation of blood group A-active oligosaccharides in human milk and feces of breast-fed infants. Journal of Pediatric Gastroenterology and Nutrition 12, 474–479.

Saito, T., Itoh, T., Adachi, S., 1984. Presence of two neutral disaccharides containing N-acetylhexosamine in bovine colostrum as free forms. Biochimica et Biophysica Acta 801, 147–150.

Saito, T., Itoh, T., Adachi, S., 1987. Chemical structures of three neutral trisaccharides isolated in free forms from bovine colostrum. Carbohydrate Research 165, 43–51.

Sakai, F., Ikeuchi, F., Urashima, T., Fujiwara, M., Ohtsuki, K., Yanahira, S., 2006. Effects of feeding sialyllactose and galactosylated N-acetylneuraminic acid on swimming learning ability and brain lipid composition in adult rats. Journal of Applied Glycoscience 53, 249–254.

Sasaki, M., Nakamura, T., Hirayama, K., Fukuda, K., Saito, T., Urashima, T., Asakuma, S., 2016. Characterization of two novel sialyl N-acetyllactosaminyl nucleotides separated from ovine colostrum. Glycoconjugate Journal. http://dx.doi.org/10.1007/s10719-016-9672-4.

Schauer, R., Srinivasan, G.V., Wipfler, D., Kniep, B., Schwartz-Albiezet, R., 2011. O-acetylated sialic acids and their role in immune defense. Advances in Experimental Medicine and Biology 705, 525–548.

Schneier, M.L., Rafelson, M.E., 1966. Isolation of two structural isomers of N-acetylneuraminyllactose from bovine colostrum. Biochimica et Biophysica Acta 130, 1–11.

Senda, A., Hatakeyama, E., Kobayashi, R., Fukuda, K., Uemura, Y., Saito, T., Packer, C., Oftedal, O.T., Urashima, T., 2010. Chemical characterization of milk oligosaccharides of an African lion (*Panthera leo*) and a clouded leopard (*Neofelis nebulosa*). Animal Science Journal 81, 687–693.

Senda, A., Kobayashi, R., Fukuda, K., Saito, T., Hood, W.R., Kunz, T.H., Oftedal, O.T., Urashima, T., 2011. Chemical characterization of milk oligosaccharides of the island flying fox (*Pteropus hypomelanus*) (Chiroptera: Pteropodidae). Animal Science Journal 82, 782–786.

Shaper, N.L., Charron, M., Lo, N.W., Shaper, J.H., 1998. β-1,4-Galactosyltransferase and lactose biosynthesis: recruitment of a housekeeping gene from the nonvertebrate gene pool for a mammary gland specific function. Journal of Mammary Gland Bioloy and Neoplasia 3, 315–324.

Shaw, D.C., Messer, M., Scrivener, A.M., Nicholas, K.R., Griffiths, M., 1993. Isolation, partial characterization, and amino acid sequence of α-lactalbumin from platypus (*Ornithorhynchus anatinus*) milk. Biochimica et Biophysica Acta 1161, 177–186.

Stewart, I.M., Messer, M., Scrivener, A.M., Nicholas, K.R., Griffiths, M., 1983. Intestinal glycosidase activities in one adult and two suckling echidnas: absence of a neutral lactase (β-D-galactosidase). Australian Journal of Biological Science 36, 139–146.

Sturman, J.A., Lin, Y.Y., Higuchi, T., Fellman, J.H., 1985. N-Acetylneuramin lactose sulfate: a newly identified nutrient in milk. Pediatric Research 19, 216–219.

Tao, N., Wu, S., Kim, J., An, H.J., Hinde, K., Power, M.L., Gagneux, P., German, B.J., Lebrilla, C.B., 2011. Evolutionary glycomics: characterization of milk oligosaccharides in primates. Journal of Proteome Research 10, 1548–1557.

Taufik, E., Fukuda, K., Senda, A., Saito, T., Williams, C., Tilden, C., Eisert, R., Oftedal, O.T., Urashima, T., 2012. Structural characterization of neutral and acidic oligosaccharides in the milks of strepsirrhine primates: greater galago, aye-aye, Coquerrel's sifaka and mongoose lemur. Glycoconjugate Journal 29, 119–134.

Taufik, E., Sekii, N., Senda, A., Fukuda, K., Saito, T., Eisert, R., Oftedal, O.T., Urashima, T., 2013. Neutral and acidic milk oligosaccharides of the striped skunk (Mephitidae: *Mephitis mephitis*). Animal Science Journal 84, 569–578.

Taufik, E., Ganzorig, K., Nansalmaa, M., Fukuda, R., Fukuda, K., Saito, T., Urashima, T., 2014. Chemical characterization of saccharides in the milk of a reindeer (*Rangifer tarandus tarandus*). International Dairy Journal 34, 104–108.

Terabayashi, T., Morita, M., Ueno, M., Nakamura, T., Urashima, T., 2006. Inhibition of influenza-virus-induced cytopathy by sialylconjugates. Carbohydrate Research 341, 2246–2253.

Thurl, S., Munzert, M., Henker, J., Bohem, G., Muller-Werner, B., Jelinek, J., Stahl, B., 2010. Variation of human milk oligosaccharides in relation to milk groups and lactation periods. British Journal of Nutrition 104, 1261–1271.

Uemura, Y., Asakuma, S., Nakamura, T., Arai, I., Taki, M., Urashima, T., 2005. Occurrence of a unique sialyl tetrasaccharide in colostrum of a bottlenose dolphin (*Tursiops truncatus*). Biochimica et Biophysica Acta 1725, 290–297.

Uemura, Y., Asakuma, S., Yon, L., Saito, T., Fukuda, K., Arai, I., Urashima, T., 2006. Structural determination of the oligosaccharides in the milk of an Asian elephant (*Elephas maximus*). Comparative Biochemistry and Physiology A145, 468–478.

Uemura, Y., Takahashi, S., Senda, A., Fukuda, K., Saito, T., Oftedal, O.T., Urashima, T., 2009. Chemical characterization of milk oligosaccharides of a spotted hyena (*crocuta crocuta*). Comparative Biochemistry and Physiology A152, 158–161.

Urashima, T., Saito, T., Nishimura, J., Ariga, H., 1989a. New galactosyllactose containing α-glycosidic linkage isolated from ovine (*Booroola dorset*) colostrum. Biochimica et Biophysica Acta 992, 375–378.

Urashima, T., Sakamoto, T., Ariga, H., Saito, T., 1989b. Structure determination of three neutral oligosaccharides obtained from horse colostrum. Carbohydrate Research 194, 280–287.

Urashima, T., Saito, T., Kimura, T., 1991a. Chemical structures of three neutral oligosaccharides obtained from horse (Thoroughbred) colostrum. Comparative Biochemistry and Physiology B100, 177–183.

Urashima, T., Saito, T., Ohmisya, K., Shimazaki, K., 1991b. Structural determination of three neutral oligosaccharides in bovine (Holstein-Friesian) colostrum, including the novel trisaccharide; GalNAcα1-3Galβ1-4Glc. Biochimica et Biophysica Acta 1073, 225–229.

Urashima, T., Messer, M., Bubb, W.A., 1992. Biosynthesis of marsupial milk oligosaccharides II: characterization of a β6-N-acetylglucosaminyltransferase in lactating mammary glands of the tammar wallaby, *Macropus eugenii*. Biochimica et Biophysica Acta 1117, 223–231.

Urashima, T., Bubb, W.A., Messer, M., Tsuji, Y., Taneda, Y., 1994a. Studies of the neutral trisaccharides of goat (*Capra hircus*) colostrum and of the one- and two-dimensional ^{1}H and ^{13}C NMR spectra of 6′-*N*-acetylglucosaminyllactose. Carbohydrate Research 262, 173–184.

Urashima, T., Saito, T., Tsuji, Y., Taneda, Y., Takasawa, T., Messer, M., 1994b. Chemical characterization of sialyl oligosaccharides isolated from tammar wallaby (*Macropus eugenii*) milk. Biochimica et Biophysica Acta 1200, 64–72.

Urashima, T., Hiramatsu, Y., Murata, S., Nakamura, T., Messer, M., 1997a. Identification of 2′-fucosyllactose in milk of the crabeater seal (*Lobodon carcinophagus*). Comparative Biochemistry and Physiology B116, 311–314.

Urashima, T., Kusaka, Y., Nakamura, T., Saito, T., Maeda, N., Messer, M., 1997b. Chemical characterization of milk oligosaccharides of the brown bear, *Ursus arctos yesoensis*. Biochimica et Biophysica Acta 1334, 247–255.

Urashima, T., Murata, S., Nakamura, T., 1997c. Structural determination of monosialyl trisaccharides obtained from caprine colostrum. Comparative Biochemistry and Physiology B116, 431–435.

Urashima, T., Kawai, Y., Nakamura, T., Arai, I., Saito, T., Namiki, M., Yamaoka, K., Kawahara, K., Messer, M., 1999a. Chemical characterisation of six oligosaccharides in a sample of colostrum of the brown capuchin, *Cebus apella* (Cebidae: Primate). Comparative Biochemistry and Physiology C124, 295–300.

Urashima, T., Sumiyoshi, W., Nakamura, T., Arai, I., Saito, T., Komatsu, T., Tsubota, T., 1999b. Chemical characterization of milk oligosaccharides of the Japanese black bear, *Ursus thibetanus japonicus*. Biochimica et Biophysica Acta 1472, 290–306.

Urashima, T., Yamamoto, M., Nakamura, T., Arai, I., Saito, T., Namiki, M., Yamaoka, K., Kawahara, K., 1999c. Chemical characterisation of the oligosaccharides in a sample of milk of a white-nosed coati, *Nasua narica* (Procyonidae: Carnivora). Comparative Biochemistry and Physiology A123, 187–193.

Urashima, T., Yamashita, T., Nakamura, T., Arai, I., Saito, T., Derocher, A.E., Wiig, O., 2000. Chemical characterization of milk oligosaccharides of the polar bear, *Ursus maritimus*. Biochimica et Biophysica Acta 1475, 395–408.

Urashima, T., Arita, M., Yoshida, M., Nakamura, T., Arai, I., Saito, T., Arnould, J.P.Y., Kovacs, K.M., Lydersen, C., 2001a. Chemical characterization of the oligosaccharides in hooded seal (*Cystophora cristata*) and Australian fur seal (*Arctocephalus pusillus doriferus*) milk. Comparative Biochemistry and Physiology B128, 307–323.

Urashima, T., Saito, T., Nakamura, T., Messer, M., 2001b. Oligosaccharides of milk and colostrum in non-human mammals. Glycoconjugate Journal 18, 357–371.

Urashima, T., Sato, H., Munakata, J., Nakamura, T., Arai, I., Saito, T., Tetsuka, M., Fukui, Y., Ishikawa, H., Lydersen, C., Kovacs, K.M., 2002. Chemical characterization of the oligosaccharides in beluga (*Delphinapterus leucas*) and minke whale (*Balaenoptera acutorostrata*) milk. Comparative Biochemistry and Physiology B132, 611–624.

Urashima, T., Nagata, H., Nakamura, T., Arai, I., Saito, T., Imazu, K., Hayashi, T., Derocher, A.E., Wiig, O., 2003a. Differences in oligosaccharides pattern of a sample of polar bear colostrum and mid-lactation milk. Comparative Biochemistry and Physiology B136, 887–896.

Urashima, T., Nakamura, T., Yamaguchi, K., Munakata, J., Arai, I., Saito, T., Lydersen, C., Kovacs, K.M., 2003b. Chemical characterization of the oligosaccharides in milk of high Arctic harbour seal (*Phoca vitulina vitulina*). Comparative Biochemistry and Physiology A135, 549–563.

Urashima, T., Nakamura, T., Nakagawa, D., Noda, M., Arai, I., Saito, T., Lydersen, C., Kovacs, K.M., 2004a. Characterization of oligosaccharides in a milk of bearded seal (*Erignathus barbatus*). Comparative Biochemistry and Physiology B138, 1–18.

Urashima, T., Nakamura, T., Teramoto, K., Arai, I., Saito, T., Komatsu, T., Tsubota, T., 2004b. Chemical characterization of sialyl oligosaccharides in milk of the Japanese black bear, *Ursus thibetanus japonicus*. Comparative Biochemistry and Physiology B139, 587–595.

Urashima, T., Nakamura, T., Ikeda, A., Asakuma, S., Arai, I., Saito, T., Oftedal, O.T., 2005. Characterization of oligosaccharides in milk of a mink, *Mustela vison*. Comparative Biochemistry and Physiology A142, 461–471.

Urashima, T., Asakuma, S., Messer, M., 2007a. Milk oligosaccharides. In: Kamerling, J.P.Y. (Ed.), Comprehensive Glycoscience. Elsevier, Amsterdam, pp. 695–724.

Urashima, T., Kobayashi, M., Asakuma, S., Uremura, Y., Arai, I., Fukuda, K., Saito, T., Mogoe, T., Ishikawa, H., Fukui, Y., 2007b. Chemical characterization of the oligosaccharides in Bryde's whale (*Balaenoptera edeni*) and Sei whale (*Balaenoptera borealis lesson*) milk. Comparative Biochemistry and Physiology B146, 153–159.

Urashima, T., Komoda, M., Asakuma, S., Uemura, Y., Fukuda, K., Saito, T., Oftedal, O.T., 2008. Structural determination of the oligosaccharides in the milk of a giant anteater (*Myrmecophaga tridatyla*). Animal Science Journal 79, 699–709.

Urashima, T., Kitaoka, M., Asakuma, S., Messer, M., 2009a. Milk oligosaccharides. In: McSweeney, P.H.L., Fox, P.F. (Eds.), Advanced Dairy Chemistry, Lactose, Water, Salts and Minor Constituents, vol. 3. third ed. Springer Science + Business Media, New York, pp. 295–349.

Urashima, T., Odaka, G., Asakuma, S., Uemura, Y., Goto, K., Senda, A., Saito, T., Fukuda, K., Messer, M., Oftedal, O.T., 2009b. Chemical characterization of oligosaccharides in chimpanzee, bonobo, gorilla, orangutan, and siamang milk or colostrum. Glycobiology 19, 499–508.

Urashima, T., Asakuma, S., Kitaoka, M., Messer, M., 2011a. Indigenous oligosaccharides in milk. In: Fuquay, J.W., Fox, P.F., McSweeney, P.L.H. (Eds.), Encyclopedia of Dairy Science, Vol. 3. second ed. Academic Press, San Diego, pp. 241–273.

Urashima, T., Kitaoka, M., Terabayashi, T., Fukuda, K., Ohnishi, M., Kobata, A., 2011b. Milk oligosaccharides. In: Gorden, N.S. (Ed.), Oligosaccharides: Sources, Properties and Applications. Nova Science Publishers Inc., New York, pp. 1–58.

Urashima, T., Asakuma, S., Leo, F., Fukuda, K., Messer, M., Oftedal, O.T., 2012a. The predominance of type I oligosaccharides is a feature specific to human breast milk. Advances in Nutrition 3, 473S–482S.

Urashima, T., Fukuda, K., Messer, M., 2012b. Evolution of milk oligosaccharides and lactose: a hypothesis. Animal 6, 369–374.

Urashima, T., Taufik, E., Fukuda, K., Asakuma, S., 2013a. Recent advances in studies on milk oligosaccharides of cows and other domestic farm animals. Bioscience, Biotechnology and Biochemistry 77, 455–466.

Urashima, T., Taufik, E., Fukuda, R., Nakamura, T., Fukuda, K., Saito, T., Messer, M., 2013b. Chemical characterization of milk oligosaccharides of the koala (*Phascolarctos cinereus*). Glycoconjugate Journal 30, 801–811.

Urashima, T., Fujita, S., Fukuda, K., Nakamura, T., Saito, T., Cowan, P., Messer, M., 2014a. Chemical characterization of milk oligosaccharides of the common brushtail possum (*Trichosurus vulpecula*). Glycoconjugate Journal 31, 387–399.

Urashima, T., Messer, M., Oftedal, O.T., 2014b. Comparative biochemistry and evolution of milk oligosaccharides of monotremes, marsupials, and eutherians. In: Pontarotti, P. (Ed.), Evolutionary Biology: Genome Evolution, Speciation, Coevolution and Origin of Life. Springer, Switzerland, pp. 1–33.

Urashima, T., Inamori, H., Fukuda, K., Saito, T., Messer, M., Oftedal, O.T., 2015a. 4-O-acetyl-sialic acid (Neu4,5Ac_2) in acidic milk oligosaccharides of the platypus (*Ornithorhynchus anatinus*) and its evolutionary significance. Glycobiology 25, 683–697.

Urashima, T., Sun, Y., Fukuda, K., Hirayama, K., Taufik, E., Nakamura, T., Saito, T., Merchant, J., Green, B., Messer, M., 2015b. Chemical characterization of milk oligosaccharides of the eastern quoll (*Dasyurus viverrinus*). Glycoconjugate Journal 32, 361–370.

Veh, R.W., Michalski, J.C., Corfield, A.P., Sander-Wewer, M., Gies, D., Schauer, R., 1981. New chromatographic system and the rapid analysis and preparation of colostrum and sialyloligosaccharides. Journal of Chromatography 212, 313–322.

Viverge, D., Grimmonprez, I., Solere, M., 1997. Chemical characterization of sialyl oligosaccharides isolated from goat (*Capra hircus*) milk. Biochimica et Biophysica Acta 1336, 157–164.

Wang, B., McVeagh, P., Petocz, P., Brand-Miller, J., 2003. Brain ganglioside and glycoprotein sialic acid in breastfed compared with formula-fed infants. American Journal of Clinical Nutrition 78, 1024–1029.

Wang, B., Yu, B., Karim, M., Hu, H., Sun, Y., McGreevy, P., Petocz, P., Held, S., Brand-Miller, J., 2007. Dietary sialic acid supplementation improves learning and memory in piglets. American Journal of Clinical Nutrition 85, 561–569.

Watanabe, Y., Kimura, K., Matsumotom, K., Miyagi, A., 2006. Concentrations and compositions of the bovine milk oligosaccharides. In: Proceeding of the 23th International Carbohydrate Symposium. Wistler, Canada, p. 78.

CHAPTER

Analytical Methods to Characterize Human Milk Oligosaccharides

4

David F. Smith[1], Richard D. Cummings[2]

[1]*Emory University School of Medicine, Atlanta, GA, United States;* [2]*Harvard Medical School, Boston, MA, United States*

1. INTRODUCTION

Human milk oligosaccharides or glycans (HMOs or HMGs) represent a unique subset or metaglycome of the human glycome. This human milk metaglycome is composed of the free (reducing) glycans that are present at 10–20 g per liter of milk, contain lactose as their precursor, and are considered nonnutrient components since they are not readily degraded by the acid conditions of the stomach or by glycosidases in the intestine (Gnoth et al., 2000; Engfer et al., 2000). These glycans, which represent a convenient source of relatively abundant and biologically relevant glycans from humans, have been the subject of intense investigation since the early 20th century. The prebiotic effect of human milk was first suggested by the observation that a fraction of human milk contained a factor that stimulated growth of *Lactobacillus bifidus*, a major intestinal bacterium of breastfed infants (Schönfeld, 1926). The "bifidus factor" was later associated with a nitrogen-containing oligosaccharide isolated from human milk that was termed "gynolactose" (Polonovski and Lespagnol, 1933). As methods for separation and isolation of oligosaccharides improved, this oligosaccharide was found to actually be a mixture of many glycans containing fucose, as well as *N*-acetylhexosamine (Polonovski and Lespagnol, 1954). Two major carbohydrate chemistry groups in Europe headed by Montreuil in France and Kuhn in Germany focused on the identification of bifidus factor and were responsible for isolating and defining the structures of many HMOs. By 1965, the complete structures of 14 neutral and sialylated glycans had been reported, as reviewed by Kobata (2010).

An early finding that also led to interest in HMOs was the discovery of the inhibitory effects of sialic acid–containing milk glycans on influenza virus infectivity and replication (Kuhn and Brossmer, 1956). This represented very early evidence for the potential role of milk glycans as decoy receptors for pathogens. Since the initial step in many bacterial, viral, and parasitic infections involves attachment of the organism to glycans on the surface of epithelial cells (the glycocalyx), it is reasonable to predict that the glycans of human milk might have structures similar to the glycans of cell surface glycoconjugates, such that HMOs could mimic the glycan receptor to inhibit the

Prebiotics and Probiotics in Human Milk. http://dx.doi.org/10.1016/B978-0-12-802725-7.00004-X

first step in infection (Zopf and Roth, 1996). In addition to influenza virus, rotavirus (RV) and norovirus (Jiang et al., 2004) are thought to infect via initial protein–glycan interactions. Examples of bacterial infections that use adhesins and host cell receptors are *Streptococcus pneumoniae* (Andersson et al., 1986), *Listeria monocytogenes* (Coppa et al., 2003), *Campylobactor jejuni* (Ruiz-Palacios et al., 2003), and enteropathogenic *Escherichia coli* (Manthey et al., 2014); a number of antiadhesin mechanisms have been reviewed (Shoaf-Sweeney and Hutkins, 2009). More recently, HMOs were shown to reduce in vitro attachment and cytotoxicity of *Entamoeba histolytica* (Jantscher-Krenn et al., 2012). While the potential involvement of HMOs as prebiotic agents and decoy receptors stimulated much of the structural analyses of HMOs during the mid and late 20th century, the field of glycobiology is currently receiving increased attention by the biomedical community in recognition of the key roles of glycans and glycoconjugates in many physiological processes and diseases.

More recent investigations strongly suggest that HMOs are much more bioactive than had originally been considered. Accumulating evidence indicates that HMOs provide significant benefits to health of neonates through both their probiotic effects and potential ability to enhance cognitive development. It is clear now that from the large concentration of HMOs ingested by an infant that a small but significant amount of HMOs are absorbed and enter the circulation, where they may have systemic effects (Rudloff et al., 1996, 2006, 2012). Interestingly, cells may be directly affected by interactions with HMOs (ten Bruggencate et al., 2014; Ballard and Morrow, 2013; Hennet et al., 2014; Bode, 2012, 2015; Andreas et al., 2015; Hsieh et al., 2015). Examples of this include stimulation of peripheral blood mononuclear cells (PBMCs) with HMOs, which caused cells to produce interleukin (IL)-10 and reduced their proliferation, but proliferation was stimulated by sialylated HMOs when added with bacterial lipopolysaccharide (Comstock et al., 2014). In a mouse model, 3-sialyl-lactose directly stimulated dendritic cells and induced cytokine production, associated with a TLR4-dependent pathway (Kurakevich et al., 2013). Finally, recent evidence indicates that HMOs may strongly influence the intestinal microbiota in premature infants (Underwood et al., 2015).

2. FUNCTIONAL GLYCOMICS OF HUMAN MILK OLIGOSACCHARIDES

Thus, accumulating evidence suggests that HMOs are recognized by glycan-binding proteins, expressed by the infant cells as well as by microbes. A functional approach to glycomics and one that provides insight into glycan recognition is "shotgun glycomics," where libraries of glycans representing a specific metaglycome or selected glycome from a cell, tissue, or organ are isolated, derivatized, printed on a microarray, and interrogated for function based on their interactions with GBP (Song et al., 2011). This approach allows one to focus the technically difficult structural analyses on specific glycans after having identified their biological relevance.

To prepare an HMO shotgun glycan microarray, we separated HMGs into neutral and sialylated glycans and the free sugars were labeled with a bifunctional fluorescent tag by reductive amination, where the fluorescent tag also possesses a primary amino group that is available for coupling to covalently immobilize the glycans. The mixtures of tagged glycans are then subjected to multidimensional high-performance liquid chromatography (HPLC) with the final separation being a particularized graphitized carbon (PGC) column that is very efficient in resolving isomers of HMOs. The separated glycans that have a single mass by matrix-assisted laser desorption ionization (MALDI)–mass spectrometry (MS) are cataloged and archived in a tagged glycan library (TGL), where they are reserved for later retrieval. The TGL of HMOs obtained from a pool of 10 individual milk samples (100mL each) representing all Lewis blood groups was printed on a glycan microarray representing 247 glycans from milk and 12 standard known HMOs (Yu et al., 2014). This shotgun glycan microarray was interrogated with recombinant forms of the VP8* domains of RV outer capsid spike protein VP4 from human neonatal strains and a bovine strain of RV. Glycans bound by the RV attachment proteins were selected for detailed structural analyses by using the metadata-assisted glycan sequencing (MAGS) approach (Smith and Cummings, 2013; Yu et al., 2012), which incorporates metadata on each glycan including its binding or lack of binding by antibodies and lectins before and after exoglycosidase and endoglycosidase digestion of the SGM, coupled with independent multistage MS analyses (MS^n) of each glycan. This complementary structural approach resulted in the identification of 32 glycans recognized by the spike protein domain VP8* of RV, and over 20 of the glycans were previously undescribed HMOs (Ashline et al., 2014). Remarkably, VP8* generated from different rotavirus strains recognized a specific glycan determinant within a unique subset of related glycan structures, and the differences in specificity were a function of specific but subtle differences in glycan structures.

Overall, there is strong evidence that HMOs provide significant health benefits to the neonate or infant human (Bode, 2015; Hill and Newburg, 2015) and that human milk with this highly complex complement of glycans is a richer source of potentially beneficial constituents than cow's milk, the source used for alternative formula feeding. As investigators continue to focus on HMOs as bioactive agents a major challenge that remains is to identify the specific function(s) of individual milk glycans, and this challenge is directly related the difficulty in identifying their structure. As biotechnology in the area of large-scale synthesis of glycans matures, the manufacture of the glycan structures expressed in milk in quantities sufficient to provide supplement to formula will be possible, but identifying what structures are worthy of attention requires methods that identify function and analytical methods that completely identify structure.

3. COMPLEXITY OF GLYCAN STRUCTURES

The biomedical research community is recognizing the importance of glycobiology as the key roles of glycans and glycoconjugates are being defined in many physiological processes and diseases. While investigators in molecular and cell biology, who are involved in translational medicine, recognize this relationship; few laboratories have the capability to use both classic and modern biochemical and chemical approaches in the area of glycosciences to explore the structure and function relationships of glycans in general and HMOs in particular. Despite major advances in structural analysis of glycans in recent years, the relatively new field of glycomics still stands in stark contrast with the more rapid advances that have occurred in genomics and proteomics (Cummings and Pierce, 2014). This is due largely to the slow development of the technologies for automated sequencing and synthesis of glycans compared with the ever-advancing automation and miniaturization of the techniques for proteins and nucleic acids. New genomes of organisms are added to the literature every year, and the large databases of protein sequences and three-dimensional structures of proteins continue to grow rapidly. In addition, the ability to amplify nucleic acids by polymerase chain reaction technologies and to amplify proteins by recombinant technologies in a multitude of expression systems have contributed to major advances in our understanding the function of specific sequences of nucleotides and amino acids. The area of glycomics stands at the brink of major advances in new technologies, which will hopefully be facilitated by the National Institutes of Health's designation of glycomics as a subject receiving funding from Common Fund Resources for the first time beginning in 2014. In the remainder of this review, we will discuss the history and attempt to project the future of investigations of the structures of HMOs and how structures can be associated with function.

4. GLYCANS OF HUMAN MILK

By 1965, the complete structures of 14 neutral and sialylated glycans had been reported, and these are included among the list of the most abundant HMOs shown in Fig. 4.1. To date, it is estimated that more than 180 glycans have been defined (Kobata, 2010; Ninonuevo et al., 2006; Wu et al., 2010, 2011; Urashima et al., 2011), and significant discussion continues regarding the actual number of glycans structures that might be present in human milk. While the glycans comprising the metaglycome of the free glycans in human milk present features that create unique challenges in fully defining their structures, the glycans composing the complete human glycome present a much more formidable challenge. As a prelude for attacking the human glycome in general, we reasoned that it would be advantageous to first address a metaglycome, namely the HMO, with the idea that if we can successfully address this metaglycome, it will provide guidance for the future studies on the human glycome. We first considered some general features or what might be called "guiding rules" of HMO "core" structures, and we developed five such rules. Using this principle, we reasoned that we could estimate the total repertoire of potential glycans that might be present in the free glycan metaglycome of human milk.

Rule 1—All glycans are extended lactose structures with glucose (Glc) occurring only at the reducing end of HMOs, which are composed of only five monosaccharides (Glc, galactose (Gal), N-acetylglucosamine (GlcNAc), fucose (Fuc), and N-acetylneuraminic acid (Neu5Ac)) compared with 10 monosaccharides that

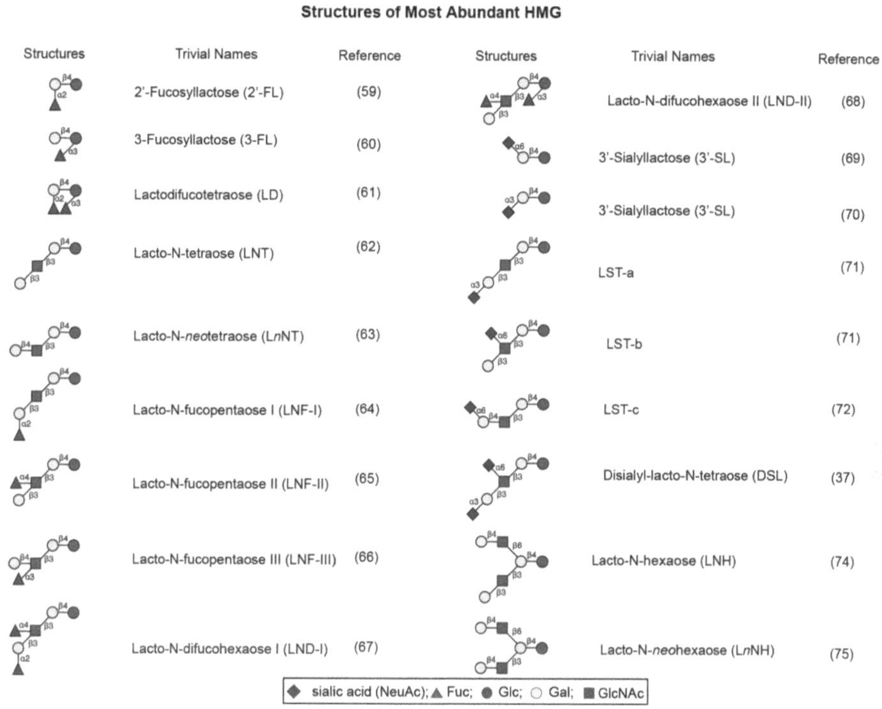

FIGURE 4.1

List of the most abundant HMOs.

compose the larger human glycome (the others being xylose, mannose, GalNAc, glucuronic acid, and iduronic acid).

Rule 2—Lactose is extended in disaccharide units of type 1 Galβ1-3GlcNAc or type 2 Galβ1-4GlcNAc sequences.

Rule 3—The only *N*-acetylhexosamine is GlcNAc is, and it does not occur as a terminal monosaccharide, because any new biosynthetic terminal GlcNAc residue is efficiently extended by one of two galactosyltransferases (either β1-3GalT or β1-4GalT) to add a β-linked Gal to either the 3 or 4 position of GlcNAc, respectively.

Rule 4—The enzyme responsible for adding GlcNAc to a lactosamine unit (Gal-GlcNAc-R) and promoting glycan extension acts only on the type 2 disaccharide acceptor, and will not extend the type 1 disaccharide acceptor (Sasaki et al., 1997; Renkonen, 2000; Mattila et al., 1998); thus, the type 1 disaccharide is a prominent terminal determinant in the HMO metaglycome (Urashima et al., 2012).

Rule 5—Glycan branching occurs only at the 6-hydroxyl on internal Gal residues within a linear sequence, and it does not occur on a terminal Gal. The enzyme responsible for this biosynthesis is presumably the developmentally regulated I-branching enzyme (Mattila et al., 1998; Bierhuizen et al., 1993). These five relatively well-defined rules are useful in completely describing what is known so far about the core structures of HMOs.

5. RULES OF HUMAN MILK GLYCAN STRUCTURE

From these guiding rules, a series of "core glycans" can be generated, which may be modified by additions of the other two monosaccharides Fuc and Neu5Ac. These additions are also governed by "rules."

Rule 6—Fuc or Neu5Ac always occurs in terminal positions.

Rule 7—Fucose addition is controlled by at least three fucosyltransferases (FuTs). A key FuT is the α(1,2)fucosyltransferase (FuT2), whose expression is genetically regulated by the "secretor" gene that is associated with the ability of an individual to produce H antigen in secretions such as saliva, mucins, and milk (Lowe, 1993). FuT2 transfers α-fucose to the 2 position of the terminal Gal only on type 1 sequences to generate H-type 1 glycans but not H-type 2 glycans (Sarnesto et al., 1992). The human secretor (*Se*) locus is on chromosome 19 at 19q13.3. Individuals known as "secretors" have an *Se/Se* or *Se/se* genotype and produce at least one copy of the *Se* gene that encodes a functional FuT2 (Kelly et al., 1995). Individuals with the genotype *se/se* ("nonsecretors") are unable to produce a soluble form of H antigen. Thus, human milk contains only traces of H-type 2 (Fucα1-2Galβ1-4GlcNAcβ1-3Galβ1-4Glc) but significant amounts of 2′-fucosyllactose (Fucα1-2Galβ1-4Glc), which is only present in milk of mothers who are secretors (Grollman and Ginsburg, 1967), indicating that FuT2 will use lactose at high concentrations as a substrate (Castanys-Munoz et al., 2013).

The so-called Lewis gene encodes an α(1,3/4)fucosyltransferase (FuT3) that is expressed by glands generating human milk and is genetically regulated by the Lewis (*Le*) locus on chromosome 19 (19q13.3) (Kukowska-Latallo et al., 1990). Fut3 expression allows an individual to generate the Lewis a antigen in secretions such as saliva, mucins, and milk. The Lewis b antigen can arise from the Lewis a precursor in individuals that also have an active Secretor gene (*Se/Se* or *Se/se*) and an active Lewis gene (*Le/Le or Le/le*) (Grollman et al., 1969). FuT3 is unique in its ability to transfer fucose from GDP-fucose to GlcNAc in both α1-3 and α1-4 linkages. This enzyme can, therefore, add fucose to either a type 1 glycan to form the Lewis a antigen or to a type 2 glycan to form the Lewis X antigen, which in concert with the H blood group α(1,2)fucosyltransferase (Larsen et al., 1990) (FuT1), can also generate the Lewis b and Lewis Y antigen, respectively. FuT3 is also responsible for transferring fucose to the 3 position of glucose, making 3-fucosyllactose and difucosyllactose dependent on the expression of this enzyme.

Since the H blood group FuT1 is not expressed or weakly expressed in cells generating human milk, there is little, if any, Lewis Y antigen present; however, relatively large amounts of the Lewis X antigen are found in human milk. This structure can obviously be synthesized by the action of Fut3, which can transfer a fucose to the GlcNAc of both type 1 and type 2 glycans.

Rule 8—The 3-fucosyl lactose can be extended as linear glycans, but based on the available known structures in HMGs, the branching enzyme will not act on lacto-*N-neo*-tetraose (LNnT) or lacto-*N*-tetraose (LNT) that possess the fucose on the 3 position of the reducing glucose. The first of the linear series of glycans with a fucose in this position are lacto-*N*-fucopentaose V and lacto-*N-neo*-fucopentaose V. It is assumed that linear glycans can have this fucose but that branched glycans will not. Of course, this guiding rule may be reconsidered in the future if branched structures with this fucose are discovered.

Since individuals with the genotype *le/le* also present significant amounts of Lewis X antigen in milk, there must be a ubiquitous α(1,3)-fucosyltransferase expressed in milk that can synthesize this structure. Analysis of the fucosyltransferase activities in human milk indicated that the α(1,3/4)fucosyltransferase activity (FuT3) could be physically separated from an α(1,3)-fucosyltransferase activity present in virtually all individuals (Johnson and Watkins, 1992) and that the α(1,3)-fucosyltransferase cannot transfer fucose to the 3 position of glucose (De Vries et al., 1997) making the presence of the 3-fucosylated glucose dependent on the expression of the Lewis fucosyltransferase [α(1,3/4)fucosyltransferase]. Thus, the α(1,3)-fucosyltransferase is distinct from the Lewis fucosyltransferase. The human gene that expresses the ubiquitous α(1,3)-fucosyltransferase (Fuc-T6) was cloned (Koszdin and Bowen, 1992; Weston et al., 1992), and the recombinant Fut6 gene product was expressed in insect cells and displayed acceptor activity identical to the ubiquitous human milk α(1,3)-fucosyltransferase (De Vries et al., 1997).

Although the amounts and distribution of sialylated glycans in milk of many species have been intensely investigated, studies on expression of the sialyltransferase genes in human milk are limited (Maksimovic et al., 2011).

Rule 9—Sialic acid addition to the soluble HMGs appears to be controlled by at least three sialyltransferases based largely on the sialic acid linkages that have been described:

Neu5Acα2-6Galβ1-4GlcNAc—This structure is presumably synthesized by the sialyltransferase that is the product of the ST6Gal I gene, which is known to be expressed in human lactating mammary gland (Maksimovic et al., 2011). This enzyme is apparently responsible for synthesis of the two major glycans in milk possessing this linkage: 6′-sialyllactose and LSTc. The α2,6 sialic acid linkage does not occur on type 1 free glycans in human milk, which is consistent with the specificity of the ST6Gal I sialyltransferase specificity for type 2 glycans (Paulson and Colley, 1989). The sialyltransferase that adds sialic acid in α2,3 linkage to type 2 glycans is apparently not expressed in human lactating mammary gland.

Neu5Acα2-3Galβ1-3GlcNAc—The Neu5Acα2-3Gal linkage occurs in human milk in several major glycan structures including 3′-sialyllactose and LSTa, but this sialic acid linkage does not occur on glycans with a terminating type 2 LacNAc (Galβ1-4GlcNAc). The gene responsible for the expression of the active α2,3-sialyltransferase in human milk has not been reported, but its specificity is very restricted for the type 1 glycan (Galβ1-3GlcNAc); however, 3′-sialylactose, which a major component of human milk soluble glycans, has a type 2–related acceptor (Galβ1-4Glc) acceptor. If this enzyme is responsible for the biosynthesis of 3′-sialylactose, its ability to use the type 2 lactose as an acceptor may be due to the high concentration of lactose available in milk or the "flexibility" of the reducing disaccharide as proposed for the addition of fucose to lactose by Fuc-T2 Fuc (Castanys-Munoz et al., 2013).

Galβ1-3(Neu5Acα2-6)GlcNAc—The Neu5Acα2-6GlcNAc is an internal structure found only on type 1 glycans and never on type 2 glycans or on the 6 position of glucose in lactose. Two major free milk glycans possessing this structure are LSTb and disialyl-lacto-*N*-tetraose (DSL). This unique α2,6-linkage has never been found in a lacto-*N*-*neo*-Tetraose (Galβ1-4GlcNAcβ1-3Galβ1-4Glc), and the gene responsible for the expression of this sialyltransferase has not been identified.

Thus, a set of rules, based on the specificity of the glycosyltransferases expressed in human milk and the defined structures documented in the literature, can be used to define all of the isomeric glycans that could possibly be synthesized by a lactating human. Because the enzymes involved transfer only four monosaccharides in different but specific linkages, the number of possible isomers is large, but not infinite, and as shown next, it is actually straightforward to then predict the structures that can exist. However, each individual mother expresses a unique "set" of free glycans that are all components within the set of glycans in this definable metaglycome. The individual variation of free glycans in milk is dependent on the genetic makeup of the individual with respect to Lewis blood group as described earlier. There are also epigenetic factors in each individual that affect enzyme expression levels and biosynthetic pathways, as well as possible environmental factors including nutrition state of the individual, time since parturition, and time of day (Ballard and Morrow, 2013; Bode, 2015; Andreas et al., 2015).

6. METHODS FOR DETERMINING HUMAN MILK OLIGOSACCHARIDE STRUCTURES

6.1 HISTORICAL PROSPECTIVE AND DEVELOPMENT OF CHEMICAL AND PHYSICAL METHODS

Initial studies on the structures of HMOs were focused on the most abundant glycans that could be obtained as pure glycans, including the structures shown in Fig. 4.1 (Kuhn et al., 1956a,b, 1958a,b; Montreuil, 1956; Kuhn and Gauhe, 1958, 1960, 1956, 1962a,b; Kuhn and Baer, 1956, 1959; Kobata and Ginsburg, 1969, 1972a,b; Kuhn, 1959; Grimmonprez and Montreuil, 1968). In most instances, the glycans were resolved as pure isomers using paper chromatography followed by crystallization to obtain large quantities of pure compounds (milligram to gram quantities) that were then structurally analyzed using classic methods such as elemental analysis, monosaccharide-specific colorimetric assays, acid hydrolysis, and separation of monosaccharides by paper chromatography to determine the molar ratios of hexose, fucose, sialic acid, and *N*-acetylhexosamines. Classic methods involving periodate consumption and identification of fragments of oligosaccharides after periodate oxidation, which preferentially cleaves vicinal hydroxyl groups, were applied to predict linkage position of monosaccharides and their sequence; however, these methods require so much material that while extremely effective in determining glycan structure, they are impractical in most of today's applications. Nevertheless, these classic methods should not be forgotten as the chemistry may have useful applications if appropriately optimized for the small quantities of material we use today.

During the 1960s and early 1970s, investigators began addressing the larger HMOs, which were present in smaller quantities. Dr. Akira Kobata, while working with Dr. Victor Ginsburg at the National Institutes of Health in Bethesda, Maryland, developed many of the isolation and purification techniques that became fundamental protocols for researchers analyzing the structures of HMOs (Kobata, 2004). These techniques were originally based on gel filtration and paper chromatography during several days of development in organic solvent mixtures (Kobata et al., 1969; Kobata, 1972). The reducing glycans were located on the dried chromatograms using silver nitrate spray reagent and then eluted from the paper with water, dried, and subjected to a variety of analyses. Many of these methods are still used but adapted to more modern separation and analytical protocols (Charlwood et al., 1999) that use more rapid HPLC methods to replace paper chromatography and gravity flow column chromatography.

Sensitive methods for compositional analysis were required, and a variety of useful chemistries and chemical "tricks" to identify monosaccharide sequences were developed. For example, monosaccharides generated by acid hydrolysis were reduced and derivatized by a variety of reagents to make them volatile and subjected to gas chromatographic methods and gas–liquid chromatographic methods (Laine et al., 1972) for qualitative and quantitative analysis to obtain monosaccharide ratios. More-sensitive techniques capitalized on the fact that the free glycans of human milk and their component monosaccharides are reducing sugars that can be conveniently reduced to the corresponding alditols by reduction with $NaBH_4$ and can be made radioactive by using $NaB[^3H]_4$ for the reduction, which is available at very high specific radioactivities (Takasaki and Kobata, 1974). For exploring sequences of HMOs, reducing oligosaccharides labeled with $NaBH_4$, which converted the reducing-end monosaccharide to an alditol, was used to confirm the reducing end glucose as sorbitol in acid hydrolyzates of the reduced glycans. Oxidation of the 6-OH group of nonreducing terminal galactose of a glycan by galactose oxidase followed by reduction with $NaB[^3H]_4$ (Morell et al., 1966) was used for HMO analysis to identify their nonreducing ends after partial acid hydrolysis (Kobata and Ginsburg, 1972a). Other techniques used in the elucidation of the structure of LNF III (Fig. 4.1), for example, included differential base stability of fucose linkages depending on the position of fucose in the glycan, differential reaction of isolated fragments with Morgan-Elson reagent that reacted with 3-substituted GlcNAc but not 4-substituted GlcNAc, differential consumption of periodate by pure glycans and subsequent identification of oxidation products, and differential inhibition of agglutination using specific antiglycan antibodies (Kobata and Ginsburg, 1969).

For determining linkage of monosaccharides in HMOs, the accepted method became methylation analysis (Lindberg, 1972; Lindberg and Lonngren, 1978), where —OH groups on sugars are converted to a methyl ether $—OCH_3$. Since this procedure remains the one of the most definitive methods for determining monosaccharide linkages within a glycan, it is briefly summarized in Fig. 4.2. The first step in this process is the methylation

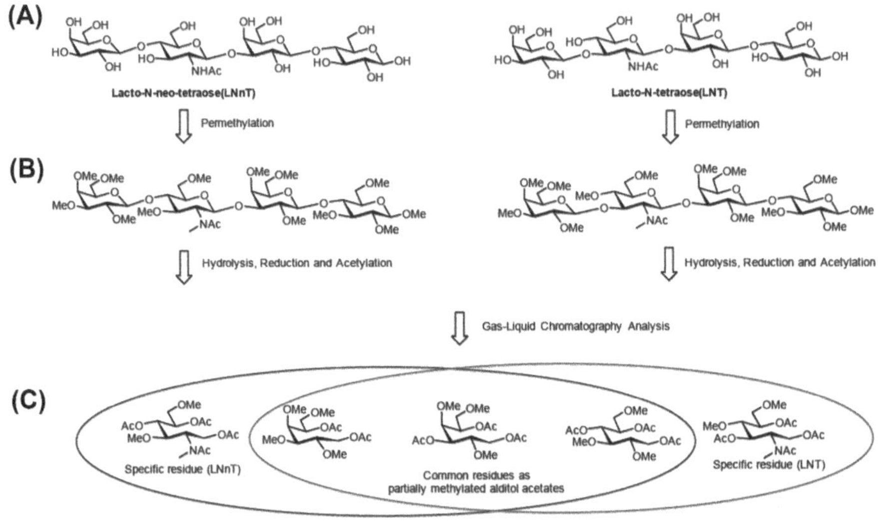

FIGURE 4.2

Methylation analysis (Lindberg, 1972; Lindberg and Lonngren, 1978) remains one of the most definitive methods for determining monosaccharide linkages within a glycan. The partially methylated alditol acetates generated from the glycan LNT are circled in red (light gray in print version) and the partially methylated alditol acetates generated from the isomeric glycan LNnT are circled in blue (dark gray in print version).

of all of the —OH groups in the glycan, which was an important reaction optimized for complete or *permethylation* of a glycan by Hakomori (Hakomori, 1964). The examples in Fig. 4.2 show the structures of LNT and LNnT (A) being permethylated to their fully methylated products (B). The permethylated glycan can be easily extracted into organic solvent to rapidly remove interfering substances, and they are subsequently hydrolyzed by HCl in methanol or by formic acid to obtain a mixture of partially methylated monosaccharides where the free hydroxyl groups on each monosaccharide mark the positions where that sugar residue was substituted. These points of substitution are revealed by reducing the mixture with $NaBH_4$, and converting the free —OH groups to acetyl esters using acetic anhydride in pyridine to obtain a mixture of partially methylated alditol acetates (C), which are identified and quantified by co-chromatography with standards using gas–liquid chromatography. The method gives information on the position of substitution of each of the monosaccharides and can identify unsubstituted monosaccharides that occur at nonreducing termini and may provide information on the reducing terminal monosaccharide. The example shown in Fig. 4.2 shows the comparison of the partially methylated alditol acetates generated from the isomeric glycans LNT (circled in red) and LNnT (circled in blue). The difference between these two structures is simply the position of the linkage of the terminal Gal residue to the penultimate GlcNAc residue, which is either 3-substituted in the case of LNT or 4-substituted in the case of LNnT. Knowing that all milk glycans have lactose (Galβ1-4Glc) at the reducing end and that Gal is the nonreducing terminal, it is easy to assign the monosaccharide sequences of LNT and LNnT. However, the arrangement of the monosaccharides in larger glycans will not be as easily determined, and methylation analysis provides no information on the anomericity (α or β configuration) of each monosaccharide.

Unequivocally determining monosaccharide sequence and the anomericity of each monosaccharide requires additional methods, and perhaps the most used was the application of glycosidases, enzymes that hydrolyzed sugar chains with specificity for not only the monosaccharide but also the anomeric configuration of the monosaccharide and, in many cases, the linkage position. The analogy of these enzymes to endonucleases for the fragmenting nucleic acids is tempting, but the analogy is only partial, since glycans are more complex than the linear polymers of nucleotides and in the case of HMOs, and the most useful glycosidases are exoglycosidases that operate at the nonreducing end of a glycan, as recently reviewed by Kobata (Kobata, 2013). Thus, labeling free glycans by reduction with $NaB[^3H]_4$, generates radioactive glycans, which are otherwise difficult to detect by nondestructive methods and can be sensitively followed during isolation and purification procedures. Gel filtration chromatography on Bio-Gel P4 was found to be a convenient medium for separating glycans based on size with excellent resolution up to approximately 24 monosaccharides (Yamashita et al., 1977a, 1982; Kobata et al., 1978). Using partial acid hydrolyzates of linear dextrans that generated a series of molecular weight standards, it was possible to estimate masses based on hexose units, and for the neutral milk glycans compositions could be estimated by assigning one hexose unit to Glc, Gal, and Fuc and two hexose units to GlcNAc. By digesting purified glycans with specific exoglycosidase and monitoring the change in apparent molecular weight by gel chromatography or paper chromatography, complete characterization of a purified HMOs was relatively straightforward especially if linkage data from permethylation analysis were available; but very labor intensive (Kobata and Ginsburg, 1972a,b; Yamashita et al., 1976a,b; Yamashita et al., 1977a,b; Tachibana et al., 1978).

By the late 1970s, it was clear that human milk contained large number of complex glycans based on the structures of approximately 40 HMOs that had been reported (Egge et al., 1983), and that these glycans were genetically regulated expressing the Lewis blood group antigens as free oligosaccharides based on the genotype of the mother (Grollman and Ginsburg, 1967; Grollman et al., 1969, 1970). Egge et al. reasoned from inspection of the known structures and information on the fucosyltransferases and sialyltransferases expressed in human milk, that an enormous number of possible structures were theoretically possible and that identification of these glycans would require more sensitive techniques (Egge et al., 1983). Starting with large quantities of pooled human milk this group prepared 15–20 g of neutral HMOs that were peracetylated and separated by multidimensional chromatography using HPLC and high-performance thin layer chromatography (HPTLC) into over 100 fractions that were analyzed by fast atom bombardment (FAB)-MS indicating structural features of glycans up to decasaccharide core structures substituted with up to five fucose residues. The fragmentation patterns and pathways of degradation of the pseudomolecular ions were interpreted to predict a variety of structural elements that were present in these glycans based on the structures of previously defined HMOs. With this demonstration of the utility of FAB-MS to detect and determine structural features of minor HMOs and the rapid advancement in instrumentation that generated increased sensitivity and resolution of mass analyses (Ninonuevo and Lebrilla, 2009), MS became an important tool in the sequence analysis of HMOs. Structural predictions were somewhat simpler since these unique glycans were composed of only five monosaccharides; however, the absolute identification of linkage and anomeric configuration of the monosaccharides was not easily identified by mass values alone. Thus, many HMO structures were determined using FAB-MS in combination with permethylation analysis to define monosaccharide linkages and specific enzyme degradation or ^{1}H and ^{13}C nuclear magnetic resonance (NMR) methods to define anomeric configurations (Wieruszeski et al., 1985; Gronberg et al., 1989, 1990, 1992; Strecker et al., 1989, 1992).

By the early 1990s, approximately 90 HMOs had been completely characterized (Stahl et al., 1994), and these glycans were available from researchers who were determining their structure; some were available from a few commercial sources, for use as standards in developing new structural methods. In particular, important advances were made in MS technology with respect to ionization methods including MALDI and electrospray ionization (ESI) and mass analyzers including Fourier transform ion cyclotron MS (FTIC-MS) and time-of-flight MS, which were reviewed (Ninonuevo and Lebrilla, 2009; Han and Costello, 2013; Reinhold et al., 1995). The sensitivity and robustness of MS methods were demonstrated in an early analysis of underivatized and permethylated neutral high-molecular-weight HMOs using MALDI-MS (Stahl et al., 1994; Pfenninger et al., 2008). These investigators identified the compositions of 146 neutral HMOs based on unique molecular weights ranging from 342 (lactose) to 6042. Unsubstituted core structures ranged from lactose (hexose 2 or H2) and lactotetraoses (hexose 3, GlcNAc 1, or H3N1) up to H17N15, and fucose substitutions ranged up to 15 fucose residues; that is, H11N9F15 has a molecular weight of 5822. The acidic glycans of human milk were similarly analyzed by MALDI-MS (Finke et al., 1999); 67 unique molecular weights of sialylated glycans larger than DSL (Fig. 4.1) with one to three sialic acid residues ranged from 1654.5 to 3628.4. The highest molecular weight sialylated glycan fraction had a composition of seven hexoses, five GlcNAcs, eight Fuc, and one SA (H7N5F8S1), and the largest core structure among the sialylated glycans was H9N7. Each molecular mass in the spectrum of the acidic and neutral glycans obviously was composed of a large number of isomers that cannot be structurally defined by this MS method, but the results clearly indicated the complexity and large number of glycans that compose this glycome.

As clinical investigations continue to demonstrate the health benefits of breastfeeding and investigators continue to unveil the functions of the components of human milk, there has been an increased interest in the structural analysis of the free glycans in human milk, and one of the most challenging aspects in identifying the specific function of individual milk oligosaccharides is to rapidly unravel their detailed structure and understand the variation in the glycan repertoires among individuals. Using the more advanced MS techniques (Ninonuevo et al., 2006; Ninonuevo and Lebrilla, 2009; Pfenninger et al., 2002a, 2008; Chai et al., 2002; Yang et al., 2011) in combination with methods such as methylation analysis for determining monosaccharide linkages, and ^{1}H and ^{13}C NMR or specific exoglycosidase digestions for determining anomeric linkages, a large number of structures for the more minor HMOs have been published (Wu et al., 2010, 2011; Pfenninger et al., 2002b; Chai et al., 2005). To date, the structures of over 200 HMOs have been completely defined and reported in the literature.

7. ALTERNATIVE METHODS FOR DETERMINING HUMAN MILK OLIGOSACCHARIDE STRUCTURE

As discussed above, more classic approaches to studies on HMOs put a premium on the collection of defined structures of glycans purified from human milk and characterization using many different methods to determine the sequence, linkage, and anomeric configurations of component monosaccharides. With the development of more-sophisticated MS methods, it is possible to produce profiles of mixtures of glycans, but due to the many isomeric structures possible, absolute structural analysis of glycans in complex mixtures using only MS is difficult.

Based on the historical development of methods for defining the structure of oligosaccharides in general and HMOs in particular, it is clear that the methods grew out of the intricate chemistry of carbohydrates; because of the complex stereochemistry and elaborate branching of glycans, the methods advanced with the development of technology capable of dealing with these complexities. Since studies of glycan structure were performed primarily by chemists with interest in physical and chemical methods, the area of carbohydrate chemistry became rather specialized and less approachable to biologists. However, the interactions of proteins with carbohydrates have been known for many years as documented by observations that isoantibodies specific for several human blood group antigens specifically bound glycan structures (Morgan and Watkins, 1951). Thus, identification of the glycan epitope for such antibodies obtained specific reagents for detecting and identifying glycan structures. In studies on the interaction of antibodies with carbohydrate, Elvin Kabat estimated that an antibody may bind glycans containing up to six monosaccharides. These studies were subsequently extended to plant lectins, which were shown to bind polysaccharides, human blood group active glycans, and other mammalian glycans, and for many decades, biologists have used specific glycan binding proteins (GBPs) to detect and identify the presence of glycan structures. Affinity chromatography is a powerful technique for the isolation of glycans based on the specificity of GBP such as lectins that can be immobilized to a solid support (Ogata et al., 1975; Tomana et al., 1976; Cummings and Kornfeld, 1982; Cummings, 1994), and this technique has been applied to studies of HMOs (Yamashita et al., 1985; Kobata et al., 1994; Tarrago et al., 1988). Antibodies directed against HMOs (Smith and Ginsburg, 1980) have been used to identify specific sequences or determinants expressed in human milk (Prieto and Smith, 1984; Smith et al., 1987) and as determinants on other free glycans (Smith et al., 1981; Prieto and Smith, 1985, 1986). A monoclonal antibody directed against the sialylated Le^a epitope was used for the isolation and subsequent purification of nine distinct glycans from human milk that possessed this determinant (Kitagawa et al., 1989, 1990, 1991, 1993).

8. ADVENT OF GLYCAN MICROARRAYS

As mentioned, glycan microarrays have been used to study biologically relevant protein–glycan interactions, which can provide clues to the function of GBPs and their corresponding glycan ligand(s) (Paulson et al., 2006; Rillahan and Paulson, 2011; Smith et al., 2010). Arrays of glycans with defined structures are extremely useful in defining the specificity of GBPs by comparing the structures of bound and unbound glycans. Large arrays such as the defined glycan microarray developed by the Consortium for Functional Glycomics (CFG) permits the simultaneous interrogation of over 600 glycan structures and the definition of the subtle differences among specificities of GBP (Rillahan and Paulson, 2011; Smith et al., 2010). Data from hundreds of analyses on this array are publically available (http://www.functionalglycomics.org/static/-consortium/consortium.shtml). Using GBPs with well-defined specificities, it is possible to identify specific glycan structures within the glycan targets printed on a shotgun glycan microarray. By collecting the metadata on the presence of glycan determinants defined by GBP binding on the microarray and by MS data from the glycan retrieved from the TGL, it is possible to define the complete glycan structures, and this approach is called MAGS (Yu et al., 2012, 2014; Smith and Cummings, 2013; Ashline et al., 2014) as summarized in Fig. 4.3. There are at least 65 plant and animal lectins and 16 antibodies with defined specificities based on the CFG glycan array that can be used for detecting specific glycan determinants. Fig. 4.4 shows five lectins and five antibodies that are particularly useful for defining determinants on arrays of HMOs. GBP binding data may also be collected after treating the glycan microarray with specific exoglycosidases, and changes in the binding profiles will indicate action of the specific enzymes and provide additional structural information. Additional determinants of HMOs can be defined by MALDI-TOF/TOF analysis of glycans retrieved from the TGL (Agravat et al., 2016). All of the metadata associated with each glycan target are stored in a database, from which structural information can be extracted.

9. THE "VIRTUAL" HUMAN MILK GLYCOME

Since this process permits analysis of large arrays composed of several 100 glycans, a novel bioinformatics approach was developed to automate the data extraction from the MAGS database. This bioinformatics approach was designed to predict structures based on matching the experimental data in the MAGS database against a knowledge

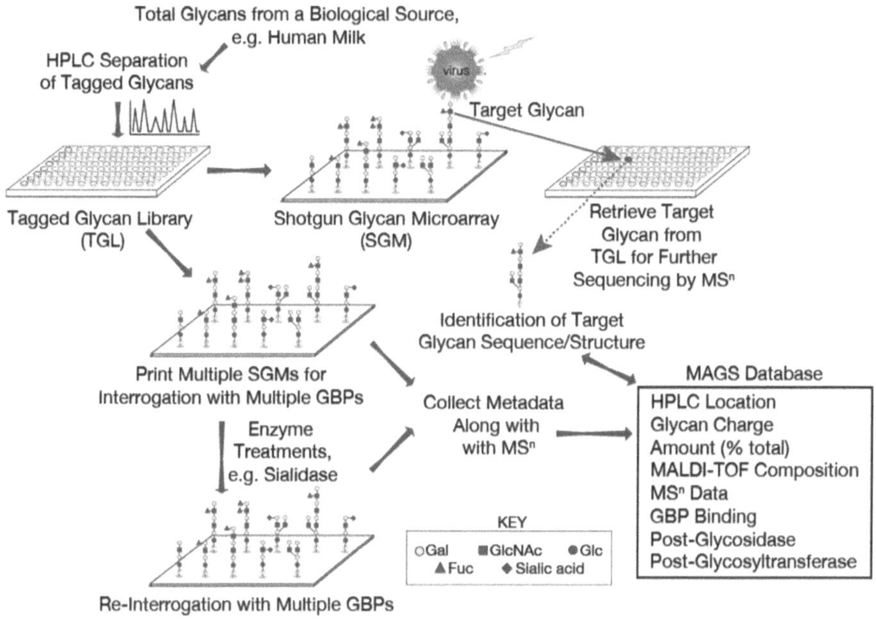

FIGURE 4.3

Metadata-assisted glycan sequencing (MAGS) is an extension of the shotgun glycan microarray concept. Beginning with the generation of the TGL, each glycan is assigned an accession number and printed on the array, and the metadata are collected for each glycan and stored in a database. Preprinted information can include the following: number of negative charges based on ion-exchange chromatography; location of the glycan in the two-dimensional HPLC separation profiles; percentage of total glycomes that each glycan represents; MALDI-TOF data to provide information on purity, composition, additional MS^n data as obtained; defined GBP binding before and after exoglycosidase digestion; and any other information deemed useful regarding the nature of the glycan.

base of all possible structures that can exist in the soluble glycans of human milk. To do this, it was first necessary to address the fundamental question of the number and the structures of the free glycans composing the human milk metaglycome. Using regular expressions (Agravat et al., 2016) to represent the biosynthetic rules for the human milk metaglycome as outlined in "Rules of Human Milk Glycan Structure," a virtual glycome generator algorithm was initialized with the core lactose structure, a threshold parameter for the maximum core size (core structures unsubstituted with fucose and sialic acid) of the glycome, and the patterns that represent the extensions and terminal modifications of HMO biosynthesis. The composition of the glycans are reported based on the numbers of residues of hexose (H), which represents the single reducing terminal Glc plus Gal, which is the only other hexose found in human milk free glycans; *N*-acetylhexosamine (N), which is GlcNAc; deoxyhexose (F), which is fucose; and sialic acid (S), which is only Neu5Ac. For example, the composition of

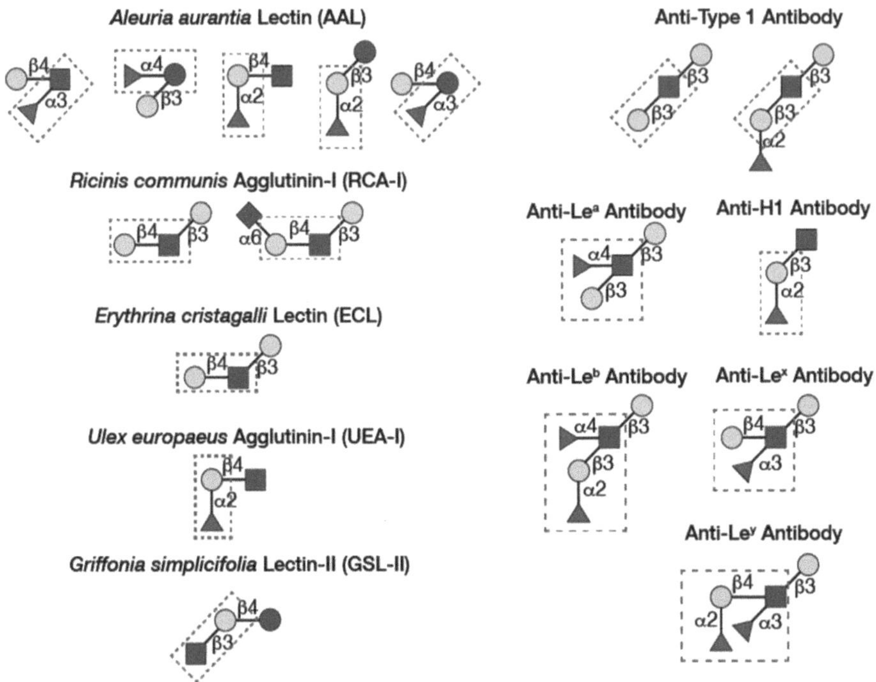

FIGURE 4.4

Glycan determinants recognized by lectins and antibodies used for MAGS of human milk glycans. The determinant of each defined glycan binding protein is outlined in each structure.

the sialyl Lewis a epitope, Neu5Acα2-3Galβ1-3(Fucα1-4)GlcNAcβ1-3Galβ1-4Glc, is H3N1F1S1; and the core structure (without fucose and sialic acid additions) would be H3N1.

The virtual glycome generator stores the virtual human milk soluble glycan glycome in a database, and Table 4.1 shows the theoretical number of glycans that can exist for each composition based on the biosynthetic rules of HMGs described earlier up to a dodecaose core structure (H7N5). While core structures as large as H17N15 have been reported, the amounts of glycans with core structures greater than H5N3 are vanishingly small. Nevertheless, the virtual glycome of human milk soluble glycans is certainly greater than 50,000 different possible structures. The web-based software tool GlycomeSeq provides the number of isomers within each composition and will display the structures of all isomers within each composition (https://glycomeseq.emory.edu/). The virtual HMO database has been shared with UniCarbKB (Campbell et al., 2014), which can be found at http://unicarbkb.org/milk. The UniCarbKB platform is a knowledgebase that allows public access to a curated database of glycan structures and associated metadata including publications and glycan structural classification by taxonomy, tissue, protein, etc.

Table 4.1 Virtual Glycome of Human Milk Free Glycans

Sialic Acid and Fucose	Core Structures (No Fucose or Sialic Acid)						
	H2	**H2N1**	**H3N1**	**H4N2**	**H5N3**	**H6N4**	**H7N5**
F0S0	1	0	2	4	10	26	72
F1S0	2	0	5	12	41	135	454
F2S0	1	0	4	13	66	291	1229
F3S0	0	0	1	6	52	335	1860
F4S0	0	0	0	1	20	220	1715
F5S0	0	0	0	0	3	81	982
F0S1	2	0	3	8	23	71	230
F1S1	2	0	7	22	91	358	1420
F2S1	0	0	5	21	140	745	3751
F3S1	0	0	1	8	104	822	5517
F4S1	0	0	0	1	37	513	4920
F5S1	0	0	0	0	5	178	2710
F0S2	0	0	1	5	19	75	299
F1S2	0	0	2	12	71	363	1794
F2S2	0	0	1	9	101	717	4578
F3S2	0	0	0	2	67	739	6454
F4S2	0	0	0	0	20	421	5460
F5S2	0	0	0	0	2	129	2814
Total glycans in each core	8	0	32	124	872	6219	46,259
Cumulative total	8	8	40	164	1036	7255	53,514
	Disaccharide core	Triaose core	Tetrtaose core	Hexaose core	Octaose core	Decaose core	Dodecaose core

Core structures, unsubstituted with fucose or sialic acid as indicated by the designation F0S0 in the top row, are designated by composition where H represents hexose (a single reducing terminal glucose and galactose residues) followed by the number of residues; that is, H2 is the lactose core structure (Galβ1-4Glc), and N represents GlcNAc residues, that is, H3N1 represents the isomers composed of a single reducing terminal glucose, two galactose residues, and a single GlcNAc. The composition H2N1 was included to be comprehensive, but this structure is not found as a free glycan in human milk. The numbers for each composition indicate the number of isomers with the indicated composition that can be biosynthetically generated in human milk based on the rules described in "Rules of Human Glycan Structures". For example, the composition H5N3F2S1 is shared among 140 isomeric structures in the virtual glycome.

The GlycomeSeq algorithm, which has been implemented in a software package that executes within a web application (http://glycomeseq.emory.edu), predicts structure from the experimental metadata. The algorithm requires a spreadsheet input file (MAGS database) that contains the identification number of the glycan with the compositions that were previously determined by MS, determinant defined by binding of each GBP and the binding data from each GBP binding each glycan target in relative fluorescence units (RFU). Given a composition for an unknown glycan target based on mass of the molecular ion by MALDI analysis, the algorithm will return all possible candidate structures from the database of virtual glycan structures matching the mass and filter candidates based on the binding metadata. The algorithm then proceeds through the remaining steps shown in Fig. 4.5. The algorithm initially selects all structures from the database that match the mass (and predicted composition) of the unknown target. It then evaluates the positive binders and selects the intersection of candidate structures from the remaining set of structures that contain the determinant for the positive binding GBPs. The selection of the candidate structures that contain the determinant is based on an XPath query defined for the GBP. Next, for each nonbinding GBP, it filters out candidate structures that contain the determinant for each nonbinding GBP using an XPath query. This step is completed for all negative binders to eliminate candidate structures for that target. Finally, if we have additional determinants as identified by MS^n reporter ions (e.g., linear lactose, branched lactose, terminal fucosylated LacNAc, etc.), we select the intersection of candidate structures in our final set of predicted structures. The utility of this approach was recently demonstrated using data obtained from the validation of the human milk

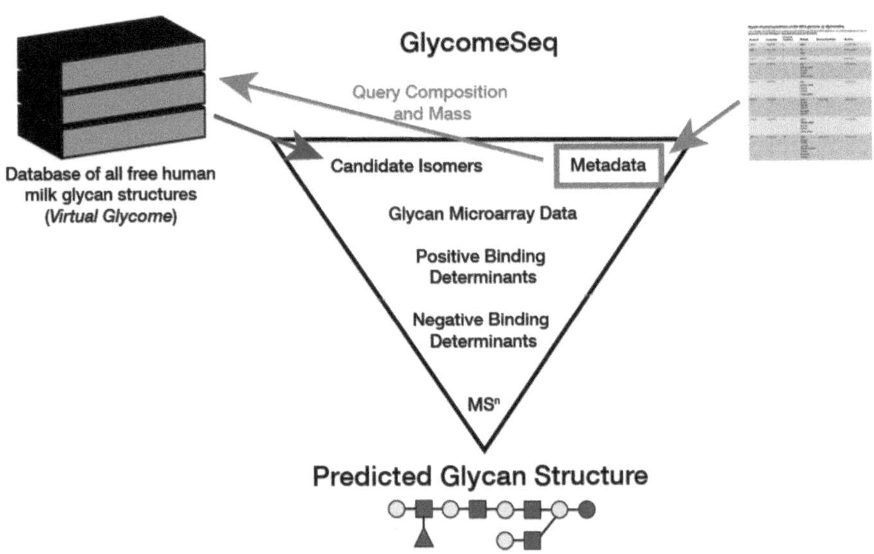

FIGURE 4.5

GlycomeSeq algorithm.

shotgun glycan microarray reported previously (Yu et al., 2014). The data from 10 GBPs with known specificities binding to 42 purified HMGs and 14 standards of known structure before and after treatment with the specific exoglycosidases, β1-3-galactosidase, β1-4-galactosidase, and α1-2-fucosidase and endo-β1-4-galactosidase provided to the algorithm and the application output a table with the predictions for each target and the associated metadata, which can be viewed on the web application. We applied the algorithm to 33 pure glycan targets, and it returned single results for 23 of the glycans, while the other 10 generated multiple candidate structures.

Thus, the MAGS approach represents a potentially high throughput, automatable method for the structural analysis of the human milk soluble glycan glycome and can potentially applied to any array of pure glycans. In addition, the concept of predicting structures based on matching the experimental data against a knowledge base of all possible structures that can exist in a virtual or latent glycome represents a valid approach to addressing the definition of any glycome.

10. SIZE AND COMPOSITION OF THE HUMAN MILK FREE GLYCAN GLYCOME

Predictions regarding the number of different glycans that can exist in human milk have varied from a few hundred to many thousands. It is clear from the work of others and from the recent application of a virtual glycome generator algorithm that number of possible HMGs could be well over 50,000 possible structures. Obviously no single individual will produce all possible glycans because the structures synthesized will depend many factors. Nevertheless, it is clear that many thousands of different glycans are synthesized and secreted into the milk of all human mothers. The compilation of lists of glycan structures has limited value since little information on function can be generated from lists of structures. However, having a compilation of all of the possible structures within a particular glycome permits some useful predictions regarding the relationship of structure and function. The total number of possible free milk glycans with disaccharide to dodecasaccharide core structures is estimated to be 53,514; however, the region of a glycoconjugate glycan that participates in recognition of a biologically relevant GBP is generally thought to reside at the nonreducing end of the glycan. This region has been termed the glycan determinant (Cummings, 2009), which is composed of disaccharides to pentasaccharides, and the number of determinants is significantly less than the total number of structures. This was demonstrated using the virtual HMG virtual glycome by identifying the number of nonreducing, terminal determinants from disaccharide to pentasaccharide determinants as a function of increasing core structure size, as shown in Fig. 4.6.

While the total number of structures in each core size increases dramatically as shown by the number of glycans in each core size (Fig. 4.6, parentheses), the number of terminal determinants increases to an apparent asymptotic value; that is, 13 terminal disaccharide determinants for all human milk free glycans, 21 terminal trisaccharide determinants, 43 terminal tetrasaccharide determinants, and 89 terminal

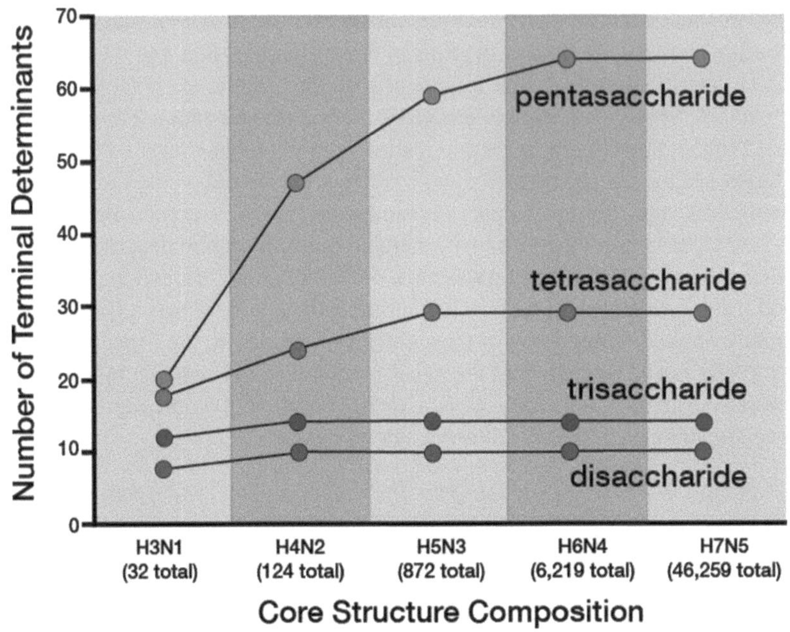

FIGURE 4.6

Number of terminal determinants in human milk glycan glycome as a function of increasing core structure size. The composition of the core structures in indicated by number of hexoses (H, galactose and reducing terminal glucose) and the number of *N*-acetylglucosamines (N) in each core structure. The number of unique glycan structures including zero to five fucose residues and zero to two sialic acid residues is indicated in parentheses under each core composition. The data show the number of di- (red *(dark gray in print versions)*), tri- (blue *(darkest gray in print versions)*), tetra- (green *(gray in print versions)*), and pentasaccharide (orange *(light gray in print versions)*) determinants found among the glycans composing each core structure.

pentasaccharide determinants. Thus, while the number of possible free glycan structures in any human milk sample may be enormous, there are a limited number of potentially relevant biologically active determinants that we would predict to be recognized by GBPs and other glycan recognition molecules. Interestingly, over 90% of the determinants in each determinant size are represented in the glycans with a core composition of H5N3, and glycans with larger core structures are found in vanishingly small amounts. These observations address the questions of how many possible free glycans can exist in human milk and how many of these structures may be biologically relevant. Although the number of possible structures of HMGs may be well over 50,000 and depends on many variables, the number of biologically relevant determinants may be less than 100. The free glycans of human milk may, therefore, present a cluster, or "bouquet," of thousands individual structures where these biosynthetic pathways may have evolved to support a relatively limited number of biologically relevant determinants. By this unique biological process, the microheterogeneity within a metaglycome is less important than the total number of relevant determinants expressed.

ACKNOWLEDGMENTS

This work was supported in part by the National Center for Functional Glycomics under NIH/NIGMS Grant P41GM103694.

REFERENCES

Agravat, S.B., Song, X., Rojsajjakul, T., Cummings, R.D., Smith, D.F., 2016. Computational approaches to define a human milk metaglycome. Bioinformatics 32, 1471–1478.

Andersson, B., Porras, O., Hanson, L.A., Lagergard, T., Svanborg-Eden, C., 1986. Inhibition of attachment of *Streptococcus pneumoniae* and *Haemophilus influenzae* by human milk and receptor oligosaccharides. The Journal of Infectious Diseases 153, 232–237.

Andreas, N.J., Kampmann, B., Mehring Le-Doare, K., 2015. Human breast milk: a review on its composition and bioactivity. Early Human Development 91, 629–635.

Ashline, D.J., Yu, Y., Lasanajak, Y., Song, X., Hu, L., Ramani, S., Prasad, V., Estes, M.K., Cummings, R.D., Smith, D.F., Reinhold, V.N., 2014. Structural characterization by multistage mass spectrometry (MSn) of human milk glycans recognized by human rotaviruses. Molecular & Cellular Proteomics 13, 2961–2974.

Ballard, O., Morrow, A.L., 2013. Human milk composition: nutrients and bioactive factors. Pediatric Clinics of North America 60, 49–74.

Bierhuizen, M.F., Mattei, M.G., Fukuda, M., 1993. Expression of the developmental I antigen by a cloned human cDNA encoding a member of a beta-1,6-N-acetylglucosaminyltransferase gene family. Genes & Development 7, 468–478.

Bode, L., 2012. Human milk oligosaccharides: every baby needs a sugar mama. Glycobiology 22, 1147–1162.

Bode, L., 2015. The functional biology of human milk oligosaccharides. Early Human Development 91, 619–622.

ten Bruggencate, S.J., Bovee-Oudenhoven, I.M., Feitsma, A.L., van Hoffen, E., Schoterman, M.H., 2014. Functional role and mechanisms of sialyllactose and other sialylated milk oligosaccharides. Nutrition Reviews 72, 377–389.

Coppa, G.V., Bruni, S., Zampini, L., Galeazzi, T., Facinelli, B., et al., 2003. Oligosaccharides of human milk inhibit the adhesion of *Listeria monocytogenes* to Caco-2 cells. Italian Journal of Pediatrics 29, 61–68.

Campbell, M.P., Peterson, R., Mariethoz, J., Gasteiger, E., Akune, Y., Aoki-Kinoshita, K.F., Lisacek, F., Packer, N.H., 2014. UniCarbKB: building a knowledge platform for glycoproteomics. Nucleic Acids Research 42, D215–D221.

Castanys-Munoz, E., Martin, M.J., Prieto, P.A., 2013. 2'-Fucosyllactose: an abundant, genetically determined soluble glycan present in human milk. Nutrition Reviews 71, 773–789.

Chai, W., Piskarev, V., Lawson, A.M., 2002. Branching pattern and sequence analysis of underivatized oligosaccharides by combined MS/MS of singly and doubly charged molecular ions in negative-ion electrospray mass spectrometry. Journal of the American Society for Mass Spectrometry 13, 670–679.

Chai, W., Piskarev, V.E., Zhang, Y., Lawson, A.M., Kogelberg, H., 2005. Structural determination of novel lacto-N-decaose and its monofucosylated analogue from human milk by electrospray tandem mass spectrometry and 1H NMR spectroscopy. Archives of Biochemistry and Biophysics 434, 116–127.

Charlwood, J., Tolson, D., Dwek, M., Camilleri, P., 1999. A detailed analysis of neutral and acidic carbohydrates in human milk. Analytical Biochemistry 273, 261–277.

Comstock, S.S., Wang, M., Hester, S.N., Li, M., Donovan, S.M., 2014. Select human milk oligosaccharides directly modulate peripheral blood mononuclear cells isolated from 10-d-old pigs. The British Journal of Nutrition 111, 819–828.

Cummings, R.D., Kornfeld, S., 1982. Fractionation of asparagine-linked oligosaccharides by serial lectin-Agarose affinity chromatography. A rapid, sensitive, and specific technique. The Journal of Biological Chemistry 257, 11235–11240.

Cummings, R.D., Pierce, J.M., 2014. The challenge and promise of glycomics. Chemistry & Biology 21, 1–15.

Cummings, R.D., 1994. Use of lectins in analysis of glycoconjugates. Methods in Enzymology 230, 66–86.

Cummings, R.D., 2009. The repertoire of glycan determinants in the human glycome. Molecular BioSystems 5, 1087–1104.

De Vries, T., Palcic, M.P., Schoenmakers, P.S., Van Den Eijnden, D.H., Joziasse, D.H., 1997. Acceptor specificity of GDP-Fuc:Gal beta 1-->4GlcNAc-R alpha 3-fucosyltransferase VI (FucT VI) expressed in insect cells as soluble, secreted enzyme. Glycobiology 7, 921–927.

Egge, H., Dell, A., Von Nicolai, H., 1983. Fucose containing oligosaccharides from human milk. I. Separation and identification of new constituents. Archives of Biochemistry and Biophysics 224, 235–253.

Engfer, M.B., Stahl, B., Finke, B., Sawatzki, G., Daniel, H., 2000. Human milk oligosaccharides are resistant to enzymatic hydrolysis in the upper gastrointestinal tract. The American Journal of Clinical Nutrition 71, 1589–1596.

Finke, B., Stahl, B., Pfenninger, A., Karas, M., Daniel, H., Sawatzki, G., 1999. Analysis of high-molecular-weight oligosaccharides from human milk by liquid chromatography and MALDI-MS. Analytical Chemistry 71, 3755–3762.

Gnoth, M.J., Kunz, C., Kinne-Saffran, E., Rudloff, S., 2000. Human milk oligosaccharides are minimally digested in vitro. The Journal of Nutrition 130, 3014–3020.

Grimmonprez, L., Montreuil, J., 1968. Physico-chemical study of 6 new oligosides isolated from human milk. Bulletin de la Societe de chimie biologique 50, 843–855.

Grollman, E.F., Ginsburg, V., 1967. Correlation between secretor status and the occurrence of 2'-fucosyllactose in human milk. Biochemical and Biophysical Research Communications 28, 50–53.

Grollman, E.F., Kobata, A., Ginsburg, V., 1969. An enzymatic basis for Lewis blood types in man. Journal of Clinical Investigation 48, 1489–1494.

Grollman, E.F., Kobata, A., Ginsburg, V., 1970. Enzymatic basis of blood types in man. Annals of the New York Academy of Sciences 169, 153–160.

Gronberg, G., Lipniunas, P., Lundgren, T., Erlansson, K., Lindh, F., Nilsson, B., 1989. Isolation of monosialyated oligosaccharides from human milk and structural analysis of three new compounds. Carbohydrate Research 191, 261–278.

Gronberg, G., Lipniunas, P., Lundgren, T., Lindh, F., Nilsson, B., 1990. Isolation and structural analysis of three new disialylated oligosaccharides from human milk. Archives of Biochemistry and Biophysics 278, 297–311.

Gronberg, G., Lipniunas, P., Lundgren, T., Lindh, F., Nilsson, B., 1992. Structural analysis of five new monosialylated oligosaccharides from human milk. Archives of Biochemistry and Biophysics 296, 597–610.

Hakomori, S., 1964. A rapid permethylation of glycolipid, and polysaccharide catalyzed by methylsulfinyl carbanion in dimethyl sulfoxide. Journal of Biochemistry 55, 205–208.

Han, L., Costello, C.E., 2013. Mass spectrometry of glycans. Biochemistry. Biokhimiia 78, 710–720.

Hennet, T., Weiss, A., Borsig, L., 2014. Decoding breast milk oligosaccharides. Swiss Medical Weekly 144, w13927.

Hill, D.R., Newburg, D.S., 2015. Clinical applications of bioactive milk components. Nutrition Reviews 73, 463–476.

Hsieh, C.C., Hernandez-Ledesma, B., Fernandez-Tome, S., Weinborn, V., Barile, D., de Moura Bell, J.M., 2015. Milk proteins, peptides, and oligosaccharides: effects against the 21st century disorders. BioMed Research International 2015, 146840.

Jantscher-Krenn, E., Lauwaet, T., Bliss, L.A., Reed, S.L., Gillin, F.D., Bode, L., 2012. Human milk oligosaccharides reduce *Entamoeba histolytica* attachment and cytotoxicity in vitro. British Journal of Nutrition 108, 1839–1846.

Jiang, X., Huang, P., Zhong, W., Tan, M., Farkas, T., Morrow, A.L., Newburg, D.S., Ruiz-Palacios, G.M., Pickering, L.K., 2004. Human milk contains elements that block binding of noroviruses to human histo-blood group antigens in saliva. The Journal of Infectious Diseases 190, 1850–1859.

Johnson, P.H., Watkins, W.M., 1992. Purification of the Lewis blood-group gene associated alpha-3/4-fucosyltransferase from human milk: an enzyme transferring fucose primarily to type 1 and lactose-based oligosaccharide chains. Glycoconjugate Journal 9, 241–249.

Kuhn, R., Brossmer, R., 1956. Über die O-Acetyl-lactamin-säure-lactose aus Kuh Colostrum und ihre Spaltbarkeit durch Influenza-Virus. Chemische Berichte 98, 2013–2035.

Kuhn, R., 1959. Biochemie der Rezeptoren und Resistenzfaktoren. Von der Widerstandsfähigkeit der Lebewesen gegen Einwirkungen der Umwelt. Naturwissenschaften 46, 43–50.

Kelly, R.J., Rouquier, S., Giorgi, D., Lennon, G.G., Lowe, J.B., 1995. Sequence and expression of a candidate for the human secretor blood group alpha(1,2)fucosyltransferase gene (FUT2). Homozygosity for an enzyme-inactivating nonsense mutation commonly correlates with the non-secretor phenotype. The Journal of Biological Chemistry 270, 4640–4649.

Kitagawa, H., Nakada, H., Kurosaka, A., Hiraiwa, N., Numata, Y., Fukui, S., Funakoshi, I., Kawasaki, T., Yamashina, I., Shimada, I., et al., 1989. Three novel oligosaccharides with the sialyl-Lea structure in human milk: isolation by immunoaffinity chromatography. Biochemistry 28, 8891–8897.

Kitagawa, H., Nakada, H., Numata, Y., Kurosaka, A., Fukui, S., Funakoshi, I., Kawasaki, T., Shimada, I., Inagaki, F., Yamashina, I., 1990. Occurrence of tetra- and pentasaccharides with the sialyl-Le(a) structure in human milk. The Journal of Biological Chemistry 265, 4859–4862.

Kitagawa, H., Nakada, H., Fukui, S., Funakoshi, I., Kawasaki, T., Yamashina, I., Tate, S., Inagaki, F., 1991. Novel oligosaccharides with the sialyl-Lea structure in human milk. Biochemistry 30, 2869–2876.

Kitagawa, H., Nakada, H., Fukui, S., Funakoshi, I., Kawasaki, T., Yamashina, I., Tate, S., Inagaki, F., 1993. Novel oligosaccharides with the sialyl-Le(a) structure in human milk. Journal of Biochemistry 114, 504–508.

Kobata, A., Ginsburg, V., 1969. Oligosaccharides of human milk. II. Isolation and characterization of a new pentasaccharide, lacto-N-fucopentaose 3. The Journal of Biological Chemistry 244, 5496–5502.

Kobata, A., Ginsburg, V., 1972a. Oligosaccharides of human milk. 3. Isolation and characterization of a new hexasaccharide, lacto-N-hexaose. The Journal of Biological Chemistry 247, 1525–1529.

Kobata, A., Ginsburg, V., 1972b. Oligosaccharides of human milk. IV. Isolation and characterization of a new hexasaccharide, lacto-N-neohexaose. Archives of Biochemistry and Biophysics 150, 273–281.

Kobata, A., Ginsburg, V., Tsuda, M., 1969. Oligosaccharides of human milk. I. Isolation and characterization. Archives of Biochemistry and Biophysics 130, 509–513.

Kobata, A., Yamashita, K., Tachibana, Y., 1978. Oligosaccharides from human milk. Methods in Enzymology 50, 216–220.

Kobata, A., Kochibe, N., Endo, T., 1994. Affinity chromatography of oligosaccharides on *Psathyrella velutina* lectin column. Methods in Enzymology 247, 228–237.

Kobata, A., 1972. Isolation of oligosaccharides from human milk. Methods in Enzymology 28, 262–271.

Kobata, A., 2004. The third chains of living organisms–a trail of glycobiology that started from the third floor of building 4 in NIH. Archives of Biochemistry and Biophysics 426, 107–121.

Kobata, A., 2010. Structures and application of oligosaccharides in human milk. Proceedings of the Japan Academy Series B Physical and Biological Sciences 86, 731–747.

Kobata, A., 2013. Exo- and endoglycosidases revisited. Proceedings of the Japan Academy Series B Physical and Biological Sciences 89, 97–117.

Koszdin, K.L., Bowen, B.R., 1992. The cloning and expression of a human alpha-1,3 fucosyltransferase capable of forming the E-selectin ligand. Biochemical and Biophysical Research Communications 187, 152–157.

Kuhn, R., Baer, H.H., 1956. Die Konstitution der Lacto-N-tetraose. Chemische Berichte 89, 504–511.

Kuhn, R., Baer, R., 1959. Über das durch Viren der Influenza-Gruppe spaltbare Trisaccharid der Milch. Chemische Berichte 92, 1667–1671.

Kuhn, R., Gauhe, A., 1956. Bestimmung der Bindungsstelle von sialinsäureresten in Oligosaccharides mit Hilfe von Periodat. Chemische Berichte 98, 395–413.

Kuhn, R., Gauhe, A., 1958. Über die lacto-difuco-tetraose der Frauenmilch. Justus Liebigs Annaien der Chemie 611, 249–252.

Kuhn, R., Gauhe, A., 1960. Über ein kristallisiertes, Lea-aktives Hexasaccharid aus Frauenmilch. Chemische Berichte 93, 647–651.

Kuhn, R., Gauhe, A., 1962a. Die Konstitution der Lacto-N-neotetraose. Chemische Berichte 95, 518–522.

Kuhn, R., Gauhe, A., 1962b. Uber drei saure pentasaccharide aus frauenmilch. Chemische Berichte 95, 513 517.

Kuhn, R., Baer, H.H., Gauhe, A., 1956a. Kristallisierte fucosido-lactose. Chemische Berichte 89, 2513.

Kuhn, R., Baer, H.H., Gauhe, A., 1956b. Kristallisation und Konstitutionsermittlung der Lacto-N-fucopentaose I. Chemische Berichte 89, 2514–2523.

Kuhn, R., Baer, H.H., Gauhe, A., 1958a. Die Konstitution der Lacto-N-fucopentaose II. Chemische Berichte 91, 364.

Kuhn, R., Baer, H.H., Gauhe, A., 1958b. 2-α-L-Fucopyranosyl-D-galaktose und 2-α-L-fucopyranosyl-D-talose. Justus Liebigs Annaien der Chemie 611, 242–249.

Kukowska-Latallo, J.F., Larsen, R.D., Nair, R.P., Lowe, J.B., 1990. A cloned human cDNA determines expression of a mouse stage-specific embryonic antigen and the Lewis blood group alpha(1,3/1,4)fucosyltransferase. Genes & Development 4, 1288–1303.

Kurakevich, E., Hennet, T., Hausmann, M., Rogler, G., Borsig, L., 2013. Milk oligosaccharide sialyl(alpha2,3)lactose activates intestinal CD11c+ cells through TLR4. Proceedings of the National Academy of Sciences of the United States of America 110, 17444–17449.

Laine, R.A., Esselman, W.J., Sweeley, C.C., 1972. Gas-liquid chromatography of carbohydrates. Methods in Enzymology 28, 159–167.

Larsen, R.D., Ernst, L.K., Nair, R.P., Lowe, J.B., 1990. Molecular cloning, sequence, and expression of a human GDP-L-fucose:beta-D-galactoside 2-alpha-L-fucosyltransferase cDNA that can form the H blood group antigen. Proceedings of the National Academy of Sciences of the United States of America 87, 6674–6678.

Lindberg, B., Lonngren, J., 1978. Methylation analysis of complex carbohydrates: general procedure and application for sequence analysis. Methods in Enzymology 50, 3–33.

Lindberg, B., 1972. Methylation analysis of polysaccharides. Methods in Enzymology 28, 178–195.

Lowe, J.B., 1993. The blood group-specific human glycosyltransferases. Bailliere's Clinical Haematology 6, 465–492.

Maksimovic, J., Sharp, J.A., Nicholas, K.R., Cocks, B.G., Savin, K., 2011. Conservation of the ST6Gal I gene and its expression in the mammary gland. Glycobiology 21, 467–481.

Manthey, C.F., Autran, C.A., Eckmann, L., Bode, L., 2014. Human milk oligosaccharides protect against enteropathogenic *Escherichia coli* attachment in vitro and EPEC colonization in suckling mice. Journal of Pediatric Gastroenterology and Nutrition 58, 165–168.

Mattila, P., Salminen, H., Hirvas, L., Niittymaki, J., Salo, H., Niemela, R., Fukuda, M., Renkonen, O., Renkonen, R., 1998. The centrally acting beta1,6N-acetylglucosaminyltransferase (GlcNAc to gal). Functional expression, purification, and acceptor specificity of a human enzyme involved in midchain branching of linear poly-N-acetyllactosamines. The Journal of Biological Chemistry 273, 27633–27639.

Montreuil, J., 1956. Structure of two triholosides isolated from human milk. Comptes rendus hebdomadaires des seances de l'Academie des sciences 242, 192–193.

Morell, A.G., Van den Hamer, C.J., Scheinberg, I.H., Ashwell, G., 1966. Physical and chemical studies on ceruloplasmin. IV. Preparation of radioactive, sialic acid-free ceruloplasmin labeled with tritium on terminal D-galactose residues. The Journal of Biological Chemistry 241, 3745–3749.

Morgan, W.T., Watkins, W.M., 1951. The inactivation of the blood group receptor on the human erythrocyte surface by the periodate ion. British Journal of Experimental Pathology 32, 34–48.

Ninonuevo, M.R., Lebrilla, C.B., 2009. Mass spectrometric methods for analysis of oligosaccharides in human milk. Nutrition Reviews 67 (Suppl. 2), S216–S226.

Ninonuevo, M.R., Park, Y., Yin, H., Zhang, J., Ward, R.E., Clowers, B.H., German, J.B., Freeman, S.L., Killeen, K., Grimm, R., Lebrilla, C.B., 2006. A strategy for annotating the human milk glycome. Journal of Agricultural and Food Chemistry 54, 7471–7480.

Ogata, S., Muramatsu, T., Kobata, A., 1975. Fractionation of glycopeptides by affinity column chromatography on concanavalin A-sepharose. Journal of Biochemistry 78, 687–696.

Paulson, J.C., Colley, K.J., 1989. Glycosyltransferases. Structure, localization, and control of cell type-specific glycosylation. The Journal of Biological Chemistry 264, 17615–17618.

Paulson, J.C., Blixt, O., Collins, B.E., 2006. Sweet spots in functional glycomics. Nat Chem Biol 2, 238–248.

Pfenninger, A., Karas, M., Finke, B., Stahl, B., 2002a. Structural analysis of underivatized neutral human milk oligosaccharides in the negative ion mode by nano-electrospray MS(n) (part 1: methodology). Journal of the American Society for Mass Spectrometry 13, 1331–1340.

Pfenninger, A., Karas, M., Finke, B., Stahl, B., 2002b. Structural analysis of underivatized neutral human milk oligosaccharides in the negative ion mode by nano-electrospray MS(n) (part 2: application to isomeric mixtures). Journal of the American Society for Mass Spectrometry 13, 1341–1348.

Pfenninger, A., Chan, S.Y., Karas, M., Finke, B., Stahl, B., Costello, C.E., 2008. Mass spectrometric detection of multiple extended series of neutral highly fucosylated -acetyllactosamine oligosaccharides in human milk. International Journal of Mass Spectrometry 278, 129–136.

Polonovski, M., Lespagnol, A., 1933. Nouvelles acquisitions sur les composés glucidiques du lai de femme. Bulletin de la Societe de Chimie Biologique 15, 320–349.

Polonovski, M., Lespagnol, A., 1954. Etude chromatographique des polyosides du lai de femme. Comptes Rendus de l'Académie des Sciences 238, 2263–2264.

Prieto, P.A., Smith, D.F., 1984. A new sialyloligosaccharide from human milk: isolation and characterization using anti-oligosaccharide antibodies. Archives of Biochemistry and Biophysics 229, 650–656.

Prieto, P.A., Smith, D.F., 1985. A new ganglioside in human meconium detected by antiserum against the human milk sialyloligosaccharide, LS-tetrasaccharide b. Archives of Biochemistry and Biophysics 241, 281–289.

Prieto, P.A., Smith, D.F., 1986. A new ganglioside in human meconium detected with antiserum against human milk sialyltetrasaccharide a. Archives of Biochemistry and Biophysics 249, 243–253.

Reinhold, V.N., Reinhold, B.B., Costello, C.E., 1995. Carbohydrate molecular weight profiling, sequence, linkage, and branching data: ES-MS and CID. Analytical Chemistry 67, 1772–1784.

Renkonen, O., 2000. Enzymatic in vitro synthesis of I-branches of mammalian polylactosamines: generation of scaffolds for multiple selectin-binding saccharide determinants. Cellular and Molecular Life Sciences 57, 1423–1439.

Rillahan, C.D., Paulson, J.C., 2011. Glycan microarrays for decoding the glycome. Annual Review of Biochemistry 80, 797–823.

Rudloff, S., Pohlentz, G., Diekmann, L., Egge, H., Kunz, C., 1996. Urinary excretion of lactose and oligosaccharides in preterm infants fed human milk or infant formula. Acta Paediatrica 85, 598–603.

Rudloff, S., Obermeier, S., Borsch, C., Pohlentz, G., Hartmann, R., Brosicke, H., Lentze, M.J., Kunz, C., 2006. Incorporation of orally applied (13)C-galactose into milk lactose and oligosaccharides. Glycobiology 16, 477–487.

Rudloff, S., Pohlentz, G., Borsch, C., Lentze, M.J., Kunz, C., 2012. Urinary excretion of in vivo (1)(3)C-labelled milk oligosaccharides in breastfed infants. The British Journal of Nutrition 107, 957–963.

Ruiz-Palacios, G.M., Cervantes, L.E., Ramos, P., Chavez-Munguia, B., Newburg, D.S., 2003. *Campylobacter jejuni* binds intestinal H(O) antigen (Fuc alpha 1, 2Gal beta 1, 4GlcNAc), and fucosyloligosaccharides of human milk inhibit its binding and infection. The Journal of Biological Chemistry 278, 14112–14120.

Sarnesto, A., Kohlin, T., Hindsgaul, O., Thurin, J., Blaszczyk-Thurin, M., 1992. Purification of the secretor-type beta-galactoside alpha 1---2-fucosyltransferase from human serum. The Journal of Biological Chemistry 267, 2737–2744.

Sasaki, K., Kurata-Miura, K., Ujita, M., Angata, K., Nakagawa, S., Sekine, S., Nishi, T., Fukuda, M., 1997. Expression cloning of cDNA encoding a human beta-1,3-N-acetylglucosaminyltransferase that is essential for poly-N-acetyllactosamine synthesis. Proceedings of the National Academy of Sciences of the United States of America 94, 14294–14299.

Schönfeld, H., 1926. Über die Beziehungen der einzelnen Bestandteile der Frauenmilch zur Bifidusflora. Jahrbuch der Kinderh 113, 19–60.

Shoaf-Sweeney, K.D., Hutkins, R.W., 2009. Adherence, anti-adherence, and oligosaccharides preventing pathogens from sticking to the host. Advances in Food and Nutrition Research 55, 101–161.

Smith, D.F., Cummings, R.D., 2013. Application of microarrays for deciphering the structure and function of the human glycome. Molecular & Cellular Proteomics 12, 902–912.

Smith, D.F., Ginsburg, V., 1980. Antibodies against sialyloligosaccharides coupled to protein. The Journal of Biological Chemistry 255, 55–59.

Smith, D.F., Magnani, J.L., Ginsburg, V., 1981. Glycolipids of cell surfaces: isolation of specific sugar sequences using carbohydrate-binding proteins. Archives of Biochemistry and Biophysics 209, 52–56.

Smith, D.F., Prieto, P.A., McCrumb, D.K., Wang, W.C., 1987. A novel sialylfucopentaose in human milk. Presence of this oligosaccharide is not dependent on expression of the secretor or Lewis fucosyltransferases. The Journal of Biological Chemistry 262, 12040–12047.

Smith, D.F., Song, X., Cummings, R.D., 2010. Use of glycan microarrays to explore specificity of glycan-binding proteins. Methods in Enzymology 480, 417–444.

Song, X., Lasanajak, Y., Xia, B., Heimburg-Molinaro, J., Rhea, J.M., Ju, H., Zhao, C., Molinaro, R.J., Cummings, R.D., Smith, D.F., 2011. Shotgun glycomics: a microarray strategy for functional glycomics. Nature Methods 8, 85–90.

Stahl, B., Thurl, S., Zeng, J., Karas, M., Hillenkamp, F., Steup, M., Sawatzki, G., 1994. Oligosaccharides from human milk as revealed by matrix-assisted laser desorption/ionization mass spectrometry. Analytical Biochemistry 223, 218–226.

Strecker, G., Wieruszeski, J.M., Michalski, J.C., Montreuil, J., 1989. Primary structure of human milk nona- and decasaccharides determined by a combination of fast atom bombardment mass spectrometry and 1H-/13C-nuclear magnetic resonance spectroscopy. Evidence for a new core structure, iso-lacto-N-octaose. Glycoconjugate Journal 6, 169–182.

Strecker, G., Fievre, S., Wieruszeski, J.M., Michalski, J.C., Montreuil, J., 1992. Primary structure of four human milk octa-, nona-, and undeca-saccharides established by 1H- and 13C-nuclear magnetic resonance spectroscopy. Carbohydrate Research 226, 1–14.

Tachibana, Y., Yamashita, K., Kobata, A., 1978. Oligosaccharides of human milk: structural studies of di-and trifucosyl derivatives of lacto-N-octaose and lacto-N-neoctaose. Archives of Biochemistry and Biophysics 188, 83–89.

Takasaki, S., Kobata, A., 1974. Microdetermination of individual neutral and amino sugars and N-acetylneuraminic acid in complex saccharides. Journal of Biochemistry 76, 783–789.

Tarrago, M.T., Tucker, K.H., Van Halbeek, H., Smith, D.F., 1988. A novel sialylhexasaccharide from human milk: purification by affinity chromatography on immobilized wheat germ agglutinin. Archives of Biochemistry and Biophysics 267, 353–362.

Tomana, M., Niedermeier, W., Mestecky, J., Schrohenloher, R.E., Porch, S., 1976. Affinity chromatography of glycopeptides using concanavalin A. Analytical Biochemistry 72, 389–399.

Underwood, M.A., Gaerlan, S., De Leoz, M.L., Dimapasoc, L., Kalanetra, K.M., Lemay, D.G., German, J.B., Mills, D.A., Lebrilla, C.B., 2015. Human milk oligosaccharides in premature infants: absorption, excretion, and influence on the intestinal microbiota. Pediatric Research 78 (6),670–677.

Urashima, T., Kitaoka, M., Terabayashi, T., Fukuda, K., Ohnishi, M., Kobata, A., 2011. Milk oligosaccharides. In: Gordon, N.S. (Ed.), Oligosaccharides: Sources, Properties and Applications. Nova Science Publishers, Inc., New York, NY, pp. 1–58.

Urashima, T., Asakuma, S., Leo, F., Fukuda, K., Messer, M., Oftedal, O.T., 2012. The predominance of type I oligosaccharides is a feature specific to human breast milk. Advances in Nutrition 3, 473S–482S.

Weston, B.W., Smith, P.L., Kelly, R.J., Lowe, J.B., 1992. Molecular cloning of a fourth member of a human alpha (1,3)fucosyltransferase gene family. Multiple homologous sequences that determine expression of the Lewis x, sialyl Lewis x, and difucosyl sialyl Lewis x epitopes. The Journal of Biological Chemistry 267, 24575–24584.

Wieruszeski, J.M., Chekkor, A., Bouquelet, S., Montreuil, J., Strecker, G., Peter-Katalinic, J., Egge, H., 1985. Structure of two new oligosaccharides isolated from human milk: sialylated lacto-N-fucopentaoses I and II. Carbohydrate Research 137, 127–138.

Wu, S., Tao, N., German, J.B., Grimm, R., Lebrilla, C.B., 2010. Development of an annotated library of neutral human milk oligosaccharides. Journal of Proteome Research 9, 4138–4151.

Wu, S., Grimm, R., German, J.B., Lebrilla, C.B., 2011. Annotation and structural analysis of sialylated human milk oligosaccharides. Journal of Proteome Research 10, 856–868.

Yamashita, K., Tachibana, Y., Kobata, A., 1976a. Oligosaccharides of human milk. Isolation and characterization of three new disialyfucosyl hexasaccharides. Archives of Biochemistry and Biophysics 174, 582–591.

Yamashita, K., Tachibana, Y., Kobata, A., 1976b. Oligosaccharides of human milk: isolation and characterization of two new nonasaccharides, monofucosyllacto-N-octaose and monofucosyllacto-N-neooctaose. Biochemistry 15, 3950–3955.

Yamashita, K., Tachibana, Y., Kobata, A., 1977a. Oligosaccharides of human milk: structures of three lacto-N-hexaose derivatives with H-haptenic structure. Archives of Biochemistry and Biophysics 182, 546–555.

Yamashita, K., Tachibana, Y., Kobata, A., 1977b. Oligosaccharides of human milk. Structural studies of two new octasaccharides, difucosyl derivatives of para-lacto-N-hexaose and para-lacto-N-neohexaose. The Journal of Biological Chemistry 252, 5408–5411.

Yamashita, K., Mizuochi, T., Kobata, A., 1982. Analysis of oligosaccharides by gel filtration. Methods in Enzymology 83, 105–126.

Yamashita, K., Kochibe, N., Ohkura, T., Ueda, I., Kobata, A., 1985. Fractionation of L-fucose-containing oligosaccharides on immobilized *Aleuria aurantia* lectin. The Journal of Biological Chemistry 260, 4688–4693.

Yang, H., Yu, Y., Song, F., Liu, S., 2011. Structural characterization of neutral oligosaccharides by laser-enhanced in-source decay of MALDI FTICR MS. Journal of the American Society for Mass Spectrometry 22, 845–855.

Yu, Y., Mishra, S., Song, X., Lasanajak, Y., Bradley, K.C., Tappert, M.M., Air, G.M., Steinhauer, D.A., Halder, S., Cotmore, S., Tattersall, P., Agbandje-McKenna, M., Cummings, R.D., Smith, D.F., 2012. Functional glycomic analysis of human milk glycans reveals the presence of virus receptors and embryonic stem cell biomarkers. The Journal of Biological Chemistry 287, 44784–44799.

Yu, Y., Lasanajak, Y., Song, X., Hu, L., Ramani, S., Mickum, M.L., Ashline, D.J., Prasad, B.V., Estes, M.K., Reinhold, V.N., Cummings, R.D., Smith, D.F., 2014. Human milk contains novel glycans that are potential decoy receptors for neonatal rotaviruses. Molecular & Cellular Proteomics 13, 2944–2960.

Zopf, D., Roth, S., 1996. Oligosaccharide anti-infective agents. Lancet 347, 1017–1021.

SECTION

B

Potential Functions and Benefits

CHAPTER

Oligosaccharide Metabolism in the Breastfed Infant

5

Silvia Rudloff[1,2], Clemens Kunz[2]

[1]*Justus-Liebig University Giessen, Giessen, Germany;* [2]*Institute of Nutritional Science, Justus-Liebig University Giessen, Giessen, Germany*

ABBREVIATIONS

Fuc Fucose
FucT Fucosyltransferase
Gal Galactose
GlcNAc *N*-acetylglucosamine
Hex Hexose
HMO Human milk oligosaccharides
HPAEC-PAD High pH anion exchange chromatography with pulsed amperometric detection
Le Lewis
MALDI-TOF-MS Matrix-assisted laser desorption/ionization time-of-flight mass spectrometry
NeuAc *N*-acetylneuraminic acid

1. BACKGROUND

Since the discovery of human milk oligosaccharides (HMOs) more than 60 years ago, research has faced major challenges including the development of methods to identify and characterize these components as well as the lack of larger quantities of single HMOs for animal and human studies. The development of methods for detailed structural analysis in very small volumes alleviates issues in addressing questions where biological samples are required. Also, large amounts of single HMOs can now be produced by chemical and biotechnological means, which are investigated in human clinical studies.

With regard to biological functions, an intriguing aspect is the susceptibility of infants to diseases associated with the amount and type of oligosaccharides they receive via their mother's milk. Depending on the mother's Lewis (Le) blood group and secretor status, the oligosaccharide pattern and the total amount of HMOs an infant receives per day vary significantly (Egge et al., 1983; Egge, 1993; Kunz et al., 1996; Le Pendu, 2004; Thurl et al., 2010; Urashima et al., 2011; Gabrielli et al., 2011; Bode, 2012; Prieto, 2012).

Prebiotics and Probiotics in Human Milk. http://dx.doi.org/10.1016/B978-0-12-802725-7.00005-1

As data support the hypotheses that there is a link between the secretor status of an individual and certain inflammatory diseases, such as of the gastrointestinal (GI) tract (McGovern et al., 2010; Morrow et al., 2011), a special focus of our review will be put on the metabolic fate of secretor- and Lewis blood group–specific components. There are some unique excretion patterns of HMOs and metabolic aspects that deserve special attention (Rudloff and Kunz, 2012). For example, why can secretor- or Lewis blood group–specific HMOs be detected in urine of infants fed nonsecretor or Lewis-negative milk. and what are the consequences for the infant? Or, why is the Lewis b–specific component LNFP I not detectable in any urine sample from infants receiving Lewis b milk from their mothers, whereas all the other major HMOs are present (Rudloff et al., 2006; Dotz et al., 2014, 2015)?

1.1 LEWIS BLOOD GROUP- AND SECRETOR-SPECIFIC COMPONENTS IN HUMAN MILK

A detailed description of the discovery of Le blood group- and secretor-specific components in human milk can be found in Chapter 2 by Akira Kobata. Here, we briefly summarize important aspects to provide a background to some new data that will be presented in the following sections.

Table 5.1 shows basic HMO structures. Their composition has been described in several recent reviews (Urashima et al., 2011; Bode, 2012; Blank et al., 2012). Of particular importance is the influence of the mothers' Lewis blood group and secretor status, which determine the presence of different neutral oligosaccharides in human milk dependent on the activity of specific fucosyltransferases (FucT) in the lactating mammary gland (Fig. 5.1) (Egge et al., 1993; Kobata, 2000; Kunz et al., 2003; Prieto, 2012). Milk of so-called "secretors" is characterized by the activity of FucT2 resulting in Fuc-α-(1→2)-Gal units (compound 1, Table 5.1) like 2′-fucosyllactose (compound 2, Table 5.1) or lacto-*N*-fucopentaose I (compound 3, Table 5.1).

In Lewis(a^+b^-) individuals, who compose about 20% of the population, FucT3 attaches Fuc residues in α-(1→4) linkages to a subterminal GlcNAc residue of type 1 chains. Therefore, in milk of Lewis(a^+b^-), non-secretors, the major fucosylated oligosaccharide is lacto-*N*-fucopentaose II (Gal-β-(1→3)-[Fuc-α-(1→4)]-GlcNAc-β-(1→3)-Gal-β-(1→4)-Glc; compound 5, Table 5.1).

In Lewis(a^-b^+) donors, who represent about 70% of the population, both FucT2 and FucT3, the secretor gene– and the Lewis gene–dependent forms of fucosyltransferases are expressed. Here, one of the major milk oligosaccharide is lacto-*N*-difucohexaose I (Fuc-α-(1→2)-Gal-β-(1→3)-[Fuc-α-(1→4)]-GlcNAc-β-(1→3)-Gal-β-(1→4)-Glc; compound 7, Table 5.1).

In about 5–10% of the population belonging to blood group Lewis(a^-b^-), FucT2 but not FucT3 is active, instead. The major oligosaccharide in their milk is lacto-*N*-fucopentaose I (Fuc-α-(1→2)-Gal-β-(1→3)-GlcNAc-β-(1→3)-Gal-β-(1→4)-Glc; compound 3, Table 5.1).

Table 5.1 Structural Elements of "HMO Prototypes" and Lewis/Secretor-Specific Components

Compound	Abbreviation	Name	Epitopes	Characteristics
1			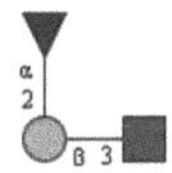	Secretor epitope
2	2′-Fuc-Lac	2′-Fucosyllactose	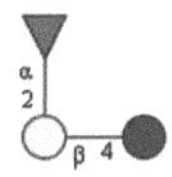	Secretor
3	LNFP I	Lacto-*N*-fucopentaose I	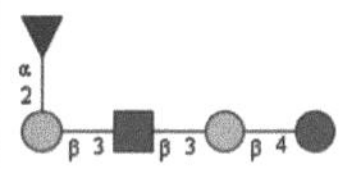	Secretor
4			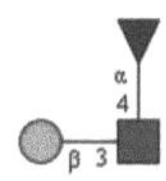	Lewis a epitope
5	LNFP II	Lacto-*N*-fucopentaose II	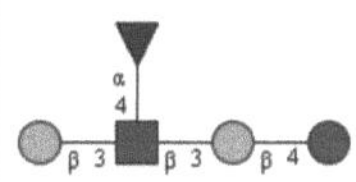	Lewis (a^+b^-)
6			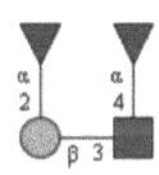	Lewis b epitope
7	LNDFH I	Lacto-*N*-difucohexaose I	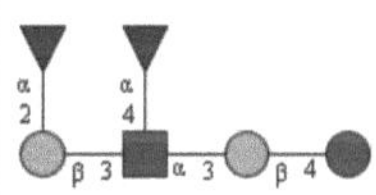	Lewis (a^-b^+)
8	LNFP III	Lacto-*N*-fucopentaose III	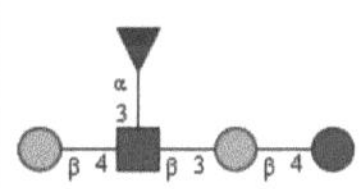	Lewis (a^-b^-)

Glycan structures are depicted according to the recommendations of the Consortium of Functional Glycomics using the GlycoWorkbench software tool (Ceroni et al., 2008). Yellow circle *(light gray in print versions), galactose;* blue circle *(dark gray in print versions), glucose;* blue square *(dark gray in print versions),* N-*acetylglucosamine;* red triangle *(gray in print versions), fucose.*

1.1.1 Total Human Milk Oligosaccharide Content and Concentrations of Single Components

To understand the magnitude of HMO excretion with feces and urine, we have to refer to the total HMO concentrations, which vary strongly within the published data for several reasons: there is no routine analytical method available and, despite of the great progress in mass spectrometry, this technique is still not the first choice for HMO quantification. Therefore, components are often quantified by high pH anion exchange chromatography with pulsed amperometric detection (HPAEC-PAD) (Kunz et al., 1996; Thurl et al., 2010; Gabrielli et al., 2011; Rudloff et al., 2012) or by HPLC separation with prior fluorescence

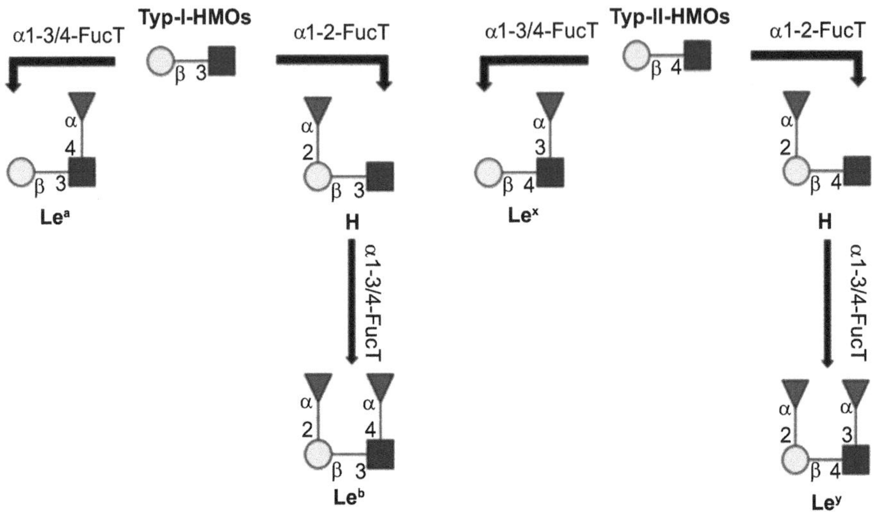

FIGURE 5.1

Biosynthesis of neutral HMO and involved fucosyltransferases.

Adapted from Blank, D., Dotz, V., Geyer, R., Kunz, C., 2012. Human milk oligosaccharides and Lewisblood group: individual high-throughput sample profiling to enhance conclusions from functional studies. Advances in Nutrition 3, 440S–449S.

labeling (Asakuma et al., 2007; Urashima et al., 2011). According to our data using HPAEC-PAD, the concentration of oligosaccharides in mature human milk is about 5–15 g/L with large variations mostly associated with the Lewis and secretor status. With regard to the concentration of major single HMOs, we refer to the contribution of Urashima et al. in Chapter 3.

2. FECAL EXCRETION OF MILK OLIGOSACCHARIDES IN TERM AND PRETERM INFANTS

In the 1980s, Lundblad and coworkers started a series of experiments analyzing feces of breastfed infants to investigate metabolic aspects of HMOs in term and preterm infants (Sabharwal et al., 1984, 1988a,b, 1991). These publications already demonstrated the unique and distinct excretion pattern depending on various factors such as the blood group and secretor status of the breastfeeding mother, the gestational age of the infant, or the time after birth when feces was collected. For example, from feces of an infant with blood group A, Lundblad's group isolated four different blood group A-active oligosaccharides (A-tetrasaccharide, A-pentasaccharide, A-hexasaccharide, and A-heptasaccharide) (Sabharwal et al., 1984). In feces of other infants with blood group A and secretor status, these components were also detected but in considerably lower amounts. As those blood group active components were not detected in the milk of the corresponding mothers, the authors' conclusion was that (1) HMOs were used as precursors to which blood group–specific epitopes were attached and (2) this modification most likely takes place in enterocytes. Today, particularly in light of the methodical progress in characterizing minute amounts of HMOs and degradation products we can now begin to address some of the questions which had previously been raised by Lundblad's group. At that time, the importance of the GI microbiota for the metabolism of HMOs had not been realized and, hence, was not investigated.

More recently, an increasing number of reports concentrating on either the fecal or the urinary excretion of oligosaccharides in infants have been published (Albrecht et al., 2010, 2011; Rudloff et al., 2006, 2012; Goehring et al., 2014; De Leoz et al., 2013;Dotz et al., 2014, 2015). In general, the developments in mass spectrometry allow a rather fast determination of a high number of molecular masses of components in biological fluids such as milk. However, a clear assignment of these masses to milk oligosaccharide structures is not always given. Hence, it needs to be shown whether they are derived from, for example the degradation of milk proteins, glycolipids, or oligosaccharides or from the turnover of intestinal mucins.

Using capillary electrophoresis with laser-induced fluorescence detection, Albrecht et al. published data on the fecal excretion of HMOs in breastfed infants (Albrecht et al., 2010, 2011). They observed a gradual change in the fecal oligosaccharide profile during the first 6 months of life. Within the first 2 months fecal oligosaccharides were subdivided into a pattern dominated by either neutral or acidic HMOs. Thereafter, fecal samples collected between 3 and 6 months of life were characterized by the absence of HMOs and the presence of a few, predominant carbohydrate structures. These carbohydrates were suggested to be GI metabolic products of HMO-carrying blood group epitopes. Then, after exclusive breastfeeding, when complementary food was introduced, predominantly oligosaccharides characteristic of the follow-up diet were found in infants' feces.

3. URINARY AND FECAL EXCRETION OF ^{13}C-LABELED HUMAN MILK OLIGOSACCHARIDES IN INFANTS

A unique way to address metabolic questions is the application of stable isotopes in humans. Some years ago, we used this technique to study the fate of oligosaccharides in breastfed infants after endogenous labeling of HMOs by applying ^{13}C-labeled glucose or galactose (^{13}C-Gal) as an oral bolus given to lactating mothers (Fig. 5.2) (Rudloff et al., 2006, 2012; Kunz et al., 2000).

We showed that a major part of ^{13}C-Gal bolus was immediately transported to the lactating mammary gland and was directly incorporated into HMOs (Fig. 5.3) (Rudloff et al., 2006). There was a rapid increase of the ^{13}C enrichment of milk fractions after the oral ^{13}C-Gal bolus was given to the mothers, followed by a decline in the second half of the day and a further increase in the morning of the

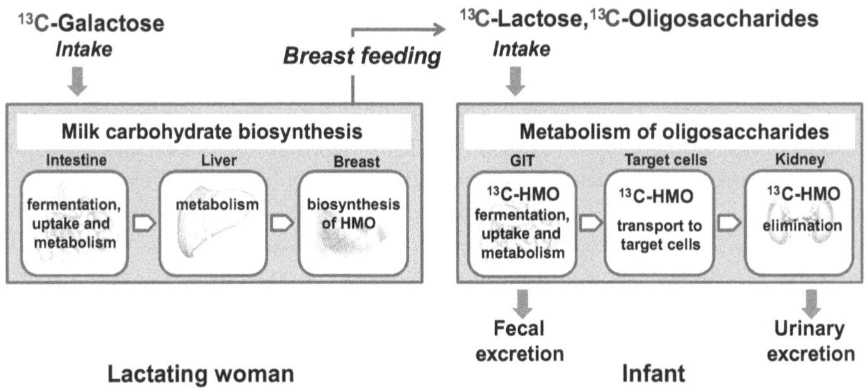

FIGURE 5.2

Scheme of in vivo ^{13}C-labeling of HMO in lactating mothers.

Reproduced from Rudloff, S., Kunz, C., 2012. Milk oligosaccharides and metabolism in infants. Advances in Nutrition 3, 398–405.

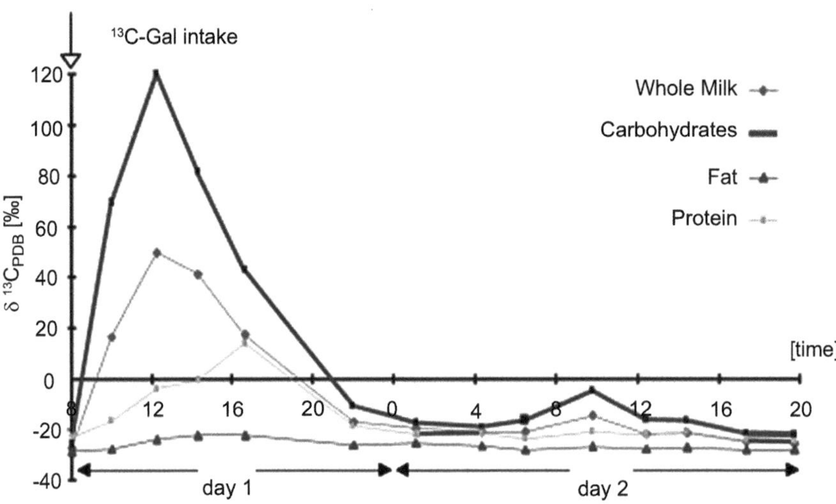

FIGURE 5.3

^{13}C-enrichment of human milk fractions with carbohydrates, fat, and protein.

Reproduced from Rudloff, S., Obermeier, S., Borsch, C., Pohlentz, G., Hartmann, R., Brosicke, H., Lentze, M.J., Kunz C., 2006. Incorporation of orally applied 13C-galactose into milk lactose and oligosaccharides. Glycobiology 16, 477–487.

next day. This pattern was found in milk of all women we have investigated so far. This ^{13}C enrichment was not restricted to the carbohydrate fraction; ^{13}C enrichment also occurred in the protein and, to a lesser degree, in the fat fraction (Fig. 5.3). Therefore, it can be expected that the ^{13}C-label was also incorporated into various glycoproteins and glycolipids.

As secretor- and Lewis blood group–specific components seem to be of particular importance with regard to individual health (see earlier), it is necessary to know whether

1. HMOs are absorbed by and circulate within the blood of infants before potentially being excreted via urine,
2. the infants' urinary oligosaccharide profile resembles the oligosaccharide pattern in their mothers' milk, and
3. HMO degradation products can be detected in urine and feces.

We observed that HMOs were present in all infant urine samples collected within 36 h after the ^{13}C-Gal bolus had been given to their mothers (Rudloff et al., 2012). As we found native, unmodified HMOs in the infants' urine, we concluded that these components can only be derived from milk as the biosynthesis of HMOs is thought to exclusively occur in the lactating mammary gland. In addition, the urinary excretion of intact HMOs in term infants at 3–6 months of life verifies our earlier data in preterm infants showing very similar results without using stable isotopes (Rudloff et al., 1996). Besides intact HMOs, we also detected cleavage products such as fucosyl-lactosamine (FucHexHexNAc) or fucosyl-lacto-*N*-triose ($FucHex_2HexNAc$) in which not, as expected, the terminal galactose but rather the glucose moiety on the reducing end had been cleaved off. This is unusual because enzymes within epithelial cells or of specific microorganisms that are capable of performing this cleavage have not been reported.

Our data so far support the general conclusion that the overall pattern of neutral oligosaccharides in urine from breastfed infants reflects those of their mothers' milk suggesting a strong association with the mothers' Lewis blood group and secretor phenotypes. MALDI-TOF-MS/MS reveals major differences between Lewis a, Lewis b, and Lewis-negative samples with a rather complex pattern in "Lewis b milk" compared with "Lewis a milk" and "Lewis-negative milk" samples (Blank et al., 2011; Dotz et al., 2014, 2015). Comparing, for example, "Lewis a" or "Lewis b milk" with the urinary oligosaccharide pattern of the infants, a similar pattern with the same molecular masses can be observed (Dotz et al., 2015). However, not only looking at molecular masses but also investigating individual structures, we found that the situation is far more complex. For example, as lacto-*N*-fucopentaose I is characteristic for "Lewis b milk," one would expect that *m/z* 876, a major mass signal in MALDI-TOF-MS, represents this component, although mass spectrometry does not directly allow a clear assignment of various isomeric structures. Analyzing the fraction by HPAEC-PAD revealing a separation of HMO isomers such as lacto-*N*-fucopentaose I and II, we were surprised to find out that there was no lacto-*N*-fucopentaose I present in any of the investigated urine samples from infants receiving "Lewis b milk" from their mothers, whereas all the other major HMOs could be identified in infants' urine (Dotz et al., 2015).

Summarizing our data comparing the HMO profile in milk with those of urine and feces of term infants, we conclude that there is no uniform pattern. For example, some components are (1) not only present in all milk samples but in all feces and urine samples collected from the receiving infant, such as *m/z* 730 (lacto-*N*-tetraose or lacto-*N*-*neo*-tetraose), (2) detectable in all milk and all urine sample but only in some fecal samples, such as *m/z* 876 (isomers of fucosyl-lacto-*N*-tetraose), or (3) present in all milk but only in some urine and fecal samples, such as *m/z* 1022 (isomers of difucosylated lacto-*N*-tetraose).

4. PARTICULAR METABOLIC ASPECTS OF SOME HUMAN MILK OLIGOSACCHARIDES AND NOVEL OLIGOSACCHARIDES

One would expect that secretor-specific HMOs would only be present, if at all, in feces or urine in infants fed milk from "secretor mothers" or "Lewis b mothers" as in the mammary gland of both the required fucosyltransferase FUT2 is active. However, we identified the secretor-specific oligosaccharides 2′-fucosyl-lactose, lacto-difuco-tetraose, and lacto-*N*-difuco-hexaose I not only in urine and feces from infants fed "secretor milk" but also in those fed "non-secretor milk" (Dotz et al., 2015). This finding is in line with reports by Lundblad's group (Sabharwal et al., 1988a,b) for feces and by De Leoz et al. (2013) for urine. The formation of lacto-*N*-difuco-hexaose I implies the consecutive activity of (1) α1-2-fucosyl- and (2) α1-4-fucosyltransferases on lacto-*N*-tetraose (Watkins, 1995). Hence, in infants fed "Lewis a milk," lacto-*N*-difuco-hexaose I can only be derived from lacto-*N*-tetraose, but not from the Lewis a–specific lacto-*N*-fucopentaose II.

Besides the detection of intact small and complex HMOs in infant urine, which had been absorbed from the GI tract, as verified via intrinsic ^{13}C-labeling, we recently detected novel HMOs such as $Hex_3HexNAc_2Fuc_3$, which might be a product of incomplete synthesis of $Hex_4HexNAc_2Fuc_3$ (Dotz et al., 2014, 2015). Even acetylated oligosaccharides such as $Ac_1Hex_2Fuc_1$, $Ac_1Hex_3HexNAc_1Fuc_1$, $Ac_1Hex_3HexNAc_1Fuc_{1/2}$, and $Ac_1Hex_4HexNAc_2Fuc_2$ have been detected for the first time. They are present mainly in infant urine but are also minor amounts of feces and even human milk.

In addition and contradictory to other publications, we detected lacto-*N*-tetraose and lacto-*N*-*neo*-tetraose, two structures commonly present in human milk (although lacto-*N*-tetraose is in much higher concentrations) in many infant urine and all infant fecal samples. Albrecht et al. (2010, 2011), however, reported the complete absence of lacto-*N*-tetraose in the feces of 10 breastfed infants at different time points.

5. OLIGOSACCHARIDES IN INFANTS' BLOOD

For ethical reasons, it is usually not possible to collect blood from term or preterm infants for research. Therefore, the few data available need special attention. Goehring et al. (2014) reported on the direct evidence of HMOs in the circulation of breastfed infants. The authors compared the content of HMOs in milk, blood, and urine of the corresponding breastfed infants with formula-fed infants as controls.

The levels of 2′-fucosyllactose, 3-fucosyllactose, and lacto-*N*-*neo*-tetraose in blood and urine significantly correlated with their concentrations in milk. The relative mounts of HMOs were low (i.e., 0.1% of the milk levels for plasma and 4% of the milk levels for urine). There is another publication from Ruhaak et al. (2014), demonstrating that mass spectrometry was able to detect relative masses in blood similar to those of HMOs. However, the infants whose blood was investigated were not exclusively breastfed; hence, no firm conclusion can be drawn from this publication with regard to the appearance of HMOs in blood and in relation to their concentration in milk.

6. INTAKE OF HUMAN MILK OLIGOSACCHARIDES THROUGH SUCKLING AND URINARY EXCRETION

Within our ongoing studies, we determined infants' intake of lacto-*N*-tetraose and its monofucosylated derivative lacto-*N*-fucopentaose II. Our data show that with each breastfeeding bout, an infant receives between 50 and 160 mg of lacto-*N*-tetraose and lacto-*N*-fucopentaose II, respectively (Table 5.2) (Rudloff et al., 2012). The renal excretion of both components varied between 1 and 3 mg per day (Table 5.3). Since the infant's intake of individual HMOs is in the range of several 100 mg per suckling bout (several grams/day), and since some of these components are excreted as intact HMOs in the urine in mg amounts, not only local but also systemic effects can be expected.

7. SUMMARY AND CONCLUSIONS

According to the available data, we conclude that there is no simple fecal or urinary HMO excretion pattern, and it is too early to suggest specific stages of an HMO metabolism. According to our own data, we simplify the results as follows.

Table 5.2 Intake of Lacto-*N*-tetraose (LNT) and Its Monofucosylated Derivative Lacto-*N*-fucopentaose II (LNFP II) by an Infant at One Feeding[a]

Milk Sample	Volume (mL)	Concentration (mg/mL)[b]		Total Intake from Milk (mg)	
		LNT	LNFP II	LNT	LNFP II
1	97	0.77±0.01	1.10±0.03	74.7	106.3
2	126	0.78±0.01	1.25±0.04	98.2	157.2
3	58	0.79±0.00	1.09±0.01	46.2	63.5
4	97	0.77±0.09	1.07±0.11	75.1	103.8
5	97	0.57±0.00	0.85±0.01	55.6	82.3

[a]*Rudloff et al. (2012).*
[b]*Concentration mg/mL is given as mean±SD (n=5 repetitions).*

Table 5.3 Urinary Excretion of Lacto-*N*-tetraose (LNT) and Its Monofucosylated Derivative Lacto-*N*-fucopentaose II (LNFP II) in One Infant[a]

Urine Sample	Urine Volume (mL)	Concentration (μg/mL)[b]		Total Excretion (mg)	
		LNT	LNFP II	LNT	LNFP II
1	35.0	13.4±0.2	13.1±0.4	0.47	0.46
2	25.0	21.2±0.5	22.6±1.5	0.53	0.56
3	22.8	15.2±0.8	17.1±0.1	0.35	0.39
4	20.0	16.6±0.9	18.2±0.4	0.33	0.36
6	26.3	11.4±0.2	12.4±0.5	0.30	0.33
7	19.7	7.3±0.1	7.0±0.1	0.14	0.14
8	23.2	11.6±0.3	13.3±0.1	0.27	0.31
9	27.0	6.7±0.1	6.6±0.3	0.18	0.18

[a]*Rudloff et al. (2012).*
[b]*Concentrations are given as mean±SD (n=4 repetitions).*

The **fecal HMO composition** is often characterized by

Pattern I: high diversity of HMOs or degraded/modified HMOs, often more complex than in human milk;
Pattern II: few oligosaccharides (lacto-*N*-tetraose/lacto-*N*-*neo*-tetraose, and derivatives) with rather low signal intensity;
Pattern III: reduced HMO diversity, but an increased number of modified HMOs.

In addition,

- secretor- or Lewis-specific HMOs are present in feces of infants fed nonsecretor or Lewis-negative milk;
- lacto-*N*-tetraose, major compound in milk, was detectable in all fecal samples; and
- in feces compared to urine: only minor amounts of acetylated HMOs or HMO degradation/modification products can be found

The **urinary composition** is characterized by

- patterns that mostly reflect milk composition (but not for all individual components);
- intestinal absorption and subsequent renal excretion of intact structures in all infants;
- rather simple HMO pattern with mainly lacto-*N*-tetraose and its monofucosylated components in some infants;
- the lack of lacto-*N*-fucopentaose I, highly abundant in secretor milk, in infants fed secretor milk (without exception);

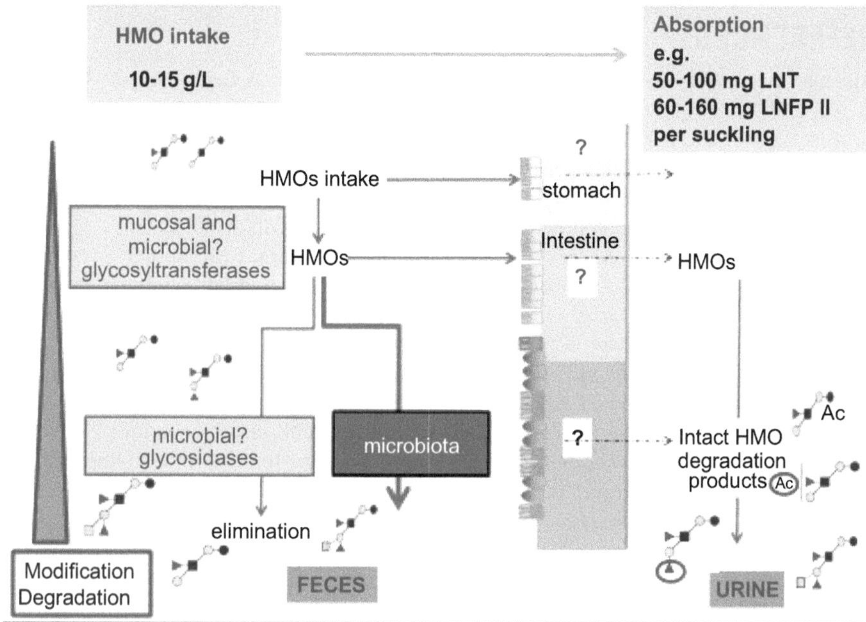

FIGURE 5.4

Schematic of the ingestion, degradation, and absorption of HMOs.

(Modified according to Dotz et al., 2015)

- secretor- or Lewis-specific HMOs in infants fed non-secretor or Lewis-negative milk; and
- HMO degradation/modification products such as acetylated HMOs.

In general, large amounts of HMOs (i.e., several grams per day) reach the GI tract of a breastfed infant (Fig. 5.4). These HMOs are considered not to be degraded by human digestive enzymes, or at least not to a large extent, and to be transported into the lower parts of the intestine where they may be metabolized by the intestinal microbiota or get excreted with feces; about 1–2% of some HMOs seem to be excreted via infants' urine (Rudloff et al., 1996, 2006, 2012; Dotz et al., 2014, 2015). Hence, several 100s of milligrams per day may circulate in the infant's blood. From our metabolic observations that intact HMOs and their degradation products can be detected in the infant urine, it is most likely that not only local effects of HMOs within the GI tract may occur but also systemic functions.

ACKNOWLEDGMENTS

We would like to appreciate the contribution of all mothers participating in our studies which were supported by the German Research Foundation DFG (grants Ku 781/8-3 and Ru 529/7-3).

REFERENCES

Albrecht, S., Schols, H.A., Van den Heuvel, E.G.H.M., Voragen, A.G.J., Gruppen, H., 2010. CE-LIF-MS^n profiling of oligosaccharides in human milk and feces of breast-fed babies. Electrophoresis 31, 1264–1273.

Albrecht, S., Schols, H.A., van den Heuvel, E.G.H.M., Voragen, A.G.J., Gruppen, H., 2011. Occurrence of oligosaccharides in feces of breast-fed babies in their first six months of life and the corresponding breast milk. Carbohydrate Research 346, 2540–2550.

Asakuma, S., Urashima, T., Akahori, M., Obayashi, H., Nakamura, T., Kimura, K., Watanabe, Y., Arai, I., Sanai, Y., 2007. Variation of major neutral oligosaccharides levels in human colostrum. European Journal of Clinical Nutrition 62, 488–494.

Blank, D., Gebhardt, S., Maass, K., Lochnit, G., Dotz, V., Blank, J., Geyer, R., Kunz, C., 2011. High-throughput mass finger printing and Lewis blood group assignment of human milk oligosaccharides. Analytical and Bioanalytical Chemistry 401, 2495–2510.

Blank, D., Dotz, V., Geyer, R., Kunz, C., 2012. Human milk oligosaccharides and Lewis blood group: individual high-throughput sample profiling to enhance conclusions from functional studies. Advances in Nutrition 3, 440S–449S.

Bode, L., 2012. Human milk oligosaccharides: every baby needs a sugar mama. Glycobiology 22, 1147–1162.

Ceroni, A., Maass, K., Geyer, H., Geyer, R., Dell, A., Haslam, S.M., 2008. GlycoWorkbench: a tool for the computer-assisted annotation of mass spectra of glycans. Journal of Proteome Research 7, 1650–1659.

De Leoz, M.L., Wu, S., Strum, J.S., Ninonuevo, M.R., Gaerlan, S.C., Mirmiran, M., German, J.B., Mills, D.A., Lebrilla, C.B., Underwood, M.A., 2013. A quantitative and comprehensive method to analyze human milk oligosaccharide structures in the urine and feces of infants. Analytical and Bioanalytical Chemistry 405, 4089–4105.

Dotz, V., Rudloff, S., Blank, D., Lochnit, G., Geyer, R., Kunz, C., 2014. ^{13}C-labeled oligosaccharides in breastfed infants' urine: individual-, structure- and time-dependent differences in the excretion. Glycobiology 24, 185–194.

Dotz, V., Rudloff, S., Meyer, C., Lochnit, G., Kunz, C., 2015. Metabolic fate of neutral human milk oligosaccharides in exclusively breast-fed infants. Molecular Nutrition and Food Research 59, 355–364.

Egge, H., Dell, A., Von Nicolai, H., 1983. Fucose containing oligosaccharides from human milk. I. Separation and identification of new constituents. Archives of Biochemistry and Biophysics 224, 235–253.

Egge, H., 1993. The diversity of oligosaccharides in human milk. In: Renner, B., Sawatzki, G. (Eds.), New Perspectives in Infant Nutrition. Thieme, Stuttgart, New York, pp. 12–26.

Gabrielli, O., Zampini, L., Galeazzi, T., Padella, L., Santoro, L., Peila, C., Giuliani, F., Bertino, E., Fabris, C., Coppa, G.V., 2011. Preterm milk oligosaccharides during the first month of lactation. Pediatrics 128 (6), e1520–e1531.

Goehring, K.C., Kennedy, A.D., Prieto, P.A., Buck, R.H., 2014. Direct evidence for the presence of human milk oligosaccharides in the circulation of breastfed infants. PLoS One 9 (1–11), e101692.

Kobata, A., 2000. A journey to the world of glycobiology. Glycoconjugate Journal 17, 443–464.

Kunz, C., Rudloff, S., Hintelmann, A., Pohlentz, G., Egge, H., 1996. High-pH anion-exchange chromatography with pulsed amperometric detection and molar response factors of human milk oligosaccharides. Journal of Chromatography B 685, 211–221.

Kunz, C., Rudloff, S., Baier, W., Klein, N., Strobel, S., 2000. Oligosaccharides in human milk. Structural, functional, and metabolic aspects. Annual Review of Nutrition 20, 699–722.

Kunz, C., Bode, L., Rudloff, S., 2003. Genetic variability of human milk oligosaccharides: are there biological consequences? In: Bachmann, C., Koletzko, B. (Eds.), Genetic Expression and Nutrition. Nestlé Nutrition Workshop Series, Pediatric Nutrition, vol. 50. Lippincott Williams & Wilkins, Philadelphia, pp. 137–149.

Le Pendu, J., 2004. Histo-blood group antigen and human milk oligosaccharides: genetic polymorphism and risk of infectious diseases. Advances in Experimental Medicine and Biology 554, 135–143.

McGovern, D.P.B., Jones, M.R., Taylor, K.D., Marciante, K., Yan, X., Dubinsky, M., Ippoliti, A., Vasiliauskas, E., Berel, D., Derkowski, C., Dutridge, D., International IDB Genetic Consortium, Fleshner, P., Shih, D.Q., Melmed, G., Mengesha, E., King, L., Pressman, S., Haritunians, T., Guo, X., Targan, S.R., Rotter, J.I., 2010. Fucosyltransferase 2 (FUT2) non-secretor status is associated with Crohn's disease. Human Molecular Genetics 19, 3468–3476.

Morrow, A.L., Meinzen-Derr, J., Huang, P., Schibler, K.R., Cahill, T., Keddache, M., Kallapur, S.G., Newburg, D.S., Tabangin, M., Warner, B.B., Jiang, X., 2011. Fucosyltransferase 2 non-secretor and low secretor status predicts severe outcomes in premature infants. The Journal of Pediatrics 158, 745–751.

Prieto, P.A., 2012. Profiles of human milk oligosaccharides and production of some human milk oligosaccharides in transgenic animals. Advances in Nutrition 3, 456S–464S.

Rudloff, S., Pohlentz, G., Diekmann, L., Egge, H., Kunz, C., 1996. Urinary excretion of lactose and oligosaccharides in preterm infants fed human milk or infant formula. Acta Paediatrica 85, 598–603.

Rudloff, S., Obermeier, S., Borsch, C., Pohlentz, G., Hartmann, R., Brosicke, H., Lentze, M.J., Kunz, C., 2006. Incorporation of orally applied 13C-galactose into milk lactose and oligosaccharides. Glycobiology 16, 477–487.

Rudloff, S., Kunz, C., 2012. Milk oligosaccharides and metabolism in infants. Advances in Nutrition 3, 398–405.

Rudloff, S., Pohlentz, G., Borsch, C., Lentze, M.J., Kunz, C., 2012. Urinary excretion of in vivo ^{13}C-labelled milk oligosaccharides in breastfed infants. British Journal of Nutrition 107, 957–963.

Ruhaak, L.R., Stroble, C., Underwood, M.A., Lebrilla, C.B., 2014. Detection of milk oligosaccharides in plasma of infants. Analytical and Bioanalytical Chemistry 406, 5775–5784.

Sabharwal, H., Nilsson, B., Chester, M.A., Sjöblad, S., Lundblad, A., 1984. Blood group specific oligosaccharides from faeces of a blood group A breast-fed infant. Molecular Immunology 21, 1105–1112.

Sabharwal, H., Nilsson, B., Chester, M.A., Lindh, F., Grönberg, G., Sjöblad, S., Lundblad, A., 1988a. Oligosaccharides from faeces of a blood-group B, breast-fed infant. Carbohydrate Research 178, 145–154.

Sabharwal, H., Nilsson, D., Grönberg, G., Chester, M.A., Dakour, J., Sjöblad, S., Lundblad, A., 1988b. Oligosaccharides from feces of preterm infants fed on breast milk. Archives of Biochemistry and Biophysics 265, 390–406.

Sabharwal, H., Sjöblad, S., Lundblad, A., 1991. Sialylated oligosaccharides in human milk and feces of preterm, full-term and weaning infants. Journal of Pediatric Gastroenterology and Nutrition 12, 480–484.

Thurl, S., Munzert, M., Henker, J., Boehm, G., Müller-Werner, B., Jelinek, J., Stahl, B., 2010. Variation of human milk oligosaccharides in relation to milk groups and lactational periods. The British Journal of Nutrition 104, 1261–1271.

Urashima, T., Kitaoka, M., Terabayashi, T., Fukuda, K., Ohnishi, M., Kobata, A., 2011. Milk oligosaccharides. In: Gordon, N.G. (Ed.), Sources, Properties and Applications. Nova Science Publishers, New York, pp. 1–77.

Watkins, W., 1995. Molecular basis of antigenic specificity in the ABO, H and Lewis blood-group systems. In: Montreuil, J.V., Schachter, H. (Eds.), Glycoproteins. Elsevier, Amsterdam, pp. 313–390.

CHAPTER

The Role of Human Milk Oligosaccharides in Host–Microbial Interactions

6

David A. Sela[1,2], Lars Bode[3]

[1]*University of Massachusetts, Amherst, MA, United States;* [2]*University of Massachusetts Medical School, Worcester, MA, United States;* [3]*University of California, San Diego, La Jolla, CA, United States*

1. INTRODUCTION

This chapter surveys the role of milk oligosaccharides in mediating interactions between the infant host and their harbored microbiota. As with many symbioses, this is a reciprocal and dynamic network of relationships that link infant homeostasis with gut microbes and their emergent functions once stably assembled in a community. In mammals, microbiota thrive within the gastrointestinal tract (GIT) and are enmeshed in a biochemical continuum with their multicellular host. Many of the recent advances in understanding the evolution of codependence between microbial commensal and mammals have been enabled by DNA sequencing technology. This has been primarily manifested in comparative and functional approaches, as well as facile culture-independent ecological tools to characterize microbial succession early in life. In addition, development of analytical instrumentation and techniques has led to the systematic characterization of milk glycan biology at the often-ambiguous interface between infant and microbe. Thus, the union of systems biology with glycochemistry has revealed exciting, albeit fundamental, scientific tenets that link lactation with microbial community structure strongly suggesting functional imperatives.

2. MILK OLIGOSACCHARIDES PROMOTE BENEFICIAL MICROBIAL POPULATIONS

2.1 AN HISTORICAL PERSPECTIVE ON THE MILK-BORNE BIFIDUS FACTOR

Consistent with their relatively high concentrations in breastfed infant stool, the first bifidobacteria were initially isolated in 1899 by Tissier and termed *Bacillus bifidus*.

Prebiotics and Probiotics in Human Milk. http://dx.doi.org/10.1016/B978-0-12-802725-7.00006-3

At the time, it was generally understood that nursing infants maintained a distinct set of bacteria relative to those that received breast milk formula (Gyorgy et al., 1954b). The observation that breastfed infants often harbor a gut microbiota replete with bifidobacteria, thus less diverse than at other developmental stages, has been since repeated using a variety of culture-independent and -dependent techniques (Yatsunenko et al., 2012; Harmsen et al., 2000). This has led to a scientific interest into the precise molecular mechanism, or "bifidus factor," as the unknown effector secreted in breast milk. Accordingly, pioneering work by Paul György and colleagues focused on the oligosaccharide fraction of milk carbohydrates as the responsible molecular agent in stimulating bifidobacterial growth (Gyorgy et al., 1954a,b; Gauhe et al., 1954). These human milk oligosaccharides (HMOs) were partially purified and used by *Bifidobacterium bifidum* var. *pennsylvanicus* in pure culture. Despite a clear provenance having been isolated from a breastfed infant, this strain has had several taxonomic iterations since these early experiments. Several decades passed until scientific interest in the prebiotic or bifidogenic effect of these soluble milk glycans were renewed, in part due to technological innovations to enable their study. HMO regulation of beneficial microbes is inexorably linked to its antimicrobial and anti-adhesive properties that guide the composition and likely function of the developing infant microbiome. Although György and contemporaries did not explore microbial community interactions, they were prescient in describing HMOs that could be potentially used by bacteria.

2.2 BIFIDOBACTERIAL ENRICHMENT WITHIN THE BREASTFED INFANT MICROBIOME

Following birth, microbes sampled from the local environment rapidly colonize niches along the infant GIT. These microbes may be associated with mother, other caregivers, and the local built environment of the hospital or home (Adlerberth and Wold, 2009; Weng and Walker, 2013). In general, microbial succession within the infant GIT typically follows a nonrandom pattern of assembly as facultative anaerobes colonize early to be replaced by strict anaerobic genera such as *Bifidobacterium* and *Bacteroides* (Matamoros et al., 2013). There are notable exceptions that are dependent on birth mode (i.e., vaginal vs caesarian) or biological variation between individuals, but the microbiome generally converges on an adult-like community composition within the first 3 years of life (Palmer et al., 2007; Groer et al., 2014; Dominguez-Bello et al., 2010). Diet has been implicated as a central driver in guiding the population structures of the infant gut microbiome with both culture-dependent and -independent approaches. Accordingly, bifidobacteria often dominate the developing breastfed neonatal distal colon relative to their distribution in adults (Yatsunenko et al., 2012; Harmsen et al., 2000; Scholtens et al., 2012). This includes several bifidobacterial species or subspecies that are repeatedly isolated from infants, hinting at adaptations to allow colonization of this ecological niche. Specifically, *Bifidobacterium breve*, *B. bifidum*, *Bifidobacterium catenulatum*, and *Bifidobacterium pseudocatenulatum* are frequently isolated from infant fecal specimens. Moreover, *Bifidobacterium longum* is a typical colonizer of the infant GIT. The taxonomic definition of this species has been revised regularly over time, but now includes a few subspecies including *B. longum* subsp. *longum* (*B. longum*) as well as *B. longum* subsp. *infantis* (*B. infantis*) (Scholtens et al., 2012; Avershina et al., 2013; Roger et al., 2010; Ruiz-Moyano et al., 2013). The former subspecies is more prevalent in adult communities, whereas the latter represents the archetypical HMO using bacterium that is believed to exclusively colonize infants (Turroni et al., 2012; Sela and Mills, 2010).

Anecdotal evidence on the geographic distribution of infant-associated bifidobacteria has been observed. Although it is currently unclear to what extent cultural or spatial separation contributes to phylogenetic variation in the bifidobacterial fraction of the infant microbiome. Yatsunenko and colleagues performed a seminal comparative study of infant microbiomes analyzed from Venezuela, rural Malawi, and US urban centers demonstrated that bifidobacteria are somewhat ubiquitous regardless of geography (Yatsunenko et al., 2012), whereas other studies suggest that infants harbor higher proportions of bifidobacteria depending on the country of isolation (Fallani et al., 2010; Grzeskowiak et al., 2012). This includes the potential for asymmetrical, and perhaps unpredictable, distribution of bifidobacterial populations that use HMOs. For example, one study documented infants born in Ghana as well as in New Zealand harbored *B. infantis*, whereas infants born in the United Kingdom did not (Young et al., 2004). Clearly more research is required to fully characterize the distribution of bifidobacterial taxa across geography.

2.3 BIFIDOBACTERIA METABOLIZE OLIGOSACCHARIDES WITHIN THEIR MAMMALIAN HOSTS

Characterization of bifidobacterial physiology has largely focused on their competence for metabolizing dietary oligosaccharides. This genus deploys a suite of transmembrane permeases to access carbohydrate polymers in their otherwise nutrient-limited habitats. As such, dietary fibers including HMOs that transit intact to the distal GIT are available to promote the growth of bifidobacteria and other microbes capable of using oligosaccharides. This attribute is exploited in nutritional interventions that seek to manipulate the endogenous microbiome to promote favorable health outcomes such as increasing short-chain fatty acid production (Moro et al., 2006; Macfarlane and Cummings, 1999). These prebiotic interventions often enrich bifidobacteria in the adult gut to address irritable bowel syndrome (O'Mahony et al., 2005) and inflammatory bowel diseases (O'Mahony et al., 2008; Furrie et al., 2005), prevent and manage diarrhea (Chouraqui et al., 2004), increase digestive efficiency of carbohydrate polymers (Flint et al., 2008), modulate the immune system (Klein et al., 2008), and erect a barrier to pathogenic colonization (Madsen et al., 2001; Lievin et al., 2000). Though it is the somewhat unique phenotype that bifidobacteria efficiently harness HMO carbon for biomass and adenosine triphosphate generation that has garnered current scientific attention. Thus, HMOs' role in the establishment of an early microbiota is the model by which other dietary oligosaccharide-based bifidogenic interventions are conceived.

2.4 STRUCTURE–FUNCTION RELATIONSHIPS ASCRIBED TO THE HUMAN MILK OLIGOSACCHARIDES

As will be discussed in greater detail elsewhere in this book, human milk contains a high concentration of soluble glycans that contribute to the third most abundant class of molecules (Coppa et al., 1993). The HMO concentrations in breast milk vary by individual and declines over the course of lactation, but it is generally understood to be present at ≥4 g/L in milk, with higher levels observed in colostrum (Chaturvedi et al., 2001; Asakuma et al., 2008). HMOs incorporate five monosaccharide residues—D-glucose, D-galactose, *N*-acetylglucosamine, L-fucose, and *N*-acetylneuraminic acid (Neu5Ac)—linked in various configurations. A lactosyl residue (Galβ1-4Glc) is typically found at the reducing end of the molecule that is elongated with several repeating *N*-acetyllactosamine units (Galβ1-3/4GlcNAc) via a β1-3 linkage. Branched isomers possess an additional β1-6 linkage. Additional structural diversity may be provided by terminal fucosylation at α1-2/3/4 linkages and α2-3 and α2-6 sialylation. To date, almost 200 distinct HMO species have been identified in pooled breast milk samples (Ninonuevo et al., 2006). When considering the combinatorial potential emanating from diverse glycosidic bonds linking five potential residues, the appearance of relatively few structures may reflect a functional constraint such as modulating specific populations within the microbial community. Accordingly, HMO biosynthesis is driven by maternal genotype such as allelic variation in Lewis and secretor status (Kunz et al., 2000). Interestingly, lactating mothers homozygous for the inactive α-1,2-fucosyltransferase gene promote a different bifidobacterial representation when compared to secretor mothers (Lewis et al., 2015).

Once consumed, HMOs largely escape hydrolysis by digestive enzymes and the acidic conditions experienced in the stomach (Gnoth et al., 2000; Engfer et al., 2000). Thus, HMOs remain intact on entry to the colon where they may exert bioactive functions such as enriching beneficial microbial populations. In addition, HMOs passively immunize against specific pathogens to be discussed in detail in subsequent sections. Briefly, some microbial pathogens or infectious particles adhere to mucins or epithelial surface glycoconjugates. Similar motifs are incorporated into the HMO structure that enable the oligosaccharide to act as a ligand mimic. HMO decoys are active in the intestinal mucosa (Ruiz-Palacios et al., 2003; Newburg et al., 2004), in the laryngopharynx (Andersson et al., 1986), as well as the urinary tract when absorbed whole and excreted by the infant (Obermeier et al., 1999). HMOs may also direct the expression of specific host glycosyltransferases that in turn remodels epithelial glycan epitopes presented to microbes (Angeloni et al., 2005; Vanmaele et al., 1999). Furthermore, there is mounting evidence that HMOs directly modulate immune responses (Velupillai and Harn, 1994; Eiwegger et al., 2004).

2.5 BIFIDOBACTERIAL USE OF HUMAN MILK OLIGOSACCHARIDE CORE STRUCTURES

There are only certain bifidobacterial taxa that efficiently use HMOs as a sole carbon source (Ward et al., 2006, 2007; LoCascio et al., 2007, 2009). Perhaps not surprisingly, these species (or subspecies) are typically isolated from the infant GIT including *B. infantis*, which is regarded as the archetypical HMO consumer (Sela et al., 2008). The HMO utilization phenotype is conserved within the *B. infantis* lineage, whereas other infant-associated bifidobacteria exhibit strain-specific variation in their ability to use host glycans (Garrido et al., 2015). This includes variation in the manner by which *B. bifidum* and *B. breve* hydrolyze and catabolize HMO constituent monosaccharides or disaccharides (Ward et al., 2007; LoCascio et al., 2009), thus, suggesting that niche partitioning has segregated bifidobacterial phylotypes with the potential for syntrophy. In this scenario, bifidobacteria may not directly access HMO carbon but are aided by heterologous species to liberate monosaccharide residues for use. This is consistent with the metatranscriptome determined from bifidobacteria that colonize the infant microbiome with an enrichment for carbohydrate utilization functions (Gonzalez et al., 2008).

Mass spectrometry–based glycoprofiling has enabled further quantitative characterization of the HMO consumption phenotype at high resolution (Ninonuevo et al., 2006; De Leoz et al., 2015). Accordingly, analyses of glycans that remain in spent culture supernatants indicate that infant-associated bifidobacteria are generally competent at using lacto-*N*-tetraose (LNT; Galβ1-3GlcNAc β1-3 Galβ1-4Glc) or lacto-*N*-neotetraose (LNnT; Galβ1-4GlcNAc β1-3 Galβ1-4Glc) (LoCascio et al., 2007, 2009), whereas *B. infantis* fully diminishes the tetrasaccharide reservoir, *B. longum*, *B. bifidum*, and *B. breve* could only partially degrade this structure, if at all (LoCascio et al., 2009). Interestingly, adult-associated bifidobacteria, such as *B. adolescentis* and *B. animalis*, are unable to use the HMO core structure.

The HMO core structure integrates a repeating lactosamine element (Galβ1-4GlcNAc) or lacto-*N*-biose (LNB; Galβ1-3GlcNAc). In order to synthesize LNB, Le Châtelier's principle could be leveraged to reverse glycolytic reactions of glycolytic enzymes to produce kilogram scale products (Nishimoto and Kitaoka, 2007; Baumgartner et al., 2015). Whereas oligosaccharide separation and purification from fluid milk may not be commercially viable, in vitro synthesis and fermentation represent a significant advance to enable HMO–microbial interaction research (Lee et al., 2012). Accordingly, the LNB disaccharide is used by a variety of bifidobacterial species that otherwise cannot catabolize the full HMO structure (Kiyohara et al., 2009). In these instances, LNB serves as a research proxy for HMOs despite not typically isolated from human milk and lacks the structure–function potential of HMOs (Bode and Jantscher-Krenn, 2012). In this regard, LNB may be functionally similar to trisaccharides such as fucosyllactose and sialyllactose. Interestingly, *B. infantis* does not metabolize fucosyllactose and sialyllactose in the same manner as pooled HMOs, purified LNT, or even lactose (Garrido et al., 2015), although the precise regulation of mechanisms deployed by *B. infantis* has yet to be characterized in full.

Contrasting with *B. infantis*, other infant-associated bifidobacteria consume HMOs by secreting extracellular enzymes prior to capturing subsequent carbohydrate degradation products. Accordingly, *B. bifidum* secretes an extracellular 1,2-α-L-fucosidase (EC 3.2.1.63) that cleaves terminal 1,2-α-fucosyl linkages that shield galactose residues in LNB, thus permitting downstream catabolism to proceed (Katayama et al., 2004; Nagae et al., 2007). In addition, a lacto-*N*-biosidase (EC 3.2.1.140) liberates LNB from lacto-*N*-tetraose and other HMO compositions that lack fucosylation or sialylation (Wada et al., 2008). Once soluble, LNB is transported across the cell membrane by a dedicated ABC transporter that integrates an LNB binding subunit (Suzuki et al., 2008; Wada et al., 2007). Interestingly, *B. longum* uses an endo-α-*N*-acetylgalactosaminidase (EC 3.2.1.97) to extract galacto-*N*-biose (GNB) from *O*-linked mucin glycans (Fujita et al., 2005). Indeed, the presence of both endo-α-*N*-acetylgalactosaminidase and fucosidase activity enables *B. bifidum* to degrade mucin, as both genes are upregulated in the presence of porcine mucin (Ruas-Madiedo et al., 2008). Once internalized, an intracellular phosphorylase cleaves LNB or GNB disaccharides derived from milk oligosaccharides or mucin glycoproteins, respectively (Kitaoka et al., 2005; Nishimoto and Kitaoka, 2007a). Finally, a modified Leloir pathway feeds LNB or GNB degradation products into the central fermentative bifid shunt in order generate adenosine triphosphate for the bifidobacterial cell (Nishimoto and Kitaoka, 2007b).

2.6 THE *B. INFANTIS* GENOME HAS EVOLVED TO USE SHORT-CHAIN HUMAN MILK OLIGOSACCHARIDE COMPOSITIONS

Although *B. infantis* is not the only bifidobacterial species isolated from infants, its evolutionary trajectory has been greatly dictated through interacting with HMOs (Sela et al., 2008). At the present, much of what is understood about microbial metabolism of HMOs has been garnered by studying *B. infantis* growth on purified HMOs as a sole carbon source (Ward et al., 2006). The direct or indirect impacts that HMOs exert on other members of the infant microbiome or as an entire community has only recently emerged (Donovan et al., 2012; Underwood et al., 2015; Frese et al., 2015; Marcobal et al., 2011). Thus, *B. infantis* is the primary model organism to study the influence of HMOs on host–microbial interactions. Moreover, *B. infantis* prominently exhibits the differentiating phenotype of consuming abundant small-mass HMO species, whereas other bifidobacteria may only use LNT-like tetrasaccharides, albeit incompletely if at all (LoCascio et al., 2007).

Accordingly, *B. infantis* ATCC 15,697 and other strains possess several discernible genomic features underlying the HMO consumption phenotype (Sela et al., 2008). The *B. infantis* genome exhibits a lineage-specific expansion of solute binding protein genes that bind and import soluble milk glycans (Garrido et al., 2011). This includes LNB and fucosylated motifs that are recognized and are embedded within the core HMO structure. In addition to oligosaccharide transport, the *B. infantis* genome integrates several glycosyl hydrolases arranged in catabolic clusters that are used to cleave HMOs once imported into the cell (Garrido et al., 2012;

Sela et al., 2011, 2012). These loci are often arranged with a transport system (e.g., ABC transporter) co-localized with glycosyl hydrolases, and in some instances genes that are involved in carbohydrate catabolism. Of particular note is 43-kbp gene cluster composed of about 30 genes that share a common transcriptional orientation with the exception of a single β-galactosidase (Sela et al., 2008; LoCascio et al., 2010). This HMO cluster includes four glycosyl hydrolases active on HMO linkages, including two α-fucosidases (i.e., GH29 and GH95), α-sialidase, β-galactosidase, and β-hexosaminidase. The aggregation of genes within a bacterial genome strongly suggests participation in a metabolic pathway under common regulation. Mechanistic studies have been performed to verify these predictions. Accordingly, *B. infantis* uses acidic HMOs through an α-sialidase gene encoded within the HMO cluster (Sela et al., 2011). There is a secondary sialic acid utilization cluster, though it is currently unclear to what extent it participates in HMO utilization. Similarly, *B. infantis* uses HMO cluster α-fucosidases to utilize fucosylated oligosaccharide compositions once tetrasaccharides (e.g., LNT) are depleted (Sela et al., 2012). Both HMO cluster β-galactosidase and β-hexosaminidase are active on milk glycans as well (Garrido et al., 2012a,b, 2013). HMO-active glycoside hydrolases are interspersed amid an array of ABC-type transporters and their associated binding proteins. These oligosaccharide-binding proteins have diverged significantly over evolutionary timescales relative to homologous bifidobacterial proteins. This is consistent with their recognition and affinity toward unique HMO epitopes (Sela et al., 2008). In addition to molecular confirmation of genomic predictions, many of these genes are transcribed and proteins expressed while *B. infantis* uses HMOs (Sela et al., 2008; Garrido et al., 2015).

B. infantis and *B. longum* possess a divergent glycan utilization strategy despite close phylogenetic origins and colonizing the human gastrointestinal (GI) tract (Sela and Mills, 2010). The genomic architecture of oligosaccharide-active loci remains conserved in *B. longum*, although the quantity and identity of specific glycolytic genes diverge appreciably. A notable difference includes the oligosaccharide binding proteins that are considerably more numerous in subspecies *infantis* (Sela et al., 2008; Garrido et al., 2011; Noll et al., 2008). In addition, several subspecies *infantis* catabolic clusters are dedicated to mammalian-type glycans that are fucosylated and sialylated including the large HMO gene cluster. This is in stark contrast to subspecies *longum* that do not possess these genes, but rather the determinants required to process plant-derived xylose and arabinose-containing oligosaccharides.

2.7 BIFIDOBACTERIAL METABOLISM OF MILK OLIGOSACCHARIDES THROUGH CENTRAL METABOLISM

Much of what is known about microbial catabolism of milk oligosaccharides is provided by studies in bifidobacteria (Marcobal et al., 2010, 2011; Hunt et al., 2012). Bifidobacteria degrade hexose monosaccharides by the fructose-6-phosphate phosphoketolase (F6PK) pathway that is commonly referred to as the *bifid shunt* (Veerkamp, 1969; de Vries and Stouthamer, 1967; Scardovi, 1986). Indeed, this fermentation mode distinguishes bifidobacteria from lactic acid bacteria (LAB) despite often linked due to historical associations (de Vries and Stouthamer, 1967). The absence of a 6-phosphogluconate intermediate distinguishes LAB heterofermentation from the bifidobacterial F6PK pathway (Kandler, 1983). Infant-associated bifidobacteria do not produce CO_2 while subsisting on HMOs except certain strains capable of using gluconate (Asano et al., 2005). The F6PK pathway terminates with a theoretical yield of 1.5:1 mol acetate to lactate secreted per mole hexose consumed (de Vries and Stouthamer, 1967; Wolin et al., 1998). When measured, this yield is variable in actively growing cells, often dependent on culture conditions and growth substrates (Ruas-Madiedo et al., 2005; Amaretti et al., 2007). This may be due to rerouting intermediates into anabolic pathways. Interestingly, acetate secreted by bifidobacteria inhibits certain enteropathogens, suggesting an indirect antimicrobial influence of HMOs within the infant microbiome (Fukuda et al., 2011).

The characteristic reaction of the bifid shunt is catalyzed by the thiamin diphosphate-dependent fructose-6-phosphate phosphoketolase (F6PPK; EC 4.1.2.22). This enzyme cleaves D-fructose-6-phosphate into erythrose-4-phosphate and acetyl-1-phosphate (Scardovi and Trovatelli, 1965). The mechanism of F6PPK is well understood is often used to screen for bifidobacterial strains capable of using HMOs (Orban and Patterson, 2000). There are two known fructose-6-phosphate phosphoketolase allozymes. One is active exclusively on fructose-6-phosphate, while a second type is maintains activity on D-xylulose-5-phosphate (EC 4.1.2.9) (Sgorbati et al., 1976; Grill et al., 1995). It was previously held that the presence of one or both allozymes is correlated to whether the isolate has descended from a human-colonizing lineage (Grill et al., 1995; Yin et al., 2005). Aside from the closely related *Gardnerella vaginalis*, F6PPK has not been biochemically characterized in anaerobic bacteria outside the bifidobacteria (Gavini et al., 1996), although sequences with high identity to the bifidobacterial F6PPK appear in public databases for other *Actinobacteria* (Markowitz et al., 2008). As *G. vaginalis* is a common member of the vaginal microbiome, it is tempting to speculate that a common ancestor to infant- and mother-associated *Actinobacteria* may have evolved to colonize these niches.

Carbon derived from HMO catabolism enters central metabolism as monosaccharides or smaller molecules. Accordingly, HMO metabolic flux has been investigated using isotopomers to verify its in vivo catabolism. Acetate produced while fermenting HMOs is either secreted or used in de novo fatty acid synthesis, the latter recruiting the multidomain fatty acid synthase I common to both *Actinobacteria* and eukaryotes (Schweizer and Hofmann, 2004). As such, metabolic flux through central metabolism is monitored by perturbing isotopomer ratios in fatty acids to be detected by gas chromatography–mass spectrometry (Price et al., 2006). After uptake of various ^{13}C-labeled sugars by bifidobacteria, the fractional distribution of ^{13}C into carbohydrate and fatty acid metabolites were analyzed by mass spectrometry. This analysis verified that both sialic acid (Neu5Ac) and a pool of HMO compositions enter the central metabolic pathway common to all bifidobacteria (Sela et al., 2008). Interestingly, the in vivo fate of fucose is less readily apparent as it does not enter the bifid shunt.

2.8 HUMAN MILK OLIGOSACCHARIDE–BOUND GALACTOSE METABOLISM IN THE BIFIDOBACTERIA

Lacto-*N*-biose phosphorylase (LNBP or GLNBP; EC 2.4.1.211) hydrolyzes LNB and GNB disaccharide subunits that repeat in HMOs and mucin glycoproteins, respectively (Kitaoka et al., 2005). First characterized in *B. longum* NCC2705, LNBP cleaves both LNB and GNB into D-galactose-1-phosphate and an *N*-acetylhexosamine with anomeric inversion. LNBP is encoded within a putative galactose operon conserved in bifidobacterial genomes that are capable of using these substrates (Kitaoka et al., 2005; Markowitz et al., 2008). Furthermore, the crystal structure of the *B. longum* JCM1217 LNBP protein has been solved while complexed with molecules secreted in milk (Hidaka et al., 2009).

2.9 REGULATION OF HUMAN MILK OLIGOSACCHARIDES AND OTHER OLIGOSACCHARIDE METABOLISM IN BIFIDOBACTERIA

The co-localization of the HMO cluster in the *B. infantis* genome suggests shared regulation in response to HMO substrates, although regulation of genes that encode HMO active proteins is poorly understood. In general, bifidobacteria exhibit a preference for lactose over glucose by tuning their transport systems (Parche et al., 2006; Kim et al., 2003; van den Bogaard et al., 2000). This is atypical for bacteria and may reflect their evolution within the breastfed infant's colon. A potential benefit of a bifidobacteria-enriched microbiome is that lactose fermentation would proceed in the absence of flatulence. However, it is unclear how much lactose would be encountered in the distal colon aside from the degradative products of HMO hydrolysis.

A global model for regulation of HMO-related functions has yet to be fully integrated despite evidence for common regulation (Garrido et al., 2015). Interestingly, certain bifidobacterial species often do not metabolize monosaccharides when presented with oligosaccharides. Again, this is unusual for host-associated microbiota unless specifically adapted to utilize polymerized carbohydrates such as HMO (Amaretti et al., 2006).

3. DIETARY OLIGOSACCHARIDES MIMIC HUMAN MILK OLIGOSACCHARIDES IN HOST–MICROBIAL INTERACTIONS

There are several nutritional strategies to rationally mimic the influence of milk oligosaccharides on infant-colonizing microbiota. This is primarily intended to enrich for bifidobacteria in a prebiotic approach. HMO mimetics are broadly classified as plant-derived fructo-oligosaccharides (FOS) or dairy-derived galacto-oligosaccharides (GOS). Both classes lack the complexity inherent to HMOs in terms of monosaccharide composition, linkage diversity and structural organization. Nevertheless, HMO mimetics represent an expanding area of scientific interest as in vitro and clinical evidence support their efficacy (Kruse et al., 1999; Roberfroid et al., 1998; Gibson et al., 1995).

These oligosaccharides are commercially distributed, as their production is currently more favorable than HMO purification or synthesis. It remains unclear, however, if molecules designed to mimic HMOs exhibit the full complement of immunological and pathogen deflection functions ascribed to milk oligosaccharides.

3.1 PLANT-DERIVED HUMAN MILK OLIGOSACCHARIDE MIMETICS

Inulin FOS are highly abundant in dietary plant material such as chicory, garlic, and sunchokes. Inulin-type FOS are a simple biopolymer (DP 2-60) of β-(2–1) linked D-fructose residues with the degree of polymerization dependent on the purification regime and plant origin (Wang et al., 1999; Roberfroid, 2005). A D-glucose moiety is often found at the terminus linked by an α-(1-2) linkage as in sucrose (Niness, 1999). Conversely, oligofructose (OF) DPs range between 2 and 10 and is derived from chicory or synthesized via transfructosylation. OF extracted from plants possess a fraction retaining terminal glucosyl moieties, whereas synthetic OF does not. Both inulin and OF are collectively referred to as FOS and differ primarily in degree of polymerization. As with soluble glucose, the theoretical ratio of acetic acid to lactic acid yield is 1.5 while growing on fructose.

OF is incorporated into formula milk and other foods impact GI microbial communities. Specifically, *Bacteroides* spp. metabolize OF well relative to bifidobacteria. Both *Bacteroides* thetaiotamicron LMG 11,262 and *B. fragilis* LMG 10,263 efficiently grow on OF. As with HMO, *B. longum* prefer shorter-chain OF fractions prior to consuming longer chains. This union of phenotypes may be indicative of overlapping physiological systems converging on oligosaccharide utilization. In contrast, *Bacteroides* strains that colonize infants do not exhibit a preference for OF species size. Glycosyl hydrolase subcellular localization may contribute to this differential phenotype. Accordingly, *Bacteroides* spp. secrete glycolytic enzymes into the periplasmic space, extracellular environment, or covalently anchor enzymes to surface molecules as is the case with *B. bifidum* (Xu et al., 2003). *B. infantis* degrades imported OF to potentially account for slower growth kinetics on these substrates (Van der Meulen et al., 2006). Efficient oligosaccharide translocation underlies an evolutionary stable strategy used by bifidobacteria to compete with *Bacteroides* within the infant GI tract. Furthermore, this may guide the development of next-generation HMO mimetics to replicate bifidogenic outcomes (Langlands et al., 2004; Kleessen et al., 2001).

3.2 DAIRY-DERIVED GALACTO-OLIGOSACCHARIDES THAT MIMIC HUMAN MILK OLIGOSACCHARIDES

GOS are nondigestible carbohydrates that possess bifidogenic function (reviewed in (Boehm and Stahl, 2007)). Briefly, GOS is stable during thermal processing and at low pH, properties that favor its incorporation in food formulations including synthetic milk. GOS is often manufactured by manipulating galactose concentrations in the presence of recombinant β-galactosidase to reverse the glycolytic reaction or *trans*-galactosylation. This process is relatively inefficient and monosaccharides and disaccharides often contaminate GOS yields unless the mixture is further purified.

The core structure of GOS incorporates a lactose residue at the reducing end from which is galactosyl units elongate ([Gal(β1-]$_{1\text{-}6}$3/4/6)Gal(β1-4)Glc). *Trans*-galactosylation is primarily performed on lactose-rich whey derivatives as the substrate (Yanahira et al., 1995). As with FOS, the structural diversity potential is markedly less than that of HMOs. Human milk lactose binds a large fraction of galactose, as do soluble oligosaccharides and glycoconjugates. This may have inadvertently perpetuated confusion that endogenous GOS is present in significant quantities in the human milk glycome (Macfarlane et al., 2008; Boehm et al., 2005). Whereas some short-chain galactosyllactose [Gal(β1-3/4/6)Gal(β1-4)Glc] has been detected in millimolar concentrations in human milk, these particular carbohydrates are three to four orders of magnitude lower than the HMO pool (Sumiyoshi et al., 2004).

In order to process GOS, bacteria deploy β-galactosidases (EC 3.2.1.23) to cleave terminal β-galactosyl linkages. Accordingly, β-galactosidases have been identified and biochemically characterized from a variety of bifidobacteria and *Bacteroides* from the infant GIT (Garrido et al., 2013; Jantscher-Krenn et al., 2012; Barboza et al., 2009; Turroni et al., 2010; Miwa et al., 2010). Species of these two genera may encode multiple isozymes in their genomes and are differentially induced by various substrates. Adult responders to GOS interventions carry more bifidobacteria, as well as certain infant populations receiving supplemented formula (Davis et al., 2011; Giovannini et al., 2014; Sierra et al., 2015).

4. ANTIADHESIVE AND ANTIMICROBIAL PROPERTIES OF HUMAN MILK OLIGOSACCHARIDES

One primary role by which HMOs influence the structure of the neonatal microbiome is through enrichment of specific bacterial taxa. Human milk guides the microbial community via antiadhesive properties inherent to HMO structures in addition to prebiotic function. Accordingly, several studies have characterized the antiadhesive attributes of milk oligosaccharides and other glycoconjugates on a variety of infectious particles or microbes. There are several review articles as of 2015 on the topic, and this constitutes an area of recent and rapid scientific advances (Bode, 2009, 2012; Ballard and Morrow, 2013; Newburg et al., 2005).

In general, human milk-fed infants experience lower incidences of gastroenteritis. Often GI pathogens bind to epithelial cell surfaces as an initial step in disease. This attachment is often mediated by glycans covalently linked to the epithelial surface including lipid and protein conjugates dissolved in the membrane. Structurally similar HMO isomers or subunits may function as an antiadhesive decoy to block pathogen binding. When pathogen lectins bind soluble HMOs, cells remain detached from the targeted tissue surface and are cleared through GIT motility. Specific bacterial pathogens have been demonstrated to interact with cognate glycan epitopes common to milk oligosaccharides. This includes *Campylobacter jejuni*, a causative agent in bacterial diarrhea, that binds α-1,2-fucosyl (H2) residues, the H2 activity blocked in vitro infections in cell culture as well as in vivo infections in a mouse model (Ruiz-Palacios et al., 2003).

Coppa et al. (2006) further ascribed this decoy activity to neutral HMOs as a molecular class as it blocks gastrointestinal pathogens including *Escherichia coli*, *Salmonella* spp., and *Vibrio cholerae*. Interestingly, sialylated HMOs conferred an antiadhesive effect against all bacteria studied in vitro, whereas neutral species exerted a size-dependent effect. This built on earlier work that demonstrated that acidic milk oligosaccharides block UPEC *E. coli* strains.

5. HUMAN MILK OLIGOSACCHARIDES IN PASSIVE ANTIVIRAL IMMUNITY

In addition to bacterial constituents of the infant microbiome, providing HMOs to the nursing infant may mitigate certain infectious particles. This includes the human immunodeficiency virus (HIV-1) that deploys a specific glycoprotein (i.e., gp120) to bind dendritic cells. Certain HMO species mimic Lewis blood groups antigens and thus compete with gp120 to bind dendritic cell receptors and thus reduce HIV-1 mother-to-child infection (Hong et al., 2009; Naarding et al., 2005). Indeed, lactating mothers infected with HIV have a higher abundance of 3'-sialyllactose in their milk compared to uninfected mothers (Van Niekerk et al., 2014). Interestingly, and in the same study, infants receiving milk containing lower concentrations of disiayl-lacto-*N*-tetraose (DSLNT) were at increased risk to develop necrotizing enterocolitis (NEC). This is consistent with a previous study in which DSLNT reduced NEC outcomes in a rat model (Jantscher-Krenn et al., 2012). Monosialylated LNT did not exhibit a similar effect, demonstrating a structure-specific influence.

Noroviruses are a major cause of gastroenteritis across geographies and human development (Glass et al., 2009; Bull et al., 2006). Interestingly, individuals who do not express the H receptor antigen have greater resistance to norovirus infections (Bull et al., 2006; Morrow et al., 2005). Thus, milk from a secretor mother blocks Norwalk virus attachment in vitro (Marionneau et al., 2002). Moreover, both secretor and Lewis antigens from human milk block norovirus from binding to cognate receptors, as later confirmed in a cohort study of infants (Jiang et al., 2004; Morrow et al., 2004). In this latter study, calicivirus-induced diarrhea was significantly lower in infants fed milk with high levels of lacto-*N*-difucohexose that display α-1,2-fucosyl moieties. Interestingly, HMOs did not significantly prevent the onset of rotavirus infection but reduced the duration of diarrhea in a piglet model through manipulating endogenous microbiota and tuning the immune response (Li et al., 2014).

Influenza viruses are of major concern to infants, who are particularly susceptible due in part to immunological immaturity (Munoz, 2003). Although clinical approaches are required to confirm antiadhesive efficacy, it is notable that human and bovine milk oligosaccharide structures may act as receptor mimics. This includes 6′-sialyllactose, 3′-sialyllactose, and 6′-sialyl-*N*-acetyllactosamine (Matrosovich et al., 1993). Finally, HMOs may also reduce susceptibility to respiratory syncytial virus (Portelli et al., 1998).

6. EVIDENCE FOR FUNGAL ANTIADHESIVE PROPERTIES OF HUMAN MILK OLIGOSACCHARIDES

There is a limited amount of studies performed to characterize the antiadhesive properties of HMOs toward fungal pathogens. This may be due in part to the relatively low concentration of commensal yeasts and fungi in the infant microbiome (Koenig et al., 2011). Nevertheless, fucosylated HMOs are known to inhibit certain *Candida* pathogens from binding to intestinal epithelia (Brassart et al., 1991). Again, antiadhesive activity was linked to an α-1,2 fucosyl determinant, suggesting that this structure acts as a host receptor for *Candida albicans* on the buccal epithelial surface. *C. albicans* is relevant as it often contributes to the etiology of NEC when colonizing the infant gut (Heisel et al., 2015; Saiman et al., 2001; Coates et al., 2005). Indeed, recent work demonstrates that HMOs reduce the invasion of premature intestinal epithelial cells by *C. albicans* in a dose-dependent manner (Gonia et al., 2015). In this study, HMOs inhibited hyphal growth and morphological development of the yeast cell. This is evidence of a structure–function antimicrobial activity, although, in general, potential interactions of HMOs and other milk glycans with the fungal fraction of the infant microbiome remain underexplored. This is despite the variety of lectins deployed by host-associated fungal microorganisms (Imberty et al., 2005).

7. HUMAN MILK OLIGOSACCHARIDES PREVENT THE ATTACHMENT OF A EUKARYOTIC PARASITE

Entamoeba histolytica infects more than 50 million people globally, causing amebiasis in mostly non-Western countries (Bode, 2015). This parasite expresses a surface lectin that enables attachment to the intestinal epithelia lining the gut and subsequent phagocytosis (Saffer and Petri Jr, 1991). Accordingly, physiological concentrations of purified HMOs detach *E. histolytica* by more than 80% and are capable of rescuing damaged epithelia cells (Jantscher-Krenn et al., 2012). Interestingly, HMOs were not observed to block *G. lamblia* attachment in the same in vitro model. This suggests that the oligosaccharides interfere with a specific adhesion mechanism such as the *E. histolytica* lectin, which is a known virulence factor.

8. CONCLUSIONS

The role of human milk in the evolution of our species and all mammals is centered on delivery of nutrition to the developing neonate. In addition, there are several bioactive molecules secreted in milk that benefit the infant beyond basal nutritive value.

This, of course, includes indigestible glycans that interact with the nascent microbiota harbored by the infant. HMOs participate in both positively and negatively regulating the composition of the infant microbiome through prebiotic and antiadhesive roles, respectively. Further scientific investigations of this important host–microbial interaction early in life will resolve fundamental biological questions regarding the developmental trajectory and metabolic homeostasis of our species. Moreover, there are several clear applications motivated by impacting infant health to be discussed in greater detail in this book. In the near term, advances in experimental models and clinical studies will likely elucidate causal linkages between specific oligosaccharide structures, microbial population and community responses, and impacts to infant physiology. Thus, linking specific HMO structures with infant physiology as transduced through the microbiome will yield diagnostic biomarkers and clear targets for clinical interventions.

REFERENCES

Adlerberth, I., Wold, A.E., 2009. Establishment of the gut microbiota in Western infants. Acta Paediatrica 98 (2), 229–238.

Amaretti, A., et al., 2006. Substrate preference of *Bifidobacterium adolescentis* MB 239: compared growth on single and mixed carbohydrates. Applied Microbiology and Biotechnology 73 (3), 654–662.

Amaretti, A., et al., 2007. Kinetics and metabolism of *Bifidobacterium adolescentis* MB 239 growing on glucose, galactose, lactose, and galactooligosaccharides. Applied and Environmental Microbiology 73 (11), 3637–3644.

Andersson, B., et al., 1986. Inhibition of attachment of *Streptococcus pneumoniae* and *Haemophilus influenzae* by human milk and receptor oligosaccharides. Journal of Infectious Diseases 153 (2), 232–237.

Angeloni, S., et al., 2005. Glycoprofiling with micro-arrays of glycoconjugates and lectins. Glycobiology 15 (1), 31–41.

Asakuma, S., et al., 2008. Variation of major neutral oligosaccharides levels in human colostrum. European Journal of Clinical Nutrition 62 (4), 488–494.

Asano, T., et al., 2005. Isolation rates of gluconate-fermenting bifidobacteria from human faeces. Microbial Ecology in Health & Disease 17 (2), 114–120.

Avershina, E., et al., 2013. Bifidobacterial succession and correlation networks in a large unselected cohort of mothers and their children. Applied and Environmental Microbiology 79 (2), 497–507.

Ballard, O., Morrow, A.L., 2013. Human milk composition: nutrients and bioactive factors. Pediatric Clinics of North America 60 (1), 49–74.

Barboza, M., et al., 2009. Glycoprofiling bifidobacterial consumption of galacto-oligosaccharides by mass spectrometry reveals strain-specific, preferential consumption of glycans. Applied and Environmental Microbiology 75 (23), 7319–7325.

Baumgartner, F., et al., 2015. Synthesis of fucosylated lacto-N-tetraose using whole-cell biotransformation. Bioorganic & Medicinal Chemistry.

Bode, L., Jantscher-Krenn, E., 2012. Structure-function relationships of human milk oligosaccharides. Advances in Nutrition 3 (3), 383S–391S.

Bode, L., 2009. Human milk oligosaccharides: prebiotics and beyond. Nutrition Reviews 67 (Suppl. 2), S183–S191.

Bode, L., 2012. Human milk oligosaccharides: every baby needs a sugar mama. Glycobiology 22 (9), 1147–1162.

Bode, L., 2015. The functional biology of human milk oligosaccharides. Early Human Development 91 (11), 619–622.

Boehm, G., et al., 2005. Prebiotic carbohydrates in human milk and formulas. Acta Paediatrica Supplement 94 (449), 18–21.

Boehm, G., Stahl, B., 2007. Oligosaccharides from milk. Journal of Nutrition 137 (3 Suppl. 2), S847–S849.

Brassart, D., et al., 1991. In vitro inhibition of adhesion of *Candida albicans* clinical isolates to human buccal epithelial cells by Fuc alpha 1---2Gal beta-bearing complex carbohydrates. Infection and Immunity 59 (5), 1605–1613.

Bull, R.A., et al., 2006. Emergence of a new norovirus genotype II.4 variant associated with global outbreaks of gastroenteritis. Journal of Clinical Microbiology 44 (2), 327–333.

Chaturvedi, P., et al., 2001. Fucosylated human milk oligosaccharides vary between individuals and over the course of lactation. Glycobiology 11 (5), 365–372.

Chouraqui, J.P., Van Egroo, L.D., Fichot, M.C., 2004. Acidified milk formula supplemented with *Bifidobacterium lactis*: impact on infant diarrhea in residential care settings. Journal of Pediatric Gastroenterology and Nutrition 38 (3), 288–292.

Coates, E.W., et al., 2005. Distinctive distribution of pathogens associated with peritonitis in neonates with focal intestinal perforation compared with necrotizing enterocolitis. Pediatrics 116 (2), e241–246.

Coppa, G.V., et al., 1993. Changes in carbohydrate composition in human milk over 4 months of lactation. Pediatrics 91 (3), 637–641.

Coppa, G.V., et al., 2006. Human milk oligosaccharides inhibit the adhesion to Caco-2 cells of diarrheal pathogens: *Escherichia coli*, *Vibrio cholerae*, and *Salmonella fyris*. Pediatric Research 59 (3), 377–382.

Davis, L.M., et al., 2011. Barcoded pyrosequencing reveals that consumption of galactooligosaccharides results in a highly specific bifidogenic response in humans. PLoS ONE 6 (9), e25200.

De Leoz, M.L., et al., 2015. Human milk glycomics and gut microbial genomics in infant feces show a correlation between human milk oligosaccharides and gut microbiota: a proof-of-concept study. Journal of Proteome Research 14 (1), 491–502.

de Vries, W., Stouthamer, A.H., 1967. Pathway of glucose fermentation in relation to the taxonomy of bifidobacteria. Journal of Bacteriology 93 (2), 574–576.

Dominguez-Bello, M.G., et al., 2010. Delivery mode shapes the acquisition and structure of the initial microbiota across multiple body habitats in newborns. Proceedings of the National Academy of Sciences of the United States of America 107 (26), 11971–11975.

Donovan, S.M., et al., 2012. Host-microbe interactions in the neonatal intestine: role of human milk oligosaccharides. Advances in Nutrition 3 (3), S450–S455.

Eiwegger, T., et al., 2004. Human milk–derived oligosaccharides and plant-derived oligosaccharides stimulate cytokine production of cord blood T-cells in vitro. Pediatric Research 56 (4), 536–540.

Engfer, M.B., et al., 2000. Human milk oligosaccharides are resistant to enzymatic hydrolysis in the upper gastrointestinal tract. American Journal of Clinical Nutrition 71 (6), 1589–1596.

Fallani, M., et al., 2010. Intestinal microbiota of 6-week-old infants across Europe: geographic influence beyond delivery mode, breast-feeding, and antibiotics. Journal of Pediatric Gastroenterology and Nutrition 51 (1), 77–84.

Flint, H.J., et al., 2008. Polysaccharide utilization by gut bacteria: potential for new insights from genomic analysis. Nature Reviews Microbiology 6 (2), 121–131.

Frese, S.A., et al., 2015. Diet shapes the gut microbiome of pigs during nursing and weaning. Microbiome 3, 28.
Fujita, K., et al., 2005. Identification and molecular cloning of a novel glycoside hydrolase family of core 1 type O-glycan-specific endo-alpha-N-acetylgalactosaminidase from *Bifidobacterium longum*. Journal of Biological Chemistry 280 (45), 37415–37422.
Fukuda, S., et al., 2011. Bifidobacteria can protect from enteropathogenic infection through production of acetate. Nature 469 (7331), 543–547.
Furrie, E., et al., 2005. Synbiotic therapy (*Bifidobacterium longum*/Synergy 1) initiates resolution of inflammation in patients with active ulcerative colitis: a randomised controlled pilot trial. Gut 54 (2), 242–249.
Garrido, D., et al., 2011. Oligosaccharide binding proteins from *Bifidobacterium longum* subsp. *infantis* reveal a preference for host glycans. PLoS ONE 6 (3), e17315.
Garrido, D., et al., 2012a. Endo-beta-N-acetylglucosaminidases from infant gut-associated bifidobacteria release complex N-glycans from human milk glycoproteins. Molecular & Cell Proteomics 11 (9), 775–785.
Garrido, D., et al., 2013. Utilization of galactooligosaccharides by *Bifidobacterium longum* subsp. *infantis* isolates. Food Microbiology 33 (2), 262–270.
Garrido, D., et al., 2015. Comparative transcriptomics reveals key differences in the response to milk oligosaccharides of infant gut-associated bifidobacteria. Scientific Reports 5, 13517.
Garrido, D., Ruiz-Moyano, S., Mills, D.A., 2012b. Release and utilization of N-acetyl-D-glucosamine from human milk oligosaccharides by *Bifidobacterium longum* subsp. *infantis*. Anaerobe 18 (4), 430–435.
Gauhe, A., et al., 1954. Bifidus factor. IV. Preparations obtained from human milk. Archives of Biochemistry and Biophysics 48 (1), 214–224.
Gavini, F., et al., 1996. Detection of fructose-6-phosphate phosphoketolase (F6PPK), a key enzyme of the bifid-shunt, in *Gardnerella vaginalis*. Anaerobe 2 (3), 191–193.
Gibson, G.R., et al., 1995. Selective stimulation of bifidobacteria in the human colon by oligofructose and inulin. Gastroenterology 108 (4), 975–982.
Giovannini, M., et al., 2014. Prebiotic effect of an infant formula supplemented with galacto-oligosaccharides: randomized multicenter trial. Journal of the American College of Nutrition 33 (5), 385–393.
Glass, R.I., Parashar, U.D., Estes, M.K., 2009. Norovirus gastroenteritis. The New England Journal of Medicine 361 (18), 1776–1785.
Gnoth, M.J., et al., 2000. Human milk oligosaccharides are minimally digested in vitro. Journal of Nutrition 130 (12), 3014–3020.
Gonia, S., et al., 2015. Human milk oligosaccharides inhibit *Candida albicans* invasion of human premature intestinal epithelial cells. Journal of Nutrition 145 (9), 1992–1998.
Gonzalez, R., et al., 2008. Differential transcriptional response of *Bifidobacterium longum* to human milk, formula milk, and galactooligosaccharide. Applied and Environmental Microbiology 74 (15), 4686–4694.
Grill, J.P., Crociani, J., Ballongue, J., 1995. Characterization of fructose 6 phosphate phosphoketolases purified from Bifidobacterium species. Current Microbiology 31 (1), 49–54.
Groer, M.W., et al., 2014. Development of the preterm infant gut microbiome: a research priority. Microbiome 2, 38.
Grzeskowiak, L., et al., 2012. Distinct gut microbiota in southeastern African and northern European infants. Journal of Pediatric Gastroenterology and Nutrition 54 (6), 812–816.

Gyorgy, P., et al., 1954a. Bifidus factor. II. Its occurrence in milk from different species and in other natural products. Archives of Biochemistry and Biophysics 48 (1), 202–208.

Gyorgy, P., Norris, R.F., Rose, C.S., 1954b. Bifidus factor. I. A variant of *Lactobacillus bifidus* requiring a special growth factor. Archives of Biochemistry and Biophysics 48 (1), 193–201.

Harmsen, H.J., et al., 2000. Analysis of intestinal flora development in breast-fed and formula-fed infants by using molecular identification and detection methods. Journal of Pediatric Gastroenterology and Nutrition 30 (1), 61–67.

Heisel, T., et al., 2015. Complementary amplicon-based genomic approaches for the study of fungal communities in humans. PLoS ONE 10 (2), e0116705.

Hidaka, M., et al., 2009. The crystal structure of galacto-N-biose/lacto-N-biose I phosphorylase: a large deformation of a TIM barrel scaffold. Journal of Biological Chemistry 284 (11), 7273–7283.

Hong, P., et al., 2009. Human milk oligosaccharides reduce HIV-1-gp120 binding to dendritic cell-specific ICAM3-grabbing non-integrin (DC-SIGN). British Journal of Nutrition 101 (4), 482–486.

Hunt, K.M., et al., 2012. Human milk oligosaccharides promote the growth of staphylococci. Applied and Environmental Microbiology 78 (14), 4763–4770.

Imberty, A., Mitchell, E.P., Wimmerova, M., 2005. Structural basis of high-affinity glycan recognition by bacterial and fungal lectins. Current Opinion in Structural Biology 15 (5), 525–534.

Jantscher-Krenn, E., et al., 2012a. Human milk oligosaccharides reduce *Entamoeba histolytica* attachment and cytotoxicity in vitro. British Journal of Nutrition 108 (10), 1839–1846.

Jantscher-Krenn, E., et al., 2012b. The human milk oligosaccharide disialyllacto-N-tetraose prevents necrotising enterocolitis in neonatal rats. Gut 61 (10), 1417–1425.

Jiang, X., et al., 2004. Human milk contains elements that block binding of noroviruses to human histo-blood group antigens in saliva. Journal of Infectious Diseases 190 (10), 1850–1859.

Kandler, O., 1983. Carbohydrate metabolism in lactic acid bacteria. Antonie Van Leeuwenhoek 49 (3), 209–224.

Katayama, T., et al., 2004. Molecular cloning and characterization of *Bifidobacterium bifidum* 1,2-alpha-L-fucosidase (AfcA), a novel inverting glycosidase (glycoside hydrolase family 95). Journal of Bacteriology 186 (15), 4885–4893.

Kim, T.B., et al., 2003. Quantitative comparison of lactose and glucose utilization in *Bifidobacterium longum* cultures. Biotechnology Progress 19 (2), 672–675.

Kitaoka, M., Tian, J., Nishimoto, M., 2005. Novel putative galactose operon involving lacto-N-biose phosphorylase in *Bifidobacterium longum*. Applied and Environmental Microbiology 71 (6), 3158–3162.

Kiyohara, M., et al., 2009. Prebiotic effect of lacto-N-biose I on bifidobacterial growth. Bioscience, Biotechnology, and Biochemistry.

Kleessen, B., Hartmann, L., Blaut, M., 2001. Oligofructose and long-chain inulin: influence on the gut microbial ecology of rats associated with a human faecal flora. British Journal of Nutrition 86 (2), 291–300.

Klein, A., et al., 2008. *Lactobacillus acidophilus* 74-2 and *Bifidobacterium animalis* subsp *lactis* DGCC 420 modulate unspecific cellular immune response in healthy adults. European Journal of Clinical Nutrition 62 (5), 584–593.

Koenig, J.E., et al., 2011. Succession of microbial consortia in the developing infant gut microbiome. Proceedings of the National Academy of Sciences of the United States of America 108 (Suppl. 1), 4578–4585.

Kruse, H.P., Kleessen, B., Blaut, M., 1999. Effects of inulin on faecal bifidobacteria in human subjects. British Journal of Nutrition 82 (5), 375–382.
Kunz, C., et al., 2000. Oligosaccharides in human milk: structural, functional, and metabolic aspects. Annual Review of Nutrition 20, 699–722.
Langlands, S.J., et al., 2004. Prebiotic carbohydrates modify the mucosa associated microflora of the human large bowel. Gut 53 (11), 1610–1616.
Lee, W.H., et al., 2012. Whole cell biosynthesis of a functional oligosaccharide, 2′-fucosyllactose, using engineered *Escherichia coli*. Microbial Cell Factories 11, 48.
Lewis, Z.T., et al., 2015. Maternal fucosyltransferase 2 status affects the gut bifidobacterial communities of breastfed infants. Microbiome 3, 13.
Li, M., et al., 2014. Human milk oligosaccharides shorten rotavirus-induced diarrhea and modulate piglet mucosal immunity and colonic microbiota. ISME Journal 8 (8), 1609–1620.
Lievin, V., et al., 2000. Bifidobacterium strains from resident infant human gastrointestinal microflora exert antimicrobial activity. Gut 47 (5), 646–652.
LoCascio, R.G., et al., 2007. Glycoprofiling of bifidobacterial consumption of human milk oligosaccharides demonstrates strain specific, preferential consumption of small chain glycans secreted in early human lactation. Journal of Agricultural and Food Chemistry 55 (22), 8914–8919.
LoCascio, R.G., et al., 2009. A versatile and scalable strategy for glycoprofiling bifidobacterial consumption of human milk oligosaccharides. Microbial Biotechnology 2 (3), 333–342.
LoCascio, R.G., et al., 2010. Broad conservation of milk utilization genes in *Bifidobacterium longum* subsp. *infantis* as revealed by comparative genomic hybridization. Applied and Environmental Microbiology 76 (22), 7373–7381.
Macfarlane, G.T., Cummings, J.H., 1999. Probiotics and prebiotics: can regulating the activities of intestinal bacteria benefit health? BMJ 318 (7189), 999–1003.
Macfarlane, G.T., Steed, H., Macfarlane, S., 2008. Bacterial metabolism and health-related effects of galacto-oligosaccharides and other prebiotics. Journal of Applied Microbiology 104 (2), 305–344.
Madsen, K., et al., 2001. Probiotic bacteria enhance murine and human intestinal epithelial barrier function. Gastroenterology 121 (3), 580–591.
Marcobal, A., et al., 2010. Consumption of human milk oligosaccharides by gut-related microbes. Journal of Agricultural and Food Chemistry 58 (9), 5334–5340.
Marcobal, A., et al., 2011. Bacteroides in the infant gut consume milk oligosaccharides via mucus-utilization pathways. Cell Host Microbe 10 (5), 507–514.
Marionneau, S., et al., 2002. Norwalk virus binds to histo-blood group antigens present on gastroduodenal epithelial cells of secretor individuals. Gastroenterology 122 (7), 1967–1977.
Markowitz, V.M., et al., 2008. The integrated microbial genomes (IMG) system in 2007: data content and analysis tool extensions. Nucleic Acids Research 36 (Database issue), D528–D533.
Matamoros, S., et al., 2013. Development of intestinal microbiota in infants and its impact on health. Trends in Microbiology 21 (4), 167–173.
Matrosovich, M.N., et al., 1993. Probing of the receptor-binding sites of the H1 and H3 influenza A and influenza B virus hemagglutinins by synthetic and natural sialosides. Virology 196 (1), 111–121.
Miwa, M., et al., 2010. Cooperation of beta-galactosidase and beta-N-acetylhexosaminidase from bifidobacteria in assimilation of human milk oligosaccharides with type 2 structure. Glycobiology 20 (11), 1402–1409.

Moro, G., et al., 2006. A mixture of prebiotic oligosaccharides reduces the incidence of atopic dermatitis during the first six months of age. Archives of Disease in Childhood 91 (10), 814–819.

Morrow, A.L., et al., 2004. Human milk oligosaccharide blood group epitopes and innate immune protection against campylobacter and calicivirus diarrhea in breastfed infants. Advances in Experimental Medicine and Biology 554, 443–446.

Morrow, A.L., et al., 2005. Human-milk glycans that inhibit pathogen binding protect breast-feeding infants against infectious diarrhea. Journal of Nutrition 135 (5), 1304–1307.

Munoz, F.M., 2003. Influenza virus infection in infancy and early childhood. Paediatric Respiratory Reviews 4 (2), 99–104.

Naarding, M.A., et al., 2005. Lewis X component in human milk binds DC-SIGN and inhibits HIV-1 transfer to CD4+ T lymphocytes. Journal of Clinical Investigation 115 (11), 3256–3264.

Nagae, M., et al., 2007. Structural basis of the catalytic reaction mechanism of novel 1,2-alpha-L-fucosidase from *Bifidobacterium bifidum*. Journal of Biological Chemistry 282 (25), 18497–18509.

Newburg, D.S., et al., 2004. Innate protection conferred by fucosylated oligosaccharides of human milk against diarrhea in breastfed infants. Glycobiology 14 (3), 253–263.

Newburg, D.S., Ruiz-Palacios, G.M., Morrow, A.L., 2005. Human milk glycans protect infants against enteric pathogens. Annual Review of Nutrition 25, 37–58.

Niness, K.R., 1999. Inulin and oligofructose: what are they? Journal of Nutrition 129 (7 Suppl.), 1402S–1406S.

Ninonuevo, M.R., et al., 2006. A strategy for annotating the human milk glycome. Journal of Agricultural and Food Chemistry 54 (20), 7471–7480.

Nishimoto, M., Kitaoka, M., 2007a. Identification of the putative proton donor residue of lacto-N-biose phosphorylase (EC 2.4.1.211). Bioscience, Biotechnology, and Biochemistry 71 (6), 1587–1591.

Nishimoto, M., Kitaoka, M., 2007b. Identification of N-acetylhexosamine 1-kinase in the complete lacto-N-biose I/galacto-N-biose metabolic pathway in *Bifidobacterium longum*. Applied and Environmental Microbiology 73 (20), 6444–6449.

Nishimoto, M., Kitaoka, M., 2007c. Practical preparation of lacto-N-biose I, a candidate for the bifidus factor in human milk. Bioscience, Biotechnology, and Biochemistry 71 (8), 2101–2104.

Noll, K.M., et al., 2008. Evolution of mal ABC transporter operons in the Thermococcales and Thermotogales. BMC Evolutionary Biology 8, 7.

Obermeier, S., et al., 1999. Secretion of ^{13}C-labelled oligosaccharides into human milk and infant's urine after an oral [^{13}C]galactose load. Isotopes in Environmental and Health Studies 35 (1–2), 119–125.

O'Mahony, L., et al., 2005. Lactobacillus and Bifidobacterium in irritable bowel syndrome: symptom responses and relationship to cytokine profiles. Gastroenterology 128 (3), 541–551.

O'Mahony, C., et al., 2008. Commensal-induced regulatory T cells mediate protection against pathogen-stimulated NF-kappaB activation. PLoS Pathogens 4 (8), e1000112.

Orban, J.I., Patterson, J.A., 2000. Modification of the phosphoketolase assay for rapid identification of bifidobacteria. Journal of Microbiological Methods 40 (3), 221–224.

Palmer, C., et al., 2007. Development of the human infant intestinal microbiota. PLoS Biology 5 (7), e177.

Parche, S., et al., 2006. Lactose-over-glucose preference in *Bifidobacterium longum* NCC2705: glcP, encoding a glucose transporter, is subject to lactose repression. Journal of Bacteriology 188 (4), 1260–1265.

Portelli, J., Gordon, A., May, J.T., 1998. Effect of compounds with antibacterial activities in human milk on respiratory syncytial virus and cytomegalovirus in vitro. Journal of Medical Microbiology 47 (11), 1015–1018.

Price, N.P., Whitehead, T.R., Cote, G.L., 2006. Gas chromatography-mass spectrometry (GC-MS) techniques for metabolic flux analysis of the Bifido shunt pathway. Biocatalysis and Biotransformation 24 (1), 95–98.

Roberfroid, M.B., Van Loo, J.A., Gibson, G.R., 1998. The bifidogenic nature of chicory inulin and its hydrolysis products. Journal of Nutrition 128 (1), 11–19.

Roberfroid, M.B., 2005. Introducing inulin-type fructans. British Journal of Nutrition 93 (Suppl. 1), S13–S25.

Roger, L.C., et al., 2010. Examination of faecal Bifidobacterium populations in breast- and formula-fed infants during the first 18 months of life. Microbiology 156 (Pt 11), 3329–3341.

Ruas-Madiedo, P., et al., 2005. A bile salt-resistant derivative of *Bifidobacterium animalis* has an altered fermentation pattern when grown on glucose and maltose. Applied and Environmental Microbiology 71 (11), 6564–6570.

Ruas-Madiedo, P., et al., 2008. Mucin degradation by Bifidobacterium strains isolated from the human intestinal microbiota. Applied and Environmental Microbiology 74 (6), 1936–1940.

Ruiz-Moyano, S., et al., 2013. Variation in consumption of human milk oligosaccharides by infant gut-associated strains of *Bifidobacterium breve*. Applied and Environmental Microbiology 79 (19), 6040–6049.

Ruiz-Palacios, G.M., et al., 2003. *Campylobacter jejuni* binds intestinal H(O) antigen (Fuc alpha 1, 2Gal beta 1, 4GlcNAc), and fucosyloligosaccharides of human milk inhibit its binding and infection. Journal of Biological Chemistry 278 (16), 14112–14120.

Saffer, L.D., Petri Jr., W.A., 1991. Role of the galactose lectin of *Entamoeba histolytica* in adherence-dependent killing of mammalian cells. Infection and Immunity 59 (12), 4681–4683.

Saiman, L., et al., 2001. Risk factors for candida species colonization of neonatal intensive care unit patients. Pediatric Infectious Disease Journal 20 (12), 1119–1124.

Scardovi, V., Trovatelli, L.D., 1965. The fructose-6-phosphate shunt as peculiar pattern of hexose degradation in the genus Bifidobacterium. Annals of Microbiology 15, 19–29.

Scardovi, V., 1986. Genus bifidobacterium. 9th ed. In: P.H.A, S., et al. (Ed.), Bergey's Manual of Systematic Bacteriology, vol. 2. Williams and Wilkins, Baltimore.

Scholtens, P.A., et al., 2012. The early settlers: intestinal microbiology in early life. Annual Review of Food Science Technology 3, 425–447.

Schweizer, E., Hofmann, J., 2004. Microbial type I fatty acid synthases (FAS): major players in a network of cellular FAS systems. Microbiology and Molecular Biology Reviews 68 (3), 501–517.

Sela, D.A., et al., 2008. The genome sequence of *Bifidobacterium longum* subsp. *infantis* reveals adaptations for milk utilization within the infant microbiome. Proceedings of the National Academy of Sciences of the United States of America 105 (48), 18964–18969.

Sela, D.A., et al., 2011. An infant-associated bacterial commensal utilizes breast milk sialyloligosaccharides. Journal of Biological Chemistry 286 (14), 11909–11918.

Sela, D.A., et al., 2012. *Bifidobacterium longum* subsp. *infantis* ATCC 15697 alpha-fucosidases are active on fucosylated human milk oligosaccharides. Applied and Environmental Microbiology 78 (3), 795–803.

Sela, D.A., Mills, D.A., 2010. Nursing our microbiota: molecular linkages between bifidobacteria and milk oligosaccharides. Trends in Microbiology 18 (7), 298–307.

Sgorbati, B., Lenaz, G., Casalicchio, F., 1976. Purification and properties of two fructose-6-phosphate phosphoketolases in Bifidobacterium. Antonie Van Leeuwenhoek 42 (1–2), 49–57.

Sierra, C., et al., 2015. Prebiotic effect during the first year of life in healthy infants fed formula containing GOS as the only prebiotic: a multicentre, randomised, double-blind and placebo-controlled trial. European Journal of Nutrition 54 (1), 89–99.

Sumiyoshi, W., et al., 2004. Galactosyllactoses in the milk of Japanese women: changes in concentration during the course of lactation. Journal of Applied Glycoscience 51 (4), 341–344.

Suzuki, R., et al., 2008. Structural and thermodynamic analyses of solute-binding protein from *Bifidobacterium longum* specific for core 1 disaccharide and lacto-N-biose I. Journal of Biological Chemistry 283 (19), 13165–13173.

Turroni, F., et al., 2010. Genome analysis of *Bifidobacterium bifidum* PRL2010 reveals metabolic pathways for host-derived glycan foraging. Proceedings of the National Academy of Sciences of the United States of America 107 (45), 19514–19519.

Turroni, F., et al., 2012. Diversity of bifidobacteria within the infant gut microbiota. PLoS ONE 7 (5), e36957.

Underwood, M.A., et al., 2015. Human milk oligosaccharides in premature infants: absorption, excretion, and influence on the intestinal microbiota. Pediatric Research.

van den Bogaard, P.T., et al., 2000. Control of lactose transport, beta-galactosidase activity, and glycolysis by CcpA in *Streptococcus thermophilus*: evidence for carbon catabolite repression by a non-phosphoenolpyruvate-dependent phosphotransferase system sugar. Journal of Bacteriology 182 (21), 5982–5989.

Van der Meulen, R., et al., 2006. In vitro kinetic analysis of oligofructose consumption by Bacteroides and Bifidobacterium spp. indicates different degradation mechanisms. Applied and Environmental Microbiology 72 (2), 1006–1012.

Van Niekerk, E., et al., 2014. Human milk oligosaccharides differ between HIV-infected and HIV-uninfected mothers and are related to necrotizing enterocolitis incidence in their preterm very-low-birth-weight infants. Journal of Nutrition 144 (8), 1227–1233.

Vanmaele, R.P., Heerze, L.D., Armstrong, G.D., 1999. Role of lactosyl glycan sequences in inhibiting enteropathogenic *Escherichia coli* attachment. Infection and Immunity 67 (7), 3302–3307.

Veerkamp, J.H., 1969. Catabolism of glucose and derivatives of 2-deoxy-2-amino-glucose in *Bifidobacterium bifidum* var. pennsylvanicus. Archives of Biochemistry and Biophysics 129 (1), 257–263.

Velupillai, P., Harn, D.A., 1994. Oligosaccharide-specific induction of interleukin 10 production by B220+ cells from schistosome-infected mice: a mechanism for regulation of CD4+ T-cell subsets. Proceedings of the National Academy of Sciences of the United States of America 91 (1), 18–22.

Wada, J., et al., 2007. Purification, crystallization and preliminary X-ray analysis of the galacto-N-biose-/lacto-N-biose I-binding protein (GL-BP) of the ABC transporter from *Bifidobacterium longum* JCM1217. Acta Crystallographica Section F Structural Biology and Crystallization 63 (Pt 9), 751–753.

Wada, J., et al., 2008. *Bifidobacterium bifidum* lacto-N-biosidase, a critical enzyme for the degradation of human milk oligosaccharides with a type 1 structure. Applied and Environmental Microbiology 74 (13), 3996–4004.

Wang, J., Sporns, P., Low, N.H., 1999. Analysis of food oligosaccharides using MALDI-MS: quantification of fructooligosaccharides. Journal of Agricultural and Food Chemistry 47 (4), 1549–1557.

Ward, R.E., et al., 2006. In vitro fermentation of breast milk oligosaccharides by *Bifidobacterium infantis* and *Lactobacillus gasseri*. Applied and Environmental Microbiology 72 (6), 4497–4499.

Ward, R.E., et al., 2007. In vitro fermentability of human milk oligosaccharides by several strains of bifidobacteria. Molecular Nutrition & Food Research 51 (11), 1398–1405.

Weng, M., Walker, W.A., 2013. The role of gut microbiota in programming the immune phenotype. Journal of Developmental Origins of Health and Disease 4 (3), 203–214.

Wolin, M.J., et al., 1998. NMR detection of $^{13}CH_3{}^{13}COOH$ from 3-^{13}C-glucose: a signature for Bifidobacterium fermentation in the intestinal tract. Journal of Nutrition 128 (1), 91–96.

Xu, J., et al., 2003. A genomic view of the human-Bacteroides thetaiotaomicron symbiosis. Science 299 (5615), 2074–2076.

Yanahira, S., et al., 1995. Formation of oligosaccharides from lactose by *Bacillus circulans* beta-galactosidase. Bioscience, Biotechnology, and Biochemistry 59 (6), 1021–1026.

Yatsunenko, T., et al., 2012. Human gut microbiome viewed across age and geography. Nature 486 (7402), 222–227.

Yin, X., et al., 2005. The gene encoding xylulose-5-phosphate/fructose-6-phosphate phosphoketolase (xfp) is conserved among Bifidobacterium species within a more variable region of the genome and both are useful for strain identification. FEMS Microbiology Letters 246 (2), 251–257.

Young, S.L., et al., 2004. Bifidobacterial species differentially affect expression of cell surface markers and cytokines of dendritic cells harvested from cord blood. Clinical and Diagnostic Laboratory Immunology 11 (4), 686–690.

CHAPTER

Potential Public Health Impact of Human Milk Oligosaccharides

7

Ardythe L. Morrow, Ying Yu

Perinatal Institute Cincinnati Children's Hospital Medical Center, Cincinnati, OH, United States

1. OVERVIEW

The human milk oligosaccharides (HMOs) are both an ancient and a nascent strategy for managing human–microbial interactions. HMOs are ancient in an evolutionary sense, but nascent in their relatively recent discovery by science, biosynthesis, and testing for public health applications. Multifunctional agents that beneficially interact with, and sustain, the microbiota, HMOs are associated with reduced infant morbidity (Morrow et al., 2004; Bode, 2012) and, potentially, mortality (Kuhn et al., 2015); support development of the infant immune system (Newburg et al., 2005; Ballard and Morrow, 2013); and enhance brain development (Tarr et al., 2015; Vazquez et al., 2015). The purpose of this chapter is to consider the biosimilarity of HMOs to endogenous gastrointestinal (GI) carbohydrates and the potential for use of HMOs to be synthesized and tested as bioactive agents to improve public health outcomes.

2. FROM ANCIENT TO NOVEL

Breastfeeding offers significant protection against infectious and inflammatory diseases of infancy and improves cognitive outcomes (Bartick and Reinhold, 2010; Dieterich et al., 2013; Kramer et al., 2009). These benefits may be due in large measure to the impact of human milk on the microbiota that colonize the infant. In an early report on the microbiome, Palmer et al. (2007) showed that infants were colonized with approximately 10^7 organisms within the first week of life. Given this microbial challenge, effective management of the microbiota and the infant's response to the microbiota are critical for survival and health, which requires reducing risk of serious infections, optimizing acquired immune response to microbes, and avoiding excessive inflammatory response. Consistent with this formidable challenge, human milk has multiple mechanisms for protecting the neonate: cells, immunoglobulins, innate defense proteins, peptides, beneficial maternal organisms, free fatty acids, cytokines and chemokines, glycans, and oligosaccharides (Ballard and Morrow, 2013).

Prebiotics and Probiotics in Human Milk. http://dx.doi.org/10.1016/B978-0-12-802725-7.00007-5

Among the various bioactive components of human milk, the oligosaccharides are the most abundant and include substantially more than 100 different bioactive carbohydrates ranging from 3 to 32 sugars in size (Newburg et al., 2005). As a class, the oligosaccharides constitute 6–12 g/L of human milk and are largely synthesized from lactose (Bode, 2012). Evolutionarily ancient molecules, many HMOs are found in the milk of all mammals as well as in "primitive milk" secretions from the sebaceous glands of premammalia (Capuco and Akers, 2009). Measurement of milk oligosaccharides from the Tasmanian echidna, a monotreme, found a modest number of neutral and acidic oligosaccharides but a low abundance of lactose as compared to the milk of modern eutherian mammalia, including humans (Oftedal et al., 2014). Thus, in evolution, the oligosaccharides appeared prior to mammals and likely contributed to management of the microbiota for the survival and developmental benefit of the offspring. The nutritional function of milk was a secondary development. However, the profile and complexity of oligosaccharides of human milk are unique to our species and are thought to provide a match to the range of pathogens that are endemic in human societies.

In the 20th century, technical advances for combating infectious diseases appeared to eclipse the evolutionary benefit of breastfeeding for protection of the offspring against infectious diseases. Municipal water treatment to ensure a safe water supply was first undertaken in New Jersey in 1908; rabies, tetanus, and typhoid vaccines were licensed in the United States in 1914; and the first modern antimicrobial medicines were available beginning in the mid-1940s. Along with the rapid development and use of safe water, vaccines, and antimicrobials, infectious diseases dramatically waned, infant mortality plummeted, and life expectancy improved during the 20th century. Nevertheless, optimal breastfeeding has in fact remained a highly effective public health strategy for infant survival, especially for the reduction of mortality due to gastroenteritis and pneumonia in developing countries (Bhutta et al., 2013). Chen and Rogan (2004) demonstrated that even in the United States, breastfeeding protects against infant mortality. Suboptimal breastfeeding in the United States also significantly contributes to morbidity, such as risk of infectious diarrhea, lower respiratory tract infections, otitis media, and sudden infant death syndrome (Bartick and Reinhold, 2010).

As infectious diseases have waned, there has been a concomitant rise in inflammatory, allergic, and autoimmune conditions. A proposed explanation for this epidemiologic pattern is known as the hygiene hypothesis, which proposes that lack of early life exposure to infectious agents and beneficial microbes dysregulates the healthy, normal development of the immune system and increases diseases of immune dysregulation (von Hertzen et al., 2011). Consistent with that view, comparative studies have shown that the GI microbiota of the US population, which has high rates of allergy and autoimmune conditions, is far less diverse than that of populations in low-income countries or traditional societies (Lin et al., 2013; De Filippo et al., 2010; Yatsunenko et al., 2012). It appears that high standards of hygiene, combined with high antibiotic use and the Western diet lacking indigestible carbohydrate and probiotic foods, may be microbial diversity in the United States and other modern societies. Antibiotic use is now understood to cause "collateral damage," resulting in less diverse microbiota, depletion of beneficial microbes, modification of the microbial–host metabolism, and selection for more antibiotic-resistant and potentially more pathogenic organisms (Modi et al., 2014; Greenwood et al., 2014). Overuse of antibiotics may also be linked to a variety of chronic conditions characterized by microbial and immune dysregulation (Blaser, 2014). Inflammation-related diseases of the GI tract, including colonic diverticulitis, inflammatory bowel disease, irritable bowel syndrome, and functional gastrointestinal disorders, are increasing worldwide (Park et al., 2015; Molodecky et al., 2012; Quigley et al., 2012; Sandberg et al., 2014; Korterink et al., 2015; Abramson et al., 2010; Hein et al., 2014; Kang et al., 2003; Tanase et al., 2015). Many of these conditions are associated with dysregulated microbiota ("dysbiosis") that can provoke GI inflammation (Rausch et al., 2011; Kashyap et al., 2013; Tong et al., 2014). Many other conditions are also linked to microbial and immune dysregulation, including allergy, autoimmunity, obesity, and neurobehavioral conditions such as anxiety, depression, and mental health problems (Cryan and Dinan, 2012; Palau-Rodriguez et al., 2015; Prince et al., 2015; Longman and Littman, 2015). The number and types of diseases associated with dysbiosis are staggering and can seem improbable. But, it can be argued that humanity coevolved with our microbiota and that we are only just becoming aware of the many functions that microbes provide to the human host.

Studies of breastfeeding demonstrate protection against many chronic and immune conditions, specifically, type 1 diabetes, necrotizing enterocolitis, asthma, and leukemia (Bartick and Reinhold, 2010). We propose that some of the protection attributable to human milk may be due to the oligosaccharides. Given the rising incidence of diseases associated with dysregulated microbiota and host immunity, there is an avidly emerging global interest in testing novel nutritional approaches and functional foods, consistent with those found in human milk, in order to optimize or restore microbial and host health.

3. HEALTH EFFECTS OF HUMAN MILK OLIGOSACCHARIDES

Research over the past decade or longer suggests that HMOs offer a novel strategy to improve health outcomes, distinct from the hygiene and anti-infectious approaches that arose in the 20th century. HMOs provide various health benefits to infants (Table 7.1). One major effect of HMOs is classified as prebiotic, that is, modifying microbial composition and function to the benefit of the host (Roberfroid et al., 2010). Another major function is the role of HMOs as antiadhesion agents, or receptor decoys. A third major function is in the direct effect of HMOs on the GI epithelium, which modulates host immune response to GI microbes. These functions are each described later.

Table 7.1 HMOs Functions for Managing Microbial–Host Interactions

• Modifying microbial composition and function
• Antiadhesion/decoy receptors
• Direct host immune-modulating effects

3.1 PREBIOTIC EFFECTS

A study of microbial populations from 12 different sites in the human body reported considerable variation in the presence of enzymes for carbohydrate metabolism from site to site; the authors proposed that local carbohydrate composition may be a major driving force that shapes each of the microbial subcommunities of the human microbiome (Cantarel et al., 2012). This is certainly true in the GI tract, as the vast majority of GI bacteria have a predominantly saccharolytic metabolism (Macfarlane and Macfarlane, 2011). Among the most recognized dietary influences on the microbiota are the carbohydrates that are indigestible by humans, but utilized by colonic bacteria for anaerobic fermentation (Gibson and Roberfroid, 1995). In infancy, the composition of colonizing microbiota is shaped by oligosaccharides from human milk (Newburg and Grave, 2014). All prebiotics, including HMOs, stimulate the growth of bifidobacteria, but individual prebiotics have other distinct effects as well, such as selection for disparate specific microbes and direct influence on discrete host inflammatory pathways (He et al., 2014, 2016). Microbes metabolize prebiotics differently, resulting in distinct bacterial growth with short-chain fatty acids (SCFAs) and lactate as metabolic products (Martens et al., 2014; Flint et al., 2012; Yu et al., 2013a). Bifidobacteria are the most efficient microbes for growth on HMOs, but the efficiency of utilization varies by strain, depending on the specific bacterial genome (LoCascio et al., 2007; Sela et al., 2008; Garrido et al., 2015; Yu et al., 2013b) The ability to use HMOs for growth depends on microbes having the requisite glycosyl hydrolase genes, either individually, or as part of the collective microbial community. Most *Bacteroidetes*, and some *Clostridia*, also possess the genome necessary to utilize HMOs efficiently (Yu et al., 2013b; Weiss et al., 2014; Crost et al., 2013). The overall impact of prebiotic carbohydrate on the GI microbiota can be profound; indeed, the GI microbial community of mice whose diet is depleted of plant polysaccharide dramatically diverges from the microbial community of mice whose diet is replete with plant polysaccharide (Kashyap et al., 2013).

3.2 ANTIADHESION AND HOST IMMUNE-MODULATION EFFECTS

In addition to their prebiotic effects, HMOs possess the distinctive ability to bind potential pathogens and/or to inhibit the inflammatory response of enterocytes to pathogens. Inhibition of pathogen binding of GI enterocytes by HMOs was elegantly demonstrated for *Campylobacter jejuni* infection and inflammation in vitro and in a murine model (Ruiz-Palacios et al., 2003). The highly abundant oligosaccharide,

2′-fucosyllactose (2′-FL), and glycans containing that motif, inhibit *Campylobacter* infection. HMOs and glycans of human milk have also been shown to bind strains of noroviruses (NoVs) (Jiang et al., 2004; Ruvoen-Clouet et al., 2006) in a strain-dependent manner. Sialyloligosaccharides may offer protection against some strains of rotaviruses that infect animals (Hester et al., 2013), but inhibition of rotavirus diarrhea in human populations may be inhibited by the glycosylated human milk innate defense proteins lactadherin and lactoferrin (Newburg et al., 1998; Moon et al., 2013).

Protection by HMOs is not limited to pathogen binding. HMOs also inhibit inflammation due to type I pili infection caused by enterotoxigenic *Escherichia coli* (ETEC), uropathogenic *E. coli* (UPEC), and adherent-invasive *E. coli* (AIEC) of human intestinal epithelial cells. Specifically, 2′-FL reduces inflammation by inhibition of CD14 expression (He et al., 2016). Another study demonstrated that HMOs protect bladder cells against invasion by the UPEC strain CFT073 (Lin et al., 2014). HMOs did not protect against binding but against internalization of these organisms into bladder cells, and sialyl HMOs were the most inhibitory.

3.3 STRUCTURE AND FUNCTION

The protective role of HMOs differs by their structure. Oligosaccharide is synthesized by a family of glycosyltransferase gene enzymes that create the linkages between the sugars. The synthesis of oligosaccharides containing fucose requires a fucosyltransferase enzyme. There are several different fucosyltransferase enzymes, but the fucosyltransferase2 (FUT2) enzyme contributes to the synthesis of half of the oligosaccharides of human milk (Fig. 7.1), the most abundant of which are 2′-FL and lacto-*N*-fucopentaose-I (LNFP-I). As shown in Fig. 7.1, these HMOs, and a number of others, are structurally similar to the terminal oligosaccharides of GI glycans, suggesting the potential for similar function.

Importantly, a number of studies demonstrate a significant association between FUT2 status and GI diseases in human populations (McGovern et al., 2010; Parmar et al., 2012), which suggests potential therapeutic opportunities for FUT2 enzyme-derived products such as 2′-FL and LNFP-I. Inactivating mutations in both alleles of the *FUT2* gene occur in 20–25% of the human population, indicating the need to understand the specific role of FUT2 and its biological end-products (Magalhaes et al., 2009).

4. PROMISING PUBLIC HEALTH TARGET POPULATIONS AND DISEASES

HMOs have not yet been produced at sufficient scale to be tested in human trials. Nevertheless, in vitro and in vivo testing and the epidemiology of HMOs strongly suggest the potential to be effective against a range of diseases, due to their potent prebiotic, pathogen binding, and antiinflammatory effects and their structural similarity to innate human GI glycans (Table 7.2).

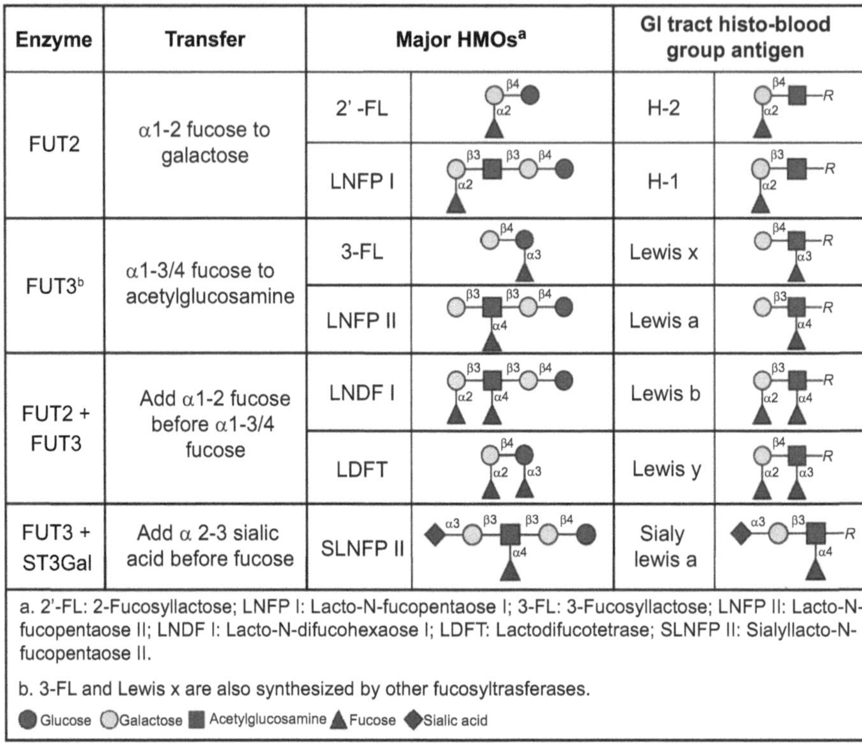

FIGURE 7.1

Major analog oligosaccharides of human milk and GI tract by the responsible glycosyltransferases.

Table 7.2 Some Potential Targets for Testing HMOs

Major Disease Targets	Major Patient Populations
Infectious diseases	**Prevention or adjunctive treatment**
• Acute diarrhea	• Immunocompromised
• Sepsis	• Outbreaks in institutions
• Urinary tract infections	• At-risk hospitalized patients
Gut dysbiosis/inflammatory conditions	
• Necrotizing enterocolitis (NEC)	• Preterm infants <32 weeks, to prevent NEC and sepsis
• Short gut syndrome	• Intestinal failure patients, to improve adaptation
• Malnutrition	• Malnourished patients—for rehabilitation
• Inflammatory bowel disease	• Irritable bowel disease (IBD) patients, to sustain remission
• Functional bowel disorders	• Functional bowel disorder patients—as treatment
• Celiac disease	• Celiac disease—primary or secondary prevention
Autoimmune conditions	
• Type 1 diabetes	• Type I diabetes—primary or secondary prevention

Table 7.3 Disease Risk Reported With *FUT2* Status

Disease	References	Risk Differs by *FUT2* Genotype
Acute gastroenteritis (AGE) • NoV • Rotavirus	Currier et al. (2015), Payne et al. (2015), and Kambpamphati et al. (2016)	Increased risk in FUT2⁺, but risk is strain specific. Based on a number of population-based studies.
Helicobacter pylori	Ikehara et al. (2001) and Magalhaes et al. (2009)	Increased risk in FUT2⁺ but only for *H. pylori* strains with the BabA adhesin.
Cholera infection	Glass et al. (1985)	Risk of cholera shown to differ by ABO blood group type. However, it is now known that expression of A or B antigen in the GI tract requires being FUT2⁺.
Graft-versus-host disease	Rayes et al. (2016)	Increased risk in FUT2⁺.
IBD–Crohn's disease	Rausch et al. (2011) and McGovern et al. (2010)	Increased risk in FUT2⁻, thus with lack of intestinal fucosylation.
NEC	Morrow et al. (2011) and Demmert et al. (2015)	Increased risk in FUT2⁻; no association.
Primary sclerosing cholangitis	Maroni et al. (2015)	Increased risk in FUT2⁻.
Type 1 diabetes	Smyth et al. (2011)	Increased risk in FUT2⁻.

There are many considerations for selection of specific disease targets for testing the use of one HMO or HMO mixtures. The fundamental criterion that we use here for consideration is that the disease or condition evidences the following: (1) gut infection or dysbiosis, (2) inflammation of the GI or urinary tract, (3) the disease or its sequelae is associated with GI glycosylation differences, such as occurs due to polymorphism in the *FUT2* gene (Table 7.3), (4) preclinical studies have identified a specific target HMO molecule or mixture to be tested, and (5) providing the HMOs can be done feasibly. The latter consideration is warranted by the primary role of the FUT2 enzyme in synthesis of HMOs and GI glycans (Fig. 7.1) as well as the high frequency of polymorphism in that gene.

Next, we consider three specific conditions and populations that by some or all of those criteria warrant consideration for testing HMOs: (1) prevention of NoV acute gastroenteritis (AGE), (2) prevention of NEC in preterm infants, and (3) prevention of relapse in patients diagnosed with IBD who are in remission.

4.1 PREVENTION OF NOROVIRUS ACUTE GASTROENTERITIS

NoV-associated AGE is a potential logical target for testing HMOs or glycoproteins for the prevention of acute or chronic NoV infections; at this time, there is no available vaccine, and NoV is the leading cause of diarrhea, including in immunocompromised patient populations. The major NoV strains, GII.4 and GII.6, and some GI strains, infect predominantly $FUT2^+$ individuals who express "secretor" histo-blood group/oligosaccharide antigens in the GI tract (Currier et al., 2015; Kambhampati et al., 2016), which have HMO analogs as that serve as the therapeutic target molecules. Based on epidemiology and in vitro studies, specific HMOs, notably lacto-di-fucotetraose, may inhibit NoV strains (Morrow et al., 2004). Unfortunately, NoV may not provide an ideal target condition for testing HMOs at this time. First, simple HMOs appear to bind some NoVs but lack the binding affinity, and specificity differs across strains and may require glycoproteins, mucins, or fragments thereof for effective binding (Ruvoen-Clouet et al., 2006; Shang et al., 2013; Tan and Jiang, 2014). Given the oligosaccharide or glycan specificity required for NoV binding, the technical and resource challenges in finding the optimal target molecules may provide too frustrating a hurdle to overcome in the near future. Furthermore, targeting acute diarrheal disease due to any pathogen presents major logistical challenges. In a free-living population, how would at-risk individuals be reached, and how could HMOs be reliably provided, in order to prevent infection or disease? Some have suggested that use of HMOs for prevention might be feasible by use of fortified weaning foods in free-living populations or could be used in institutionalized populations at high risk of disease transmission, for whom no other prophylaxis exists (e.g., immunocompromised patients under medical supervision, hospitalized patients, child day care, and nursing homes). Regardless, the goal of testing HMOs for the prevention of NoV or other causes of acute diarrhea must overcome the major hurdles of identifying and synthesizing the right target molecules.

4.2 TESTING IN PRETERM INFANTS

Preterm infants born earlier than 32 weeks gestational age are prone to excessive GI inflammation and microbial dysbiosis, and are at high risk of NEC and sepsis, diseases also associated with inflammation and microbial dysbiosis (Neu and Walker, 2011; Taft et al., 2015b; Torrazza and Neu, 2013; Morrow et al., 2013; Nanthakumar et al., 2011, 2013). We previously reported that FUT2 nonsecretors and low-secretors are at increased risk of NEC, but another study has shown that *FUT2* genotype is not reliably associated with NEC (Morrow et al., 2011; Demmert et al., 2015). In our recent cohort, we have found FUT2 phenotype but not genotype to be associated with microbial community colonization and increased risk of NEC (data unpublished), leaving the question of the relevance of GI glycosylation to risk of NEC unanswered. Be that as it may, several target HMOs have been proposed as having the potential to reduce risk of NEC, specifically, in mouse and human studies, disialyl-lacto-*N*-tetraose (DSLNT) and oligosaccharides that include an α-1,2-fucose linkage (e.g., 2′-FL) have been implicated as beneficial for reducing NEC or GI inflammation (Jantscher-Krenn et al., 2012; Yu et al., 2014; He et al., 2016; Morrow et al., March, 2015; Autran et al.,2016).

But, as preterm infants should be human milk-fed and should therefore already be consuming HMOs, is there then a point to testing these or other HMOs? We believe that there is indeed rationale for testing specific HMOs or combinations as fortification of mother's milk or donor human. Concentrations of HMOs in human milk vary from mother to mother, and this variation can have health consequences (Morrow et al., 2004; Chaturvedi et al., 2001; Lewis et al., 2015; Underwood et al., 2015). Furthermore, there is evidence that HMOs in the milk of preterm infants differs from that of mature infants (Davidson et al., 2004; De Leoz et al., 2012). Together, findings indicate the importance of testing specific HMOs or HMO mixtures as fortifiers to the infant's enteral intake. The HMOs should also be tested in relation to the growth of preterm infants, as findings to date suggest that HMOs and gut microbiota influence infant growth (Taft et al., 2015a; Alderete et al., 2015).

In summary, testing HMOs for improved health and developmental outcomes of preterm infants appears warranted, feasible, and supported by candidate HMOs and should thus be a high priority.

4.3 PREVENTION OF RELAPSE IN PATIENTS WITH IRRITABLE BOWEL DISEASE

IBD is a chronic, progressively disabling disease that affects more than 3 million individuals in Western countries, while the incidence is increasing in non-Western countries. Many of the new cases of IBD occur in children. Although the etiology of the disease is complex, IBD is an immune-mediated condition that occurs more often in genetically-susceptible individuals, including $FUT2^-$ "nonsecretor" individuals (McGovern et al., 2010; Rausch et al., 2011). In addition to IBD, several other autoimmune diseases also appear to be associated with FUT2 status (Smyth et al., 2011; Maroni et al., 2015; Rayes et al., 2016). Onset of IBD appears to be triggered by environmental factors that perturb the mucosal barrier, alter the healthy balance of the GI microbiota, and abnormally stimulate GI immune responses (Boyapati et al., 2015). In order to maintain GI homeostasis, the host actively suppresses cellular and humoral immune reactivity to common microbial commensal-derived antigens ("tolerance"). Failure to maintain tolerance contributes to the development of IBD and other autoimmune diseases.

The therapeutic goal in IBD is clinical remission and absence of mucosal ulcerations. Maintaining this deep remission is critical for prevention of bowel damage and disability. Strategies to mitigate symptoms of IBD by targeting the microbiota and immune homeostasis offer great potential. Early intervention with anti–tumor necrosis factor (TNF) agents is effective for establishing remission (Danese et al., 2014; Mandel et al., 2014), but about one-half of IBD patients suffer disease relapse (Kotze et al., 2015). In addition, treatment complications occur in one of five patients after 14 years of follow-up. Risk of tuberculosis and viral infections are also increased with TNFα inhibitor. As a consequence, discontinuation of TNFα inhibitor is often required (Freling et al., 2015). There remains a significant need for novel therapeutics in order to prevent, alter the natural history, and ultimately cure IBD.

We propose that HMOs should be tested as an adjunctive therapy to sustain remission in IBD, particularly those that contain α-1,2 fucose, such as 2′-FL, which are products of the FUT2 enzyme. FUT2 nonsecretors are deficient in innate GI carbohydrates containing fucose, and there is evidence that this lack of surface fucosylation contributes to risk of IBD by increasing susceptibility to GI inflammation and microbial dysregulation (Kashyap et al., 2013; Rausch et al., 2011; Pickard et al., 2014; Tong et al., 2013). Further, 2′-FL inhibits inflammatory response, specifically, CD14 expression, of human intestinal epithelial cells to pathogenic *E. coli* (He et al., 2016). However, prior to any potential oligosaccharide trial in IBD, dosing and safety studies in adolescents and adults, for whom the impact of HMOs and optimum dosing are not known, will be required.

5. SUMMARY AND CONCLUSIONS

HMOs contribute to the efficacy of breastfeeding in managing infection and promoting the growth of beneficial microbiota. HMOs also have significant potential to improve human health as a novel medical food. They differ from currently used prebiotic carbohydrates by their multifunctionality and biosimilarity to GI surface glycans. Options for testing HMOs include infectious diseases or chronic disease targets that are characterized by dysbiosis and GI inflammation and, potentially, genetic risk related to HMO structure and function. However, the structural and functional differences of HMOs make it critical to refine the specific HMOs to be used, and the logistics of administration should be considered. For infectious disease targets, such as NoV, testing the optimal target molecule does not appear to be close at hand; simple HMOs structures may not suffice, and complex glycoprotein structures, which are not readily synthesized, may be required. Furthermore, the timing of and route of administration of HMOs are a challenge for prevention of infectious diseases. But we believe that this may have significant potential to protect medically-managed chronic disease, immunocompromised, or institutionalized patient populations, in whom appropriate testing and use of HMOs are feasible. Testing of HMOs in preterm infants and IBD patients could occur more imminently than many other conditions, as simple HMO structures have been identified that might soon be available for human trials. We believe that the potential for use of HMOs in various conditions is such that it deserves a major public health initiative that involves both the private and public sectors.

REFERENCES

Abramson, O., Durant, M., Mow, W., et al., 2010. Incidence, prevalence, and time trends of pediatric inflammatory bowel disease in Northern California, 1996 to 2006. The Journal of Pediatrics 157 (2), 233–239 e231.

Alderete, T.L., Autran, C., Brekke, B.E., et al., 2015. Associations between human milk oligosaccharides and infant body composition in the first 6 mo of life. The American Journal of Clinical Nutrition 102 (6), 1381–1388.

Autran, C.A., Schoterman, M.H., Jantscher-Krenn, E., Kamerling, J.P., Bode, L., 2016. Sialylated galacto-oligosaccharides and 2'-fucosyllactose reduce necrotising enterocolitis in neonatal rats. British Journal of Nutrition 116 (2), 294–299. http://dx.doi.org/10.1017/S0007114516002038 [PMID: 27212112].

Ballard, O., Morrow, A.L., 2013. Human milk composition: nutrients and bioactive factors. Pediatric Clinics of North America 60 (1), 49–74.

Bartick, M., Reinhold, A., 2010. The burden of suboptimal breastfeeding in the United States: a pediatric cost analysis. Pediatrics 125 (5), e1048–e1056.

Bhutta, Z.A., Das, J.K., Walker, N., et al., 2013. Interventions to address deaths from childhood pneumonia and diarrhoea equitably: what works and at what cost? Lancet 381 (9875), 1417–1429.

Blaser, M.J., 2014. Missing Microbes. How the Overuse of Antibiotics Is Fueling Our Modern Plagues. Henry Holt and Co., LLC, New York, NY.

Bode, L., 2012. Human milk oligosaccharides: every baby needs a sugar mama. Glycobiology 22 (9), 1147–1162.

Boyapati, R., Satsangi, J., Ho, G.T., 2015. Pathogenesis of Crohn's disease. F1000Prime Reports 7, 44.

Cantarel, B.L., Lombard, V., Henrissat, B., 2012. Complex carbohydrate utilization by the healthy human microbiome. PLoS One 7 (6), e28742.

Capuco, A.V., Akers, R.M., 2009. The origin and evolution of lactation. Journal of Biology 8 (4), 37.

Chaturvedi, P., Warren, C.D., Altaye, M., et al., 2001. Fucosylated human milk oligosaccharides vary between individuals and over the course of lactation. Glycobiology 11 (5), 365–372.

Chen, A., Rogan, W.J., 2004. Breastfeeding and the risk of postneonatal death in the United States. Pediatrics 113 (5), e435–e439.

Crost, E.H., Tailford, L.E., Le Gall, G., Fons, M., Henrissat, B., Juge, N., 2013. Utilisation of mucin glycans by the human gut symbiont *Ruminococcus gnavus* is strain-dependent. PLoS One 8 (10), e76341.

Cryan, J.F., Dinan, T.G., 2012. Mind-altering microorganisms: the impact of the gut microbiota on brain and behaviour. Nature Reviews Neuroscience 13 (10), 701–712.

Currier, R.L., Payne, D.C., Staat, M.A., et al., 2015. Innate susceptibility to norovirus infections influenced by FUT2 genotype in a United States pediatric population. Clinical Infectious Diseases 60 (11), 1631–1638.

Danese, S., Fiorino, G., Fernandes, C., Peyrin-Biroulet, L., 2014. Catching the therapeutic window of opportunity in early Crohn's disease. Current Drug Targets 15 (11), 1056–1063.

Davidson, B., Meinzen-Derr, J.K., Wagner, C.L., Newburg, D.S., Morrow, A.L., 2004. Fucosylated oligosaccharides in human milk in relation to gestational age and stage of lactation. Advances in Experimental Medicine and Biology 554, 427–430.

De Filippo, C., Cavalieri, D., Di Paola, M., et al., 2010. Impact of diet in shaping gut microbiota revealed by a comparative study in children from Europe and rural Africa. Proceedings of the National Academy of Sciences of the United States of America 107 (33), 14691–14696.

De Leoz, M.L., Gaerlan, S.C., Strum, J.S., et al., 2012. Lacto-N-tetraose, fucosylation, and secretor status are highly variable in human milk oligosaccharides from women delivering preterm. Journal of Proteome Research 11 (9), 4662–4672.

Demmert, M., Schaper, A., Pagel, J., et al., 2015. FUT 2 polymorphism and outcome in very-low-birth-weight infants. Pediatric Research 77 (4), 586–590.

Dieterich, C.M., Felice, J.P., O'Sullivan, E., Rasmussen, K.M., 2013. Breastfeeding and health outcomes for the mother-infant dyad. Pediatric Clinics of North America 60 (1), 31–48.

Flint, H.J., Scott, K.P., Duncan, S.H., Louis, P., Forano, E., 2012. Microbial degradation of complex carbohydrates in the gut. Gut Microbes 3 (4), 289–306.

Freling, E., Baumann, C., Cuny, J.F., et al., 2015. Cumulative incidence of, risk factors for, and outcome of dermatological complications of anti-TNF therapy in inflammatory bowel disease: a 14-year experience. American Journal of Gastroenterology 110 (8), 1186–1196.

Garrido, D., Ruiz-Moyano, S., Lemay, D.G., Sela, D.A., German, J.B., Mills, D.A., 2015. Comparative transcriptomics reveals key differences in the response to milk oligosaccharides of infant gut-associated bifidobacteria. Scientific Reports 5, 13517.

Gibson, G.R., Roberfroid, M.B., 1995. Dietary modulation of the human colonic microbiota: introducing the concept of prebiotics. The Journal of Nutrition 125 (6), 1401–1412.

Glass, R.I., Holmgren, J., Haley, C.E., Khan, M.R., Svennerholm, A.M., Stoll, B.J., Belayet Hossain, K.M., Black, R.E., Yunus, M., Barua, D., 1985. Predisposition for cholera of individuals with O blood group. Possible evolutionary significance. Am J Epidemiol 121 (6), 791–796 [PMID: 4014172].

Greenwood, C., Morrow, A.L., Lagomarcino, A.J., et al., 2014. Early Empiric antibiotic use in preterm infants is associated with lower bacterial diversity and higher relative abundance of enterobacter. The Journal of Pediatrics 165 (1), 23–29. http://dx.doi.org/10.1016/j.jpeds.2014.01.010 [Epub 2014 February 13].

He, Y., Liu, S., Kling, D.E., Leone, S., Lawlor, N.T., Huang, Y., Feinberg, S.B., Hill, D.R., Newburg, D.S., 2016. The human milk oligosaccharide 2'-fucosyllactose modulates CD14 expression in human enterocytes, thereby attenuating LPS-induced inflammation. Gut 65 (1), 33–46. http://dx.doi.org/10.1136/gutjnl-2014-307544 [Epub 2014 November 27].

He, Y., Liu, S., Leone, S., Newburg, D.S., 2014. Human colostrum oligosaccharides modulate major immunologic pathways of immature human intestine. Mucosal Immunology 7 (6), 1326–1339.

Hein, R., Koster, I., Bollschweiler, E., Schubert, I., 2014. Prevalence of inflammatory bowel disease: estimates for 2010 and trends in Germany from a large insurance-based regional cohort. Scandinavian Journal of Gastroenterology 49 (11), 1325–1335.

Hester, S.N., Chen, X., Li, M., et al., 2013. Human milk oligosaccharides inhibit rotavirus infectivity in vitro and in acutely infected piglets. The British Journal of Nutrition 110 (7), 1233–1242.

von Hertzen, L., Hanski, I., Haahtela, T., 2011. Natural immunity. Biodiversity loss and inflammatory diseases are two global megatrends that might be related. EMBO Reports 12 (11), 1089–1093.

Ikehara, Y., Nishihara, S., Yasutomi, H., Kitamura, T., Matsuo, K., Shimizu, N., Inada, K., Kodera, Y., Yamamura, Y., Narimatsu, H., Hamajima, N., Tatematsu, M., 2001. 3. Polymorphisms of two fucosyltransferase genes (Lewis and Secretor genes) involving type I Lewis antigens are associated with the presence of anti-Helicobacter pylori IgG antibody. Cancer Epidemiol Biomarkers Prev 10 (9), 971–977 [PMID: 11535550].

Jantscher-Krenn, E., Zherebtsov, M., Nissan, C., et al., 2012. The human milk oligosaccharide disialyllacto-N-tetraose prevents necrotising enterocolitis in neonatal rats. Gut 61 (10), 1417–1425.

Jiang, X., Huang, P., Zhong, W., et al., 2004. Human milk contains elements that block binding of noroviruses to human histo-blood group antigens in saliva. The Journal of Infectious Diseases 190 (10), 1850–1859.

Kambhampati, A., Payne, D.C., Costantini, V., Lopman, B.A., 2016. Host genetic susceptibility to enteric viruses: a systematic review and metaanalysis. Clin Infect Dis 62 (1), 11–18. http://dx.doi.org/10.1093/cid/civ873 [Epub2015 October 26, PMID: 26508510].

Kang, J.Y., Hoare, J., Tinto, A., et al., 2003. Diverticular disease of the colon–on the rise: a study of hospital admissions in England between 1989/1990 and 1999/2000. Alimentary Pharmacology & Therapeutics 17 (9), 1189–1195.

Kashyap, P.C., Marcobal, A., Ursell, L.K., et al., 2013. Genetically dictated change in host mucus carbohydrate landscape exerts a diet-dependent effect on the gut microbiota. Proceedings of the National Academy of Sciences of the United States of America 110 (42), 17059–17064.

Korterink, J.J., Diederen, K., Benninga, M.A., Tabbers, M.M., 2015. Epidemiology of pediatric functional abdominal pain disorders: a meta-analysis. PLoS One 10 (5), e0126982.

Kotze, P.G., Ludvig, J.C., Teixeira, F.V., et al., 2015. Disease duration did not influence the rates of loss of efficacy of the anti-TNF therapy in Latin American Crohn's disease patients. Digestion 91 (2), 158–163.

Kramer, M.S., Matush, L., Bogdanovich, N., et al., 2009. Health and development outcomes in 6.5-y-old children breastfed exclusively for 3 or 6 mo. The American Journal of Clinical Nutrition 90 (4), 1070–1074.

Kuhn, L., Kim, H.Y., Hsiao, L., et al., 2015. Oligosaccharide composition of breast milk influences survival of uninfected children born to HIV-infected mothers in Lusaka, Zambia. The Journal of Nutrition 145 (1), 66–72.

Lewis, Z.T., Totten, S.M., Smilowitz, J.T., et al., 2015. Maternal fucosyltransferase 2 status affects the gut bifidobacterial communities of breastfed infants. Microbiome 3, 13.

Lin, A., Bik, E.M., Costello, E.K., et al., 2013. Distinct distal gut microbiome diversity and composition in healthy children from Bangladesh and the United States. PLoS One 8 (1), e53838.

Lin, A.E., Autran, C.A., Espanola, S.D., Bode, L., Nizet, V., 2014. Human milk oligosaccharides protect bladder epithelial cells against uropathogenic *Escherichia coli* invasion and cytotoxicity. The Journal of Infectious Diseases 209 (3), 389–398.

LoCascio, R.G., Ninonuevo, M.R., Freeman, S.L., et al., 2007. Glycoprofiling of bifidobacterial consumption of human milk oligosaccharides demonstrates strain specific, preferential consumption of small chain glycans secreted in early human lactation. Journal of Agricultural and Food Chemistry 55 (22), 8914–8919.

Longman, R.S., Littman, D.R., 2015. The functional impact of the intestinal microbiome on mucosal immunity and systemic autoimmunity. Current Opinion in Rheumatology 27 (4), 381–387.

Macfarlane, G.T., Macfarlane, S., 2011. Fermentation in the human large intestine: its physiologic consequences and the potential contribution of prebiotics. Journal of Clinical Gastroenterology 45 (Suppl.), S120–S127.

Magalhaes, A., Gomes, J., Ismail, M.N., et al., 2009. Fut2-null mice display an altered glycosylation profile and impaired BabA-mediated *Helicobacter pylori* adhesion to gastric mucosa. Glycobiology 19 (12), 1525–1536.

Mandel, M.D., Balint, A., Golovics, P.A., et al., 2014. Decreasing trends in hospitalizations during anti-TNF therapy are associated with time to anti-TNF therapy: results from two referral centres. Digestive and Liver Disease 46 (11), 985–990.

Maroni, L., van de Graaf, S.F., Hohenester, S.D., 2015. Oude Elferink RP, Beuers U. Fucosyltransferase 2: a genetic risk factor for primary sclerosing cholangitis and Crohn's disease–a comprehensive review. Clinical Reviews in Allergy & Immunology 48 (2–3), 182–191.

Martens, E.C., Kelly, A.G., Tauzin, A.S., Brumer, H., 2014. The devil lies in the details: how variations in polysaccharide fine-structure impact the physiology and evolution of gut microbes. Journal of Molecular Biology 426 (23), 3851–3865.

McGovern, D.P., Jones, M.R., Taylor, K.D., et al., 2010. Fucosyltransferase 2 (FUT2) non-secretor status is associated with Crohn's disease. Human Molecular Genetics 19 (17), 3468–3476.

Modi, S.R., Collins, J.J., Relman, D.A., 2014. Antibiotics and the gut microbiota. Journal of Clinical Investigation 124 (10), 4212–4218.

Molodecky, N.A., Soon, I.S., Rabi, D.M., et al., 2012. Increasing incidence and prevalence of the inflammatory bowel diseases with time, based on systematic review. Gastroenterology 142 (1), 46–54 e42; quiz e30.

Moon, S.S., Tate, J.E., Ray, P., et al., 2013. Differential profiles and inhibitory effect on rotavirus vaccines of nonantibody components in breast milk from mothers in developing and developed countries. The Pediatric Infectious Disease Journal 32 (8), 863–870.

Morrow, A.L., Ruiz-Palacios, G.M., Altaye, M., et al., 2004. Human milk oligosaccharides are associated with protection against diarrhea in breast-fed infants. The Journal of Pediatrics 145 (3), 297–303.

Morrow, A.L., Meinzen-Derr, J., Huang, P., et al., 2011. Fucosyltransferase 2 non-secretor and low secretor status predicts severe outcomes in premature infants. The Journal of Pediatrics 158 (5), 745–751.

Morrow, A.L., Lagomarcino, A.J., Schibler, K.R., et al., 2013. Early microbial and metabolomic signatures predict later onset of necrotizing enterocolitis in preterm infants. Microbiome 1 (1), 13.

Morrow, A.L., Newburg, D.S., Ruiz-Palacios, G.M., March 2015. Inventors: The General Hospital Corporation Instituto Nacional de Ciencias Medicas Y Nutricion Children's Hospital Medical Center, assignee. Use of secretor, Lewis and sialyl antigen levels in clinical samples as predictors of risk for disease.

Nanthakumar, N., Meng, D., Goldstein, A.M., et al., 2011. The mechanism of excessive intestinal inflammation in necrotizing enterocolitis: an immature innate immune response. PLoS One 6 (3), e17776.

Nanthakumar, N.N., Meng, D., Newburg, D.S., 2013. Glucocorticoids and microbiota regulate ontogeny of intestinal fucosyltransferase 2 requisite for gut homeostasis. Glycobiology 23 (10), 1131–1141.

Neu, J., Walker, W.A., 2011. Necrotizing enterocolitis. The New England Journal of Medicine 364 (3), 255–264.

Newburg, D.S., Grave, G., 2014. Recent advances in human milk glycobiology. Pediatric Research 75 (5), 675–679.

Newburg, D.S., Peterson, J.A., Ruiz-Palacios, G.M., et al., 1998. Role of human-milk lactadherin in protection against symptomatic rotavirus infection. Lancet 351 (9110), 1160–1164.

Newburg, D.S., Ruiz-Palacios, G.M., Morrow, A.L., 2005. Human milk glycans protect infants against enteric pathogens. Annual Review of Nutrition 25, 37–58.

Oftedal, O.T., Nicol, S.C., Davies, N.W., et al., 2014. Can an ancestral condition for milk oligosaccharides be determined? Evidence from the Tasmanian echidna (*Tachyglossus aculeatus setosus*). Glycobiology 24 (9), 826–839.

Palau-Rodriguez, M., Tulipani, S., Isabel Queipo-Ortuno, M., Urpi-Sarda, M., Tinahones, F.J., Andres-Lacueva, C., 2015. Metabolomic insights into the intricate gut microbial-host interaction in the development of obesity and type 2 diabetes. Frontiers in Microbiology 6, 1151.

Palmer, C., Bik, E.M., DiGiulio, D.B., Relman, D.A., Brown, P.O., 2007. Development of the human infant intestinal microbiota. PLoS Biology 5 (7), e177.

Park, R., Mikami, S., LeClair, J., et al., 2015. Inpatient burden of childhood functional GI disorders in the USA: an analysis of national trends in the USA from 1997 to 2009. Neurogastroenterology and Motility 27 (5), 684–692.

Parmar, A.S., Alakulppi, N., Paavola-Sakki, P., et al., 2012. Association study of FUT2 (rs601338) with celiac disease and inflammatory bowel disease in the Finnish population. Tissue Antigens 80 (6), 488–493.

Payne, D.C., Currier, R.L., Staat, M.A., et al., 2015. Epidemiologic association between FUT2 secretor status and severe rotavirus gastroenteritis in children in the United States. JAMA Pediatr 169 (11), 1040–1045. http://dx.doi.org/10.1001/jamapediatrics.2015.2002.

Pickard, J.M., Maurice, C.F., Kinnebrew, M.A., et al., 2014. Rapid fucosylation of intestinal epithelium sustains host-commensal symbiosis in sickness. Nature 514 (7524), 638–641.

Prince, B.T., Mandel, M.J., Nadeau, K., Singh, A.M., 2015. Gut microbiome and the development of food allergy and allergic disease. Pediatric Clinics of North America 62 (6), 1479–1492.

Quigley, E.M., Abdel-Hamid, H., Barbara, G., et al., 2012. A global perspective on irritable bowel syndrome: a consensus statement of the World Gastroenterology Organisation Summit Task Force on irritable bowel syndrome. Journal of Clinical Gastroenterology 46 (5), 356–366.

Rausch, P., Rehman, A., Kunzel, S., et al., 2011. Colonic mucosa-associated microbiota is influenced by an interaction of Crohn disease and FUT2 (Secretor) genotype. Proceedings of the National Academy of Sciences of the United States of America 108 (47), 19030–19035.

Rayes, A., Morrow, A.L., Payton, L.R., Lake, K.E., Lane, A., Davies, S.M., 2016. A genetic modifier of the gut microbiome influences the risk of graft-versus-host disease and bacteremia after hematopoietic stem cell transplantation. Biol Blood Marrow Transplant 22 (3), 418–422. http://dx.doi.org/10.1016/j.bbmt.2015.11.017 [Epub 2015 November 28, PMID: 26643031].

Roberfroid, M., Gibson, G.R., Hoyles, L., et al., 2010. Prebiotic effects: metabolic and health benefits. The British Journal of Nutrition 104 (Suppl. 2), S1–S63.

Ruiz-Palacios, G.M., Cervantes, L.E., Ramos, P., Chavez-Munguia, B., Newburg, D.S., 2003. *Campylobacter jejuni* binds intestinal H(O) antigen (Fuc alpha 1, 2Gal beta 1, 4GlcNAc), and fucosyloligosaccharides of human milk inhibit its binding and infection. The Journal of Biological Chemistry 278 (16), 14112–14120.

Ruvoen-Clouet, N., Mas, E., Marionneau, S., Guillon, P., Lombardo, D., Le Pendu, J., 2006. Bile-salt-stimulated lipase and mucins from milk of ‘secretor’ mothers inhibit the binding of Norwalk virus capsids to their carbohydrate ligands. The Biochemical Journal 393 (Pt 3), 627–634.

Sandberg, K.C., Davis, M.M., Gebremariam, A., Adler, J., 2014. Increasing hospitalizations in inflammatory bowel disease among children in the United States, 1988–2011. Inflammatory Bowel Diseases 20 (10), 1754–1760.

Sela, D.A., Chapman, J., Adeuya, A., et al., 2008. The genome sequence of *Bifidobacterium longum* subsp. infantis reveals adaptations for milk utilization within the infant microbiome. Proceedings of the National Academy of Sciences of the United States of America 105 (48), 18964–18969.

Shang, J., Piskarev, V.E., Xia, M., et al., 2013. Identifying human milk glycans that inhibit norovirus binding using surface plasmon resonance. Glycobiology 23 (12), 1491–1498.

Smyth, D.J., Cooper, J.D., Howson, J.M., et al., 2011. FUT2 nonsecretor status links type 1 diabetes susceptibility and resistance to infection. Diabetes 60 (11), 3081–3084.

Taft, D., Ward, D., Ollberding, N., Schibler, K., Ambalavanan, N., Yu, Z., Newburg, D., Davidson, B., Morrow, A. 2015a. Preterm infant gut microbiome and weight at 36 weeks corrected gestational age. The FASEB Journal 29 (1), (601.6 Suppl. pp.).

Taft, D.H., Ambalavanan, N., Schibler, K.R., et al., 2015b. Center variation in intestinal microbiota prior to late-onset sepsis in preterm infants. PLoS One 10 (6), e0130604.

Tan, M., Jiang, X., 2014. Histo-blood group antigens: a common niche for norovirus and rotavirus. Expert Reviews in Molecular Medicine 16, e5.

Tanase, I., Paun, S., Stoica, B., Negoi, I., Gaspar, B., Beuran, M., 2015. Epidemiology of diverticular disease – systematic review of the literature. Chirurgia (Bucur) 110 (1), 9–14.

Tarr, A.J., Galley, J.D., Fisher, S.E., Chichlowski, M., Berg, B.M., Bailey, M.T., 2015. The prebiotics 3′Sialyllactose and 6′Sialyllactose diminish stressor-induced anxiety-like behavior and colonic microbiota alterations: evidence for effects on the gut-brain axis. Brain Behavior and Immunity 50, 166–177.

Tong, M., Li, X., Wegener Parfrey, L., et al., 2013. A modular organization of the human intestinal mucosal microbiota and its association with inflammatory bowel disease. PLoS One 8 (11), e80702.

Tong, M., McHardy, I., Ruegger, P., et al., 2014. Reprograming of gut microbiome energy metabolism by the FUT2 Crohn's disease risk polymorphism. ISME Journal 8 (11), 2193–2206.

Torrazza, R.M., Neu, J., 2013. The altered gut microbiome and necrotizing enterocolitis. Clinics in Perinatology 40 (1), 93–108.

Underwood, M.A., Gaerlan, S., De Leoz, M.L., Dimapasoc, L., Kalanetra, K.M., Lemay, D.G., German, J.B., Mills, D.A., Lebrilla, C.B., 2015. Human milk oligosaccharides in premature infants: absorption, excretion and influence on the intestinal microbiota. Pediatric Research 8 (6), 670–677. http://dx.doi.org/10.1038/pr.2015.162 [Epub 2015 August 31, PMID: 26322410].

Vázquez, E., Barranco, A., Ramírez, M., Gruart, A., Delgado-García, J.M., Martínez-Lara, E., Blanco, S., Martín, M.J., Castanys, E., Buck, R., Prieto, P., Rueda, R., 2015. Effects of a human milk oligosaccharide, 2′-fucosyllactose, on hippocampal long-term potentiation and learning capabilities in rodents. The Journal of Nutritional Biochemistry 26 (5), 455–465. http://dx.doi.org/10.1016/j.jnutbio.2014.11.016 [Epub 2015 January 15, PMID: 25662731].

Weiss, G.A., Chassard, C., Hennet, T., 2014. Selective proliferation of intestinal *Barnesiella* under fucosyllactose supplementation in mice. The British Journal of Nutrition 111 (9), 1602–1610.

Yatsunenko, T., Rey, F.E., Manary, M.J., et al., 2012. Human gut microbiome viewed across age and geography. Nature 486 (7402), 222–227.

Yu, Z.T., Chen, C., Kling, D.E., et al., 2013a. The principal fucosylated oligosaccharides of human milk exhibit prebiotic properties on cultured infant microbiota. Glycobiology 23 (2), 169–177.

Yu, Z.T., Chen, C., Newburg, D.S., 2013b. Utilization of major fucosylated and sialylated human milk oligosaccharides by isolated human gut microbes. Glycobiology 23 (11), 1281–1292.

Yu, H., Lau, K., Thon, V., et al., 2014. Synthetic disialyl hexasaccharides protect neonatal rats from necrotizing enterocolitis. Angewandte Chemie (International Edition) 53 (26), 6687–6691.

CHAPTER

8

Human Milk Oligosaccharides as Modulators of Intestinal and Systemic Immunity

Sarah S. Comstock[1], Sharon M. Donovan[2]

[1]*Michigan State University, East Lansing, MI, United States;* [2]*University of Illinois, Urbana, IL, United States*

1. INTRODUCTION

The immune system of the newborn is functionally naïve and is quantitatively and qualitatively different from that of the adult in terms of immune cellularity (Belderbos et al., 2012; Hassan and Reen, 2000; Hawkes et al., 1999), immunoglobulin production (Siegrist et al., 1998; Splawski and Lipsky, 1991), and cytokine response (Chheda et al., 1996; Gibbons et al., 2014; Upham et al., 2002). This state has been described as a "physiological immunodeficiency" that encompasses all arms of the host response, as reflected by the increased risk for common infections like otitis media, upper respiratory tract infections, or gastroenteritis, and serious infections, such as sepsis or meningitis (Jaspan et al., 2006; Lawrence and Pane, 2007). Immune maturation is driven by microbial and antigenic exposures and human milk has evolved to protect the infant during this high-risk period through a number of mechanisms (Turfkruyer and Verhasselt, 2015; Verhasselt, 2015). Human milk contains bioactive lipids, proteins, and carbohydrates that stimulate intestinal development (Donovan, 2006), actively protect the infant from pathogenic infection (Andreas et al., 2015), promote immune tolerance (Verhasselt, 2010), and facilitate the establishment of the microbiota (Walker and Iyengar, 2015).

Emerging evidence has revealed the bidirectional communication between the gut microbiota and the host immune system, in which the microbiota stimulates maturation and specificity of the neonatal mucosal and systemic immune systems (Kaplan et al., 2011; Walker, 2014). The immune system, in turn, ensures that commensal gut microbes are tolerated, while remaining responsive to pathogenic infections (Brown et al., 2013; Kaplan et al., 2011). Moreover, the immune system (Thompson et al., 1996) and microbiota (Herich et al., 2004; Wang et al., 2015) are essential for normal intestinal development. Early nutrition can be viewed as a key regulator of these interactions by directly influencing intestinal growth and barrier function, microbial

Prebiotics and Probiotics in Human Milk. http://dx.doi.org/10.1016/B978-0-12-802725-7.00008-7

composition, and the function of the immune system (Catassi et al., 1995; Donovan, 2006; Kaplan et al., 2011). Human milk oligosaccharides (HMOs), described in Chapters 1 and 2, have the potential to influence immune development and function by affecting gut growth and maturation (Hester and Donovan, 2012; Holscher et al., 2014), immune function (Bode, 2015; Comstock et al., 2014; He et al., 2016; Newburg and He, 2015), and the development of the microbiota (Chichlowski et al., 2011; Wang et al., 2015). This chapter will review the evidence for HMOs as modulators of the infant's gastrointestinal and systemic immune systems.

2. OVERVIEW OF THE IMMUNE SYSTEM

Because this chapter focuses on immunity, we will provide a brief primer on immunity and the immune system to set the stage. Immunology, as with many fields within biology, has its own set of associated vocabulary. For detailed information about the immune system, the reader is directed to immunology textbooks such as *Cellular and Molecular Immunology* (Abbas et al., 2014), *Immunobiology* (Murphy, 2011), or *Fundamental Immunology* (Paul, 2012).

The human immune system consists of organized tissues as well as single cells. Organized tissues of the immune system include the thymus, spleen, lymph nodes, and Peyer's patches. Specialized immune cells are numerous and include basophils, eosinophils, neutrophils, mast cells, monocytes/macrophages, dendritic cells (DCs), natural killer (NK) cells, T cells, and B cells. Also, due to their expression of the major histocompatibility complex (MHC) I molecule, nearly every cell in the body can be considered part of the immune system. The MHC I molecules on the cell surface hold pieces of cytoplasmic constituents. This provides a mechanism by which any cell in the body can notify nearby immune cells that it currently contains nonself (e.g., a virus) or damaged self (e.g., oxidized molecules).

2.1 SYSTEMIC VERSUS PERIPHERAL IMMUNITY

The immune system consists of systemic immune factors that broadly survey and protect the body, as well as peripheral immune factors that are important for protection in peripheral tissues, such as the gastrointestinal tract. These arms of the immune system are in nearly constant communication with one another. This communication occurs as cells and molecules travel from the site of infection or damage to the local immune tissue (such as a lymph node or Peyer's patch) or from one peripheral location through the blood and lymphatic systems to other peripheral locations.

Systemic immunity is composed of the spleen and circulating immune cells. The spleen constantly filters the blood so that its resident immune cells can survey the challenges and immune responses occurring throughout the body. Within the spleen, phagocytes clear dead/damaged cells, bacteria, and other debris from the blood. It is here in the spleen that immune responses to blood-borne pathogens are mounted. The pool of circulating immune cells includes peripheral blood mononuclear cells

(PBMCs) and polymorphonuclear cells (PMNs). PBMCs include T cells, B cells, NK cells, monocytes, and DCs. These cells may be conducting surveillance of the systemic environment, or they may be on their way to, or from, immune response sites in the body.

PBMCs isolated from adult humans (Jentsch-Ullrich et al., 2005) are typically about 70–90% lymphocytes (T, B, and NK cells), 10–30% monocytes, and 1–2% DCs. Within the lymphocytes, 70–85% are T cells (45–70% of PBMCs), 5–20% are B cells (up to 15% of PBMCs), and 5–20% are NK cells (up to 15% of PBMCs). T cells are often divided into T helper (Th) cells and cytotoxic T cells on the basis of their cell surface expression of the molecules CD4 and CD8. CD4-expressing cells, the Th cells, compose about 25–60% of PBMCs, while cytotoxic CD8-expressing T cells make up about 5–30% of PBMCs. CD4 and CD8 T cells exist in an about 2:1 ratio. All of these percentages vary with age and illness.

In infants (Comans-Bitter et al., 1997; Hawkes et al., 1999), PBMCs are typically about 50–85% T cells, 30–60% CD4-expressing Th cells, and 9–25% CD8-expressing cytotoxic T cells, with CD4:CD8 T-cell ratios being anywhere from 2 to 6 depending on the exact age of the infant (Denny et al., 1992). B cells account for 10–19% of an infant's PBMCs. PMNs include neutrophils, basophils, and eosinophils. The majority of PMNs are neutrophils. Healthy infants typically have between 1800 and 5400 neutrophils per 1 mL of blood (Manroe et al., 1979). Basophils and eosinophils make up a small proportion (0.01–10%) of PMNs.

Circulating immune cells offer insight into the overall immune status of an individual but do not predict how immune cells are functioning in local environments, such as the gastrointestinal tissues. To characterize peripheral immune responses, these tissues must be directly sampled. In the case of gastrointestinal tract immune responses, the peripheral immune tissues include the mesenteric lymph nodes (MLNs) and Peyer's patches.

2.2 INNATE AND ADAPTIVE IMMUNE RESPONSES

The human immune system has the capacity to immediately respond to threats, such as pathogens, using innate immune responses. These responses are specific for conserved regions of known nonhuman and potentially dangerous threats. With time, typically 5–7 days, a more specific immune response develops. This response is called the adaptive immune response, which is targeted to the specific threat and to the region(s) of the body where the threat has localized. Once the threat is cleared, the memory immune response continues to survey the body so that a quick, adaptive response can be mounted if the threat should reappear.

There are several ways the immune system can respond to molecules in the body. Pathogen recognition receptors of the innate immune response are proteins that are expressed on many cell types. These receptors bind to molecules commonly expressed by bacteria, viruses, or parasites or molecules that are homologous to those expressed by microbes. They have names such as Toll-like receptors (TLRs) or nucleotide-binding oligomerization domain (NOD)-like receptors. Immune cells, such as T and B cells, have variable receptors that are generated stochastically and are not targeted to any one specific threat and are not self-reactive. These receptors bind to protein, lipid, or carbohydrate domains of pathogens or other nonself molecules. The engagement of the T- or B-cell receptor causes the cell to rapidly proliferate, which results in an army of cells specific for that threat. There are two types of T cells: Th and cytotoxic T cells. The Th cells produce molecules to educate the cytotoxic T cells and B cells about the type and location of the threat. If the Th cells primarily stimulate the cytotoxic T-cell response, then a cellular immune response is mounted. If the Th cells primarily stimulate the B-cell response, then a humoral immune response is mounted.

The newborn immune system is developmentally naïve but undergoes rapid maturation upon exposure to environmental antigens. PBMC gene expression in human infants shifts from humoral to cellular immunity in the first 6 months of life (Donovan et al., 2014a). As part of a clinical trial in infants aimed at assessing how diet impacts the PBMC transcriptome, genes that were developmentally regulated independent of diet were observed. From 4 to 6 months of age, genes associated with humoral immunoglobulin-mediated immunity as well as those associated with interferon (IFN) and interleukin (IL)-4 signaling predominated. These data illustrate the changing gene expression in circulating immune cells of human infants. Neonatal immune development and the impact of diet on immune development in the neonate will be discussed next.

3. IMMUNE DEVELOPMENT OF BREASTFED VERSUS FORMULA-FED INFANTS

In the early postnatal period, the neonate faces a vast array of new and potentially pathogenic microorganisms. The neonatal innate immune system plays a crucial role in both protecting the neonate from pathogenic infection and shaping the adaptive immune system for further protection. For example, NK cells contribute to early protective responses against a variety of infections before pathogen-specific cytotoxic T cells are developed (Levy, 2007). NK cells also secrete inflammatory cytokines to induce the activation of neighboring cells or the adaptive immune cells (Biron et al., 1999). In addition, infants are born with an impaired production of Th1-cell–associated cytokines due to a maternal Th2 bias during pregnancy that protects the fetus from immune response or rejection (Calder et al., 2006). This Th2 bias creates a Th2 dominance in the fetus. Because this comes at the expense of Th1 cytokine production, it leaves the newborn susceptible to microbial infection. Additionally, if the neonate is not able to effectively downregulate the preexisting Th2 dominance, an allergic phenotype may develop (Calder et al., 2006).

How and what the infant is fed influence the development and competence of the immune system (Volman et al., 2008; West et al., 2010), and there is abundant evidence that breastfeeding provides a protective effect in the first 4–6 months of life (Golding et al., 1997; Stuebe and Schwarz, 2010). Furthermore, infants who are breastfed (BF) have increased NK cell counts (Grimble and Westwood, 2001), higher antibody titers (Grimble and Westwood, 2001), more rapid cytotoxic T-cell phenotype development (Andersson et al., 2009; Hawkes et al., 1999), increased vaccination response (Dorea, 2009), and lower morbidity and mortality rates (Kelly and Coutts, 2000) than their formula-fed (FF) peers (reviewed in Stuebe and Schwarz, 2010).

Human milk may confer immune protection by providing factors that contribute to innate immune defense (Turfkruyer and Verhasselt, 2015; Verhasselt, 2015), signaling the immune system and initiating immune development (Kelly and Coutts, 2000), or stimulating the establishment of the microbiome, which in turn influences immune development (Kaplan et al., 2011; Walker, 2014; Walker and Iyengar, 2015). Human milk is a rich source of immune components including immunoglobulins, cytokines, bioactive proteins such as lactoferrin, osteopontin and lysozyme, and bioactive lipids that benefit the infant. Additionally, a strong case can be made for a key role of HMOs in neonatal immune defense and maturation. HMOs are present in high concentrations in human milk, exist in an incredible structural diversity (Bode, 2009) and confer host protection and mediate immune response through a number of mechanisms as will be outlined below.

Chapter 2 of this book (Structures, Classification, and Biosynthesis of Human Milk Oligosaccharides) provides a description of the building blocks, major structural themes, and general biosynthetic machine of the human glycome. Thus, the next topic in this chapter is the interaction of glycans with the immune system.

4. IMPORTANCE OF GLYCANS IN IMMUNE RESPONSES

Carbohydrates and carbohydrate-binding proteins play an important role in immune responses. Mammalian cells have a carbohydrate-containing coating called the glycocalyx (Maverakis et al., 2015). The glycocalyx is engaged when a cell contacts another cell or other components of its environment (Matzinger, 1994). Cells have unique glycan signatures made from combinations of specific glycan motifs. However, many of the glycan motifs found on mammalian cells are also found on microbes and in food.

The carbohydrate-binding proteins associated with mammalian cells translate recognition of specific motifs and the spatial presentation of those motifs into actions (Gabius et al., 2015). This class of proteins is the lectins. Selectins, galectins, and siglecs are just a few types of mammalian lectins (Schnaar, 2015; Taylor and Drickamer, 2014). The reader is directed to a recent review article (Gabius et al., 2015) for a survey of immune lectins.

Lectins are grouped according to their carbohydrate recognition domains (CRDs). Although there are at least a dozen CRDs identified in mammals, three are of particular significance for immune responses: C-type, I-type, and P-type. C-type CRDs require calcium ions for glycan binding. I-type CRD have an immunoglobulin-like structure and P-type CRD bind to mannose-6-phosphate units. Interactions between lectins and glycans are dependent on the structural features of the glycan as well as the density of lectin-reactive groups. Neither the presence of a specific CRD on the receptor nor a specific glycan on the ligand can alone predict the receptor–ligand interaction, because both structures are affected by the other domains of the molecules. Therefore, it is difficult to predict these interactions. However, it is known that glycosylation and lectin expression are coregulated during immune responses (Sperandio, 2006; Zarbock et al., 2011).

The glycans in human milk contain motifs that can bind to these types of receptors. In some cases, HMOs bind directly to glycan-specific cell surface receptors on immune cells. These cases are presented later in this chapter. In other cases, HMO may bind to cell surface receptors on microbes preventing those microbes from binding to their human cell ligands. Examples of this mechanism of action are presented in Chapters 6 and 9 of this book. One example is the rolling of immune cells along blood vessels and lymphatics while waiting to be targeted to infected tissues. Immune cell rolling relies on selectins, highly regulated glycan-binding lectins. The high endothelial venules of lymph nodes constitutively express glycosylation-dependent cell adhesion molecule-1 (GlyCAM-1). GlyCAM-1 is the ligand for L-selectin. Since L-selectin (also known as CD62L) is expressed by naïve and central memory T cells, binding of L-selectin to GlyCAM-1 enables naïve and central memory T cells to enter the lymph nodes. In contrast, effector memory T cells lack L-selectin and thus stay in the periphery (Sallusto et al., 1999). Therefore, the lack of a specific glycoconjugate can prevent cells from accessing specific tissues (Sallusto et al., 1999). Furthermore, blockage of the selectin molecule by free glycans could also prevent rolling leukocytes from extravasation into tissues. HMOs have been shown to affect the rolling of immune cells along endothelial cell monolayers in cell culture experiments (Bode et al., 2004a) and in dynamic flow chambers (Schumacher et al., 2006).

Sometimes glycan signatures are inducible on mammalian cells, and this signature enables trafficking to specific locations within the body. For instance, the cutaneous lymphocyte-associated antigen (CLA) is expressed on skin-associated T cells and enables these cells to access the skin microenvironment through interactions with E-selectin. CLA differs from another selectin, P-selectin glycoprotein ligand-1 (PSGL-1), a glycoprotein expressed by all human T cells (Fuhlbrigge et al., 1997), only in its carbohydrate motifs. Thus, changes in the carbohydrate molecules associated with a protein can trigger T cells to home to the skin. In the same way, association of specific HMOs with particular proteins or cells can target those complexes to specific locations in the infant's gastrointestinal track or other tissues of the infant. Because these complexes must transit the gastrointestinal epithelial barrier, these complexes likely affect other tissues only during the earliest perinatal period when the infant's intestinal barrier is permeable (Catassi et al., 1995). However, circulating HMOs have been detected in the blood of BF human infants up to 6 months of age (Rudloff et al., 2012). Thus, HMOs could complex with proteins or lipids after intestinal absorption. These associations could direct trafficking of associated cells or molecules to specific locations within the infant's body.

Although some examples of glycan-specific immune signatures are known (see examples given earlier), many of the glycan structures and receptor–ligand interactions between glycan structures and the components of the immune system have yet to be characterized (Maverakis et al., 2015). Furthermore, the mechanism(s) by which these glycan moieties are modified remain to be fully elucidated. Although it is known that cytokines can influence the expression of glycosidases, sialidases, and glycosyltransferases and thus impact glycan structure (Azuma et al., 2000), the full ramifications of these modifications need to be catalogued. However, it is clear that oligosaccharide structure is indeed important in immune responses.

Humans express nearly 100 lectins that have been separated into structural families on the basis of their CRDs. Lectins are used by host cells and microbes to interpret the messages encoded in the glycome (Smith and Cummings, 2013). They have complex specificities that not only incorporate select sugar monomers, such as galactose, mannose, and fucose, but also recognize carbohydrate branching, spacing, and multivalency. In some cases, lectins also have secondary or extended binding sites for hydrophobic acyl chains or sulfate groups associated with the oligosaccharides (Taylor and Drickamer, 2014). Examples include the soluble mannose-binding lectins (MBLs), which recognize glycan patterns of microbes and injured host cells. MBLs form complexes with MBL-associated serine proteases (MASPs), which in turn activate complement to destroy the microbial pathogen or potentially dangerous host cell (Banda et al., 2011). The α-defensins have similar carbohydrate-binding properties (Lehrer et al., 2009). Several recent reviews comprehensively discuss sugars and receptors on immune cells (Gabius et al., 2015; Marth and Grewal, 2008; Rabinovich et al., 2012; Schnaar, 2015; van Kooyk and Rabinovich, 2008).

Three important classes of lectins related to the influence of HMO on immune responses will be discussed here: c-type lectins, siglecs, and galectins.

4.1 C-TYPE LECTINS

These lectins are called C-type lectins because they require calcium to function. This group includes selectins, mannose-binding lectin, and DC-specific intercellular adhesion molecule 3-grabbing nonintegrin (DC-SIGN). C-type lectin receptors (CLRs) on the surface of DCs determine whether the cell will induce tolerance rather than lymphocyte activation (Geijtenbeek et al., 2004; Steinman et al., 2003).

The C-type lectin DC-SIGN is of particular interest with regard to mechanisms by which HMO can influence immunity because it has CRD specific for fucose units (Becker and Lowe, 2003; Bogoevska et al., 2006). Furthermore, DC-SIGN is expressed by cells in the gastrointestinal tracts of infants (Koning et al., 2015). These intestinal cells are likely antigen presenting cells as DC-SIGN is expressed by antigen presenting cells, specifically DCs (Garcia-Vallejo and van Kooyk, 2013). Although interactions between fucosylated ligands and DC-SIGN contribute to immune tolerance (Conde et al., 2015), the full story is more complicated with the cellular response to DC-SIGN ligation being dependent on the other ligand–receptor actions occurring simultaneously (Garcia-Vallejo and van Kooyk, 2015).

4.2 SIGLECS

Siglecs (sialic acid–binding Ig-like lectins) are sialic acid–binding lectins most commonly found on subsets of immune cells (Bochner and Zimmermann, 2015; Macauley et al., 2014). Some siglecs are conserved across mammals. These include sialoadhesin (siglec-1), CD22 (siglec-2), myelin-associated glycoprotein (MAG, siglec-4), and siglec-15. Others, specifically the CD33-related siglecs exhibit variation across mammals. Siglec specificity derives from differences in secondary binding sites (Schnaar, 2015). There are at least 16 siglecs expressed by different leukocyte populations (Pillai et al., 2012). Because siglecs are endocytic cell surface receptors that carry their cargo between the cell surface and intracellular vesicles, these receptors are mainly expressed on cells involved in antigen processing and presentation (Crocker et al., 2007; Macauley et al., 2014). Furthermore, sialic acid–containing molecules can gain entry to macrophages by binding to siglecs on the cell surface (Izquierdo-Useros et al., 2014).

Mammalian cells can express self-associated molecular patterns (SAMPs) to prevent immune responses to nonpathogenic stimuli (Varki and Gagneux, 2009). Some sialic acid–containing glycans function as SAMPs. Therefore, siglecs (e.g., CD33) are potential SAMP-recognizing receptors that can repress immune responses as they contain immunoreceptor tyrosine-based inhibitory motifs (ITIMs) (Chen et al., 2009; Crocker et al., 2007). Furthermore, ligation of some siglecs stimulates the production of the immunoregulatory cytokine IL-10 (Stephenson et al., 2014).

4.3 GALECTINS

The CRD of galectins is specific for β-galactosides (Ebrahim et al., 2014). This class of lectins is important for cell turnover and immune regulation. Sialic acid groups, or rather, the removal of sialic acid groups, are important for triggering cellular turnover. Sialyation of red blood cells is a good example. As a red blood cell ages, it becomes progressively desialylated, increasing the density of exposed galactose moieties on its surface. This allows for asialoglycoprotein receptors expressed by the liver to recognize the aged red blood cells and signal for their destruction (Aminoff et al., 1977). As another example, naïve T cells express CD45 with an α-2,6–linked sialic acid. The amount of α-2,6–linked sialic acid is reduced following T-cell activation. This decrease in α-2,6–linked sialic acid renders the activated T cells susceptible to galectin-1–mediated apoptosis (Earl et al., 2010). Furthermore, differential sialyation of Th1 and Th2 effector cells selectively regulates their susceptibility to cell death (Toscano et al., 2007).

Given these brief primers on the immune system, infant immunity, and the importance of glycans in immune responses, the specific roles of HMOs in immunity will now be presented.

5. HUMAN MILK OLIGOSACCHARIDES AS MODULATORS OF SYSTEMIC AND MUCOSAL IMMUNITY

Potential mechanisms whereby HMOs influence host immune function are summarized in Fig. 8.1. The overall structure of the intestine is shown in panel A, and a higher detail of the intestinal lumen is shown in panel B. Intestinal health and barrier

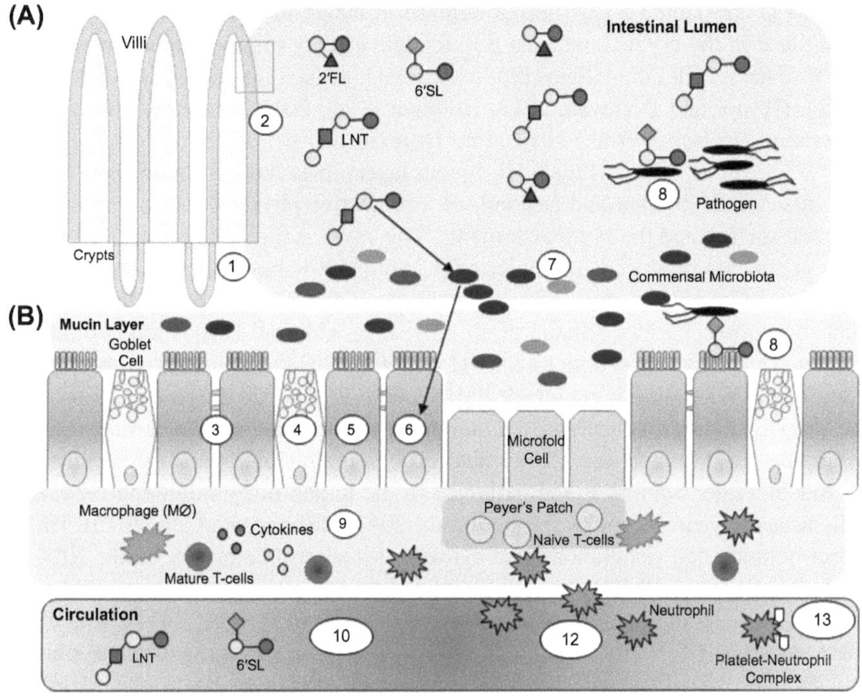

FIGURE 8.1

Potential mechanisms whereby human milk oligosaccharides (HMOs) influence host immune function. The overall structure of the intestine is shown in panel A, and a higher detail of the intestinal lumen is shown in panel B. HMOs affect innate immunity through the epithelial barrier: HMOs reduce intestinal crypt cell proliferation (1) (Hester and Donovan, 2012; Holscher et al., 2014), increase intestinal cell maturation (2) (Holscher et al., 2014), increase barrier function (3) (Holscher et al., 2014), and may influence goblet cell function (4), as has been shown for galacto-oligosaccharides (Bhatia et al., 2015). In addition, HMOs affect epithelial immune gene expression both directly (5) (Lane et al., 2013) and indirectly through the microbiota (6) (Wickramasinghe et al., 2015). HMOs serve as prebiotics to promote the growth of healthy bacteria, including bifidobacterial and *Bacteroides* species (7) (Marcobal and Sonnenburg, 2012), and HMOs inhibit infections by bacteria and viruses by either binding to the pathogen in the lumen or by inhibiting binding to cell-surface glycan receptors (8) (Hester et al., 2013; Newburg and He, 2015). HMOs affect immune cell populations and cytokine secretion (9) (Comstock et al., 2014; Li et al., 2014). HMOs are also absorbed into the bloodstream (10) (Goehring et al., 2014; Obermeier et al., 1999; Rudloff et al., 2012; Ruhaak et al., 2014) where they affect binding of monocytes, lymphocytes, and neutrophils to endothelial cells (11) (Bode et al., 2004a) and formation of platelet–neutrophil complexes (12) (Bode et al., 2004b).

function is considered a first line of defense in innate immunity. Cell proliferation takes place in the crypts, and cells differentiate as they migrate up or down (in the case of Paneth cells) the villus–crypt axis. HMOs reduce intestinal crypt cell proliferation (Hester and Donovan, 2012; Holscher et al., 2014), increase intestinal cell maturation (Holscher et al., 2014), and increase barrier function (Holscher et al., 2014). A layer of mucus (Fig. 8.1B, mucin layer) lines the gastrointestinal tract. It acts, first, as a lubricant and, second, as a protective physical barrier between the mucosal surface and the luminal contents. This layer is formed by mucus glycoproteins or mucins produced by goblet cells. Although it has not been demonstrated experimentally, HMOs may influence goblet cell function, as has been shown for galacto-oligosaccharides (Bhatia et al., 2015). In addition, HMOs affect epithelial immune gene expression both directly (Lane et al., 2013) and indirectly through the microbiota (Wickramasinghe et al., 2015). HMOs serve as prebiotics to promote the growth of healthy bacteria, including bifidobacterial and *Bacteroides* genera (Marcobal and Sonnenburg, 2012), and HMOs inhibit infections by bacteria and viruses by either binding to the pathogen in the lumen or by inhibiting binding to cell-surface glycan receptors (Hester et al., 2013; Newburg and He, 2015). HMOs affect immune cell populations and cytokine secretion (Comstock et al., 2014; Li et al., 2014). Some HMOs are also absorbed into the bloodstream (Goehring et al., 2014; Obermeier et al., 1999; Rudloff et al., 2012; Ruhaak et al., 2014), where they exert systemic effects by binding of monocytes, lymphocytes, and neutrophils to endothelial cells (Bode et al., 2004a) and formation of platelet–neutrophil complexes (Bode et al., 2004a).

5.1 METHODS

Before further discussing the effects of HMOs on systemic and mucosal immunity, a brief overview of key methods is needed. When analyzing immune responses of any type, careful attention must be paid to timing. An immune response is a highly kinetic occurrence with expected results varying based on the timing of the analysis. Furthermore, the reader is cautioned that dietary effects on immunity are more detectable in situations where immune homeostasis is perturbed. As a general reference for immunology-related protocols, we direct the reader to *Current Protocols in Immunology* (Strober, 2015).

5.1.1 Ex Vivo Methods

Common methods of assessing the effects of a compound on immune cells include isolation and stimulation of mixed cell types, isolation and stimulation of pure populations of specific cell types, and immediate analysis of isolated cells. These cells can be analyzed for cell surface expression of particular glycans or cell surface receptors, presence of key glycosylation-related proteins, glycan- or immune-related gene expression, or production of specific immune signaling molecules such as cytokines (van Kooyk et al., 2013). Important glycosylation-related proteins include enzymes, cofactors, transporters, and activated sugar donor molecules needed for glycan synthesis. These methods can be used with cells of human or animal origin. These methods are particularly of benefit for assessing the behavior of human cells because other human tissue is not readily available for study.

5.1.2 In Vitro Methods

In vitro and ex vivo analyses differ in the cell types available for use. In vitro methods rely on cell lines or transformed primary cells. In some instances, cell lines may not provide appropriate responses because long-term culture and passage can result in changes to the glycocalyx (Barratt et al., 1978) and changes to glycosylation patterns of the produced proteins (Restelli et al., 2006). Furthermore, the performance of immune cell lines is unlikely to mirror that of freshly isolated cells or cells analyzed from in vivo feeding experiments.

5.1.3 Animal Models

Until recently, securing sufficient quantities of HMOs had been difficult. Within the last 5 years, laboratory workers have begun to feed HMOs to rodents as well as use them in large animal models such as pigs. Animals models are beneficial for a variety of reasons that have been reviewed elsewhere (Puiman and Stoll, 2008). When conducting experiments with a focus on the immune response, it is important to consider the similarity of the animal's immune system to that of the human. Neonatal pigs are a highly suitable animal model for human infants (Odle et al., 2014). The percentage (6–12%) of NK cells found in piglets (Thorum et al., 2013) is close to that reported in human infants (Andersson et al., 2009; Hawkes et al., 1999). Previous studies have shown that BF infants had a higher percentage of NK cells in PBMCs than did FF infants (Andersson et al., 2009; Hawkes et al., 1999). NK cell population size in the blood and tissues of SR pigs is also larger than that of FF pigs (Liu et al., 2013). Lymphocytes from FF infants proliferate more in response to mitogens (Juto et al., 1982; Stephens et al., 1986). Additionally, FF infants have more Th cells than do BF infants (Carver et al., 1991), and the CD4:CD8 ratio in PBMCs isolated from BF infants is lower than that in FF infants (Andersson et al., 2009; Hawkes et al., 1999). These differences are similar to results obtained from PBMCs isolated from piglets where cells from FF piglets proliferated more, consisted of more Th cells, and had greater Th:cytotoxic T-cell ratios than those isolated from the sow-reared (SR) piglets (Comstock et al., 2014). One caveat to using a larger animal model, such as pigs, is that larger amounts of HMOs must be obtained to conduct a feeding trial in neonatal pigs compared to rodents.

5.1.4 Human Studies

Although it is possible to enroll humans in dietary consumption trials, difficulties in truly randomizing participants to treatment and accessing human tissue make objective conclusions from these studies challenging. These difficulties limit the research to systemic immune parameters as the only easily obtainable and isolatable immune cells are those from cord blood or peripheral blood. Recent progress in obtaining noninvasive molecular fingerprints of host gene expression is beginning to enable the study of in vivo localized intestinal immune responses (Donovan et al., 2014b). Furthermore, some researchers are making progress by using tissues from discarded human fetuses (He et al., 2014). Although not yet applied to this field, newer methods of analysis requiring smaller blood volumes likely will be used soon as mass cytometry, where cellular targets are labeled with metal-tagged antibodies and detected and quantified by time-of-flight mass spectrometry, becomes more popular and available (Fessenden, 2015).

5.2 SYSTEMIC IMMUNITY

5.2.1 Direct Effects on Immune Cells

To directly affect systemic immune cells, HMOs must be absorbed into the neonate's bloodstream. Because of their structural complexity and the high concentrations of HMOs found in the feces of BF infants (Coppa et al., 2001; Goehring et al., 2014), it had been assumed that these complex oligosaccharides were not absorbed. However, between 1 and 3 mg of single HMOs has been shown to be excreted in the urine (24-h collection) of infants fed mother's milk (Rudloff et al., 2012). Urinary excretion of intact HMOs indicates that these compounds are not only absorbed but also present in the blood in their typical conformation. This is supported by work that identified HMOs (1–133 mg/L) in plasma of infants fed human milk (Goehring et al., 2014; Marriage et al., 2015; Radzanowski et al., 2013). Combined, this evidence confirms that HMOs have the potential to exert systemic effects.

As discussed earlier, many immune receptors recognize the oligosaccharide structures of their glycoprotein ligands (Rabinovich et al., 2012). Oligosaccharides can affect binding to, the quality of or the length of association between cell surface receptors and their ligands, thereby altering signaling from the surface to nucleus of a cell (Rana and Haltiwanger, 2011). Selectins are one class of cell-surface proteins that bind glycan moieties (Bevilacqua and Nelson, 1993; Ley, 2003). Because some HMOs are structurally similar to selectin ligands (Bevilacqua and Nelson, 1993; Bode, 2006; Kunz and Rudloff, 2008; Rudloff et al., 2002), it is likely that HMOs can bind directly to immune cells and trigger signaling that results in changes to immune cell populations and functions. For instance, the P- and E-selectins recognize sialyl-Lewis X (sLeX), a glycan moiety found on several HMOs (Huang et al., 2002). Additionally, fucosylation and sialylation, two enzymatic modifications commonly found on HMOs, enable binding to selectins (Luhn and Wild, 2012).

Immune protein–carbohydrate interactions, such as those mediated by selectins, have been shown to be modulated by HMOs. These studies are summarized in Table 8.1. Interruption of immune protein–carbohydrate interactions reduced neutrophil rolling (Bode et al., 2004a; Schumacher et al., 2006) and activation (Bode et al., 2004b). HMOs have also been demonstrated to have direct effects on immune cell proliferation and cytokine production in ex vivo experiments with PBMCs from neonatal pigs (Comstock et al., 2014). In this study, isolated HMOs triggered PBMCs to produce more of the regulatory cytokine IL-10. These isolated HMOs also enhanced proliferation of PBMCs stimulated with a T-cell mitogen, phytohemagglutinin (PHA).

Table 8.1 Immune-Related Outcomes of HMO Cell Stimulation Assays

Cells Types	Study Design	Major Findings	References
PBMCs isolated from sow-reared and colostrum-deprived formula-fed piglets	• cells stimulated ex vivo for 72 h • HMOs studied: iHMO, 2′-FL, 3′-FL, 3′-SL, 6′-SL, LNnT • Dose: 125 μg/mL • outcomes: cell proliferation, cytokine secretion, cell phenotypes	• iHMO: Increased IL-10 • PHA + LNnT: Increased TNFα • 2′-FL: Less proliferation • PHA + iHMO: More proliferation • LPS + sialylated HMOs: More proliferation • LPS + iHMO: Fewer $CD4^+$ T cells • LPS + sialylated HMOs: Fewer $CD4^+$ T cells • LPS + fucosylated HMOs: Fewer $CD4^+$ T cells	Comstock et al. (2014)
Human CBMCs and allergen-specific $CD4^+$ T cells isolated from adult human blood	• Cells stimulated ex vivo for 72 h • HMO studied: aHMO, pectin-derived oligosaccharides, GOS/FOS • Dose: 100 μg/mL • Outcomes: Cytokine production	• aHMO: Increased CBMC IFNγ • aHMO: Increased CBMC IL-10 • aHMO: Decreased allergen-specific T-cell IL-4 • aHMO: Increased allergen-specific T-cell IFNγ:IL-4 ratio	Eiwegger et al. (2010)
U937 human myeloid cell line	• Ex vivo flow chamber coated with P-selectin • HMOs studied: iHMO, nHMO, aHMO, GOS, sLeX • Dose: 100 μg/mL • Outcomes: cell adhesion and rolling	• aHMO: Decreased adhesion • sLeX: Decreased adhesion	Schumacher et al. (2006)
Monocytes, lymphocytes, and neutrophils isolated from human blood	• Ex vivo flow chamber coated with TNFα-activated HUVECs • Preincubated with oligosaccharides for 1 h • HMOs studied: iHMO, aHMO, 3′-SL, 6′-SL, 3′-sialyl-3-fucosyl-lactose, sLeX • Dose: 12.5–125 μg/mL • Outcomes: cell rolling and adhesion	• aHMO: Inhibited cell rolling and adhesion • sLeX: Inhibited cell adhesion • 3′-Sialyl-3-fucosyl-lactose: Inhibited cell rolling and adhesion	Bode et al. (2004a)
Human whole blood	• Cells activated ex vivo with ADP • HMOs studied: aHMO, nHMO, sLeX • Dose: 6.25–125 μg/mL • Outcomes: PNC formation and neutrophil β2-integrin expression	• aHMO: Reduced PNC formation and neutrophil β2-integrin expression • sLeX: Reduced PNC formation and neutrophil β2-integrin expression	Bode et al. (2004b)
Human CBMC	• Cells stimulated ex vivo for 5–20 day • HMOs studied: aHMO, nHMO • Dose: 1 μg/mL (aHMO), 10 μg/mL (nHMO) • outcomes: Cell phenotypes (day 5) and cytokine production (day 20)	• aHMO: Increased CBMC $CD4^+$ IFNγ-expressing cells • aHMO: Increased CBMC $CD8^+$ IFNγ-expressing cells • aHMO: Increased CBMC $CD8^+$ IL-13–expressing cells • aHMO: Increased T regulatory cells	Eiwegger et al. (2004)

2′-FL, *2-fucosyllactose;* 3′-SL, *3-sialylactose;* 6′-SL, *6-sialylactose;* ADP, *adenosine 5′-diphosphate;* aHMO, *acidic HMO;* CBMC, *cord blood mononuclear cell;* FOS, *fructo-oligosaccharide;* GOS, *galacto-oligosaccharide;* HMO, *human milk oligosaccharide;* HUVEC, *human umbilical vein endothelial cell;* iHMO, *fraction of HMOs isolated from human milk;* IL, *interleukin;* LNnT, *lacto-N-neo-tetraose;* LPS, *lipopolysaccharide;* nHMO, *neutral HMO;* PHA, *phytohemagglutinin;* PNC, *platelet–neutrophil complex;* sLeX, *sialyl-Lewis*^{x}.

When analyzed separately, the fucosylated HMOs, 2-fucosyllactose (2′-FL), inhibited proliferation of unstimulated PBMCs cultured for 3 days. The sialylated HMOs enhanced proliferation of PBMCs stimulated with the B-cell mitogen lipopolysaccharide (LPS). Others have observed that the acidic HMOs induce IL-10 production; additionally, they find that acidic HMOs induce IFNγ from ex vivo stimulated human cord blood mononuclear cells (Eiwegger et al., 2010).

5.2.2 Effects in Animal Models

To date, very few studies in which HMOs were fed to animals and immune outcomes were analyzed (Castillo-Courtade et al., 2015; He et al., 2016; Kurakevich et al., 2013; Li et al., 2014) (Table 8.2). Marriage et al. (2015) fed 2′-FL to human infants, but immune outcomes have not yet been reported. Another group fed 2′-FL to baby piglets but reported only growth and toxicological outcomes (Hanlon and Thorsrud, 2014). In an additional study, although the mice were not fed 2′-FL, rather *Fut2* gene expression and therefore fucosylation of the intestinal epithelial cell layer was induced via systemic LPS administration, the presence of these fucosylated molecules on the epithelium and in the gut lumen reduced colonic cell proliferation and weight loss (Pickard et al., 2014). The studies in which pigs and human infants were fed the HMOs have focused on 2′-FL, This is likely because it is readily available in large quantities for a reasonable cost, but it is also because the fucosylated oligosaccharides have been shown to feed specific beneficial classes of bacteria during intestinal inflammatory events (Kashyap et al., 2013; Pickard et al., 2014). Given what is known about the effects of other HMOs, these compounds also should be used in feeding studies.

Only one in vivo study has used a complex mixture of HMOs and assessed immune outcomes. In that report, neonatal pigs fed a diet containing 4 g/L HMOs consisting of 40% 2′-FL, 10% 6′-sialyllactose (SL), 35% lacto-*N-neo*-tetraose (LNnT), 5% 3′-SL, and 10% free sialic acid had a shorter duration of diarrhea, in response to rotavirus (RV) infection than did pigs fed formula containing little prebiotic (Li et al., 2014). Ileal tissue from the pigs fed HMOs contained greater IFNγ (produced by Th1 cells) and IL-10 (an antiinflammatory cytokine) mRNA than that from pigs fed formula. Another report of neonatal piglets fed only 2′-FL was recently published, but no immune-related end points were reported (Hanlon and Thorsrud, 2014). In mice, the milk oligosaccharides lacto-*N*-fucopentaose III (LNFPIII) and LNnT are Th2-biasing and suppress Th1 responses (Okano et al., 2001; Terrazas et al., 2001; Velupillai et al., 1997).

In a mouse model of food allergy, 2′-FL and 6′-SL administered via oral gavage reduced symptoms in mice sensitized to ovalbumin, an egg protein (Castillo-Courtade et al., 2015). Specifically, ovalbumin-stimulated splenocytes from mice treated with 6′-SL produced more IL-10 and less IFNγ than those from untreated mice. Furthermore, 2′-FL– or 6′-SL–treated mice had more regulatory immune cells in their intestinal immune tissues than untreated mice. Interestingly, neither 2′-FL nor 6′-SL affected intestinal T regulatory cells when administered to nonsensitized mice. This exemplifies the necessity of identifying an appropriate challenge model to assess the effects of dietary compounds on the immune system.

Table 8.2 Immune-Related Outcomes of HMO Feeding Studies

Species	Study Design	Major Findings	References

Colostrum-deprived piglets	• 15-day feeding study
	  ◦ Formula
	  ◦ Formula + 4 g/L HMO (40% 2′-FL; 35% LNnT; 10% 6′-SL; 5% 3′-SL; 10% free SA)
	  ◦ Formula prebiotic (PRE; 90% scGOS; 10% scFOS)
	• Infected with OSU strain RV on day 10
	• Analyzed day 15
		• HMOs and PREs: Shorter duration of diarrhea
		• HMOs: Higher ileal IFNγ and IL-10 mRNA expression than formula
		• HMOs: Similar concentrations of RV-specific IgG and IgM as formula
		• PREs: Higher RV-specific IgM than formula
			Li et al. (2014)

Adult male BALB/c mice	• Food allergy treatment model
	  ◦ i.p. sensitized to OVA
	  ◦ 2 week later (day 27), oral gavage daily (1 mg in 200 μL PBS)
	    - 2′-FL
	    - 6′-SL
	    - Lactose
	  ◦ Day 28 oral challenge with OVA (50 mg) every 3 day until day 43
	  ◦ Analyzed day 43
		• 2′-FL and 6′-SL attenuated the diarrhea and hypothermia induced by OVA challenge
		• 2′-FL and 6′-SL reduced intestinal mast cell numbers
		• 6′-SL increased OVA-specific IgG2a
		• 6′-SL splenocytes produced more IFNγ and IL-10 but less TNF
		• 2′-FL splenocytes produced less IFNγ
		• 2′-FL and 6′-SL increased Peyer's patch T regulatory cells and CD11c⁺ CD103⁺ DCs
		• 6′-SL increased MLN T regulatory cells
		• Intestinal immune cell populations were not affected by feeding nonsensitized mice with oligosaccharides
		• 2′-FL and 6′-SL reduced passive cutaneous anaphylaxis
			Castillo-Courtade et al. (2015)

Adult female C57BL/6 mice	• *E. coli* infection model
	  ◦ 0.25% dextran sodium sulfate (DSS) orally for day 0–3
	  ◦ 2′-FL (100 mg/200 μL) or vehicle by oral gavage day 0–4
	  ◦ 20 mg streptomycin by oral gavage day 4
	• Infected with AIEC on day 5
	• Analyzed day 9
		• 2′-FL prevented body weight loss
		• 2′-FL reduced AIEC colonization
		• 2′-FL reduced colonic crypt cell CD14 expression
		• 2′-FL reduced colon inflammation
		• 2′-FL reduced colonic IL-6, IL-17, and TNFα production in response to AIEC infection
			He et al. (2016)

2′-FL, *2-fucosyllactose;* 6′-SL, *6-sialylactose;* AIEC, *adherent-invasive* E. coli; DC, *dendritic cell;* HMO, *human milk oligosaccharide;* IFN, *interferon;* IL, *interleukin;* LNnT, *lacto-N-neo-tetraose;* MLN, *mesenteric lymph nodes;* OSU, *Ohio State University;* OVA, *ovalbumin;* PRE, *prebiotic;* RV, *rotavirus;* SA, *sialic acid;* scGOS, *short-chain galacto-oligosaccharides;* scFOS, *short-chain fructo-oligosaccharide;* TNF, *tumor necrosis factor.*

Another approach using knock out mice has shown that SL-containing compounds can directly affect gastrointestinal mucosal immunity (Fuhrer et al., 2010; Huang et al., 2015; Kurakevich et al., 2013). In one study, the presence of 3′-SL in the milk increased the number of immune cells infiltrating the gut in IL-10 null mice (Kurakevich et al., 2013). Furthermore, supplementation with 3′-SL increased colitis severity in newborn IL-10 and St3gal4 (the enzyme that synthesizes 3′-SL) null mice and cross-fostering wildtype mice to deficient dams reduced colitis severity. One caveat of this work is that it was conducted in the absence of endogenous IL-10 production, whereas other in vivo studies have demonstrated that some HMOs increase intestinal IL-10 (Castillo-Courtade et al., 2015; Li et al., 2014). 3′-SL is a product of several pathogenic bacteria (Severi et al., 2007), and the conformation on pathogenic bacteria and in human milk is the same α2,3-link between sialic acid and galactose (Audry et al., 2011). 3′-SL is recognized by DCs and generates an immune response through the toll-like receptor 4 (TLR4) signaling pathway (Kuijf et al., 2010). These results suggest that the presence of 3′-SL increases the inflammatory response. This report also presents evidence that 3′-SL alters the immune response through direct effects on DCs. The authors show that 3′-SL was less effective at inducing DC activation when TLR4 was absent. However, those DC also demonstrated a minimal increase in CD40 expression, suggesting at least one other 3′-SL–sensing mechanism, albeit much less efficient than the TLR4 pathway, exists on DC. TLR4 is the receptor for *Escherichia coli* LPS. Another link between 3′-SL and TLR4 is explained in a more recent report, where it is demonstrated that 3′-SL stimulates the proliferation of the intestinal *E. coli* population and that this overgrowth of *E. coli* is responsible for exacerbation of dextran sodium sulfate (DSS) colitis through release of proinflammatory cytokines from intestinal DCs (Huang et al., 2015). These examples demonstrate the complexity of the relationships between oligosaccharides, the gut bacteria, and the immune system.

5.3 INTESTINAL MUCOSAL IMMUNITY

5.3.1 Effects Observed In Vitro and In Situ

Intestinal cell lines have been used to determine effects of HMOs on immune-related gene expression and protein production. Some studies have used direct coincubation with oligosaccharides (Lane et al., 2013), others have coincubated intestinal cells with bacteria (Wickramasinghe et al., 2015), and still others have tested incubation of intestinal cell lines with LPS as a bacterial infection model (He et al., 2016). One limitation of all of these reports is the failure to publish the final oligosaccharide composition of the HMO fraction used. Coincubation of *Bifidobacterium* with cells of the Caco-2 intestinal cell line and HMOs resulted in downregulation of intestinal cell genes related to chemokine activity compared to coincubation in the presence of the simpler sugars glucose or lactose (Wickramasinghe et al., 2015). Conversely, in the absence of a bacterial costimulant, HMOs increased expression of several chemokines by the HT-29 cell line (Lane et al., 2013). Additional work in T84 and HCT8 intestinal cell lines also demonstrates the ability of complex mixtures of HMO as well as 2′-FL to reduce signatures of intestinal inflammation (He et al., 2016).

HMOs have been demonstrated to affect the course of a gastrointestinal viral infection. In an acute RV infection model where a 21-day-old piglet's ileum is isolated in situ, intestinal loops cotreated with HMO and RV had reduced nonstructural protein-4 (NSP-4) mRNA expression, indicating that HMOs can reduce RV replication (Hester et al., 2013). Intestinal cytokine and chemokine expression, however, was not affected. Both neutral and acidic HMOs decreased NSP4 intestinal mRNA expression, whereas only acidic HMOs effectively inhibited RV infectivity of an in vitro cell line.

5.3.2 Effects on Tissues

Immunological consequences of feeding HMOs may result from a change in intestinal barrier function mediated through altered intestinal cell proliferation and changes in the gut bacterial populations brought about by feeding HMOs. Diet-induced changes in the gut microbial populations would also affect gut development and barrier function (Andrade et al., 2015; Huang et al., 2013). HMOs are known to affect intestinal cell proliferation (Hester and Donovan, 2012; Holscher et al., 2014; Kuntz et al., 2009). Additionally, dietary HMOs decorate the intestinal lining contributing to the intestinal glycome (Kavanaugh et al., 2015). HMOs also contribute to epithelial barrier function by supporting the growth of *Bifidobacterium longum* subspecies infantis (*B. infantis*) bacteria in the infant gut (Underwood et al., 2015). *B. infantis* produces peptides that have been shown to normalize intestinal permeability through enhanced tight junction protein expression in a mouse model of colitis (Ewaschuk et al., 2008). It is likely that HMOs support other bacterial species that are important for the maintenance of gut integrity. These changes in intestinal barrier function would, in turn, alter both the local and systemic immune system (Macpherson et al., 2005; Nalle and Turner, 2015).

5.3.3 Effects on the Microbiota

Another immunological consequence of feeding HMOs is altered immune response due to alteration of intestinal bacterial populations. Dietary complex oligosaccharides are important food for intestinal bacteria because bacteria have enzymatic systems capable of breaking glycolytic bonds which the host cannot. Therefore, the composition of the intestinal bacterial population depends on which complex oligosaccharides are fed. In this way, HMOs affect gut microbial populations. Previously, we have shown that HMO fermentation by neonatal pig microbiota produced short-chain fatty acids and promoted the growth of beneficial bacteria in vitro (Li et al., 2012) and in vivo (Li et al., 2014). Gut bacteria and the immune response, particularly the gastrointestinal immune response, are tightly interrelated (Goto and Kiyono, 2012). Thus, in this animal model, HMO-induced changes in the gut bacterial populations of the pigs could alter the course of an intestinal infection, which in turn would alter the immune response (Lacroix-Lamande et al., 2014; Pickard and Chervonsky, 2015; Sassone-Corsi and Raffatellu, 2015). Alternatively, the change in the gut bacteria could directly affect the immune system of these animals (Walker, 2014).

6. SUMMARY AND CONCLUSIONS

The rich diversity of HMOs has the potential to modulate both innate and adaptive arms of the neonatal immune system. Data generated through in vitro experiments and preclinical animal models have shown that HMOs directly interact with the epithelial cells lining the gastrointestinal tract as well as immune cells located in mucosal immune tissues and the circulation to modulate immune function. HMOs also beneficially shape the microbiome of the BF infant. With the increased availability of HMOs from commercial sources and research demonstrating that formula supplemented with HMOs is safe and may confer benefits for human infants, it is possible that in the near future infant formula will contain HMOs alone or in combination with other prebiotics. In addition, due to their beneficial effects on immune function and host defense, HMOs may also be beneficial for other segments of the population who are immune compromised or may be at high risk for infection. There are limited studies in which animals or humans have been fed HMOs. Additionally, few studies have assessed the effects of feeding complex mixtures of HMOs on the immune response. Most studies feed a single HMO and assess a single immunological situation. Clearly, this is an area of research that is only in its infancy.

REFERENCES

Abbas, A.K., Lichtman, A.H., Pillai, S., 2014. Cellular and Molecular Immunology, eighth ed. Saunders, Philadelphia, PA.

Aminoff, D., Bruegge, W.F., Bell, W.C., Sarpolis, K., Williams, R., 1977. Role of sialic acid in survival of erythrocytes in the circulation: interaction of neuraminidase-treated and untreated erythrocytes with spleen and liver at the cellular level. Proceedings of the National Academy of Sciences of the United States of America 74, 1521–1524.

Andersson, Y., Hammarstrom, M.L., Lonnerdal, B., Graverholt, G., Falt, H., Hernell, O., 2009. Formula feeding skews immune cell composition toward adaptive immunity compared to breastfeeding. Journal of Immunology 183, 4322–4328.

Andrade, M.E., Araujo, R.S., de Barros, P.A., Soares, A.D., Abrantes, F.A., Generoso, S.V., Fernandes, S.O., Cardoso, V.N., 2015. The role of immunomodulators on intestinal barrier homeostasis in experimental models. Clinical Nutrition.

Andreas, N.J., Kampmann, B., Mehring Le-Doare, K., 2015. Human breast milk: a review on its composition and bioactivity. Early Human Development 91, 629–635.

Audry, M., Jeanneau, C., Imberty, A., Harduin-Lepers, A., Delannoy, P., Breton, C., 2011. Current trends in the structure-activity relationships of sialyltransferases. Glycobiology 21, 716–726.

Azuma, Y., Murata, M., Matsumoto, K., 2000. Alteration of sugar chains on alpha(1)-acid glycoprotein secreted following cytokine stimulation of HuH-7 cells in vitro. Clinica Chimica Acta 294, 93–103.

Banda, N.K., Takahashi, M., Takahashi, K., Stahl, G.L., Hyatt, S., Glogowska, M., Wiles, T.A., Endo, Y., Fujita, T., Holers, V.M., Arend, W.P., 2011. Mechanisms of mannose-binding lectin-associated serine proteases-1/3 activation of the alternative pathway of complement. Molecular Immunology 49, 281–289.

Barratt, D.G., Rogers, J.D., Sharom, F.J., Grant, C.W., 1978. Direct modification of the glycocalyx of a cultured muscle cell line by incorporation of foreign gangliosides and an integral membrane glycoprotein. Journal of Supramolecular Structure 8, 119–128.

Becker, D.J., Lowe, J.B., 2003. Fucose: biosynthesis and biological function in mammals. Glycobiology 13, 41R–53R.

Belderbos, M.E., Houben, M.L., van Bleek, G.M., Schuijff, L., van Uden, N.O., Bloemen-Carlier, E.M., Kimpen, J.L., Eijkemans, M.J., Rovers, M., Bont, L.J., 2012. Breastfeeding modulates neonatal innate immune responses: a prospective birth cohort study. Pediatric Allergy and Immunology 23, 65–74.

Bevilacqua, M.P., Nelson, R.M., 1993. Selectins. Journal of Clinical Investigation 91, 379–387.

Bhatia, S., Prabhu, P.N., Benefiel, A.C., Miller, M.J., Chow, J., Davis, S.R., Gaskins, H.R., 2015. Galacto-oligosaccharides may directly enhance intestinal barrier function through the modulation of goblet cells. Molecular Nutrition & Food Research 59, 566–573.

Biron, C.A., Nguyen, K.B., Pien, G.C., Cousens, L.P., Salazar-Mather, T.P., 1999. Natural killer cells in antiviral defense: function and regulation by innate cytokines. Annual Review of Immunology 17, 189–220.

Bochner, B.S., Zimmermann, N., 2015. Role of siglecs and related glycan-binding proteins in immune responses and immunoregulation. Journal of Allergy and Clinical Immunology 135, 598–608.

Bode, L., Kunz, C., Muhly-Reinholz, M., Mayer, K., Seeger, W., Rudloff, S., 2004a. Inhibition of monocyte, lymphocyte, and neutrophil adhesion to endothelial cells by human milk oligosaccharides. Thrombosis and Haemostasis 92, 1402–1410.

Bode, L., Rudloff, S., Kunz, C., Strobel, S., Klein, N., 2004b. Human milk oligosaccharides reduce platelet-neutrophil complex formation leading to a decrease in neutrophil beta 2 integrin expression. Journal of Leukocyte Biology 76, 820–826.

Bode, L., 2006. Recent advances on structure, metabolism, and function of human milk oligosaccharides. Journal of Nutrition 136, 2127–2130.

Bode, L., 2009. Human milk oligosaccharides: prebiotics and beyond. Nutrition Reviews 67 (2), S183–S191.

Bode, L., 2015. The functional biology of human milk oligosaccharides. Early Human Development 91, 619–622.

Bogoevska, V., Horst, A., Klampe, B., Lucka, L., Wagener, C., Nollau, P., 2006. CEACAM1, an adhesion molecule of human granulocytes, is fucosylated by fucosyltransferase IX and interacts with DC-SIGN of dendritic cells via Lewis x residues. Glycobiology 16, 197–209.

Brown, E.M., Sadarangani, M., Finlay, B.B., 2013. The role of the immune system in governing host-microbe interactions in the intestine. Nature Immunology 14, 660–667.

Calder, P.C., Krauss-Etschmann, S., de Jong, E.C., Dupont, C., Frick, J.S., Frokiaer, H., Heinrich, J., Garn, H., Koletzko, S., Lack, G., Mattelio, G., Renz, H., Sangild, P.T., Schrezenmeir, J., Stulnig, T.M., Thymann, T., Wold, A.E., Koletzko, B., 2006. Early nutrition and immunity – progress and perspectives. British Journal of Nutrition 96, 774–790.

Carver, J.D., Pimentel, B., Wiener, D.A., Lowell, N.E., Barness, L.A., 1991. Infant feeding effects on flow cytometric analysis of blood. Journal of Clinical Laboratory Analysis 5, 54–56.

Castillo-Courtade, L., Han, S., Lee, S., Mian, F.M., Buck, R., Forsythe, P., 2015. Attenuation of food allergy symptoms following treatment with human milk oligosaccharides in a mouse model. Allergy 70, 1091–1102.

Catassi, C., Bonucci, A., Coppa, G.V., Carlucci, A., Giorgi, P.L., 1995. Intestinal permeability changes during the first month: effect of natural versus artificial feeding. Journal of Pediatric Gastroenterology and Nutrition 21, 383–386.

Chen, H.Y., Fermin, A., Vardhana, S., Weng, I.C., Lo, K.F., Chang, E.Y., Maverakis, E., Yang, R.Y., Hsu, D.K., Dustin, M.L., Liu, F.T., 2009. Galectin-3 negatively regulates TCR-mediated CD4+ T-cell activation at the immunological synapse. Proceedings of the National Academy of Sciences of the United States of America 106, 14496–14501.

Chheda, S., Palkowetz, K.H., Garofalo, R., Rassin, D.K., Goldman, A.S., 1996. Decreased interleukin-10 production by neonatal monocytes and T cells: relationship to decreased production and expression of tumor necrosis factor-alpha and its receptors. Pediatric Research 40, 475–483.

Chichlowski, M., German, J.B., Lebrilla, C.B., Mills, D.A., 2011. The influence of milk oligosaccharides on microbiota of infants: opportunities for formulas. Annual Review of Food Science and Technology 2, 331–351.

Comans-Bitter, W.M., de Groot, R., van den Beemd, R., Neijens, H.J., Hop, W.C., Groeneveld, K., Hooijkaas, H., van Dongen, J.J., 1997. Immunophenotyping of blood lymphocytes in childhood. Reference values for lymphocyte subpopulations. Journal of Pediatrics 130, 388–393.

Comstock, S.S., Wang, M., Hester, S.N., Li, M., Donovan, S.M., 2014. Select human milk oligosaccharides directly modulate peripheral blood mononuclear cells isolated from 10-d-old pigs. British Journal of Nutrition 111, 819–828.

Conde, P., Rodriguez, M., van der Touw, W., Jimenez, A., Burns, M., Miller, J., Brahmachary, M., Chen, H.M., Boros, P., Rausell-Palamos, F., Yun, T.J., Riquelme, P., Rastrojo, A., Aguado, B., Stein-Streilein, J., Tanaka, M., Zhou, L., Zhang, J., Lowary, T.L., Ginhoux, F., Park, C.G., Cheong, C., Brody, J., Turley, S.J., Lira, S.A., Bronte, V., Gordon, S., Heeger, P.S., Merad, M., Hutchinson, J., Chen, S.H., Ochando, J., 2015. DC-SIGN(+) macrophages control the induction of transplantation tolerance. Immunity 42, 1143–1158.

Coppa, G.V., Pierani, P., Zampini, L., Bruni, S., Carloni, I., Gabrielli, O., 2001. Characterization of oligosaccharides in milk and feces of breast-fed infants by high-performance anion-exchange chromatography. Advances in Experimental Medicine and Biology 501, 307–314.

Crocker, P.R., Paulson, J.C., Varki, A., 2007. Siglecs and their roles in the immune system. Nature Reviews Immunology 7, 255–266.

Denny, T., Yogev, R., Gelman, R., Skuza, C., Oleske, J., Chadwick, E., Cheng, S.C., Connor, E., 1992. Lymphocyte subsets in healthy children during the first 5 years of life. JAMA 267, 1484–1488.

Donovan, S., Monaco, M., Drnevich, J., Lönnerdal, B., Kvistgaard, A., Peng, Y.-M., 2014a. Peripheral blood mononuclear cell (PBMC) gene expression in human infants shifts from innate to adaptive immunity in the first six months of life (247.5). FASEB Journal 28.

Donovan, S.M., Wang, M., Monaco, M.H., Martin, C.R., Davidson, L.A., Ivanov, I., Chapkin, R.S., 2014b. Noninvasive molecular fingerprinting of host-microbiome interactions in neonates. FEBS Letters 588, 4112–4119.

Donovan, S.M., 2006. Role of human milk components in gastrointestinal development: current knowledge and future needs. Journal of Pediatrics 149, S49–S61.

Dorea, J.G., 2009. Breastfeeding is an essential complement to vaccination. Acta Paediatrica 98, 1244–1250.

Earl, L.A., Bi, S., Baum, L.G., 2010. N- and O-glycans modulate galectin-1 binding, CD45 signaling, and T cell death. Journal of Biological Chemistry 285, 2232–2244.

Ebrahim, A.H., Alalawi, Z., Mirandola, L., Rakhshanda, R., Dahlbeck, S., Nguyen, D., Jenkins, M., Grizzi, F., Cobos, E., Figueroa, J.A., Chiriva-Internati, M., 2014. Galectins in cancer: carcinogenesis, diagnosis and therapy. Annals of Translational Medicine 2, 88.

Eiwegger, T., Stahl, B., Schmitt, J., Boehm, G., Gerstmayr, M., Pichler, J., Dehlink, E., Loibichler, C., Urbanek, R., Szépfalusi, Z., 2004. Human milk-derived oligosaccharides stimulate cytokine production of cord-blood T-cells in vitro. Pediatric Research 56, 536–540.

Eiwegger, T., Stahl, B., Haidl, P., Schmitt, J., Boehm, G., Dehlink, E., Urbanek, R., Szepfalusi, Z., 2010. Prebiotic oligosaccharides: in vitro evidence for gastrointestinal epithelial transfer and immunomodulatory properties. Pediatric Allergy and Immunology 21, 1179–1188.

Ewaschuk, J.B., Diaz, H., Meddings, L., Diederichs, B., Dmytrash, A., Backer, J., Looijer-van Langen, M., Madsen, K.L., 2008. Secreted bioactive factors from *Bifidobacterium infantis* enhance epithelial cell barrier function. American Journal of Physiology – Gastrointestinal and Liver Physiology 295, G1025–G1034.

Fessenden, M., 2015. The cell menagerie: human immune profiling. Nature 525, 409–411.

Fuhlbrigge, R.C., Kieffer, J.D., Armerding, D., Kupper, T.S., 1997. Cutaneous lymphocyte antigen is a specialized form of PSGL-1 expressed on skin-homing T cells. Nature 389, 978–981.

Fuhrer, A., Sprenger, N., Kurakevich, E., Borsig, L., Chassard, C., Hennet, T., 2010. Milk sialyllactose influences colitis in mice through selective intestinal bacterial colonization. World Journal of Experimental Medicine 207, 2843–2854.

Gabius, H.J., Kaltner, H., Kopitz, J., Andre, S., 2015. The glycobiology of the CD system: a dictionary for translating marker designations into glycan/lectin structure and function. Trends in Biochemical Sciences 40, 360–376.

Garcia-Vallejo, J.J., van Kooyk, Y., 2013. The physiological role of DC-SIGN: a tale of mice and men. Trends in Immunology 34, 482–486.

Garcia-Vallejo, J.J., van Kooyk, Y., 2015. DC-sign: the strange case of Dr. Jekyll and Mr. Hyde. Immunity 42, 983–985.

Geijtenbeek, T.B., van Vliet, S.J., Engering, A., t Hart, B.A., van Kooyk, Y., 2004. Self- and nonself-recognition by C-type lectins on dendritic cells. Annual Review of Immunology 22, 33–54.

Gibbons, D., Fleming, P., Virasami, A., Michel, M.L., Sebire, N.J., Costeloe, K., Carr, R., Klein, N., Hayday, A., 2014. Interleukin-8 (CXCL8) production is a signatory T cell effector function of human newborn infants. Nature Medicine 20, 1206–1210.

Goehring, K.C., Kennedy, A.D., Prieto, P.A., Buck, R.H., 2014. Direct evidence for the presence of human milk oligosaccharides in the circulation of breastfed infants. PLoS ONE 9, e101692.

Golding, J., Emmett, P.M., Rogers, I.S., 1997. Breast feeding and infant mortality. Early Human Development 49 (Suppl.), S143–S155.

Goto, Y., Kiyono, H., 2012. Epithelial barrier: an interface for the cross-communication between gut flora and immune system. Immunological Reviews 245, 147–163.

Grimble, G.K., Westwood, O.M., 2001. Nucleotides as immunomodulators in clinical nutrition. Current Opinion in Clinical Nutrition and Metabolic Care 4, 57–64.

Hanlon, P.R., Thorsrud, B.A., 2014. A 3-week pre-clinical study of 2′-fucosyllactose in farm piglets. Food and Chemical Toxicology 74, 343–348.

Hassan, J., Reen, D.J., 2000. T-cell function in the human newborn. Immunology Today 21, 107–108.

Hawkes, J.S., Neumann, M.A., Gibson, R.A., 1999. The effect of breast feeding on lymphocyte subpopulations in healthy term infants at 6 months of age. Pediatric Research 45, 648–651.

He, Y., Liu, S., Kling, D.E., Leone, S., Lawlor, N.T., Huang, Y., Feinberg, S.B., Hill, D.R., Newburg, D.S., 2016. The human milk oligosaccharide 2'-fucosyllactose modulates CD14 expression in human enterocytes, thereby attenuating LPS-induced inflammation. Gut 65, 33–46.

He, Y., Liu, S., Leone, S., Newburg, D.S., 2014. Human colostrum oligosaccharides modulate major immunologic pathways of immature human intestine. Mucosal Immunology 7, 1326–1339.

Herich, R., Levkut, M., Bomba, A., Gancarcikova, S., Nemcova, R., 2004. Differences in the development of the small intestine between gnotobiotic and conventionally bred piglets. Berliner und Münchener tierärztliche Wochenschrift 117, 46–51.

Hester, S.N., Donovan, S.M., 2012. Individual and combined effects of nucleotides and human milk oligosaccharides on proliferation, apoptosis and necrosis in a human fetal intestinal cell line. Food and Nutrition Sciences 3, 1567–1576.

Hester, S.N., Chen, X., Li, M., Monaco, M.H., Comstock, S.S., Kuhlenschmidt, T.B., Kuhlenschmidt, M.S., Donovan, S.M., 2013. Human milk oligosaccharides inhibit rotavirus infectivity in vitro and in acutely infected piglets. British Journal of Nutrition 110, 1233–1242.

Holscher, H.D., Davis, S.R., Tappenden, K.A., 2014. Human milk oligosaccharides influence maturation of human intestinal Caco-2Bbe and HT-29 cell lines. Journal of Nutrition 144, 586–591.

Huang, M.C., Laskowska, A., Vestweber, D., Wild, M.K., 2002. The alpha(1,3)-fucosyltransferase Fuc-TIV, but not Fuc-TVII, generates sialyl Lewis X-like epitopes preferentially on glycolipids. Journal of Biological Chemistry 277, 47786–47795.

Huang, X.Z., Zhu, L.B., Li, Z.R., Lin, J., 2013. Bacterial colonization and intestinal mucosal barrier development. World Journal of Pediatrics 2, 46–53.

Huang, Y.L., Chassard, C., Hausmann, M., von Itzstein, M., Hennet, T., 2015. Sialic acid catabolism drives intestinal inflammation and microbial dysbiosis in mice. Nature Communications 6, 8141.

Izquierdo-Useros, N., Lorizate, M., McLaren, P.J., Telenti, A., Krausslich, H.G., Martinez-Picado, J., 2014. HIV-1 capture and transmission by dendritic cells: the role of viral glycolipids and the cellular receptor Siglec-1. PLoS Pathogens 10, e1004146.

Jaspan, H.B., Lawn, S.D., Safrit, J.T., Bekker, L.G., 2006. The maturing immune system: implications for development and testing HIV-1 vaccines for children and adolescents. AIDS 20, 483–494.

Jentsch-Ullrich, K., Koenigsmann, M., Mohren, M., Franke, A., 2005. Lymphocyte subsets' reference ranges in an age- and gender-balanced population of 100 healthy adults–a monocentric German study. Clinical Immunology 116, 192–197.

Juto, P., Moller, C., Engberg, S., Bjorksten, B., 1982. Influence of type of feeding on lymphocyte function and development of infantile allergy. Clinical & Experimental Allergy 12, 409–416.

Kaplan, J.L., Shi, H.N., Walker, W.A., 2011. The role of microbes in developmental immunologic programming. Pediatric Research 69, 465–472.

Kashyap, P.C., Marcobal, A., Ursell, L.K., Smits, S.A., Sonnenburg, E.D., Costello, E.K., Higginbottom, S.K., Domino, S.E., Holmes, S.P., Relman, D.A., Knight, R., Gordon, J.I., Sonnenburg, J.L., 2013. Genetically dictated change in host mucus carbohydrate landscape exerts a diet-dependent effect on the gut microbiota. Proceedings of the National Academy of Sciences of the United States of America 110, 17059–17064.

Kavanaugh, D., O'Callaghan, J., Kilcoyne, M., Kane, M., Joshi, L., Hickey, R.M., 2015. The intestinal glycome and its modulation by diet and nutrition. Nutrition Reviews 73, 359–375.

Kelly, D., Coutts, A.G., 2000. Early nutrition and the development of immune function in the neonate. Proceedings of the Nutrition Society 59, 177–185.

Koning, N., Kessen, S.F., Van Der Voorn, J.P., Appelmelk, B.J., Jeurink, P.V., Knippels, L.M., Garssen, J., Van Kooyk, Y., 2015. Human milk blocks DC-SIGN-pathogen interaction via MUC1. Frontiers in Immunology 6, 112.

Kuijf, M.L., Samsom, J.N., van Rijs, W., Bax, M., Huizinga, R., Heikema, A.P., van Doorn, P.A., van Belkum, A., van Kooyk, Y., Burgers, P.C., Luider, T.M., Endtz, H.P., Nieuwenhuis, E.E., Jacobs, B.C., 2010. TLR4-mediated sensing of *Campylobacter jejuni* by dendritic cells is determined by sialylation. Journal of Immunology 185, 748–755.

Kuntz, S., Kunz, C., Rudloff, S., 2009. Oligosaccharides from human milk induce growth arrest via G2/M by influencing growth-related cell cycle genes in intestinal epithelial cells. British Journal of Nutrition 101, 1306–1315.

Kunz, C., Rudloff, S., 2008. Potential anti-inflammatory and anti-infectious effects of human milk oligosaccharides. Advances in Experimental Medicine and Biology 606, 455–465.

Kurakevich, E., Hennet, T., Hausmann, M., Rogler, G., Borsig, L., 2013. Milk oligosaccharide sialyl(alpha2,3)lactose activates intestinal CD11c+ cells through TLR4. Proceedings of the National Academy of Sciences of the United States of America 110, 17444–17449.

Lacroix-Lamande, S., Guesdon, W., Drouet, F., Potiron, L., Lantier, L., Laurent, F., 2014. The gut flora is required for the control of intestinal infection by poly(I: C) administration in neonates. Gut Microbes 5, 533–540.

Lane, J.A., O'Callaghan, J., Carrington, S.D., Hickey, R.M., 2013. Transcriptional response of HT-29 intestinal epithelial cells to human and bovine milk oligosaccharides. British Journal of Nutrition 110, 2127–2137.

Lawrence, R.M., Pane, C.A., 2007. Human breast milk: current concepts of immunology and infectious diseases. Current Problems in Pediatric and Adolescent Health Care 37, 7–36.

Lehrer, R.I., Jung, G., Ruchala, P., Andre, S., Gabius, H.J., Lu, W., 2009. Multivalent binding of carbohydrates by the human alpha-defensin, HD5. Journal of Immunology 183, 480–490.

Levy, O., 2007. Innate immunity of the newborn: basic mechanisms and clinical correlates. Nature Reviews Immunology 7, 379–390.

Ley, K., 2003. The role of selectins in inflammation and disease. Trends in Molecular Medicine 9, 263–268.

Li, M., Bauer, L.L., Chen, X., Wang, M., Kuhlenschmidt, T.B., Kuhlenschmidt, M.S., Fahey Jr., G.C., Donovan, S.M., 2012. Microbial composition and in vitro fermentation patterns of human milk oligosaccharides and prebiotics differ between formula-fed and sow-reared piglets. Journal of Nutrition 142, 681–689.

Li, M., Monaco, M.H., Wang, M., Comstock, S.S., Kuhlenschmidt, T.B., Fahey Jr., G.C., Miller, M.J., Kuhlenschmidt, M.S., Donovan, S.M., 2014. Human milk oligosaccharides shorten rotavirus-induced diarrhea and modulate piglet mucosal immunity and colonic microbiota. ISME Journal 8, 1609–1620.

Liu, K.Y., Comstock, S.S., Shunk, J.M., Monaco, M.H., Donovan, S.M., 2013. Natural killer cell populations and cytotoxic activity in pigs fed mother's milk, formula, or formula supplemented with bovine lactoferrin. Pediatric Research 74, 402–407.

Luhn, K., Wild, M.K., 2012. Human deficiencies of fucosylation and sialylation affecting selectin ligands. Seminars in Immunopathology 34, 383–399.

Macauley, M.S., Crocker, P.R., Paulson, J.C., 2014. Siglec-mediated regulation of immune cell function in disease. Nature Reviews Immunology 14, 653–666.

Macpherson, A.J., Geuking, M.B., McCoy, K.D., 2005. Immune responses that adapt the intestinal mucosa to commensal intestinal bacteria. Immunology 115, 153–162.

Manroe, B.L., Weinberg, A.G., Rosenfeld, C.R., Browne, R., 1979. The neonatal blood count in health and disease. I. Reference values for neutrophilic cells. Journal of Pediatrics 95, 89–98.

Marcobal, A., Sonnenburg, J.L., 2012. Human milk oligosaccharide consumption by intestinal microbiota. Clinical Microbiology and Infection 18 (Suppl. 4), 12–15.

Marriage, B.J., Buck, R.H., Goehring, K.C., Oliver, J.S., Williams, J.A., 2015. Infants fed a lower calorie formula with 2′-fucosyllactose (2′FL) show growth and 2′FL uptake like breast-fed infants. Journal of Pediatric Gastroenterology and Nutrition.

Marth, J.D., Grewal, P.K., 2008. Mammalian glycosylation in immunity. Nature Reviews Immunology 8, 874–887.

Matzinger, P., 1994. Tolerance, danger, and the extended family. Annual Review of Immunology 12, 991–1045.

Maverakis, E., Kim, K., Shimoda, M., Gershwin, M.E., Patel, F., Wilken, R., Raychaudhuri, S., Ruhaak, L.R., Lebrilla, C.B., 2015. Glycans in the immune system and the altered glycan theory of autoimmunity: a critical review. Journal of Autoimmunity 57, 1–13.

Murphy, K., 2011. Immunobiology, eighth ed. Garland Science.

Nalle, S.C., Turner, J.R., 2015. Intestinal barrier loss as a critical pathogenic link between inflammatory bowel disease and graft-versus-host disease. Mucosal Immunology 8, 720–730.

Newburg, D.S., He, Y., 2015. Neonatal gut microbiota and human milk glycans cooperate to attenuate infection and inflammation. Clinical Obstetrics and Gynaecology 58, 814–826.

Obermeier, S., Rudloff, S., Pohlentz, G., Lentze, M.J., Kunz, C., 1999. Secretion of 13C-labelled oligosaccharides into human milk and infant's urine after an oral [13C] galactose load. Isotopes in Environmental and Health Studies 35, 119–125.

Odle, J., Lin, X., Jacobi, S.K., Kim, S.W., Stahl, C.H., 2014. The suckling piglet as an agrimedical model for the study of pediatric nutrition and metabolism. Annual Review of Animal Biosciences 2, 419–444.

Okano, M., Satoskar, A.R., Nishizaki, K., Harn Jr., D.A., 2001. Lacto-N-fucopentaose III found on *Schistosoma mansoni* egg antigens functions as adjuvant for proteins by inducing Th2-type response. Journal of Immunology 167, 442–450.

Paul, W.E., 2012. Fundamental Immunology, seventh ed. Wolters Kluwer.

Pickard, J.M., Chervonsky, A.V., 2015. Intestinal fucose as a mediator of host-microbe symbiosis. Journal of Immunology 194, 5588–5593.

Pickard, J.M., Maurice, C.F., Kinnebrew, M.A., Abt, M.C., Schenten, D., Golovkina, T.V., Bogatyrev, S.R., Ismagilov, R.F., Pamer, E.G., Turnbaugh, P.J., Chervonsky, A.V., 2014. Rapid fucosylation of intestinal epithelium sustains host-commensal symbiosis in sickness. Nature 514, 638–641.

Pillai, S., Netravali, I.A., Cariappa, A., Mattoo, H., 2012. Siglecs and immune regulation. Annual Review of Immunology 30, 357–392.

Puiman, P., Stoll, B., 2008. Animal models to study neonatal nutrition in humans. Current Opinion in Clinical Nutrition and Metabolic Care 11, 601–606.

Rabinovich, G.A., van Kooyk, Y., Cobb, B.A., 2012. Glycobiology of immune responses. Annals of the New York Academy of Sciences 1253, 1–15.

Radzanowski, G.G., Garrett, P.N., Li, X., Anita, M., 2013. Short-chain milk oligosaccharide levels in human milk and infant plasma. FASEB Journal 27.

Rana, N.A., Haltiwanger, R.S., 2011. Fringe benefits: functional and structural impacts of O-glycosylation on the extracellular domain of notch receptors. Current Opinion in Structural Biology 21, 583–589.

Restelli, V., Wang, M.D., Huzel, N., Ethier, M., Perreault, H., Butler, M., 2006. The effect of dissolved oxygen on the production and the glycosylation profile of recombinant human erythropoietin produced from CHO cells. Biotechnology and Bioengineering 94, 481–494.

Rudloff, S., Stefan, C., Pohlentz, G., Kunz, C., 2002. Detection of ligands for selectins in the oligosaccharide fraction of human milk. European Journal of Nutrition 41, 85–92.
Rudloff, S., Pohlentz, G., Borsch, C., Lentze, M.J., Kunz, C., 2012. Urinary excretion of in vivo (1)(3)C-labelled milk oligosaccharides in breastfed infants. British Journal of Nutrition 107, 957–963.
Ruhaak, L.R., Stroble, C., Underwood, M.A., Lebrilla, C.B., 2014. Detection of milk oligosaccharides in plasma of infants. Analytical and Bioanalytical Chemistry 406, 5775–5784.
Sallusto, F., Lenig, D., Forster, R., Lipp, M., Lanzavecchia, A., 1999. Two subsets of memory T lymphocytes with distinct homing potentials and effector functions. Nature 401, 708–712.
Sassone-Corsi, M., Raffatellu, M., 2015. No vacancy: how beneficial microbes cooperate with immunity to provide colonization resistance to pathogens. Journal of Immunology 194, 4081–4087.
Schnaar, R.L., 2015. Glycans and glycan-binding proteins in immune regulation: a concise introduction to glycobiology for the allergist. Journal of Allergy and Clinical Immunology 135, 609–615.
Schumacher, G., Bendas, G., Stahl, B., Beermann, C., 2006. Human milk oligosaccharides affect P-selectin binding capacities: in vitro investigation. Nutrition 22, 620–627.
Severi, E., Hood, D.W., Thomas, G.H., 2007. Sialic acid utilization by bacterial pathogens. Microbiology 153, 2817–2822.
Siegrist, C.A., Cordova, M., Brandt, C., Barrios, C., Berney, M., Tougne, C., Kovarik, J., Lambert, P.H., 1998. Determinants of infant responses to vaccines in presence of maternal antibodies. Vaccine 16, 1409–1414.
Smith, D.F., Cummings, R.D., 2013. Application of microarrays for deciphering the structure and function of the human glycome. Molecular & Cellular Proteomics 12, 902–912.
Sperandio, M., 2006. Selectins and glycosyltransferases in leukocyte rolling in vivo. FEBS Journal 273, 4377–4389.
Splawski, J.B., Lipsky, P.E., 1991. Cytokine regulation of immunoglobulin secretion by neonatal lymphocytes. Journal of Clinical Investigation 88, 967–977.
Steinman, R.M., Hawiger, D., Nussenzweig, M.C., 2003. Tolerogenic dendritic cells. Annual Review of Immunology 21, 685–711.
Stephens, S., Brenner, M.K., Duffy, S.W., Lakhani, P.K., Kennedy, C.R., Farrant, J., 1986. The effect of breast-feeding on proliferation by infant lymphocytes in vitro. Pediatric Research 20, 227–231.
Stephenson, H.N., Mills, D.C., Jones, H., Milioris, E., Copland, A., Dorrell, N., Wren, B.W., Crocker, P.R., Escors, D., Bajaj-Elliott, M., 2014. Pseudaminic acid on *Campylobacter jejuni* flagella modulates dendritic cell IL-10 expression via Siglec-10 receptor: a novel flagellin-host interaction. Journal of Infectious Diseases 210, 1487–1498.
Strober, W., 2015. Current protocols in immunology. In: Coico, R. (Ed.), Current Protocols. Wiley, Wiley Online Library.
Stuebe, A.M., Schwarz, E.B., 2010. The risks and benefits of infant feeding practices for women and their children. Journal of Perinatology 30, 155–162.
Taylor, M.E., Drickamer, K., 2014. Convergent and divergent mechanisms of sugar recognition across kingdoms. Current Opinion in Structural Biology 28, 14–22.
Terrazas, L.I., Walsh, K.L., Piskorska, D., McGuire, E., Harn Jr., D.A., 2001. The schistosome oligosaccharide lacto-N-neotetraose expands Gr1(+) cells that secrete anti-inflammatory cytokines and inhibit proliferation of naive CD4(+) cells: a potential mechanism for immune polarization in helminth infections. Journal of Immunology 167, 5294–5303.

Thompson, F.M., Mayrhofer, G., Cummins, A.G., 1996. Dependence of epithelial growth of the small intestine on T-cell activation during weaning in the rat. Gastroenterology 111, 37–44.

Thorum, S.C., Comstock, S.S., Hester, S.N., Shunk, J.M., Monaco, M.H., Donovan, S.M., 2013. Impact of diet on development of bronchial-associated immunity in the neonatal piglet. Veterinary Immunology and Immunopathology 151, 63–72.

Toscano, M.A., Bianco, G.A., Ilarregui, J.M., Croci, D.O., Correale, J., Hernandez, J.D., Zwirner, N.W., Poirier, F., Riley, E.M., Baum, L.G., Rabinovich, G.A., 2007. Differential glycosylation of TH1, TH2 and TH-17 effector cells selectively regulates susceptibility to cell death. Nature Immunology 8, 825–834.

Turfkruyer, M., Verhasselt, V., 2015. Breast milk and its impact on maturation of the neonatal immune system. Current Opinion in Infectious Diseases 28, 199–206.

Underwood, M.A., German, J.B., Lebrilla, C.B., Mills, D.A., 2015. *Bifidobacterium longum* subspecies *infantis*: champion colonizer of the infant gut. Pediatric Research 77, 229–235.

Upham, J.W., Lee, P.T., Holt, B.J., Heaton, T., Prescott, S.L., Sharp, M.J., Sly, P.D., Holt, P.G., 2002. Development of interleukin-12-producing capacity throughout childhood. Infection and Immunology 70, 6583–6588.

van Kooyk, Y., Rabinovich, G.A., 2008. Protein-glycan interactions in the control of innate and adaptive immune responses. Nature Immunology 9, 593–601.

van Kooyk, Y., Kalay, H., Garcia-Vallejo, J.J., 2013. Analytical tools for the study of cellular glycosylation in the immune system. Frontiers in Immunology 4, 451.

Varki, A., Gagneux, P., 2009. Human-specific evolution of sialic acid targets: explaining the malignant malaria mystery? Proceedings of the National Academy of Sciences of the United States of America 106, 14739–14740.

Velupillai, P., Secor, W.E., Horauf, A.M., Harn, D.A., 1997. B-1 cell (CD5+B220+) outgrowth in murine schistosomiasis is genetically restricted and is largely due to activation by polylactosamine sugars. Journal of Immunology 158, 338–344.

Verhasselt, V., 2010. Neonatal tolerance under breastfeeding influence: the presence of allergen and transforming growth factor-beta in breast milk protects the progeny from allergic asthma. Journal of Pediatrics 156, S16–S20.

Verhasselt, V., 2015. Is infant immunization by breastfeeding possible? Philosophical Transactions of the Royal Society of London 370.

Volman, J.J., Ramakers, J.D., Plat, J., 2008. Dietary modulation of immune function by beta-glucans. Physiology & Behavior 94, 276–284.

Walker, W.A., Iyengar, R.S., 2015. Breast milk, microbiota, and intestinal immune homeostasis. Pediatric Research 77, 220–228.

Walker, A., 2014. Intestinal colonization and programming of the intestinal immune response. Journal of Clinical Gastroenterology 48 (Suppl. 1), S8–S11.

Wang, M., Li, M., Wu, S., Lebrilla, C.B., Chapkin, R.S., Ivanov, I., Donovan, S.M., 2015. Fecal microbiota composition of breast-fed infants is correlated with human milk oligosaccharides consumed. Journal of Pediatric Gastroenterology and Nutrition 60, 825–833.

West, C.E., Videky, D.J., Prescott, S.L., 2010. Role of diet in the development of immune tolerance in the context of allergic disease. Current Opinion in Pediatrics 22, 635–641.

Wickramasinghe, S., Pacheco, A.R., Lemay, D.G., Mills, D.A., 2015. Bifidobacteria grown on human milk oligosaccharides downregulate the expression of inflammation-related genes in Caco-2 cells. BMC Microbiology 15, 172.

Zarbock, A., Ley, K., McEver, R.P., Hidalgo, A., 2011. Leukocyte ligands for endothelial selectins: specialized glycoconjugates that mediate rolling and signaling under flow. Blood 118, 6743–6751.

SECTION

C

Challenges and Opportunities

CHAPTER

Making Human Milk Oligosaccharides Available for Research and Application – Approaches, Challenges, and Future Opportunities

9

Lars Bode[1], Stewart Campbell[2], Richard Furneaux[3], Joeri Beauprez[4], Andrew Muscroft-Taylor[5]

[1]University of California, San Diego, La Jolla, CA, United States; [2]CordenPharma International, Inc., Woburn, MA, United States; [3]Victoria University of Wellington, Lower Hutt, New Zealand; [4]Inbiose NV, Ghent, Belgium; [5]University of Canterbury, Christchurch, New Zealand

Human milk contains 5–15 g/L of free oligosaccharides, rivaling milk-based protein levels, and nearly 200 human milk oligosaccharide (HMO) structures have been identified (Bode, 2009; Boehm and Stahl, 2003; Newburg et al., 2005). Many of the plethora of the well-documented health benefits of breastfeeding have been attributed to HMOs (Bode, 2009; Blamk et al., 2012), but in most cases the evidence is still only correlative. Over 90% of HMOs pass through the infant gastrointestinal (GI) tract unaltered (Chaturvedi et al., 2001), and given the energy required by the mother to produce and secrete HMOs, it is reasonable to expect that the majority of HMOs must therefore serve a role beyond prebiotics. While it is attractive to hypothesize that human milk has evolved such that each HMO provides a specific benefit to the infant, it will only be through access to structurally defined, homogeneous HMO that their specific functional roles can be elucidated.

HMOs have been established or implicated as (1) prebiotics that aid in the development of healthy GI microbiota; (2) antiadhesion molecules that act as inhibitory ligands to prevent GI colonization with and/or invasion of pathogenic bacteria such as *Escherichia coli* (Manthey et al., 2014) and viruses such as HIV (Bode et al., 2012); and (3) immune modulators believed to impact immune responses in both infants (Jantscher-Krenn et al., 2011) and adults (Zhu et al., 2012; Vellupillai and Harn, 1994), although it has not been until very recently that specific immune modulation functions have been attributed to specific HMOs. It was recently shown that disialyllacto-*N*-tetraose (DSLNT), an oligosaccharide uniquely found in human milk, can prevent necrotizing enterocolitis-like outcomes when administered to neonatal

Prebiotics and Probiotics in Human Milk. http://dx.doi.org/10.1016/B978-0-12-802725-7.00009-9

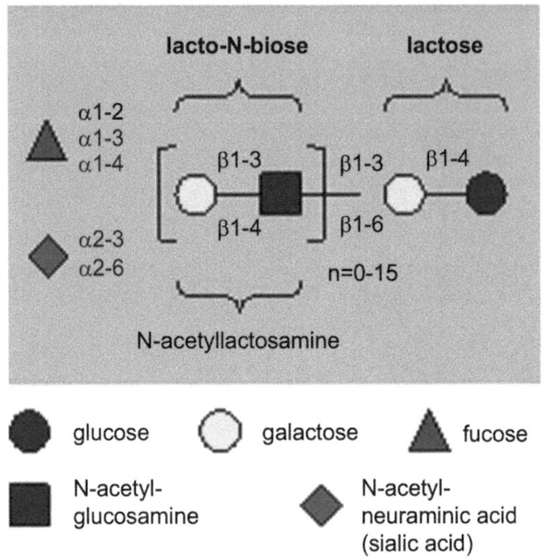

FIGURE 9.1

General structure of HMOs and related glycolipid glycans, including Lewis antigens. Key: *Blue circle*: D-glucose (Glc), *blue square*: *N*-acetylglucosamine (GlcNAc), *purple diamond*: 5-*N*-acetylneuraminic (sialic) acid (Neu5Ac), *red triangle*: L-fucose (Fuc), *yellow circle*: D-galactose (Gal).

rats (Jantscher-Krenn et al., 2011). Critical to the success of this research was access to a reasonably homogeneous sample of DSLNT, which allowed direct testing of the hypothesis. This work demonstrates both the value of and the need for homogeneous, structurally-defined HMOs and serves as evidence that access to such carbohydrate content has the potential to yield new insight into glycobiology and give rise to therapeutic development opportunities.

Structurally, HMOs are composed of a reducing end lactose unit that is further elaborated at the 3- or 6-position of the terminal galactose residue with one of two cores (Fig. 9.1):

- Type 1 core: lactosaminyl-lactose (LNT) [Galβ(1-**3**)-GlcNAcβ] containing
- Type 2 core: *neo*-lactosaminyl-lactose (LNnT) [Galβ(1-**4**)-GlcNAcβ] containing

The vast structural diversity among HMOs comes from further variable fucosylation and/or sialylation of each core (Bode, 2009; Boehm and Stahl, 2003; Newburg et al., 2005).

HMOs share significant structural homology with the Lewis blood group determinants and related glycolipid glycans ("Lewis antigens"), but in contrast to HMOs, the complete Lewis antigen glycans persist in membrane-bound forms at epithelial and red blood cell surfaces where they play a significant role in the following

1. Selectin-dependent inflammatory processes such as leukocyte rolling and adhesion (Kawashima, 2006; Etzioni, 1996);

2. Tumor cell migration and adhesion (Heimburg-Molinaro et al., 2011). Lewis antigens such as Lewis y (Le^y), sialyl Lewis a (SLe^a), and SLe^x are overexpressed in many invasive and metastatic cancers including mammary (Urgorskim and Laskowska, 2002), colon, prostate, ovarian, and liver cancers (Ravindranath et al., 1997). Indeed, overexpression of SLe^a correlates positively with tumor metastasis and negatively with outcome prognosis (Ragupathi et al., 2009). It has therefore been proposed that Lewis antigens may serve as potential biomarkers for cancer diagnosis and progression and perhaps even form the basis of cancer vaccine targets.
3. Adhesion of pathogenic and commensal bacteria such as *Helicopbacter pylori* and *Lactobacillus* spp. (Kinoshita et al., 2008).

The structural homology between HMOs and Lewis antigens is likely biologically significant and the functional roles of Lewis antigens may serve as a leading guide for elucidation of the structure–function relationship of HMOs. Indeed, soluble forms of Lewis antigens that share the same or similar nonreducing end structural variability with HMOs but lack the reducing end lactose moiety, formally known as the Lewis blood group antigens or determinants, are secreted in bodily fluids such as saliva and plasma. Critical to progress in this field is routine access to homogeneous, structurally defined HMOs. This chapter presents a brief survey of a wide range of approaches to such HMO materials through chemical synthesis, enzymatic/chemoenzymatic synthesis, and expression in engineered cells.

1. CHEMICAL SYNTHESIS APPROACHES TO HUMAN MILK OLIGOSACCHARIDES

Initial reports on the isolation and characterization of HMOs began to appear in the literature nearly a half-century ago (Kobata et al., 1969), but it has only been in the past 20–25 years that structure–activity relationships has begun to emerge (Bode, 2009). Rapid progress has been hindered by limitations in access to significant quantities of structurally defined HMO materials. Historically, structure–function studies have used HMO pools enriched in structurally similar HMOs (Bode et al., 2004a,b; Morrow et al., 2004; Jiang et al., 2004) or have focused on smaller, simpler HMOs such as the fucosyl- and sialyl-lactoses that are accessible via isolation methodologies or engineered bioprocess approaches (Michalak et al., 2014; Chin et al., 2015). Comprehensive elucidation of HMO structure–activity relationships in principle requires access to all HMO content. Chemical synthesis, enzymatic, and fermentation approaches have the potential to provide full access to HMOs, and this section focuses on chemical synthesis approaches with high potential for achieving structural diversity.

1.1 SYNTHESIS APPROACH AND RETROSYNTHESIS

The broader goal of elucidating the biological function of specific HMOs requires the development of a versatile synthetic approach that will enable rapid access to the entire HMO structural space. Ideally, access to both type 1 and type 2 cores (Fig. 9.1), with these cores variably substituted with L-fucose, sialic acid, and sulfate residues will be possible; therefore the strategy must accommodate systematic structural changes, which will allow for probing the relevance and characteristics of both major and subtle HMO structural variations. Furthermore, the most useful synthesis approach also will grant access to a variety of defined Lewis antigen structures to enable comparative studies between HMOs and Lewis antigens.

The retrosynthesis of the HMO glycan type 1 and type 2 cores presents a need for three main components: a lactose disaccharide differentiated on the 3′-position (3-position of the Gal residue) and the 2-position (2-position of the reducing end Glc residue), a fully differentiated GlcNAc unit, and a fully differentiated Gal unit. Critical to the successful implementation of the strategy is identification of building blocks that can be prepared cost-effectively on large scale and are shelf stable. Using the approach outlined in Fig. 9.2, both core types may be accessed from a set of only three building blocks, all of which are amenable to large-scale production. The Fuc and Neu5Ac monosaccharide components that decorate the HMO cores are most frequently terminal moieties devoid of further substitution; therefore, the only two relatively simple building blocks suffice (Fig. 9.2). Significantly, all of these five building blocks are useful for synthesis of the Lewis antigen core sequences as well.

1.2 BUILDING BLOCK SYNTHESIS

Facile access to a wide range of HMO structures requires that the building block synthesis routes be scalable and cost-effective, with particular emphases on minimizing reaction times and volumes, minimizing chromatographic separations and identifying crystalline intermediates. Per-*O*-acetylation offers one commonly used general approach for scalable production of stable, crystalline early stage intermediates that often enable controlled further elaboration. Examples of syntheses of the three core building blocks are shown in Fig. 9.3.

The Lac building block process proceeds via a stable 1,2-benzyl orthoester intermediate, and through 2-position neighboring group participation results in as a single reducing end anomer (β-*O*-benzyl) important for simplifying isolation and characterization of downstream intermediates. The 3′-position is temporarily protected as an allyl ether can be removed for subsequent installation of a GlcNAc building block for more complex HMOs or a Neu5Ac building block for simpler HMOs (e.g., 3′-sialyllactose). The use of the PMB ether at the 2-position enables future regiospecific introduction of a Fuc residue (e.g., 2-fucosyl-lactose).

The GlcNAc building block comprises an allyl glycoside for subsequent removal and activation as a trichloroacetimidate donor, a 2-*N*-trifluoracetyl group for subsequent β-coupling products and a 4,6-acetonide group, which enables differentiation of the 3-, 4-, and 6-positions of the GlcNAc unit (Christ et al., 1996). Glycosylation or protection at the 3-position followed by removal of the 4,6-acetonide and regioselective introduction of a 6-*O*-protecting group accommodates access to both type 1 and type 2 cores, thus allowing access to the full HMO structural space from a single

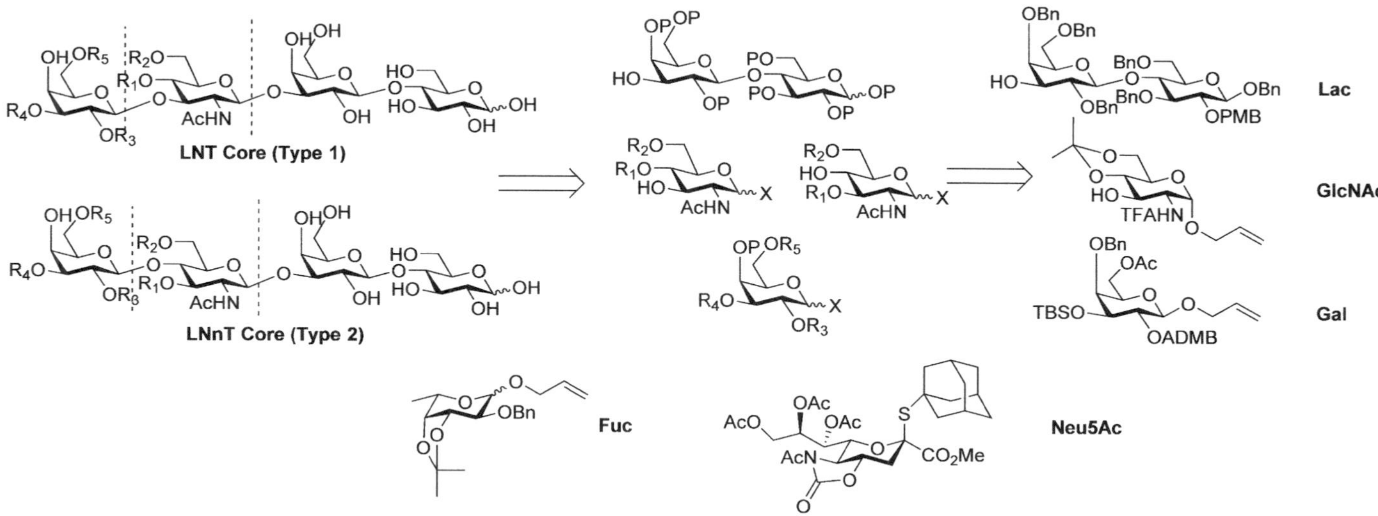

FIGURE 9.2

Retrosynthesis of HMO LNT and LNnT glycans and identification of component building blocks. Key: *Ac*: Acetyl, *ADMB*: 4-*O*-acetyl-2,2-dimethylbutyryl, *P*: semipermanent protecting group (e.g., benzyl ether, Bn), *PMB*: *p*-methoxybenzyl, R_n: temporary protecting groups with orthogonal reactivity, *TBS*: *tert*-butyldimethylsilyl, *TFA*: trifluoroacetyl, *X*: reactive anomeric group for coupling units together.

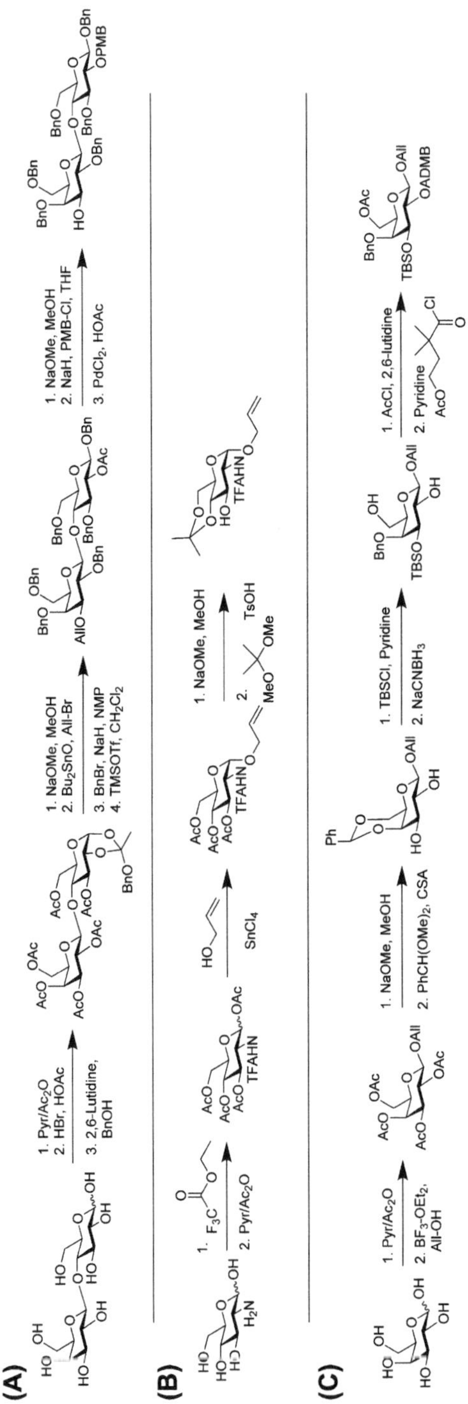

FIGURE 9.3

Synthesis of (A) Lac, (B) GlcNAc, and (C) Gal building blocks.

GlcNAc building block. The 6-OH group may be liberated for installation of Fuc and Neu5Ac moieties as necessary.

Due to its highly substituted nature within HMOs, the Gal unit is a key moiety for achieving diversity in HMOs. A versatile building block therefore requires full differentiation with multiple orthogonal protecting groups. The Gal building block in Fig. 9.3 is designed with protecting groups with different reactivities at each position. The allyl glycoside allows for conversion into a trichloroacetimidate donor. The ADMB ester at the 2-position is a strong participating group, which ensures high β-glycoside selectivity when coupled to the GlcNAc 3-porition (type 1 core) or 4-position (type 2 core). Subsequently, each of the remaining positions may be accessed selectively for installing Fuc or Neu5Ac residues or larger oligosaccharides as necessary.

The Fuc and Neu5Ac monosaccharide building blocks are shown in Fig. 9.4. Due to their terminal nature in HMO structures, in principle these building blocks could be uniformly protected with the same groups at each position. Indeed, a per-*O*-benzylated Fuc building block was used in a recent efficient large-scale synthesis of the Lewis^x trisaccharide (Munneke et al., 2015). However, the imidate donor of this Fuc building block is known to be unstable on mid- to long-term storage, which has led to the more common strategy of preparing the 2-*O*-benzyl-3,4-di-*O*-acetyl derivative (Fig. 9.4; Flowers, 1981), which offers the desired higher α-selectivity due to the nonparticipating 2-*O*-benzyl group but is shelf stable due to the electron-withdrawing (disarming) 3,4-di-*O*-acetyl groups. Thus, the differentially protected, more-stable Fuc building block shown is preferred for producing a wide range of HMO structures.

As with Fuc residues in HMOs, the Neu5Ac is usually a terminal residue; therefore, the hydroxyl groups and 5-NHAc may be uniformly protected, which potentially simplifies the Neu5Ac building block. The key aspect of Neu5Ac building block design is a donor that gives very high α-selectivity when coupled to an HMO core acceptor to establish the common α-2,3 and α-2,6 linkages. Both glycosyl phosphate and thioglycosides are most commonly used as donor groups for Neu5Ac, and exceptional α-selectivity and high coupling yields to a variety of acceptors have been demonstrated (Crich and Li, 2007a,b; Chu et al., 2011). Achieving high α-selectivity is also highly dependent on other groups in the Neu5Ac building block, with the 4,5-oxazolidine ring protecting group serving as a notable example (Crich and Li, 2007a,b). The selected Neu5Ac building block (Fig. 9.4) is readily available from a scalable eight-step process requiring little chromatography.

1.3 CONVERGENT MODULAR ASSEMBLY

Starting with the reducing end Lac disaccharide, HMO glycans may be assembled through a variety of approaches, including (1) iterative addition of monosaccharide building blocks to a growing oligosaccharide chain (Roussel et al., 2001); (2) assembly of the linear LacNAc-Lac or *neo*-LacNAc-Lac cores followed by addition of Fuc and Neu5Ac residues; or (3) preassembly of oligosaccharide blocks (e.g., Le^x, SLe^x, Le^y, Le^a oligosaccharides) that are added to the Lac disaccharide. For synthesis of simple

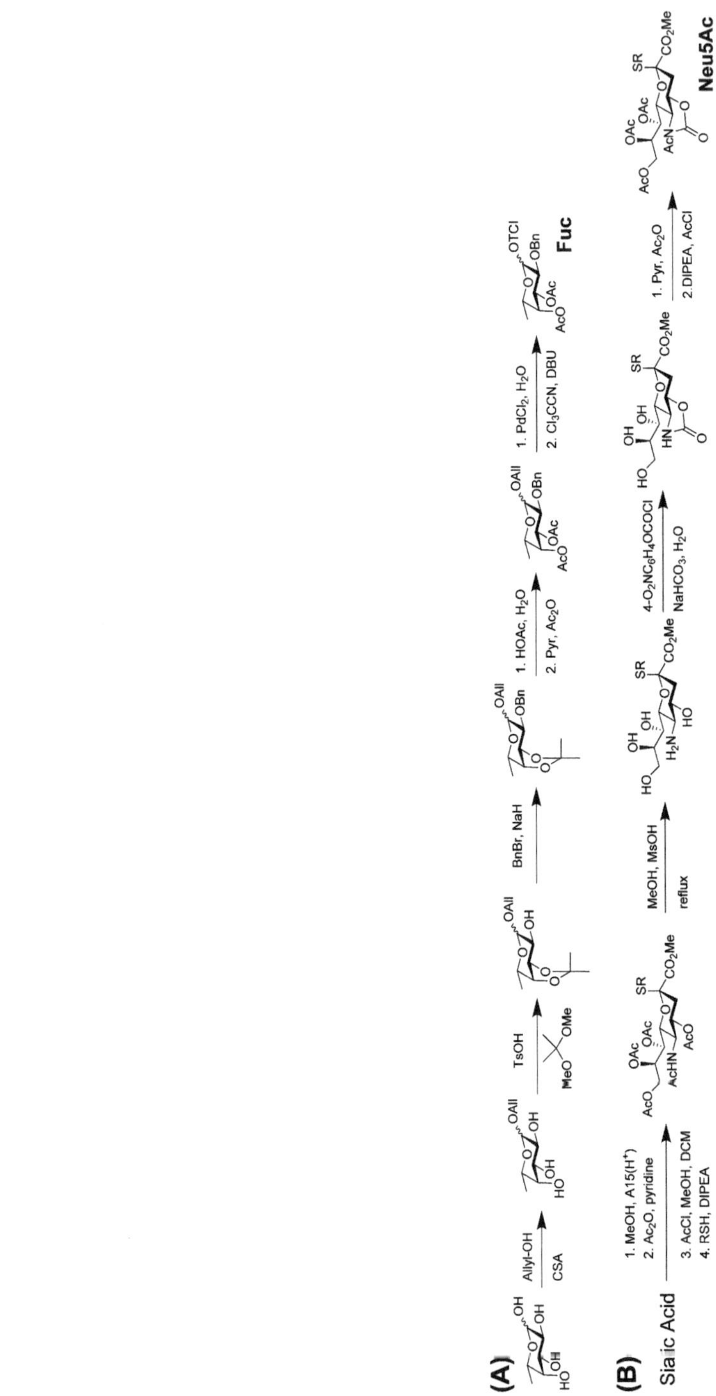

FIGURE 9.4

Synthesis of (A) Fuc and (B) Neu5Ac building blocks.

HMOs such as the fucosyllactoses or sialyllactoses, iterative addition of the Fuc or Neu5Ac to the Lac disaccharide is the preferred approach (Rencurosi et al., 2002). In contrast, the most commonly used option for synthesis of complex HMOs is the addition of preassembled oligosaccharides to the Lac disaccharide (Lubineau et al., 1994; Aly et al., 1999). Two case studies are provided next to demonstrate use of a block assembly strategy to produce type 1 and type 2 HMOs of biological interest.

1.4 TYPE 2 CORE CASE STUDY

Synthesis of the Le^x pentasaccharide LNFPIII. Fig. 9.5 illustrates the synthesis of the immunomodulatory HMO LNFP-III (Zhu et al., 2012), implemented at Corden Pharma on multigram scale, from the aforementioned common set of building blocks. The assembly method made use of a "3+2" block coupling of the Le^x-like trisaccharide donor with a differentiated lactose acceptor, a strategy reported by many other groups for the synthesis of Le^x-containing oligosaccharides (Munneke et al., 2015; Roussel et al., 2001; Lubineau et al., 1994; Ellervik and Magnusson, 1998). The Le^x trisaccharide donor was assembled by first fucosylating the 3-position of the GlcNAc building block. Subsequent removal of the GlcNAc 4,6-acetonide and differentiation provided the disaccharide acceptor to be glycosylated with the Gal donor building block. At this stage, the reducing end allyl group was removed and converted into its trichloroacetimidate donor. The Le^x trisaccharide donor was coupled to the Lac acceptor with high β-stereoselectivity to establish the full LNFP-III pentasaccharide framework. Deprotection and purification were effected via a three-step sequence commencing with removal of all ester and amide protecting groups using KOH (Christ et al., 1996). Subsequent *N*-acetylation gave the partially protected *O*-benzyl intermediate. At this stage it was best to purify the material to homogeneity using size exclusion chromatography on Sephadex LH-20. Final purification on Sephadex G-10 provided LNFP-III in multigram quantities.

1.5 TYPE 1 CORE CASE STUDY

Synthesis of 3′-sulfated Le^a pentasaccharide. Fig. 9.6 summarizes an early example of the synthesis of a sulfated Le^a pentasaccharide antigen, a type 1 core containing structure (Lubineau et al., 1994). This synthesis serves as an example of the structural homology between HMOs and blood group antigens and of how the Lewis trisaccharide unit, Le^a in this case, is preassembled and then coupled to the Lac disaccharide. The Le^a trisaccharide was prepared by first glycosylating the GlcNAc acceptor with a per-*O*-acetylated Gal donor at the 3-position followed by introduction of the per-*O*-benzylated Fuc donor using halide-assisted coupling conditions to enhance the α-selectivity (Lemieux et al., 1975). The optional 3′-sulfate ester was introduced very late in the synthesis using SO_3-trimethylamine, which demonstrates the versatility of the building blocks design.

These examples illustrate that chemical synthesis of a wide variety of HMOs is feasible from only a few well-designed building blocks. The processes are

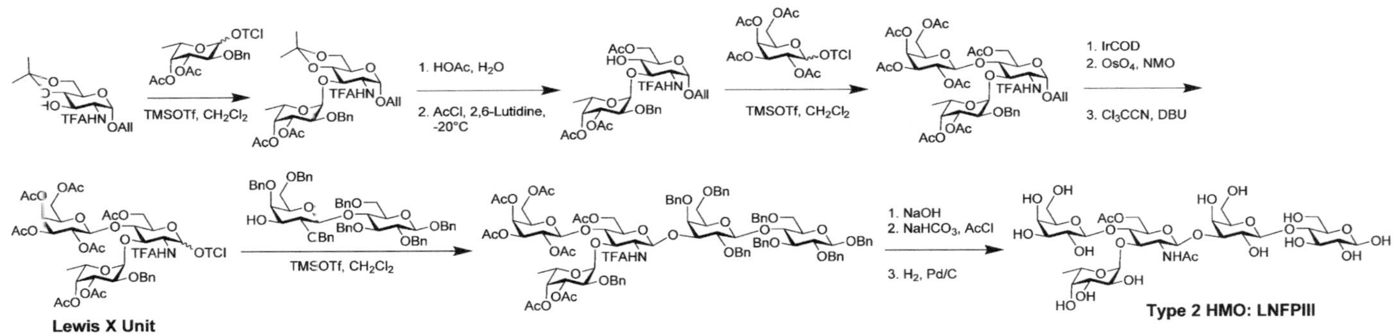

FIGURE 9.5

Assembly and deprotection of type 2 HMO LNFP-III.

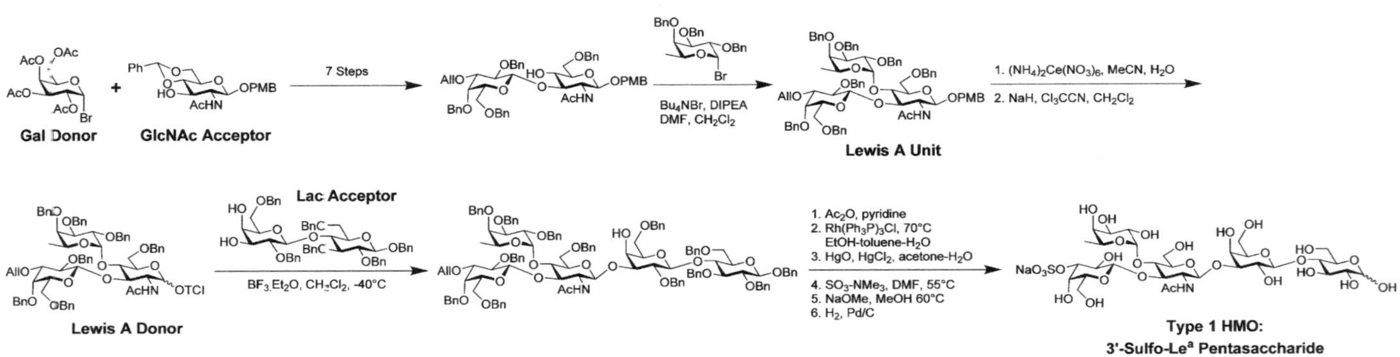

FIGURE 9.6

Synthesis of Le^a pentasaccharide, a type 1 HMO (Lubineau et al., 1994).

scalable and can lead to defined HMO libraries wherein the core type and fucosylation, sialylation, and sulfation sites are systematically varied to enable elucidation of the structure–function relationship of HMOs. Chemical synthesis represents but one viable approach, and ultimately the best overall, most economical solution may be a combination of chemical synthesis of the LacNAc-Lac/*neo*-LacNAc-Lac backbone followed by enzyme-catalyzed substitution with Neu5Ac and Fuc residues using well-characterized recombinant enzymes. Once a specific HMO is identified as a potential nutritional or pharmaceutical product, development of an engineered bacterial or cell-free expression system may provide economical access on industrial scale.

2. CHEMOENZYMATIC SYNTHESIS OF HUMAN MILK OLIGOSACCHARIDES

Despite the complexity of HMOs (Bode, 2009), common structural features enable chemoenzymatic routes to be developed using a relatively restricted portfolio of enzymes to mediate the attachment of glycosyl donors to acceptors. Enzymatic reactions are noted to proceed with complete chemoselectivity and stereoselectivity, often with high regioselectivity and efficiency, and are usually performed on substrates in the absence of protection groups in mild aqueous conditions (Schmaltz et al., 2011). In many cases, an enzyme-mediated transformation can substitute for a number of chemical reactions within a chemical synthetic scheme. The individual enzymes required to perform specific transformations may be combined in multienzyme systems to recapitulate biosynthetic pathways enabling realistic and scalable methods to synthesize complex oligosaccharides on a milligram-to-kilogram scale (Johnson, 1999).

2.1 ENZYMATIC SYNTHESIS OF OLIGOSACCHARIDES

Specific enzymes of interest for synthesis of HMOs are glycosyltransferases (GTs), in particular galactosyltransferases (GalTs), *N*-acetylglucosaminyltransferases (GlcNAcTs), fucosyltransferases (FucTs), sialyltransferases (STs), and glycohydrolases (GHs), in particular β-galactosidases and sialidases, and modified GHs termed glycosynthases (GSs), Fig. 9.7 (Schmaltz et al., 2011).

Mammalian glycan synthesis is performed in vivo predominantly within the endoplasmic reticulum and Golgi apparatus where GTs transfer sugar moieties from glycosyl donors to an acceptor. Prokaryotes achieve a similar process in the bacterial periplasm or at the cytosolic face of the inner membrane where the enzymes can access the nucleotide sugar donors as well as the acceptor substrates (Whitfield et al., 2014). Glycosyl donors for GTs can be either activated nucleotide sugars (Leloir type) or sugar monophosphates (non-Leloir type) donors (Lairson et al., 2008). GT enzymes are advantageous in chemoenzymatic syntheses due to the complete stereocontrol and regiocontrol achieved with an almost quantitative yield for formation of

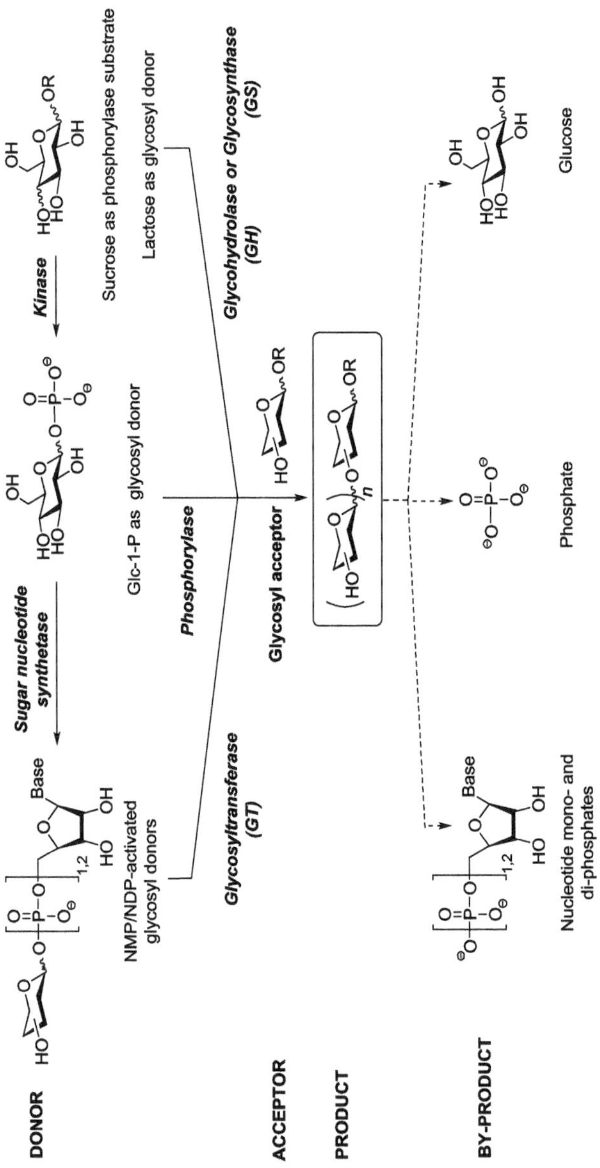

FIGURE 9.7

Enzymatic synthesis of oligosaccharides by Leloir GTs, non-Leloir GHs, and GSs.

the glycosidic linkage. Their requirement for high-cost donor substrates, however, has hampered exploitation of GTs for large-scale synthetic glycochemistry.

GHs, which usually cleave glycosidic linkages, can be applied to synthesis by manipulating the reaction equilibrium to achieve bond formation in a process called *trans*-glycosylation. They are frequently cytoplasmically located and have greater stability compared to GTs. GHs have less stringent substrate specificity and lower cost donor substrates, which make them synthetically attractive. The main limitations, however, are: reduced specificity that can lead to regioisomer formation; competitive hydrolysis, since the generated products are frequently also substrates, so yields are rarely greater than 30%; and product isolation being complicated by the excess donor required to favor *trans*-glycosylation (Schmaltz et al., 2011).

The invention of GSs, engineered GHs that lacked the ability to hydrolyze the formed glycosidic bond through mutation of the active site nucleophilic residue, enables near quantitative yields for glycan bond formation. The challenges with the GS approach, however, remain the need to provide activated glycosyl donors, frequently glycosyl fluorides, azides or nitrophenols, and the production of regioisomers depending on the acceptor structure.

2.2 CHALLENGES IN ENZYMATIC HUMAN MILK OLIGOSACCHARIDE SYNTHESIS

The three problems often cited for enzymatic approaches are the following.

1. The requisite enzymes are not readily available.
2. The sugar nucleotide donors are expensive and available from limited commercial sources, precluding their use as stoichiometric reagents for large-scale synthesis.
3. The enzymatic reactions are limited by the inherent biological capability of the enzymes which may include constraints imposed by enzyme stability, low catalytic turnover, substrate and acceptor tolerances, and product inhibition caused by products, substrates, and/or released nucleoside phosphates or pyrophosphates.

Many of these challenges have been overcome. Microbial enzymes have been demonstrated to perform enzymatic reactions analogous to their mammalian homologues but often with improved expression characteristics, enzyme stabilities, and broader substrate scope, which make them more amenable to industrial implementation. The substrate specificity of the native GTs and GHs can also be modified or improved in order to create enzymes that tolerate unnatural acceptor and/or donor substrates. Cofactor recycling systems have been developed that minimize the stoichiometric requirements for expensive sugar nucleotide donor substrates. Indeed, many chemical synthetic approaches to oligosaccharide targets, including HMOs, use chemoenzymatic processes at key junctures to overcome particularly challenging glycoside bond formations. For example, STs have been extensively adopted to install the sialic acid moieties at the terminal position of synthesized glycoforms due to the complex protection group and stereoselectivity issues associated with a purely chemical approach (Tsai et al., 2013).

2.3 SOURCING ENZYMES

Enzymes required for enzymatic reactions can be sourced from their native host organisms through a process of selective precipitation and iterative purification or, more commonly, through recombinant technology in which the target gene is specifically overexpressed and isolated from a heterologous host, which may be of a mammalian, insect, or microbial origin.

2.3.1 Mammalian Sources of Enzymes

Mammalian GTs are often integral membrane glycoproteins with the catalytic center localized in the lumen of the Golgi apparatus. This membrane association frequently results in difficulties in isolation requiring solubilization with detergents to ensure stability and to prevent denaturation and aggregation. Recombinant mammalian GTs often express poorly in microbial host species such as *E. coli*, due to absence of comparable organelle membrane structures, or express as inactive enzymes potentially due to the absence of posttranslational modifications or differences in the oxidative environment during the folding processes (Skretas et al., 2009). Truncated bovine β1,3GalT is a noted exception, being capable of expression in a conventional *E. coli* BL21(DE3) host (Fang et al., 1998). The soluble human β1,4GalT, a 55-kDa sialoglycoprotein, can be purified from human milk following proteolytic cleavage of the membrane-associating stem as a mix of at least 13 distinct heterogeneous glycoforms (Shibatani et al., 2001). The heterologous expression of mammalian GTs can benefit from truncation of membrane binding domains (Weinstein et al., 1987) and attachment of protein fusion tags such as glutathione-*S*-transferase (GST), transcription termination/antitermination protein NusA, maltose binding protein, thioredoxin, or polyhistidine to assist with enzyme folding and soluble expression and for purification (Liu et al., 2009). Coexpression of chaperones and heat shock proteins that assist with protein folding, solubilization, and disaggregation often assist in production in microbial systems. For many mammalian GTs, baculovirus-mediated insect cell expression is used to achieve functional expression (Skretas et al., 2009).

2.3.2 Microbial Sources of Enzymes

The costs associated with large-scale expression of GTs using mammalian or insect cell lines has led to an emphasis on identifying novel microbial GTs that can catalyze the same reactions but that are more conveniently expressed in soluble, active form. This is feasible, for despite the fact that bacteria do not synthesis HMOs, they do express a wide array of lipo-oligosaccharide (LOS) and lipopolysaccharide (LPS) structures on their surface, many of which mimic mammalian carbohydrate structures, including LNT, LNnT, and globotriose, fucosylated structures such as Le^x

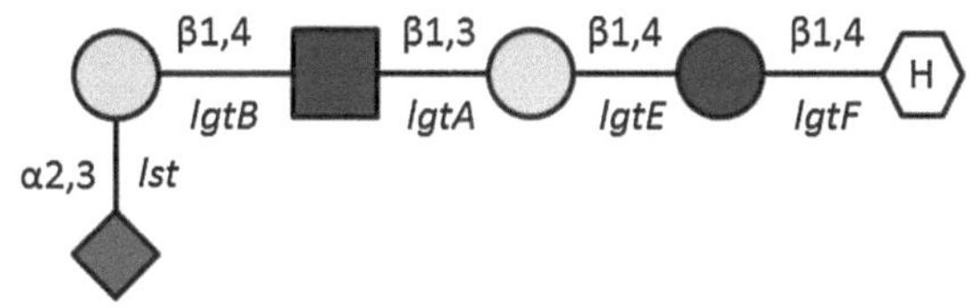

FIGURE 9.8

Microbial glycosyltransferase enzymes catalyze identical glycan bond formations to those observed in LNnT synthesis. Thus, *N. gonorrhoeae* enzymes *lgtE, lgtA,* and *lgtB* consecutively functionalise the heptose (H) residue in LOS to generate an LNnT core, which is sialylated by *lst.*

and Le^a, and sialylated motifs such as sLe^x (Brockhausen, 2014). Genes responsible for LOS and LPS synthesis often have catalytic domains that resemble mammalian homologues and are clustered in loci, which facilitate identification and isolation. *Neisseria gonorrhoeae* LOS glycosyl*t*ransferase genes (designated *lgt*) encode all the GT enzymes necessary to generate an LNnT-like structure, which is a mimic of the human glycosphingolipid paragloboside (Fig. 9.8; Zhu et al., 2006). Similarly, *Streptococcus pneumoniae* serotype 14 *c*apsular *p*oly*s*accharide locus (designated *cps*) encodes 12 enzymes (*cps14A–cps14L*), including all the glycosyltransferases necessary to generate LNT (Kolkman et al., 1997).

In general, microbial GTs are relatively easily expressed in *E. coli*, a common expression system, and are soluble, active, and stable and frequently either not or only weakly inhibited by sugar nucleotide by-products compared to their mammalian homologues, making them better suited for scaled production of HMOs (Johnson, 1999; Brockhausen, 2014). As the vast bacterial gene pool continues to be sequenced, new enzymes involved in oligosaccharide synthesis continue to be identified, expanding the repertoire of available enzymes to use in chemoenzymatic applications.

2.4 GLYCOSYLTRANSFERASES

GTs are responsible for the synthesis of most glycoconjugates in mammals and bacteria. Mammalian glycosyltransferases tend to have narrowly defined acceptor specificities, whereas microbial GTs such as β1,3GlcNAcT (lgtA) and β1,4GalT (lgtB) can accept a wide range of acceptors including HMO core structures such as LNT and LNT-2 (Zhang et al., 2002). An excellent comparison of mammalian and bacterial glycosyltransferases can be found in a recent review (Brockhausen, 2014).

Glycosyltranferases with applications in HMO core synthesis include β1,4-galactosyltransferase (β4GalT1), which catalyzes the transfer of Gal from UDP-Gal to free or bound GlcNAc, producing *N*-acetyllactosamine (Galβ1-4GlcNAc, LacNAc). β4GalT1 in the presence of α-lactalbumin constitutes lactose synthase, which transfers Gal from UDP-Gal to free Glc to form lactose, the major milk carbohydrate

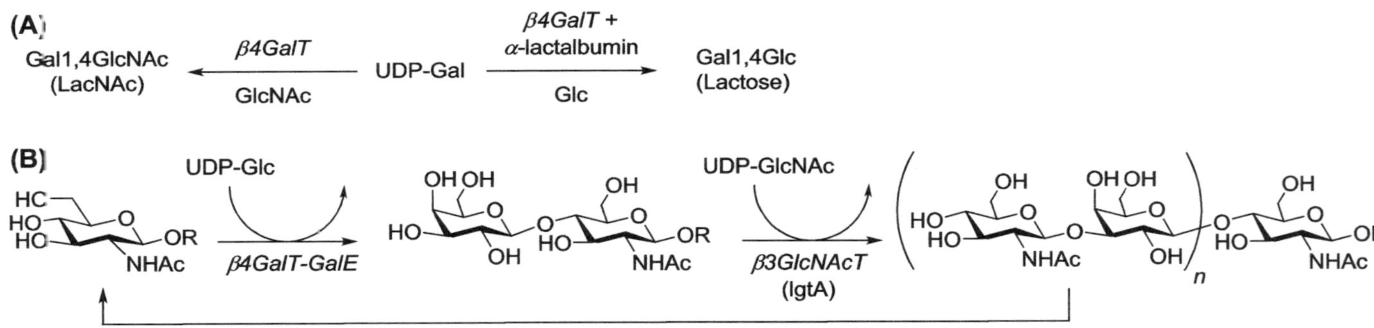

FIGURE 9.9

(A) Divergent enzymatic synthesis of LacNAc and lactose by β4GalT-GalE and (B) iterative synthesis of poly-LacNAc motif by concerted action of β4GalT and β3GlcNAcT.

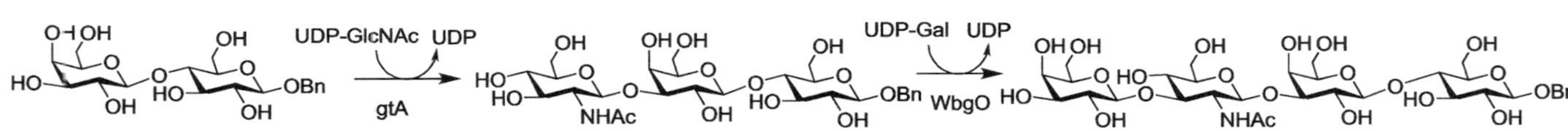

FIGURE 9.10

Iterative coupling of GlcNAc and Gal to lactose to generate LNT core structure.

(Fig. 9.9). The relatively flexible substrate specificity of bovine and human β4GalTs has been exploited in the synthesis of HMOs cores and neoglycoconjugates using non-natural donor and acceptor substrates (Shibatani et al., 2001). Recombinant human α1,3GalT has been use to prepare Le^c (Baisch et al., 1998), and mutant versions have been prepared with altered specificity (Tumbale et al., 2008).

Microbial enzymes that produce LPS and LOS have been used to synthesize HMOs. For example, both *N. meningitidis* and *H. pylori* LOS contain the LNnT structure (Wakarchuk et al., 1996). β3GlcNAcT LgtA is expressed to high levels in *E. coli* and catalyzes the transfer of a GlcNAc from UDP-GlcNAc to the lactose unit in the extending LOS. Its broad acceptor specificity enables transfer from both UDP-GlcNAc and UDP-GalNAc to terminal α- and β-anomeric Gal residues in acceptors (Blixt et al., 1999). The β4GalT LgtB has been used in the synthesis of LacNAc and backbone of Le structures (Endo et al., 2000a,b). β4GalT LgtC can transfer Gal from UDP-Gal to a variety of acceptor substrates and has been used in the synthesis of Globo-H, globotrihexose and a range of precursors for use in glycan arrays (Zhang et al., 2002; Zhou et al., 2011). Chemoenzymatic synthesis of poly-*N*-acetyllactosamine on a multigram scale used an iterative elongation comprising Gal addition, arising from UDP-Glc in the presence of a β4GalT-UDPGalE fusion enzyme (Chen et al., 2000) and then GalNAc addition from UDP-GalNAc in the presence of LgtA (Vasiliu et al., 2006).

β3GalT has been identified in humans, higher eukaryotes, and microbial species (Brockhausen, 2014). The benzyl β-glycoside of LNT was prepared from benzyl β-lactoside in two steps via the iterative coupling of GlcNAc mediated by *N. meningitidis* LgtA (86% yield) and then Gal mediated by *E. coli* O55:H7 β3GalT (WbgO) (87% yield) (Fig. 9.10; Liu et al., 2009).

2.5 GLYCOSYLTRANSFERASE GLYCOSYL DONORS

Efficient use of GTs requires practical and high yielding preparations of the activated nucleotide sugar (Leloir) donors. Mammalian systems use eight sugar nucleotides of which five—UDP-galactose (UDP-Gal), UDP-*N*-acetylglucosamine (UDP-GlcNAc), UDP-*N*-acetylgalactosamine (UDP-GalNAc), GDP-L-fucose (GDP-Fuc), and CMP-*N*-acetylneuraminic acid (CMP-NeuAc)—are the donors predominantly used in HMO synthesis. Commercially available sugar nucleotides are too expensive to be used in stoichiometric amount on a large scale, and chemical methods of preparation are laborious and difficult. Thus, multienzyme sugar nucleotide regeneration processes have been developed, which enable the use of catalytic amounts of these sugar nucleotides, reducing the cost and eliminating the problem of nucleoside-diphosphate–based inhibition. Subordinate recycle systems use readily available enzymes (with inexpensive substrates): pyruvate kinase (with phosphoenolpyruvate (PEP, Fig. 9.11), polyphosphate kinase (with polyphosphate), or acetyl kinase (with acetyl phosphate) (Schmaltz et al., 2011).

Non-Leloir GTs that use monosaccharide-1-phosphates as glycosyl donors that are called phosphorylases (Fig. 9.7). Sucrose phosphorylase has been used to access Glc-1-phosphate directly from inexpensive sucrose and inorganic phosphate (PPi),

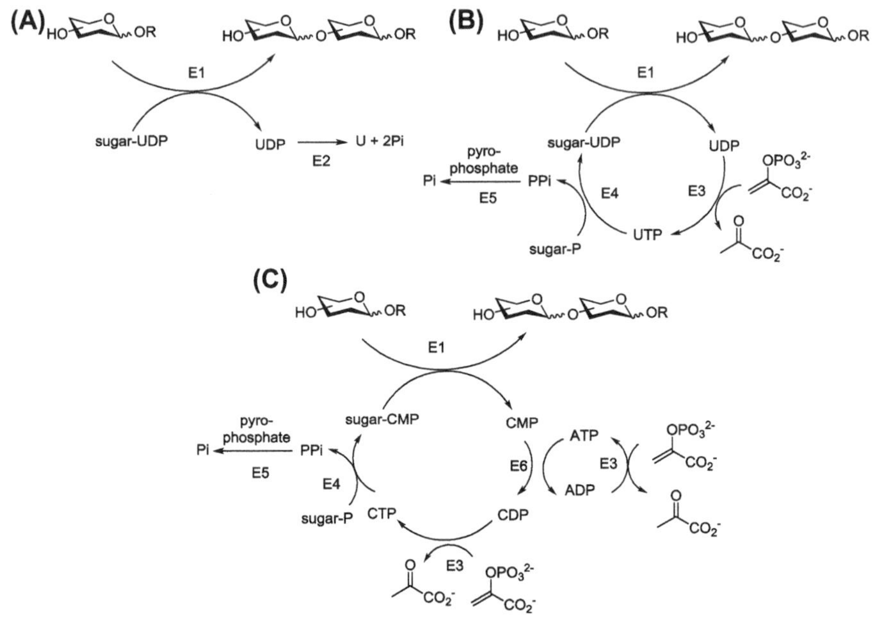

FIGURE 9.11

Strategies to regenerate sugar nucleotide donors in glycosyltransferase-catalyzed syntheses: (A) nonrecycling process is which alkaline phosphatase decomposes nucleotides; (B) nucleotide diphosphate recycling; (C) nucleotide monophosphate (CMP-NeuAc) recycling; E1, glycosyltransferase; E2, alkaline phosphatase; E3, pyruvate kinase; E4, sugar nucleotide synthetase; E5, pyrophosphorylase; E6, myokinase.

which overcomes the requirement for stoichiometric adenosine triphosphate (ATP) in kinase-based approaches (Nishimoto et al., 2009; Nakai et al., 2013).

2.5.1 *UDP-Gal*

UDP-Gal can be generated from UDP-Glc using UDP-Gal 4-epimerase (UDP-GalE) (Chen et al., 2000). Precursor UDP-Glc is in turn accessed from Glc via sequential reactions of glucose 6-phosphatase (G6Pase) or hexokinase (HK), phosphoglucomutase (PGM), and UDP-Glc pyrophosphorylase (UDPGP), Fig. 9.12.

UDP-Gal may also be accessed through a salvage mechanism in which Gal is converted Gal-1-P by galactose kinase (GK) and then via a nucleotide exchange reaction to UDP-Gal, with UDP-Glc being converted to Glc-1-P mediated by Gal-1-P uridyltransferase (GalPUT). As both the UDPGalE and the GalPUT equilibria favor UDP-Glc over UDP-Gal, it is often necessary to couple the UDP-Gal synthesis to a GalT-catalyzed reaction to drive the equilibrium to product formation (Wong et al., 1992). The UDP by-product arising from the coupling of UDP-Glc or UDP-Gal is recycled through conversion to UTP with PEP and

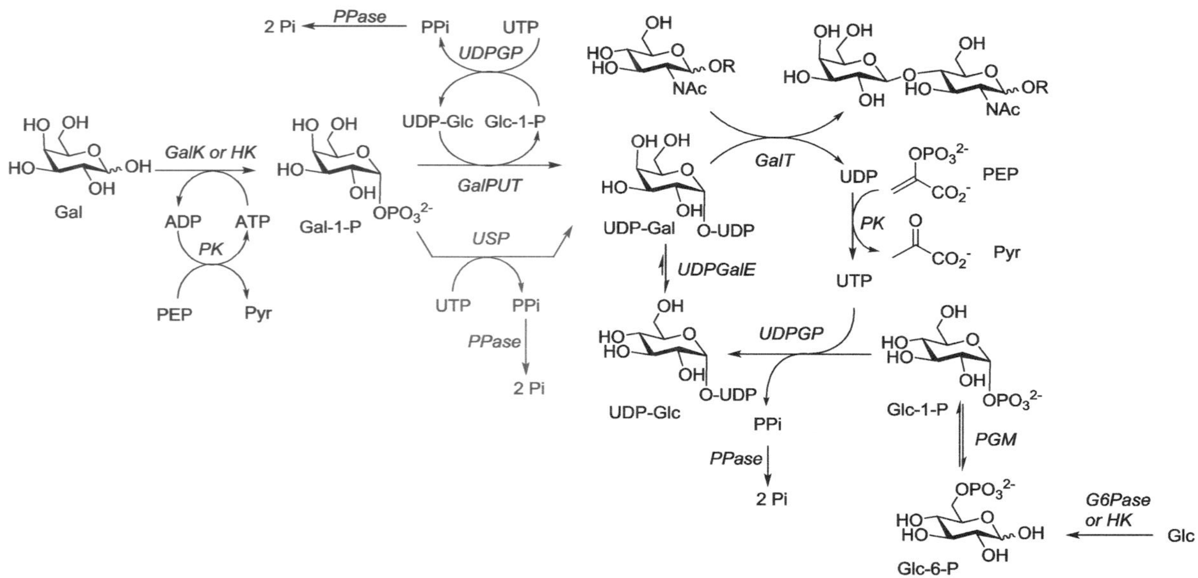

FIGURE 9.12

Synthesis of LacNAc with in situ cofactor regeneration using UDPGP and UDPGalE to regenerate UDP-Gal from Glc-1-P (black). Alternatively, UDP-Gal can be generated from Gal using GalK and GalPUT through a Gal-1-P intermediate (blue), or via promiscuous USPs, which convert Gal-1-P to UDP-Gal with UTP without the need for involvement of UDP-Glc in the recycle system.

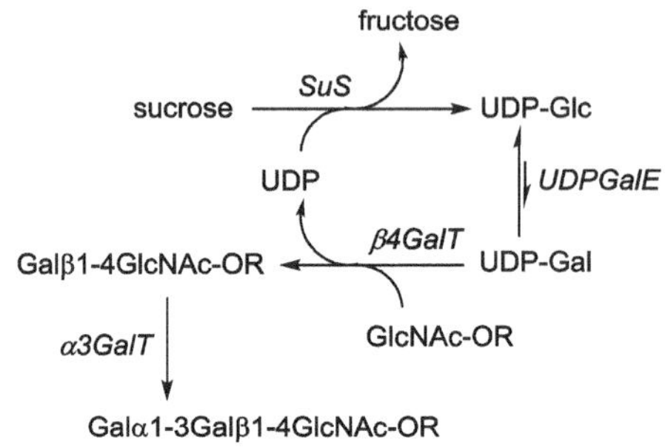

FIGURE 9.13

Enzymatic synthesis of LacNAc and Galα1-3LacNAc derivatives using four enzymes in one pot.

pyruvate kinase (PK), and the PPi is decomposed by inorganic pyrophosphatase (PPase).

The recent discovery of UDP-sugar pyrophosphorylases (USP) with broad substrate specificities enables a further salvage route for direct synthesis of UDP-monosaccharides, including those of Glc, Gal, Man, Fuc, GlcN, GalN, GlcNAc, and Xyl from their precursor sugar phosphates. Many of the enzymes have sufficient substrate promiscuity to enable preparation of 2- or 6-azido, or 6-sulfo- or *N*-sulfo-modified NDP-monosaccharides, enabling the production of HMO mimics (Muthana et al., 2012; Zou et al., 2013).

The enzymes required to generate UDP-monosaccharide donors are commonly combined in a one-pot synthesis approach or immobilized on agarose beads ("superbeads") to enable reuse. Superbeads containing the enzymes GalK, UDPGP, and GalPUT for UDP-Gal formation, UMP kinase (UMK), and nucleotide diphosphate kinase (NDK) for UTP formation from UMP, polyphosphate kinase (PpK) for ATP recycling, and finally PPase for hydrolysis of the inorganic pyrophosphate were reported to convert 50% of the UMP into UDP-Gal and to be effective in the preparative synthesis of HMOs (Chen et al., 2001).

Sucrose-UDP glucosyltransferase, referred to as sucrose synthase (SuS), generates UDP-Glc from sucrose and UDP. Combined with UDPGalE, this allows generation of UDP-Gal from sucrose (Fig. 9.13). SuS, UDPGalE, and β4GalT have been used in a three-enzyme reaction cycle to synthesize LacNAc in 57% average yield over 10 repetitive batch cycles (Zervosen et al., 1996). The system avoids the need for NTPs and NTP regeneration and does not generate potentially inhibitory phosphate. Addition of bovine α3GalT to the system generates LNT derivatives in 44% yield based on the GlcNAc-OR acceptor (Hokke et al., 1996). SuS, UDPGalE, and β4GalT have been used in a three-enzyme reaction cycle to synthesize LacNAc in 57% average yield over 10 repetitive batch cycles (Zervosen et al., 1996). The system avoids the need for NTPs and NTP regeneration and does not generate potentially inhibitory phosphate. Addition of bovine α3GalT to the system generates LNT derivatives in 44% yield based on the GlcNAc-OR acceptor (Hokke et al., 1996).

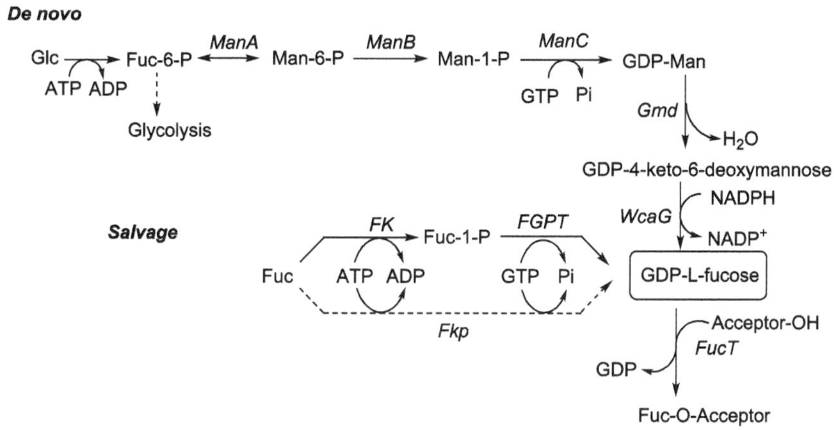

FIGURE 9.14

Routes to GDP-Fuc depicting the de novo pathway from endogenous Glc via mannose-6-phosphate isomerase (ManA), phosphomannomutase (ManB), Gmd and WcaG, and the salvage pathways, converting exogenous Fuc to GDP-Fuc through a Fuc-1-P intermediate catalyzed by FK and FPGT or with bifunctional FKP.

2.5.2 GDP-Fuc

FucTs catalyze the transfer of L-fucose from a GDP-L-fucose donor to an acceptor molecule. Although some chemical and enzymatic routes have been developed, the cost and general unavailability of both fucose and GDP-L-fucose have limited large-scale production of fucosylated oligosaccharides.

Two different pathways for GDP-Fuc production have been applied in chemoenzymatic synthesis: the de novo pathway and the salvage pathway (Fig. 9.14). The de novo pathway present in mammals and bacteria commences with fructose-6-phosphate (Fuc-6-P), an intermediate in the glycolysis pathway, and passes through GDP-D-mannose (GDP-Man) using GDP-D-mannose 4,6-dehydratase (Gmd) and GDP-L-fucose synthase (WcaG in *E. coli*) as key enzymes to generate GDP-Fuc (Albermann et al., 2000).

In the mammalian salvage pathway, extracellular L-fucose is transferred into cells, phosphorylated by L-fucose kinase (FK) using ATP to generate L-Fuc-1-phosphate (Fuc-1-P) and combined with GTP by L-fucose-1-phosphate guanylyltransferase (FPGT) to produce GDP-L-fucose. Deletion of the de novo *Gmd/WcaG* genes in *Bacteroides fragilis* led to identification of a comparable microbial salvage pathway mediated by a single bifunctional L-fucokinase/GDP-L-Fuc pyrophosphorylase enzyme (Fkp), which can scavenge Fuc from host organisms and convert L-fucose into GDP-fucose via a Fuc-1-P intermediate (Coyne et al., 2005).

GDP-Fuc production has been demonstrated using both the de novo and salvage pathways. The heterologous expression and isolation of the genes encoding *E. coli* Gmd and WcaG enzymes enabled conversion of GDP-Man to GDP-Fuc by a two-step enzymatic reaction in a yield of 78%. This process was complicated, however,

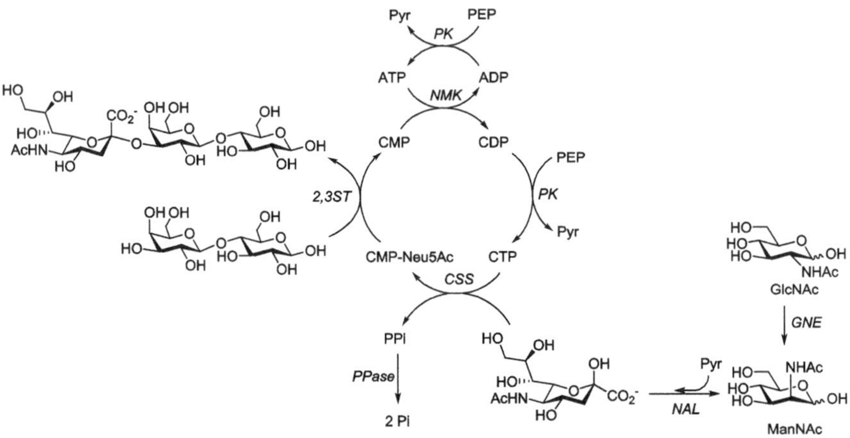

FIGURE 9.15

Synthesis of 3′-sialyllactose using cofactor regeneration.

by strong product inhibition of Gmd by GDP-Fuc, which means the two enzyme steps need to be performed separately (Albermann et al., 2001). Fkp has been successfully used to prepare modified Le^x derivatives (Wang et al., 2009).

2.5.3 CMP-NeuAc

A CMP-Neu5Ac regeneration system has been developed for use in the ST-catalyzed synthesis of a sialyloligosaccharide (Fig. 9.15). Bacterial CMP-sialic acid synthetase (CSS) catalyzes the reaction of CTP with Neu5Ac to form CMP-Neu5Ac, and the coproduced PPi is broken down by PPase to drive the reaction toward completion (Mizanur et al., 2008). The sialylation by-product CMP is recycled to CTP using nucleoside monophosphate kinase and PK. The system requires only catalytic amounts of CMP and ATP but stoichiometric amounts of PEP, acetyl phosphate, or inorganic polyphosphate as phosphate sources to regenerate CTP and ATP (Ichikawa et al., 1992). Addition of *N*-acetylneuraminic acid lyase (NAL) enables formation of Neu5Ac from *N*-acetylmannosamine (ManNAc) and pyruvate (Yu et al., 2015) or, with inclusion of GlcNAc-2-epimerase (GNE), the formation of Neu5Ac from GlcNAc as a precursor substrate (Lee et al., 2007).

2.5.4 Monosaccharide-1-phosphates

Phosphorylases catalyze reversible transfer of a glycosyl moiety from a polysaccharide (such as sucrose) onto PPi to generate monosaccharide-1-phosphates. These can be used as donors in glycosidation reactions. For example, the combination of sucrose phosphorylase (SP) and galacto-*N*-biose/lacto-*N*-biose phosphorylase (GLNBP) provides efficient preparations of HMOs (Fig. 9.16; Nakai et al., 2013). GLNBP derived from *Bifidobacterium longum* JCM1217 combined with SP enabled production of LNB on a kilogram scale from sucrose and GlcNAc or of

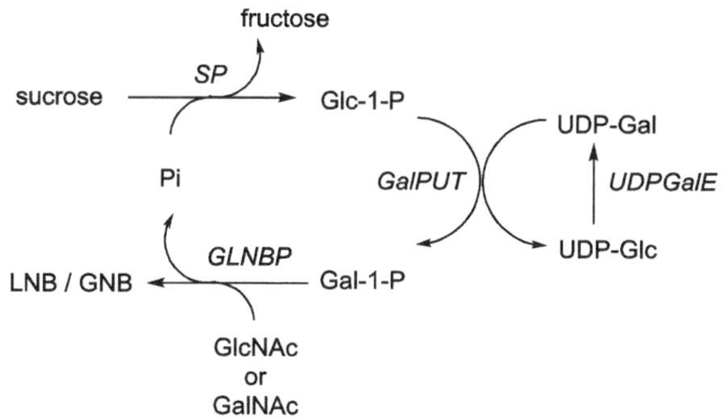

FIGURE 9.16

One-pot enzymatic synthesis of LNB and GNB from sucrose with addition of GlcNAc or GalNAc, respectively.

galacto-*N*-biose (GNB) from sucrose and GalNAc (Nishimoto et al., 2007, 2009). Directed evolution of *B. longum*–derived GLNBP using error-prone polymerase chain reaction (PCR) mutagenesis identified amino acid substitutions C235Y/D576V as providing a 20°C improvement in thermostability (Koyama et al., 2013). GLNBP derived from *B. longum* subsp. *infantis* was capable of the efficient coupling of Gal-1-P to a diverse range of acceptors including the production of LNB and GNB in 95% yield. In this instance, the donor substrate Gal-1-P was generated from ATP and Gal (1.2 or 1.5 equiv.) to drive the reaction toward disaccharide formation (Yu et al., 2010).

2.6 GLYCOHYDROLASES AND GLYCOSYNTHASES

GH-catalyzed synthesis of HMOs can occur under thermodynamically controlled reverse hydrolysis conditions with excess monosaccharide donor substrates or under kinetically controlled transglycosylation conditions, where an activated donor such as a disaccharide or a *p*-nitrophenyl (pNP) glycoside is sed. In both cases, the synthetic reaction takes place in competition with hydrolysis of both the substrate and product, Fig. 9.17 GHs are often explored as alternatives to GTs because GHs are easier to produce or purchase and do not require expensive nucleotide sugars as glycosyl donors, making them attractive from an industrial perspective. The regioselectivity of GH-mediated transglycosylations can be less than absolute, however, yields are generally ~5–30%, and high substrate concentrations are required to outcompete water-based hydrolysis (Schmaltz et al., 2011). Commercially, galacto-oligosaccharides (GOS) are synthesized from lactose mediated by β-galactosidases, and fructo-oligosaccharides (FOS) from sucrose mediated by β-fructosidases, in exemplars of the thermodynamically mediated process, in which yields of 50% can be achieved at substrate concentrations (Nath et al., 2014; Nobre et al., 2015).

GSs, in contrast, are engineered GHs with mutations within the active site that preserve the ability to form glycosidic bonds but abolish the subsequently capacity to

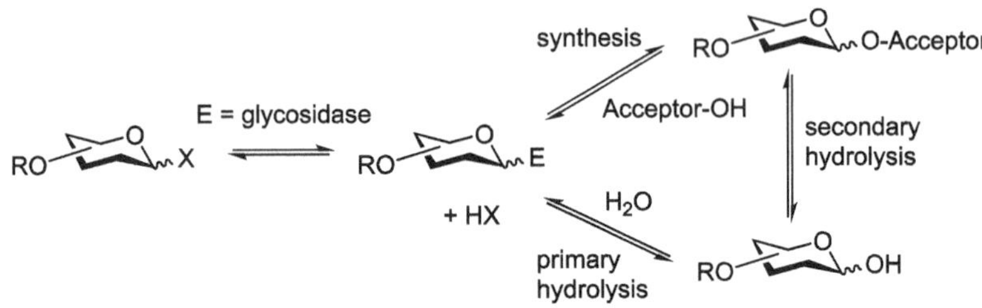

FIGURE 9.17

General mechanism for glycosidase (sialidase, fucosidase, galactosidase)-mediated trans-glycosylation and competing hydrolysis. An activated donor species forms a glycosyl-enzyme intermediate, which may undergo productive synthesis with a glycosyl acceptor or nonproductive hydrolysis with water. The glycosylglycoside may also undergo secondary hydrolysis.

hydrolyze the resultant glycosidic bond. GSs have been demonstrated as useful tools for chemoenzymatic synthesis of carbohydrates in high yields, as alternatives to more expensive GT routes, and have been recently reviewed (Schmaltz et al., 2011). A challenge with the GS approach is a need to provide activated glycosyl donors frequently nitrophenol glycosides, or glycosyl fluorides or azides. This approach is feasible for small-scale synthesis of high-value intermediates, but for large-scale synthesis, the price of the donor becomes an important consideration and the toxicity of the released nitrophenol, hydrofluoric acid (HF) or hydrazoic acid (HN_3) by-product is an issue in the approval of such processes for use in food applications (Zeuner et al., 2014).

GH and GS enzymes used for the synthesis of HMOs include β-galactosidases, α-L-fucosidases, and sialidases. Lactose is commonly used donor for *trans*-galactosylation, especially in the production of GOS under thermodynamic conditions. pNP β-Gal is primarily used as the donor substrate under kinetic conditions (Zeuner et al., 2014). LNB was synthesized regiospecifically in a 55% yield using pNP β-Gal as donor and GlcNAc as acceptor (in a 1:10 ratio) catalyzed by *Xanthomonas manihotis* β-galactosidase with respect to the donor (Vetere et al., 2000). 3′-Sialyl-LNB was then obtained in 35% yield form LNB using 4-methylumbellyferyl Neu5Ac as a donor (in a 1:1 ratio) catalyzed by *Trypanosoma cruzi* sialidase (Fig. 9.18; Vetere et al., 2000).

Fucosidases, classified as α-1,2-, α-1,3-, or α-1,6-fucosidases, catalyze the release of terminal fucose residues α-linked to glycans and glycoproteins resulting in hydrolysis or *trans*-fucosylation. Similar to glycohydrolases, fucosidases have been used to effect *trans*-fucosylations in the presence of fucopyranoside donors such as pNP Fuc, fucosyl fluoride, or fucosyl azides to yield fucosylated oligosaccharides. A mixture of 2′-, 3′-, and 6′-fucosyl-lactose (2′-FL, 3′-FL, and 6′-FL) was obtained in 13% yield using porcine fucosidase–catalyzed reactions of pNP Fuc with LacNAc. In contrast, *Alcaligene* sp. KSF-9687 FucT generated 3′-FL in 54% (Murata et al., 1999a,b). Fucosidases alfB and alfC from *Lactobacillus casei* produced Fucα3GlcNAc (23%) and Fucα6GlcNAc (56%), respectively, in the presence of pNP Fuc and GlcNAc (Rodriguez-Diaz et al., 2013), and α-L-fucosidase extracted from *Penicillium multicolor* generated Fucα1-3Glc (49%) and Fucα1-3GlcNAc (28%) in the presence of Glc and GlcNAc, respectively (Ajisaka et al., 1998). In a process analogous to the glycosynthase approach, it

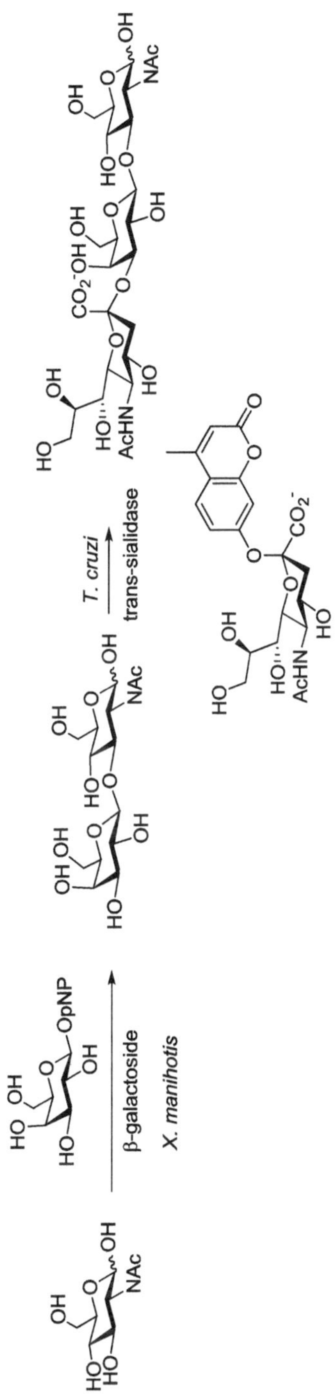

FIGURE 9.18
Synthesis of LNB and 3′-sialyl-LNB using only *trans*-glycosylation methodology.

has been reported that *B. bifidum* BbAfcA and BbAfcB can be engineered as fucosynthases to generate 2′-FL with Fuc fluoride (Wada et al., 2008) and to generate Le^a and Le^x epitopes with LNB and LacNAc chains (Sakurama et al., 2012).

Sialidases catalyze the release of terminal sialic acid residues α-linked to glycolipids, glycoproteins, and polysaccharides, resulting in either hydrolysis or *trans*-sialylation. Typical *trans*-sialylation donors include pNP NeuAc, 4-methylumbelliferyl NeuAc, 3′-SL, dimers and polymers of α2,8-linked sialic acid, as well as the fetal calf serum glycoprotein fetuin. Recently, casein glycomacropeptide (cGMP), produced during cheese manufacture, has been explored as a sialyl donor for *trans*-sialylation. cGMP contains 5–11% (w/w) sialic acid, approximately half is α2,3-linked to Gal and half α2,6-linked to GalNAc. The well-studied α2,3-*trans*-sialidases from *Trypanosoma cruzi* and *Trypanosoma rangeli* (Tr6) expressed in *Pichia pastoris* have been used in the production of 3′-sialyllactose in 20–90% yield, dependent on the cGMP donor to acceptor ratios employed (Holck et al., 2014; Michalak et al., 2014), with 3.6g of 3′-SL obtained in a 50% yield based on cGMP on a 5-L scale. Several sialyltranferases from microbial sources possess sialidase activity including *Photobacterium damsela* α2,6-ST displaying 2,6-sialidase activity, multifunctional *Campylobacter jejuni* sialyltransferase CstII displaying 2,8-*trans*-sialidase activity, and *Pasteurella multocida* PmST displaying α-2,3/2,6-*trans*-sialidase activities (Yu et al., 2015). These sialyltransferases have been used to catalyze the synthesis of 3′SL and 6′SL by *trans*-sialylation of lactose using cGMP as donor (Guo et al., 2015).

2.6.1 Fucosyl Transferases

In mammals, FucT catalyzes the transfer of the Fuc moiety from GDP-Fuc to a variety of acceptors. α1,2FucT transfers Fuc to the 2-position of the Gal moiety LNB or LacNAc, and α1,3/4FucTs add Fuc to the 3- or 4-position of the GlcNAc moiety. In eukaroytes, FucTs are transmembrane proteins with an N-terminal cytosolic tail, a hydrophobic transmembrane domain, a variable-length stem region, and a C-terminal catalytic domain, most of which are located in the Golgi apparatus. Their microbial counterparts, however, are usually soluble proteins without transmembrane segments (Ma et al., 2006). For expression of microbial FucTs, it has been found necessary to truncate the problematic C-terminal tails rich in hydrophobic and positively charged amino acids and/or to create fusion proteins with peptide sequences that enhance expression of soluble, active protein and aid purification (Albermann et al., 2001; Engels et al., 2014).

The α1,2FucT from *H. pylori* (FutC) and from *E. coli* O128:B12 (WbsJ) have broad substrate specificities that include the type I and II motifs, LNT, lactose, and the monofucosylated species Galβ1-3(α1-3Fuc)GlcNAc and Galβ1-4(α1-3Fuc) GlcNAc (Stein et al., 2008; Engels et al., 2014). When expressed as a fusion with either polyhistidine or GST, they transferred Fuc onto lactose to produce 2′-FL and onto the Le^a trisaccharide to generate a difucosylated species (Wang et al., 1999; Albermann et al., 2001; Stein et al., 2008). The α1,3-FucT3 from *H. pylori* displayed a strong preference for type II structures with the LNnT preferred over LacNAc (Fig. 9.19; Martin et al., 1997).

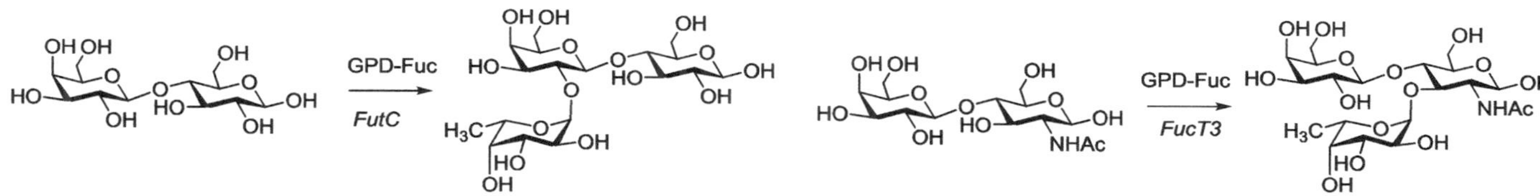

FIGURE 9.19

Chemoenzymatic syntheses of 2′-FL from lactose with FutC and of Lewis x from LacNAc with FucT3 using GDP-Fuc as a donor.

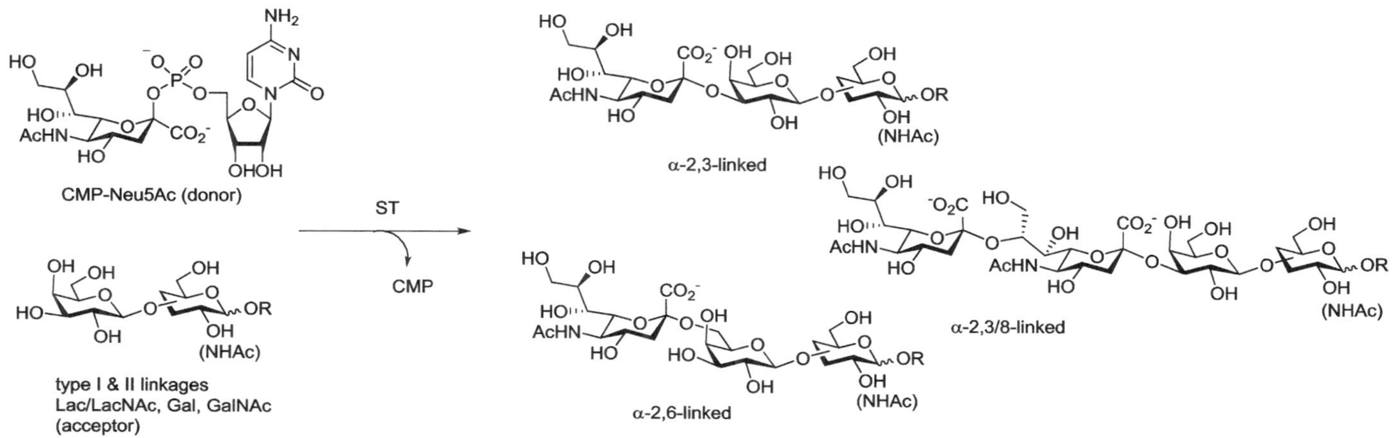

FIGURE 9.20

Sialyltransferase-mediated addition of sialic acid.

2.7 SIALYLTRANSFERASES

STs catalyze the transfer of Neu5Ac from the activated sugar donor CMP-NeuAc to a variety of acceptors. Four linkage patterns are commonly observed: NeuAcα2-3-Gal, NeuAcα2-6Gal, NeuAcα2-6GalNAc, and NeuAcα2-8NeuAc. Consequently, the STs that make them are classified as α2,3ST, α2,6ST, α2,8ST, and polysialyltransferases, respectively Fig. 9.20.

Mammalian ST are membrane proteins localized in the Golgi with an N-terminal cytoplasmic domain, a single transmembrane domain, a variable size stem region, and a C-terminal catalytic domain in the Golgi lumen. The substrate specificity of mammalian STs is strictly determined by the nature and linkage of the terminal and subterminal sugars of the acceptor. Mammalian STs have been cloned and studied in detail, and some are commercially available, yet bacterial STs have been more frequently used in preparative synthesis due to their more facile expression, robust character, broader substrate tolerance, and lower cost. Bacterial STs from more than 20 species have been produced, following the cloning of α2,3-ST from *N. meningitidis* and *N. gonorrhoeae* (Gilbert et al., 1996) and α2,6-ST from *Photobacterium damselae* (Yamamoto et al., 1998). They have broader substrate specificities and are reported to be multifunctional, having ST, sialidase, and *trans*-sialidase activities (Yu et al., 2005). A recent review provides an excellent coverage of bacterial ST donor and acceptor substrate specificities (Yu et al., 2015).

Marine bacteria are a particularly productive source of ST for HMO synthesis. *P. damsela* JT0160 2,6ST (Pd2,6ST) accepts β-Gal and β-GalNAc moieties as substrates and retains moderate activity toward the corresponding α-glycosides. Transfer of sialic acid to type II oligosaccharides such as Lac, LacNAc, Sia-Lac, and Fuc-Lac has been achieved in good yield (Yamamoto et al., 1998). *Vibrio* sp. JT-FAJ-16, an α2,3ST with a wide acceptor specificity and no intrinsic sialidase activity, has been used in the large-scale synthesis of Globo H and SSEA4 for clinical trials (Tsai et al., 2013). *P. multocida* PM0188 encodes a multifunctional ST (PmST1) with α2,3ST, α2,6ST, and α2,3-sialidase activity and has been used synthetically for preparation of Sia-LNT (Yao et al., 2015), Sia-GNB (Li et al., 2015), and diverse sialoside libraries (Yu et al., 2005). Selective mutations can modify the ST inherent reaction profiles, with the P34H mutation of PmST1 leading to a 980-fold increase in α2,6-ST activity while abolishing α2,3ST activity, whereas the mutants E271F and R313Y lead to preferential α2,3ST over α2,6-ST activity when applied to the synthesis of 3′SL (Guo et al., 2015). Similarly, the structure-guided mutations P7H-M117A swapped the acceptor specificity of *Pasteurella dagmatis* ST from α2,3 to α2,6 (Choi et al., 2014). A fusion construct in which the CSS and α2,3ST from *N. meningitides* (NmST) were linked was expressed in high yield in *E. coli* and enabled the synthesis of sialylated oligosaccharides, including 3′-SL at 100-g scale, starting from lactose and sialic and using a CMP-Neu5Ac recycle system (Gilbert et al., 1998). A one-pot multienzyme (OPME) synthesis of sialyloligosaccharides using GlcNAc or ManNAc as the source of the sialic acid donor has been used to generate sialyl-GNB (Li et al., 2015), sialyl-T-MUC1 glycopeptides (Malekan et al., 2013), and sialoside libraries (Yu et al., 2005).

2.8 CHEMOENZYMATIC PROCESSES TO PREPARE HUMAN MILK OLIGOSACCHARIDES

The chemoenzymatic synthesis of HMOs most commonly uses heterologously expressed and purified enzymes that are combined in the presence of substrates, cofactors, and donors. Immobilization of the enzymes on solid surface supports or beads facilitates product purification and enables recycling of enzymes (Chen et al., 2001). Isolation of target oligosaccharide can involve relatively simple removal of protein by centrifugation with passage through an anion exchange column to chelate nucleotide materials. Subsequent chromatography on activated charcoal, ion-exchange resins, or polyacrylamide columns is required to separate the acceptor from the glycosylated material if the conversion has been incomplete. Immobilized yeast cells (*Saccharomyces cerevisiae*) both in isolation and in combination with β-galactosidase have been reported as an efficient way to remove unwanted monosaccharide, disaccharide, and trisaccharide by-products, facilitating downstream purification (Zhou et al., 2011). The following examples are of the production of the dominant HMOs using GT, GS, and GH enzyme-mediated conversions, often using recycle systems as described earlier.

2.8.1 N-Acetyllactosamine (LacNAc, Galβ1-4GalNAc)

The success of chemoenzymatic methods for the production of HMOs was first demonstrated as early as 1982 with conversion of Gal-6-P and GlcNAc into LacNAc mediated by bovine β4GalT on a greater than 10-g scale in 85% yield (Wong et al., 1982). The system used an in situ regeneration of UDP-Gal from UDP-Glc using UDPGP and UDPGalE to avoid the cost of the nucleotide sugar donor and to minimize β1,4GalT inhibition. The enzymes, which were immobilized on a PAN-resin, were recovered at the conclusion of the 4-day process and shown to retain greater than 80% activity. A subsequent variation to this system used GK and GalPUT to convert Gal to UDP-Gal for subsequent β4GalT-mediated coupling to GlcNAc provided LacNAc in 45% yield on the milligram scale (Wong et al., 1992). PK and PEP were used for in situ UTP regeneration, although subsequently, polyphosphate kinase and polyphosphate have been used (Noguchi et al., 1998).

2.8.2 Lacto-N-biose (LNB, Galβ1-3GalNAc)

Recombinantly expressed human β3GalT with stoichiometric UDP-Gal was effective in synthesizing LNB in 74% on a milligram scale (Baisch et al., 1998). In contrast, an OPME synthesis with four *Bifidobacteria*-derived enzymes (SP, GalPUT, UDPGalE, and GLNBP), and sucrose and GlcNAc as substrates yielded 190 g/L of LNB when conducted at 10-L scale, 83% based on consumed GlcNAc. Yeast treatment was used to remove the fructose and unreacted sucrose, and LNB was crystallized from the reaction mixture to give 1.8 kg of LNB in 95% purity. A second recrystallization of LNB yielded 1.4 kg of crystalline LNB (99.6% purity) (Nishimoto et al., 2007). This method can be used in the production of GNB by substituting GlcNAc for GalNAc (Kitaoka, 2012).

GH-based routes to LNB and GNB include the synthesis of LNB using *Xanthomonas manihotis*–derived β-galactosidase to mediate glycosylation of GlcNAc with pNP Gal as donor in a 52% yield with respect to the donor on 70-mg scale (Fig. 9.12; Vetere et al., 2000). *Trans*-Glycosylation using lactose as a donor with β-galactosidase from bovine testes gave LNB in 21% yield based on GlcNAc acceptor (Hedbys et al., 1989). GS enzymes prepared from *Thermus thermophilus* β-glycosidase catalyzed formation of LNB derivatives using Gal-F as a donor and GlcNAc-SPh as acceptor, with LNB being obtained in 80% yield following cleavage of the thiophenyl group (D'Almeida et al., 2009).

2.8.3 Lacto-N-triose (LNT-2, GlcNAcβ1-3Galβ1-4Glc) and Lacto-N-neotetraose (LNnT, Galβ1-4GlcNAcβ1-3Galβ1-4Glc)

Neose Technologies achieved the synthesis of LNT-2 on a 250-g scale by combining lactose, UDP-GlcNAc, and recombinantly expressed *N. meningitides lgtA* (β3GlcNAcT) in a 100-L reactor at 25°C for 16h. The yield was 85% based on the UDP-GlcNAc substrate (Johnson, 1999). Subsequent reaction of LNT-2 with UDP-Gal and recombinantly expressed *N. meningitides lgtB* (β4GalT) at 25°C for 16h generated more than 300g of LNnT, in >85% yield based on LNT-2 substrate. Alternative GT- and GH-mediated preparations of LNT-2, LNT, and LNnT by consecutive additions of GlcNAc and Gal residues to lactose have been reported. Thus, bovine serum–derived β3GlcNAcT catalyzed the reaction of UDP-GlcNAc with lactose to provide LNT-2 in 26% yield, and this was subsequently converted to LNT (20%) or LNnT (19%) using β-galactosidase from *Bacillus circulans* ATCC31382 to introduce Gal to the 3-position or *B. circulans* β-galactosidase (Biolacta) to introduced Gal to the 4-position (Fig. 9.21; Murata et al., 1999a,b).

2.8.4 Globotriose (Gb3, Galα1-4Galβ1-4Glc) and Globotetraose (Gb4, GalNAcβ1-3Galα1-4Galβ1-4Glc)

Globotriose (Gb3) was synthesized from lactose and UDP-Gal in 90% yield on a 2.2-g scale using a truncated *N. meningitidis* α4GalT (lgtC) (Zhang et al., 2002) or in 75% yield on a 5-g scale when using a truncated *N. gonorrhoeae* lgtC (Johnson, 1999). Globotetraose (Gb4) (1.5g) was subsequently synthesized from Gb3 in 60% yield using UDP-GlcNAc and *N. gonorrhoeae* lgtD.

2.8.5 2′-Fucosyllactose (2′-FL, Fucα1-3Galβ1-4Glc)

2′-FL (18mg, 65% yield) was synthesized from lactose using recombinant *H. pylori* FucT2 and GDP-Fuc, but the requirement to purify the GDP-Fuc made using sequential Gmd-WcaG–mediated enzyme reactions complicated this approach (Albermann et al., 2001). More recently, the OPME synthesis of 2′-FL was demonstrated using the bifunctional Fkp from *Bacteroides fragilis* in conjunction with the α1,2-FucT from *E. coli* O126, WbgL (Fig. 9.22; Engels et al., 2014). In this approach, fucose was converted quantitatively to Fuc-1-P and then to GDP-Fuc by Fkp, consuming 1 equivalent each of ATP and GTP. Alkaline phosphatase was used to cleave the

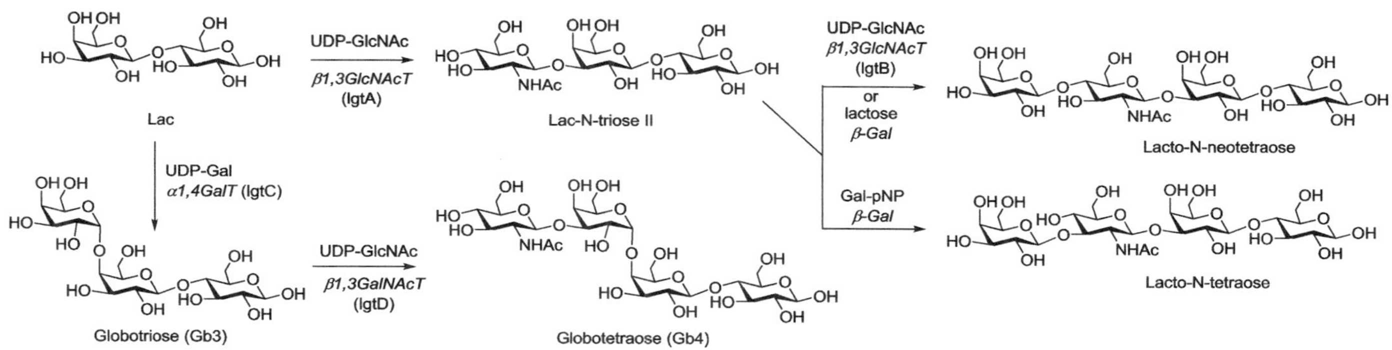

FIGURE 9.21

Galactosyltransferase- and galactosidase-mediated preparation of LNT-II, LNT, LNnT, Gb3, and Gb4.

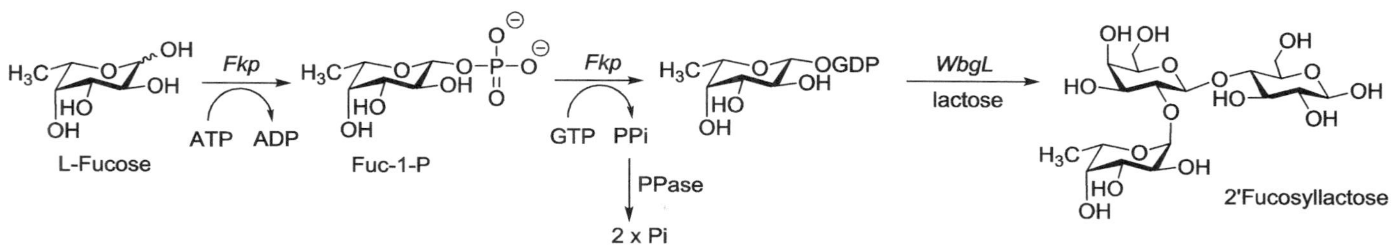

FIGURE 9.22

One-pot multienzyme preparation of 2′-FL.

nucleotide by-products and drive the equilibrium to GDP-Fuc. In the presence of added lactose, WbgL generated 2′-FL in near quantitative yield. The integration of an in situ GDP-Fuc recycling system has been demonstrated in the synthesis of Globo H and SSEA4 (Tsai et al., 2013).

2.8.6 *Sialyllactose and Sialyloligosaccharides*

Enzymatic synthesis of 3′-SL and/or 6′-SL from lactose has been demonstrated with STs including Pd2,6ST (Yamamoto et al., 1998), PmST1 (Guo et al., 2015), NmST (Priem et al., 2002), and PST6-224 (Drouillard et al., 2010) and with mutant ST enzymes generated from Pd2,6ST and PmST1 with the objective of changing the inherent regioselectivity (Choi et al., 2014; Guo et al., 2015).

An OPME sialylation system containing PmST1, NmCSS, and *E. coli* NAL in the presence of lactose, mannose, CTP, and pyruvate generated 3′-SL in 79% on a 100- to 200-mg scale enabling the synthesis of 3′-SL mimics as part of a sialoside library (Yu et al., 2005). Sialyl T-antigens and derivatives, such as 3′-sialyl-LNB and 3′-sialyl-GNB, have been prepared via sequential reactions that use the enzymes GalK and GLNBP to phosphorylate and then couple Gal donors to GlcNAc or GalNAc moieties in acceptors. The resulting β1,3-linked galactosides underwent α2,3-sialylation mediated by PmST1 to yield α2,3-sialyl-galactosides in greater than 85% yield on a preparative scale (Lau et al., 2011; Li et al., 2015). The *T. cruzi trans*-sialidase–mediated *trans*-glycosylation has recently been demonstrated to be a cost-effective method to produce sialyllactose in gram quantities from low-cost dairy-sourced substrates (Zeuner et al., 2014). A yield of 1.54 g/L of 3′-SL was attained using *T. cruzi* sialidase under optimized conditions with cGMP as a donor, equivalent to 64% of theoretical conversion yield (Holck et al., 2014).

2.9 PERSPECTIVE

The use of enzymes for the synthesis of HMOs has a particular benefit in comparison to chemical synthesis as the inherent donor and acceptor preferences of the enzymes circumvent the requirements for multistep protecting group strategies, while the anomeric specificity of the glycosidic bond formation eliminates the need to physically separate anomeric mixtures. The development of OPME reactions systems has further shortened enzymatic syntheses. But challenges remain, especially for the large-scale production of HMOs in relation to technical issues such as enzyme expression, stability, activity, and inhibition. Economic considerations incentivize the development of reactor-format compatible enzymes and development of effective in situ regeneration systems for donors, cofactors, and nucleotides to translate nucleotide use from a stoichiometric to a catalytic basis. The continued development of improved chemoenzymatic pathways to achieve scalable synthesis of HMOs promises access to related glycoprotein materials, including glycoproteins, glycolipids, and glycoconjugates, with diverse application in the fields of human nutrition, diagnostics, and therapeutics.

3. BIOTECHNOLOGICAL PRODUCTION OF HUMAN MILK OLIGOSACCHARIDES

One of the main problems for the synthesis of HMOs is the sourcing of the building blocks. Glucose and galactose are common building blocks; however, *N*-acetylglucosamine, L-fucose, and *N*-acetylneuramic acid are more difficult to come by, especially from sources compatible with end applications such as infant nutrition. A second hurdle to overcome is the specific assembly of these monosaccharides into an oligosaccharide. Specific enzymes such as glycosyltransferases are needed to enable such synthesis, but these enzymes require nucleotide sugars that are even more rare and expensive than the monosaccharides. In order to solve these issues, some strategies have been developed over the years (Fig. 9.23).

One of the first strategies was to produce the needed nucleotide sugars first via in vivo synthesis and then assemble HMOs via biocatalysis. The solution proposed by Prieto and coworkers is to have yeasts such as *Candida famata* synthetize nucleotide

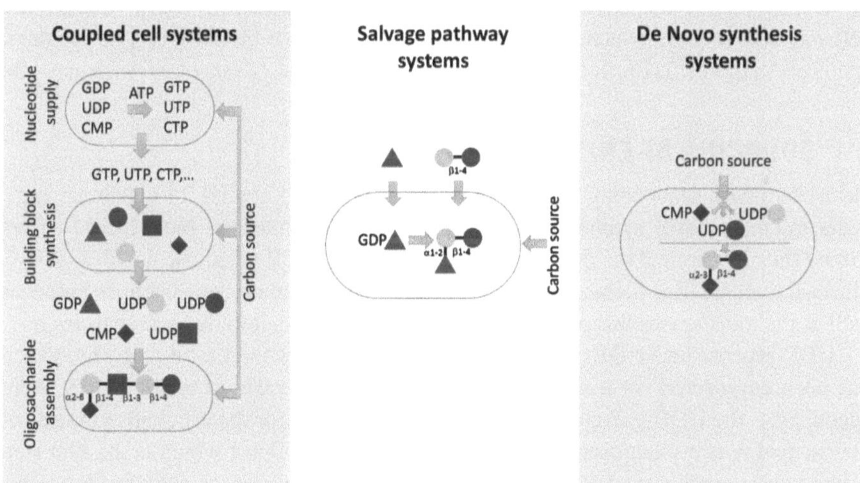

FIGURE 9.23

Biotechnological strategies for HMO synthesis (*blue circle*: glucose, *blue square*: *N*-acetylglucosamine, *purple diamond*: *N*-acetylneuraminic acid, *red triangle*: L-fucose, *yellow circle*: galactose). The coupled cell systems are based on combinations of bacterial and yeast hosts providing nucleotides and building blocks to an assembly host that expresses the transferases required to assemble the HMO. In the salvage pathway system, specific building blocks such as *N*-acetylglucosamine, *N*-acetylneuraminic acid, or L-fucose are fed to the microorganism, which converts these building blocks into their activated form via a salvage pathway and heterologous transferase then forms the final HMO. Finally, in the single cell system, all building blocks are synthesized by the production host itself, which converts these building blocks into HMO.

sugars (Prieto et al., 1999). These yeasts were combined with recombinant *E. coli* that express specific transferases that catalyze the synthesis of HMOs. The methodology resulted in the first amounts of HMOs, for instance LNT-2 (30 g/L), LNnT (13 g/L), and LNF-III (4 g/l), obtained via recombinant microorganisms.

This concept was further expanded by combining multiple (recombinant) microorganisms, mainly *E. coli* and *Corynebactrium* sp., in cell coupling reactions. DeFrees and Koizumi successfully synthesized a whole range of HMOs in this manner (DeFrees et al., 2001; Endo et al., 2000a,b) and were the first to synthetize recombinant 3′-sialyllactose (4 and 33 g/L respectively).

The logical next step was to combine the enzymes and pathways used for the aforementioned microbial host into a single production host. With the dawn of metabolic engineering and synthetic biology, the cloning and optimization of multiple biosynthesis pathway enzymes have become increasingly easy, allowing relative fast development of single-cell production organisms. It was Samain and coworkers who described the first single production host systems for the synthesis of 3′-sialyllactose and 2′-fucosyllactose (Fierfort et al., 2008; Drouillard et al., 2006). In some processes, the precursors such as *N*-acetylneuraminic acid were added to the medium, to be converted into HMOs (via so-called salvage pathways); in other systems, the cell was engineered in such a way that it supplied its own building blocks (de novo synthesis pathways) (Fierfort et al., 2008; Drouillard et al., 2006).

3.1 SOURCING OF ENZYMES AND PATHWAYS

Next-generation sequencing and metagenomics have been crucial for metabolic engineers to create novel synthetic pathways. Knowledge about the biochemical routes toward the biochemical building blocks, UDP-glucose, UDP-galactose, UDP-*N*-acetylglucosamine, GDP-L-fucose, and CMP-*N*-acetylneuraminate, has been essential as well as the transferases that assemble these building blocks into oligosaccharides.

UDP-glucose and UDP-galactose are intermediates of the Leloir pathway, which has been engineered for a wide variety of purposes (De Bruyn et al., 2015). More specifically, the UDP-galactose pool has been optimized for the efficient synthesis of lactose and *N*-acetyllactosamine in *E. coli* (Mao et al., 2006), which is the first step in the whole synthesis of HMOs. To this end, the expression of galactosyltransferase *lgtB* originating from *N. meningitides* (Wkarchuk et al., 1998) was optimized in concert with the endogenous phosphoglucomutase gene and the UDP-glucose pyrophosphorylase gene (Mao et al., 2006).

Building further on lactose, lacto-*N*-triose II is synthetized by introducing the *lgtA* gene from *Neisseria*, which transfers *N*-acetylglucosamine on lactose (Priem et al., 2002). Efficient synthesis requires, as stated by Priem et al., an optimized UDP-*N*-acetylglucosamine pool, which was achieved by pathway engineering (Jin et al., 2016; Rodriguez-Diaz et al., 2012a,b).

As mentioned, the lactose and lacto-*N(n)*-tetraose backbone are mainly functionalized with L-fucose and *N* acetylneuraminic acid (sialic acid). To incorporate these two building blocks into HMOs, both the salvage pathway and the de novo synthesis pathway have been used efficiently. In both cases, multiple competing reactions had to be knocked out and heterologous genes had to be introduced into the production hosts (Fierfort et al., 2008; Priem et al., 2002; Baumgartner et al., 2014). To enable the conversion of L-fucose into GDP-fucose, the introduction of fucokinase and guanidyltransferase activities is required. This activity used to be only known in higher eukaryotic cells, but these have recently been found in human symbiotic bacteria (Coyne et al., 2005). The alternative de novo L-fucose pathway is well known in bacteria, namely as part of biosynthesis of capsular polysaccharide pathways (Stevenseon et al., 1996) of which *N*-acetylneuraminic acid biosynthesis pathway also is part in some microorganisms (Vimr et al., 2004). Both have been applied for the synthesis of sialyllactoses and fucosyllactoses (Drouillard et al., 2006; Priem et al., 2002).

To assemble the different building blocks into specific oligosaccharides, several transferases are required. These transferases could be sourced from mammalia; however, difficult expression in microbial hosts hampers the efficiency of the production hosts. Alternatively, many capsular polysaccharide form microorganisms; in many cases pathogenic organisms, such as *Neisseria*, *Campylobacter*, etc. (Weijers et al., 2008), have the necessary glycosyltransferases that can be easily expressed into an HMO production host. It is probably not coincidental that the pathogens toward which HMOs are active form an excellent source for enzymes and pathways.

4. CONCLUSION

Technological advances in oligosaccharide production, isolation and purification have provided an exciting opportunity to study the many potential benefits of HMOs. HMO mixtures and individual HMOs have become available in unprecedented quantities that allow us to assess their metabolic fate, efficacy, and structure–function relationships using the entire spectrum from in vitro and in vivo models to human intervention studies.

This chapter outlines several different approaches to synthesize or isolate HMOs; each one of them comes with a set of advantages and challenges. Chemical and chemoenzymatic synthesis can create structurally defined HMOs and HMO libraries to facilitate initial research studies for target identification. Bioengineered microorganisms have the advantage of ostensibly ceilingless scale-up opportunities. A better understanding of how HMOs are produced in the human mammary gland would both guide chemoenzymatic synthesis and educate the bioengineering process.

With the improvement in technologies for synthesizing or isolating the oligosaccharide structures in human milk comes the exciting possibility of improving infant formulas by providing a composition closer to human milk, creating personalized supplementation for human milk, and potentially using these compounds as ingredients in dietary supplements for use in adult populations.

Therefore, it will become increasingly important to determine both the efficacy and safety of HMOs.

As we move to confirming the many benefits and safety of HMOs in human populations as well as the production of commercial supplies of HMOs, it will be important to be specific about which structures (or groups of structures) are responsible for which benefits and to avoid the trap of attributing all of the observed benefits of HMOs to a single structure. The advancement of technologies for the identification, purification, and scaled-up production of HMOs promises to bring a "bench-to-beside" translation of the many potential benefits of HMOs.

REFERENCES

Ajisaka, K., Fujimoto, H., Miyasato, M., 1998. An α-l-fucosidase from Penicillium multicolor as a candidate enzyme for the synthesis of α (1→3)-linked fucosyl oligosaccharides by transglycosylation. Carbohydrate Research 309 (1), 125–129.

Albermann, C., Distler, J., Piepersberg, W., 2000. Preparative synthesis of GDP-beta-L-fucose by recombinant enzymes fronterobacterial sources. Glycobiology 10 (9), 875–881.

Albermann, C., Piepersberg, W., Wehmeier, U.F., 2001. Synthesis of the milk oligosaccharide 2′-fucosyllactose using recombinant bacterial enzymes. Carbohydrate Research 334 (2), 97–103.

Aly, M.R.E., Ibrahim, E.-S.I., Ashry, E.-S.H., Schmidt, R.R., 1999. Synthesis of lacto-N-neotetraose and lacto-N-tetraose using the dimethylmaleoyl group as amino protective group. Carbohydrate Research 316, 121–132.

Baisch, G., Ohrlein, R., Streiff, M., Kolbinger, F., 1998. On the preparative use of recombinant beta(1→3)galactosyl-transferase. Bioorganic & Medicinal Chemistry Letters 8 (7), 751–754.

Baumgartner, F., Seitz, L., Sprenger, G., Albermann, C., 2014. Construction of *Escherichia coli* strains with chromosomally integrated expression cassettes for the synthesis of 2′-fucosyllactose. Microbial Cell Factories 12, 40.

Blank, D., Dotz, V., Geyer, R., Kunz, C., 2012. Human milk oligosaccharides and Lewis blood group: individual high-throughput sample profiling to enhance conclusions from functional studies. Advances in Nutrition 3, 440S–449S.

Blixt, O., van Die, I., Norberg, T., van den Eijnden, D.H., 1999. High-level expression of the Neisseria meningitidis lgtA gene in *Escherichia coli* and characterization of the encoded N-acetylglucosaminyltransferase as a useful catalyst in the synthesis of GlcNAc beta 1→3Gal and GalNAc beta 1-->3Gal linkages. Glycobiology 9 (10), 1061–1071.

Bode, L., 2009. Human milk oligosaccharides: prebiotics and beyond. Nutrition Reviews 67 (Suppl. 2), S183–S191.

Bode, L., Kuhn, L., Kim, H.-Y., Hsiao, L., Nissan, C., Sinkala, M., Kankasa, C., Mwiya, M., Thea, D.M., Aldrovandi, G.M., 2012. Human milk oligosaccharide concentration and risk of postnatal transmission of HIV through breastfeeding. American Journal of Clinical Nutrition 96, 831–839.

Bode, L., Muhly-Reinholz, M., Pohlentz, G., Seeger, W., Kunz, C., Rudloff, S., 2004. Human milk oligosaccharides as inhibitors of monocyte and lymphocyte adhesion to endothelial cells. Thrombosis and Haemostasis 92, 1402–1410.

Bode, L., Rudloff, S., Kunz, C., Strobel, S., Klein, N., 2004. Human milk oligosaccharides reduce platelet-neutrophil complex-formation leading to a decrease in neutrophil beta 2 integrin expression. Journal of Leukocyte Biology 76, 820–826.

Boehm, G., Stahl, B., 2003. Oligosaccharides. In: Mattila-Sandholm, T., Saarela, M. (Eds.), Functional Dairy Products. CRC Press LLC, Boca Raton, FL, pp. 203–243.

Brockhausen, I., 2014. Crossroads between bacterial and mammalian glycosyltransferases. Frontiers in Immunology 5, 492.

Chaturvedi, P., Warren, C.D., Buescher, C.R., Pickering, L.K., Newburg, D.S., 2001. Bioactive components of human milk. Advances in Experimental Medicine and Biology 501, 315–323.

Chen, X., Fang, J., Zhang, J., Liu, Z., Shao, J., Kowal, P., Andreana, P., Wang, P.G., 2001. Sugar nucleotide regeneration beads (Superbeads): a versatile tool for the practical synthesis of oligosaccharides. Journal of the American Chemical Society 123 (9), 2081–2082.

Chen, X., Liu, Z., Wang, J., Fang, J., Fan, H., Wang, P.G., 2000. Changing the donor cofactor of bovine alpha 1, 3-galactosyltransferase by fusion with UDP-galactose 4-epimerase. More efficient biocatalysis for synthesis of alpha-Gal epitopes. Journal of Biological Chemistry 275 (41), 31594–31600.

Chin, Y.W., Kim, J.Y., Lee, W.H., Seo, J.H., 2015. Enhanced production of 2′-fucosyllactose in engineered *Escherichia coli* BL21star(DE3) by modulation of lactose metabolism and fucosyltransferase. Journal of Biotechnology 210, 107–115.

Choi, Y.H., Kim, J.H., Park, J.H., Lee, N., Kim, D.H., Jang, K.S., Park, I.H., Kim, B.G., 2014. Protein engineering of alpha2,3/2,6-sialyltransferase to improve the yield and productivity of in vitro sialyllactose synthesis. Glycobiology 24 (2), 159–169.

Christ, W.J., Rossignol, D.P., Kobayashi, S., Kawata, T., 1996. Substituted Liposaccharides Useful in the Treatment and Prevention of Endotoxemia PCT/US96/09578.

Chu, K.C., Ren, C.-T., Lu, C.-P., Hsu, C.-H., Sun, T.-H., Han, J.-L., Pal, B., Chao, T.-A., Lin, Y.-F., Wu, S.-H., Wong, C.-H., Wu, C.-Y., 2011. Efficient and stereoselective synthesis of α(2→9) oligosialic acids: from monomers to dodecamers. Angewandte Chemie International Edition 50, 9391–9395.

Coyne, M.J., Reinap, B., Lee, M.M., Comstock, L.E., 2005. Human symbionts use a host-like pathway for surface fucosylation. 80 Science 307 (5716), 1778–1781.

Crich, D., Li, W., 2007. O-sialylation with N-acetyl-5-N,4-O-carbonyl-protected thiosialoside donors in dichloromethane: facile and selective cleavage of the oxazolidinone ring. Journal of Organic Chemistry 72, 2387.

Crich, D., Li, W., 2007. α-Selective sialylations at −78°C in nitrile solvents with a 1-Adamantanyl thiosialoside. Journal of Organic Chemistry 72, 7794.

D'Almeida, A., Ionata, M., Tran, V., Tellier, C., Dion, M., Rabiller, C., 2009. An expeditious and efficient synthesis of β-d-galactopyranosyl-(1→3)-d-N-acetylglucosamine (lacto-N-biose) using a glycosynthase from *Thermus thermophilus* as a catalyst. Tetrahedron-Asymmetry 20 (11), 1243–1246.

De Bruyn, F., Maertens, J., Beauprez, J., Soetaert, W., De Mey, M., 2015. Biotechnological advances in UDP-sugar based glycosylation of small molecules. Biotechnology Advances 33, 288–302.

DeFrees, S., Johnson, K., 2001. Low Cost Manufacture of Oligosaccharides US Pat. App. 09/757289.

Drouillard, S., Driguez, H., Samain, E., 2006. Large-scale synthesis of H-antigen oligosaccharides by expressing *Helicobacter pylori* alpha1,2-fucosyltransferase in metabolically engineered *Escherichia coli* cells. Angewandte Chemie International Edition England 45, 1778–1780.

Drouillard, S., Mine, T., Kajiwara, H., Yamamoto, T., Samain, E., 2010. Efficient synthesis of 6′-sialyllactose, 6,6′-disialyllactose, and 6′-KDO-lactose by metabolically engineered *E. coli* expressing a multifunctional sialyltransferase from the Photobacterium sp. JT-ISH-224. Carbohydrate Research 345 (10), 1394–1399.

Ellervik, U., Magnusson, G., 1998. A high yielding chemical synthesis of sialyl Lewis x tetrasaccharide and Lewis x trisaccharide; examples of regio- and stereodifferentiated glycosylations. Journal of Organic Chemistry 63, 9314–9322.

Endo, T., Koizumi, S., Tabata, K., Ozaki, A., 2000. Large-scale production of CMP-NeuAc and sialylated oligosaccharides through bacterial coupling. Applied Microbiology and Biotechnology 53, 257–261.

Endo, T., Koizumi, S., Tabata, K., Ozaki, A., 2000. Cloning and expression of β1,4-galactosyltransferase gene from *Helicobacter pylori*. Glycobiology 10 (8), 809–813.

Engels, L., Elling, L., 2014. WbgL: a novel bacterial alpha1,2-fucosyltransferase for the synthesis of 2′-fucosyllactose. Glycobiology 24 (2), 170–178.

Etzioni, A., 1996. Adhesion molecules-their role in health and disease. Pediatric Research 39, 191–198.

Fang, J., Li, J., Chen, X., Zhang, Y., Wang, J., Guo, Z., Zhang, W., Yu, L., Brew, K., Wang, P.G., 1998. Highly efficient chemoenzymatic synthesis of α-galactosyl epitopes with a recombinant α(1→3)-galactosyltransferase. Journal of the American Chemical Society 120 (27), 6635–6638.

Fierfort, N., Samain, E., 2008. Genetic engineering of *Escherichia coli* for the economical production of sialylated oligosaccharides. Journal of Biotechnology 134, 261–265.

Flowers, H.M., 1981. Chemistry and Biochemistry of d- and l-Fucose. Advances in Carbohydrate Chemistry and Biochemistry 39, 279.

Gilbert, M., Watson, D.C., Cunningham, A.M., Jennings, M.P., Young, N.M., Wakarchuk, W.W., 1996. Cloning of the lipooligosaccharide alpha-2,3-sialyltransferase from the bacterial pathogens *Neisseria meningitidis* and *Neisseria gonorrhoeae*. Journal of Biological Chemistry 271 (45), 28271–28276.

Gilbert, M., Bayer, R., Cunningham, A.M., DeFrees, S., Gao, Y., Watson, D.C., Young, N.M., Wakarchuk, W.W., 1998. The synthesis of sialylated oligosaccharides using a CMP-Neu5Ac synthetase/sialyltransferase fusion. Nature Biotechnology 16 (8), 769–772.

Guo, Y., Jers, C., Meyer, A.S., Li, H., Kirpekar, F., Mikkelsen, J.D., 2015. Modulating the regioselectivity of a *Pasteurella multocida* sialyltransferase for biocatalytic production of 3′- and 6′-sialyllactose. Enzyme and Microbial Technology 78, 54–62.

Hedbys, L., Johansson, E., Mosbach, K., Larsson, P.O., 1989. Synthesis of 2-acetamido-2-deoxy-3-O-beta-D-galactopyranosyl-D-galacto se by the sequential use of beta-D-galactosidases from bovine testes and *Escherichia coli*. Carbohydrate Research 186 (2), 217–223.

Heimburg-Molinaro, J., Lum, M., Vijay, G., Jain, M., Almogren, A., Rittenhouse-Olson, K., 2011. Cancer vaccines and carbohydrate epitopes. Vaccine 29, 8802–8826.

Hokke, C.H., Zervosen, A., Elling, L., Joziasse, D.H., van den Eijnden, D.H., 1996. One-pot enzymatic synthesis of the Gal alpha 1→3Gal beta 1→4GlcNAc sequence with in situ UDP-Gal regeneration. Glycoconjugate Journal 13 (4), 687–692.

Holck, J., Larsen, D.M., Michalak, M., Li, H., Kjaerulff, L., Kirpekar, F., Gotfredsen, C.H., Forssten, S., Ouwehand, A.C., Mikkelsen, J.D., Meyer, A.S., 2014. Enzyme catalysed production of sialylated human milk oligosaccharides and galactooligosaccharides by *Trypanosoma cruzi* trans-sialidase. New Biotechnology 31 (2), 156–165.

Ichikawa, Y., Lin, Y.C., Dumas, D.P., Shen, G.J., Garcia-Junceda, E., Williams, M.A., Bayer, R., Ketcham, C., Walker, L.E., 1992. Chemical-enzymic synthesis and conformational analysis of sialyl Lewis X and derivatives. Journal of the American Chemical Society 114 (24), 9283–9298.

Jantscher-Krenn, E., Zherebtsov, M., Nissan, C., Goth, K., Guner, Y.S., Naidu, N., Choudhury, B.P., Grishin, A.V., Ford, H.R., Bode, L., 2011. The human milk oligosaccharide disialyllacto-N-tetraose prevents necrotizing enterocolitis in neonatal rats. Gut 61, 1417–1425.

Jiang, X., Huang, P., Zhong, W., Tan, M., Farkas, T., Morrow, A.L., Newburg, D.S., Ruiz-Palacios, G.M., Pickering, L.K., 2004. Human milk contains elements that block binding of noroviruses to human Histo—Blood group antigens in saliva. Journal of Infectious Diseases 190, 1850–1859.

Jin, P., Kang, Z., Yuan, P., Du, G., Chen, J., 2016. Production of specific-molecular-weight hyaluronan by metabolically engineered *Bacillus subtilis* 168. Metabolic Engineering 35, 21–30.

Johnson, K.F., 1999. Synthesis of oligosaccharides by bacterial enzymes. Glycoconjugate Journal 16 (2), 141–146.

Kawashima, H., 2006. Roles of sulfated glycans in lymphocyte homing. Biological and Pharmaceutical Bulletin 29, 2343–2349.

Kinoshita, H., Wakahara, N., Watanabe, M., Kawasaki, T., Matsuo, H., Kawai, Y., Kitazawa, H., Ohnuma, S., Miura, K., Horii, A., Saito, T., 2008. Cell surface glyceraldehyde-3-phosphate dehydrogenase (GAPDH) of *Lactobacillus plantarum* LA 318 recognizes human A and B blood group antigens. Research in Microbiology 159, 685–691.

Kitaoka, M., 2012. Bifidobacterial enzymes involved in the metabolism of human milk oligosaccharides. Advances in Nutrition 3 (3), 422S–429S.

Kobata, A., Ginsburg, V., Tsuda, M., 1969. Oligosaccharides of human milk: I. Isolation and characterization. Archives in Biochemistry and Biophysics 130, 509–513.

Kolkman, M.A., Wakarchuk, W., Nuijten, P.J., van der Zeijst, B.A., 1997. Capsular polysaccharide synthesis in *Streptococcus pneumoniae* serotype 14: molecular analysis of the complete cps locus and identification of genes encoding glycosyltransferases required for the biosynthesis of the tetrasaccharide subunit. Molecular Microbiology 26 (1), 197–208.

Koyama, Y., Hidaka, M., Nishimoto, M., Kitaoka, M., 2013. Directed evolution to enhance thermostability of galacto-N-biose/lacto-N-biose I phosphorylase. PEDS 26 (11), 755–761.

Lairson, L.L., Henrissat, B., Davies, G.J., Withers, S.G., 2008. Glycosyltransferases: structures, functions, and mechanisms. Annual Review of Biochemistry 77, 521–555.

Lau, K., Yu, H., Thon, V., Khedri, Z., Leon, M.E., Tran, B.K., Chen, X., 2011. Sequential two-step multienzyme synthesis of tumor-associated sialyl T-antigens and derivatives. Organic & Biomolecular Chemistry 9 (8), 2784–2789.

Lee, Y.C., Chien, H.C., Hsu, W.H., 2007. Production of N-acetyl-D-neuraminic acid by recombinant whole cells expressing Anabaena sp. CH1 N-acetyl-D-glucosamine 2-epimerase and *Escherichia coli* N-acetyl-D-neuraminic acid lyase. Journal of Biotechnology 129 (3), 453–460.

Lemieux, R.U., Hendriks, K.B., Stick, R.V., James, K., 1975. Halide ion catalyzed glycosidation reactions. Syntheses of.alpha.-linked disaccharides. Journal of the American Chemical Society 97, 4056–4062.

Li, L., Liu, Y., Li, T., Wang, W., Yu, Z., Ma, C., Qu, J., Zhao, W., Chen, X., Wang, P.G., 2015. Efficient chemoenzymatic synthesis of novel galacto-N-biose derivatives and their sialylated forms. Chemical Communications (Cambridge) 51 (51), 10310–10313.

Liu, X.W., Xia, C., Li, L., Guan, W.Y., Pettit, N., Zhang, H.C., Chen, M., Wang, P.G., 2009. Characterization and synthetic application of a novel beta1,3-galactosyltransferase from *Escherichia coli* O55:H7. Bioorganic & Medicinal Chemistry 17 (14), 4910–4915.

Lubineau, A., Le Gallic, J., Lemoine, R., 1994. First synthesis of the 3′ - sulfated Lewis^{a} pentasaccharide, the most potent human E-selectin ligand so far. Bioorganic and Medicinal Chemistry 2, 1143–1151.

Ma, B., Simala-Grant, J.L., Taylor, D.E., 2006. Fucosylation in prokaryotes and eukaryotes. Glycobiology 16 (12), 158R–184R.

Malekan, H., Fung, G., Thon, V., Khedri, Z., Yu, H., Qu, J., Li, Y., Ding, L., Lam, K.S., Chen, X., 2013. One-pot multi-enzyme (OPME) chemoenzymatic synthesis of sialyl-Tn-MUC1 and sialyl-T-MUC1 glycopeptides containing natural or non-natural sialic acid. Bioorganic & Medicinal Chemistry 21 (16), 4778–4785.

Manthey, C.F., Autran, C.A., Eckmann, L., Bode, L., 2014. Human Milk Oligosaccharides protect against enteropathogenic *E.coli* attachment *in vitro* and colonization in suckling mice. Journal of Pediatric Gastroenterology and Nutrition 58, 167–170.

Mao, Z., Shin, H.-D., Chen, R.R., 2006. Engineering the *E. coli* UDP-glucose synthesis pathway for oligosaccharide synthesis. Biotechnology Progress 22, 369–374.

Martin, S.L., Edbrooke, M.R., Hodgman, T.C., van den Eijnden, D.H., Bird, M.I., 1997. Lewis X biosynthesis in *Helicobacter pylori*. Molecular cloning of an alpha(1,3)-fucosyltransferase gene. Journal of Biological Chemistry 272 (34), 21349–21356.

Michalak, M., Larsen, D.M., Jers, C., Almeida, J.R.M., Willer, M., Li, H., Kirpekar, F., Kjærulff, L., Gotfredsen, C.H., Nordvang, R.T., Meyer, A.S., Mikkelsen, J.D., 2014. Biocatalytic production of 3′-sialyllactose by use of a modified sialidase with superior trans-sialidase activity. Process Biochemistry 49 (2), 265–270.

Mizanur, R.M., Pohl, N.L., 2008. Bacterial CMP-sialic acid synthetases: production, properties, and applications. Applied Microbiology and Biotechnology 80 (5), 757–765.

Morrow, A.L., Ruiz-Palacios, G.M., Altaye, M., Jiang, X., Guerrero, M.L., Meinzen-Derr, J.K., Farkas, T., Chaturvedi, P., Pickering, L.K., Newburg, D.S., 2004. Human milk oligosaccharides are associated with protection against diarrhea in breast-fed infants. Journal of Pediatrics 145, 297–303.

Munneke, S., Painter, G.F., Gainsford, G.J., Stocker, B.L., Timmer, M.S.M., 2015. Total synthesis of Lewis^X using a late-stage crystalline intermediate. Carbohydrate Research 414, 1–7.

Murata, T., Morimoto, S., Zeng, X., Watanabe, S., Usui, T., 1999. Enzymatic synthesis of alpha-L-fucosyl-N-acetyllactosamines and 3′-O-alpha-L-fucosyllactose utilizing alpha-L-fucosidases. Carbohydrate Research 320 (3–4), 192–199.

Murata, T., Inukai, T., Suzuki, M., Yamagishi, M., Usui, A.T., 1999. Facile enzymatic conversion of lactose into lacto-N-tetraose and lacto-N-neotetraose. Glycoconjugate Journal 16 (3), 189–195.

Muthana, M.M., Qu, J., Li, Y., Zhang, L., Yu, H., Ding, L., Malekan, H., Chen, X., 2012. Efficient one-pot multienzyme synthesis of UDP-sugars using a promiscuous UDP-sugar pyrophosphorylase from *Bifidobacterium longum* (BLUSP). Chemical Communications (Cambridge) 48 (21), 2728–2730.

Nakai, H., Kitaoka, M., Svensson, B., Ohtsubo, K., 2013. Recent development of phosphorylases possessing large potential for oligosaccharide synthesis. Current Opinion in Chemical Biology 17 (2), 301–309.

Nath, A., Mondal, S., Chakraborty, S., Bhattacharjee, C., Chowdhury, R., 2014. Production, purification, characterization, immobilization, and application of β-galactosidase: a review. Asia-Pacific Journal of Chemical Engineering 9 (3), 330–348.

Newburg, D.S., Ruiz-Palacios, G.M., Morrow, A.L., 2005. Human milk glycans protect infants against enteric pathogens. Annual Review of Nutrition 25, 37–58.

Nishimoto, M., Kitaoka, M., 2007. Practical preparation of lacto-N-biose I, a candidate for the bifidus factor in human milk. Bioscience, Biotechnology, and Biochemistry 71 (8), 2101–2104.

Nishimoto, M., Kitaoka, M., 2009. One-pot enzymatic production of beta-D-galactopyranosyl-(1-->3)-2-acetamido-2-deoxy-D-galactose (galacto-N-biose) from sucrose and 2-acetamido-2-deoxy-D-galactose (N-acetylgalactosamine). Carbohydrate Research 344 (18), 2573–2576.

Nobre, C., Teixeira, J.A., Rodrigues, L.R., 2015. New trends and technological challenges in the industrial production and purification of fructo-oligosaccharides. Critical Reviews in Food Science and Nutrition 55 (10), 1444–1455.

Noguchi, T., Shiba, T., 1998. Use of *Escherichia coli* polyphosphate kinase for oligosaccharide synthesis. Bioscience, Biotechnology, and Biochemistry 62 (8), 1594–1596.

Priem, B., Gilbert, M., Wakarchuk, W., Heyraud, A., Samain, E., 2002. A new fermentation process allows large-scale production of human milk oligosaccharides by metabolically engineered bacteria. Glycobiology 12 (4), 235–240.

Prieto, P., Kleman-Leyer, K., 1999. Process for Synthesizing Oligosaccharides US Pat. 5945314.

Ragupathi, G., Damani, P., Srivastava, G., Srivastava, O., Sucheck, S.J., Ichikawa, Y., Livingston, P.O., 2009. Synthesis of sialyl Lewis^a (sLe^a, CA19-9) and construction of an immunogenic sLe^a vaccine. Cancer Immunology. Immunotherapy 58, 1397–1405.

Ravindranath, M.H., Amiri, A.A., Bauer, P.M., Kelley, M.C., Essner, R., Morton, D.L., 1997. Endothelial-selectin ligands sialyl Lewis^x and sialyl Lewis^a are differentiation antigens immunogenic in human melanoma. Cancer 79, 1686–1697.

Rencurosi, A., Poletti, L., Guerrini, M., Russo, G., Lay, L., 2002. Human milk oligosaccharides: an enzymatic protection step simplifies the synthesis of 3′- and 6′-O-sialyllactose and their analogues. Carbohydr. Res. 337, 473–483.

Rodriguez-Diaz, J., Carbajo, R.J., Pineda-Lucena, A., Monedero, V., Yebra, M.J., 2013. Synthesis of fucosyl-N-acetylglucosamine disaccharides by transfucosylation using alpha-L-fucosidases from *Lactobacillus casei*. Applied and Environmental Microbiology 79 (12), 3847–3850.

Rodríguez-Díaz, J., Rubio-del-Campo, A., Yebra, M.J., 2012. Metabolic engineering of *Lactobacillus casei* for production of UDP-N-acetylglucosamine. Biotechnology and Bioengineering 109, 1704–1712.

Rodríguez-Díaz, J., Rubio-del-Campo, A., Yebra, M.J., 2012. Regulatory insights into the production of UDP-N-acetylglucosamine by *Lactobacillus casei*. Bioengineered 3, 339–342.

Roussel, F., Takhi, M., Schmidt, R.R., 2001. Solid-phase synthesis of a branched hexasaccharide using a highly efficient synthetic strategy. Journal of Organic Chemistry 66, 8540–8548.

Sakurama, H., Fushinobu, S., Hidaka, M., Yoshida, E., Honda, Y., Ashida, H., Kitaoka, M., Kumagai, H., Yamamoto, K., Katayama, T., 2012. 1,3–1,4-alpha-L-fucosynthase that specifically introduces Lewis a/x antigens into type-1/2 chains. Journal of Biological Chemistry 287 (20), 16709–16719.

Schmaltz, R.M., Hanson, S.R., Wong, C.H., 2011. Enzymes in the synthesis of glycoconjugates. Chemical Reviews 111 (7), 4259–4307.

Shibatani, S., Fujiyama, K., Nishiguchi, S., Seki, T., Maekawa, Y., 2001. Production and characterization of active soluble human beta1,4-galactosyltransferase in *Escherichia coli* as a useful catalyst in synthesis of the Gal beta1→4 GlcNAc linkage. Journal of Bioscience and Bioengineering 91 (1), 85–87.

Skretas, G., Carroll, S., DeFrees, S., Schwartz, M.F., Johnson, K.F., Georgiou, G., 2009. Expression of active human sialyltransferase ST6GalNAcI in *Escherichia coli*. Microbial Cell Factories 8, 50.

Stein, D.B., Lin, Y.-N., Lin, C.-H., 2008. Characterization of *Helicobacter pylori* α1,2-fucosyltransferase for enzymatic synthesis of tumor-associated antigens. Advanced Synthesis & Catalysis 350 (14–15), 2313–2321.

Stevenson, G., Andrianopoulos, K., Hobbs, M., Reeves, P.R., 1996. Organization of the *Escherichia coli* K-12 gene cluster responsible for production of the extracellular polysaccharide colanic acid. Journal of Bacteriology 178, 4885–4893.

Tsai, T.I., Lee, H.Y., Chang, S.H., Wang, C.H., Tu, Y.C., Lin, Y.C., Hwang, D.R., Wu, C.Y., Wong, C.H., 2013. Effective sugar nucleotide regeneration for the large-scale enzymatic synthesis of Globo H and SSEA4. Journal of the American Chemical Society 135 (39), 14831–14839.

Tumbale, P., Jamaluddin, H., Thiyagarajan, N., Acharya, K.R., Brew, K., 2008. Screening a limited structure-based library identifies UDP-GalNAc-specific mutants of alpha-1,3-galactosyltransferase. Glycobiology 18 (12), 1036–1043.

Urgorskim, M., Laskowska, A., 2002. Sialyl Lewis[a]: a tumor-associated carbohydrate antigen involved in adhesion and metastatic potential of cancer cells. Acta Biochimica Polonica 49, 303–311.

Vasiliu, D., Razi, N., Zhang, Y., Jacobsen, N., Allin, K., Liu, X., Hoffmann, J., Bohorov, O., Blixt, O., 2006. Large-scale chemoenzymatic synthesis of blood group and tumor-associated poly-N-acetyllactosamine antigens. Carbohydrate Research 341 (10), 1447–1457.

Velupillai, P., Harn, D.A., 1994. Oligosaccharide-specific induction of interleukin 10 production by B220+ cells from schistosome-infected mice: a mechanism for regulation of CD4+ T-cell subsets. Proceedings of the National Academy of Sciences USA 91, 18–22.

Vetere, A., Miletich, M., Bosco, M., Paoletti, S., 2000. Regiospecific glycosidase-assisted synthesis of lacto-N-biose I (Galbeta1-3GlcNAc) and 3′-sialyl-lacto-N-biose I (NeuAcalpha2-3Galbeta1-3GlcNAc). Eur. J. Biochem. 267 (4), 942–949.

Vimr, E.R., Kalivoda, K.A., Deszo, E.L., Steenbergen, S.M., 2004. Diversity of microbial sialic acid metabolism. Microbiology and Molecular Biology Reviews 68, 132–153.

Wada, J., Honda, Y., Nagae, M., Kato, R., Wakatsuki, S., Katayama, T., Taniguchi, H., Kumagai, H., Kitaoka, M., Yamamoto, K., 2008. 1,2-alpha-l-Fucosynthase: a glycosynthase derived from an inverting alpha-glycosidase with an unusual reaction mechanism. FEBS Letters 582 (27), 3739–3743.

Wakarchuk, W.W., Cunningham, A., Watson, D.C., Young, N.M., 1998. Role of paired basic residues in the expression of active recombinant galactosyltransferases from the bacterial pathogen *Neisseria meningitidis*. Protein Engineering 11, 295–302.

Wakarchuk, W., Martin, A., Jennings, M.P., Moxon, E.R., Richards, J.C., 1996. Functional relationships of the genetic locus encoding the glycosyltransferase enzymes involved in expression of the lacto-N-neotetraose terminal lipopolysaccharide structure in *Neisseria meningitidis*. Journal of Biological Chemistry 271 (32), 19166–19173.

Wang, G., Boulton, P.G., Chan, N.W., Palcic, M.M., Taylor, D.E., 1999. Novel *Helicobacter pylori* alpha1,2-fucosyltransferase, a key enzyme in the synthesis of Lewis antigens. Microbiology 145 (Pt 11), 3245–3253.

Wang, W., Hu, T., Frantom, P.A., Zheng, T., Gerwe, B., del Amo, D.S., Garret, S., Seidel, R.D., Wu, P., 2009. Chemoenzymatic synthesis of GDP-l-fucose and the Lewis X glycan derivatives. Proceedings of the National Academy of Sciences of the United States of America 106 (38), 16096–16101.

Weijers, C.A., Franssen, M.C.R., Visser, G.M., 2008. Glycosyltransferase-catalyzed synthesis of bioactive oligosaccharides. Biotechnology Advances 26, 436–456.

Weinstein, J., Lee, E.U., McEntee, K., Lai, P.H., Paulson, J.C., 1987. Primary structure of beta-galactoside alpha 2,6-sialyltransferase. Conversion of membrane-bound enzyme to soluble forms by cleavage of the NH2-terminal signal anchor. Journal of Biological Chemistry 262 (36), 17735–17743.

Whitfield, C., Trent, M.S., 2014. Biosynthesis and export of bacterial lipopolysaccharides. Annual Review of Biochemistry 83, 99–128.

Wong, C.H., Wang, R., Ichikawa, Y., 1992. Regeneration of sugar nucleotide for enzymic oligosaccharide synthesis: use of Gal-1-phosphate uridyltransferase in the regeneration of UDP-galactose, UDP-2-deoxygalactose, and UDP-galactosamine. Journal of Organic Chemistry 57 (16), 4343–4344.

Wong, C.H., Haynie, S.L., Whitesides, G.M., 1982. Enzyme-catalyzed synthesis of N-acetyllactosamine with in situ regeneration of uridine 5′-diphosphate glucose and uridine 5′-diphosphate galactose. Journal of Organic Chemistry 47 (27), 5416–5418.

Yamamoto, T., Nagae, H., Kajihara, Y., Terada, I., 1998. Mass production of bacterial alpha 2,6-sialyltransferase and enzymatic syntheses of sialyloligosaccharides. Bioscience, Biotechnology, and Biochemistry 62 (2), 210–214.

Yao, W., Yan, J., Chen, X., Wang, F., Cao, H., 2015. Chemoenzymatic synthesis of lacto-N-tetrasaccharide and sialyl lacto-N-tetrasaccharides. Carbohydrate Research 401, 5–10.

Yu, C.-C., Withers, S.G., 2015. Recent developments in enzymatic synthesis of modified sialic acid derivatives. Advanced Synthesis & Catalysis 357 (8), 1633–1654.

Yu, H., Chokhawala, H., Karpel, R., Yu, H., Wu, B., Zhang, J., Zhang, Y., Jia, Q., Chen, X., 2005. A multifunctional *Pasteurella multocida* sialyltransferase: a powerful tool for the synthesis of sialoside libraries. Journal of the American Chemical Society 127 (50), 17618–17619.

Yu, H., Thon, V., Lau, K., Cai, L., Chen, Y., Mu, S., Li, Y., Wang, P.G., Chen, X., 2010. Highly efficient chemoenzymatic synthesis of beta1-3-linked galactosides. Chemical Communications (Cambridge) 46 (40), 7507–7509.

Zervosen, A., Elling, L., 1996. A novel three-enzyme reaction cycle for the synthesis of N-Acetyllactosamine with in situ regeneration of uridine 5′-Diphosphate glucose and uridine 5′-Diphosphate galactose. Journal of the American Chemical Society 118 (8), 1836–1840.

Zeuner, B., Jers, C., Mikkelsen, J.D., Meyer, A.S., 2014. Methods for improving enzymatic trans-glycosylation for synthesis of human milk oligosaccharide biomimetics. Journal of Agricultural and Food Chemistry 62 (40), 9615–9631.

Zhang, J., Kowal, P., Fang, J., Andreana, P., Wang, P.G., 2002. Efficient chemoenzymatic synthesis of globotriose and its derivatives with a recombinant alpha-(1-->4)-galactosyltransferase. Carbohydrate Research 337 (11), 969–976.

Zhou, G., Liu, X., Su, D., Li, L., Xiao, M., Wang, P.G., 2011. Large scale enzymatic synthesis of oligosaccharides and a novel purification process. Bioorganic & Medicinal Chemistry Letters 21 (1), 311–314.

Zhu, B., Trikudanathan, S., Zozulya, A.L., Sandoval-Garcia, C., Kennedy, J.K., Atochina, O., Norberg, T., Castagner, B., Seeberger, P., Fabry, Z., Harn, D., Khoury, S.J., Guleri, I., 2012. Immune modulation by Lacto-N-fucopentaose III in experimental autoimmune encephalomyelitis. Clinical Immunology 142, 351–361.

Zhu, P., Boykins, R.A., Tsai, C.M., 2006. Genetic and functional analyses of the lgtH gene, a member of the beta-1,4-galactosyltransferase gene family in the genus Neisseria. Microbiology 152 (Pt 1), 123–134.

Zou, Y., Xue, M., Wang, W., Cai, L., Chen, L., Liu, J., Wang, P.G., Shen, J., Chen, M., 2013. One-pot three-enzyme synthesis of UDP-Glc, UDP-Gal, and their derivatives. Carbohydrate Research 373, 76–81.

SECTION

D

Background, Methods, Origin, and Interpretation

CHAPTER

Isn't Milk Sterile? A Historical Perspective on Microbes in Milk

10

Michelle K. McGuire[1], Mark A. McGuire[2]
[1]*Washington State University, Pullman, WA, United States;* [2]*University of Idaho, Moscow, ID, United States*

1. INTRODUCTION

Despite the fact that we have, in all likelihood, coexisted with microbes since the beginning of human existence, our appreciation of microbial ecology complexity and particularly its relationship to human health is relatively rudimentary. Indeed, our understanding of the relationship between microbes and food—be it in terms of fermentation, preservation, infectious disease, or spoilage—is understood in substantially more detail than how the microbes in foods—particularly milk—positively impact physiologic health.

Indeed, aside from a growing literature related to how a small subset of intentionally fermented or microbially fortified foods (often referred to as *probiotic* foods[1]) impact health (e.g., as reviewed by Astrup, 2014; Le Bar et al., 2015; Tapsell, 2015), most written work on this topic is related to the health *risks* of microbially contaminated foods. Beginning with the first visual description of microbes by Antony van Leeuwenhoek (often referred to as the "father of microbiology"; Snyde, 2015; Fig. 10.1), and extending through Louis Pasteur and Ignaz Semmelweis' mid-19th century elucidation of the "germ theory" (Gayne, 2011), Armauer Hansen's late 19th century discovery that the bacterium *Mycobacterium leprae* caused leprosy (Han and Silva, 2014), and Ilya Mechnikov's early 20th century theory that consumption of fermented foods could protect the intestinal tract from toxic substances (Schmalstieg and Goldman, 2008), we have had a "love–hate" relationship with bacteria in terms of whether they help or harm human health.

Here, we will provide a brief history of the evolution of thought related to the microbial content (or lack, thereof) of the only food ever truly "designed" to nourish *Homo sapiens*: human milk. To place this in the context of a much larger and more

[1] It is historically noteworthy that origination of the term "probiotic" is generally attributed to Lilly and Stillwell who, in 1965, used it to describe "growth promoting factors produced by microorganisms," not the actual organisms themselves. Today, the internationally endorsed definition of probiotics is "live microorganisms that, when administered in adequate amounts, confer a health benefit on the host" (Food and Agriculture Organization and World Health Organization, 2002).

Prebiotics and Probiotics in Human Milk. http://dx.doi.org/10.1016/B978-0-12-802725-7.00010-5

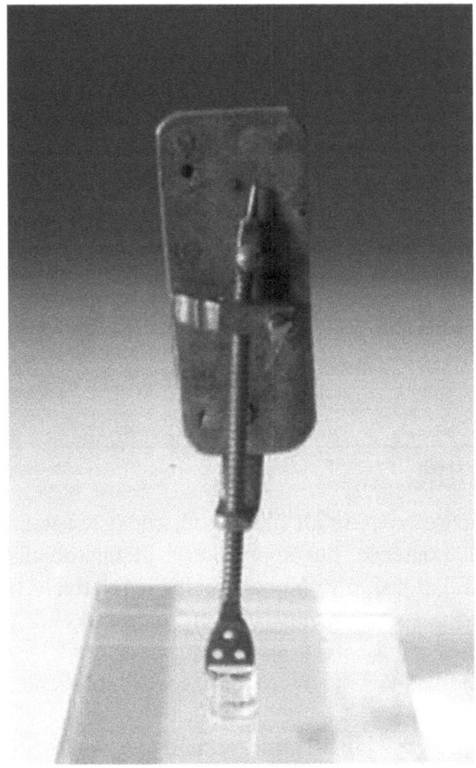

FIGURE 10.1

van Leeuwenhoek's original microscope.

Courtesy of Museum Boerhaave, Leiden, Netherlands.

long-standing literature on microbes in milk, we will also address the parallel evolution of this topic as it relates to bovine milk. It is noteworthy and essential to understand that this chapter is not meant to be an exhaustive history of the topic but rather a retrospective justification for the recent (and initially controversial) paradigm shift and allied, newly emerging questions related to microbes in milk. The chapters following this one will delve much more deeply into the state-of-the-science as it relates to the origin of milk bacteria, how they are characterized, and what researchers currently know and do not know about factors related to their community composition and diversity.

2. BRIEF HISTORY OF MICROBES IN BOVINE MILK: THE GOOD, THE BAD, AND THE USEFUL

Although there is no doubt that *human* milk has forever been the quintessential dairy product intended to nourish humans (at least during infancy), *bovine* milk is thought to have entered the human diet only about 11,000 years ago when farmers (predominantly cattle herders) residing in the Middle East's fertile crescent developed ways to lower the lactose content of otherwise lactose-rich dairy products by converting liquid milk into cheeses and yogurts via bacterial fermentation (Curry, 2013). This outcome is due to the catabolism of lactose into its monosaccharides (glucose and galactose) by bacteria. This development in food processing was important because, until relatively recently and at least in most human populations, transcription of the lactase gene predictably and naturally has been universally downregulated sometime during late childhood (Rasinpera et al., 2005; Wang et al., 1998). As such, discovery and use of these bacterially driven fermentation methods rendered previously "harmful" milk safe for human consumption throughout the lifespan.

Indeed, experts believe that cultural acceptance and consumption of *fresh* (unfermented) milk from birth until old age did not occur until after the emergence of a persistent lactase gene as recently as only 6500 years ago, most prevalently in northern Germany where the ability to consume fresh dairy products year-round likely conferred significant and selective nutritional benefit to adults in addition to infants and toddlers (Itan et al., 2009). Until that time, fermented dairy products, rather than their fresh counterparts, likely constituted more substantial sources of essential nutrients while not contributing excessive amounts of lactose to the diet.

Aside from being tolerable to populations unable to digest lactose, the coagulation of dairy foods (either via intestinal rennet or lactic acid production from dairy-intrinsic bacteria) also served as an important form of food preservation—again allowing continuous, year-round sources of macronutrients and micronutrients with minimal lactose. Evidence for long-standing, historical cheese production is supported by numerous discoveries of earthen vessels apparently designed to separate whey from curds during cheese making; these ancient cheese presses often contain residues of milk fat (Copley et al., 2003; Dunne et al., 2012; Evershed et al., 2008; Salque et al., 2013). In summary, the natural fermentation of bovine (and other) milk into yogurts and, more recently cheeses, provides some (albeit limited) historical and cultural evidence that milk has been bacterially fermented for literally thousands of years. However, there are several questions related to this fact that might be of interest to the reader—most importantly, "From where did the bacteria used in these food preservation processes originate? " "Were the bacteria of environmental or mammary origin?" The likelihood that the bacteria were historically derived from those inherently in milk is described briefly next.

2.1 NATURAL FERMENTATION OF RAW MILK

Raw milk has, in fact, for generations been fermented using its endogenous bacteria. For instance, traditionally cultured buttermilk is made by first allowing fresh raw (unheated) milk to sit uncovered at room temperature until it has clabbered—a process that typically takes several days (Mendelson, 2013). This process is typically followed by repeated and sequential mixing of a portion of the clabbered milk with additional fresh milk (which can be pasteurized) until the resultant mixture (which can then be used as a starter culture) reliably clabbers within 24 h. It is now known that methods of traditional buttermilk production handed down from one generation to the next all rely on the presence and growth of lactic acid–producing *Streptococcus lactis* and *Leuconostoc citrovorum*, which also convert lactic acid to specific aldehydes and ketones, uniquely endowing buttermilk with its distinct flavor and fragrance.

Similarly, Montel et al. (2014) have shown that "traditional" French cheeses crafted with raw (unheated) milk involved long-held, intergenerational "know-how" ranging from agricultural methods to cheese-processing steps that coordinately maintain both the richness of endogenous microbial taxa within an individual cheese variety and microbial diversity among the vast selection of cheeses. Reviewing dozens of previously published studies mostly relying on culture-dependent methods (and thus providing underestimations of bacterial taxa present), these researchers list more than 400 species of lactic acid bacteria, gram- and catalase-positive bacteria, gram-negative bacteria, yeasts, and molds in raw milk; standard plate counts appear to range from 5000 to 10,000 colony forming units per milliliter of milk (CFU/mL). They have also published convincing evidence that whereas bacterial biodiversity decreases with time within the interior of raw milk–derived cheese (where lactic acid bacteria species dominate), there are wide variations in the dynamics of the same species in different cheese types. Importantly, a cheese's flavor appears to be intensified if it is made with raw rather than pasteurized milk, and these authors attribute this to the presence of *live native microbiota* (emphasis added) that interact with each other, starter cultures, and the myriad milk components as the cheese ages.

In summary, although we tend to think of fermented dairy products as being made from an "external" starter culture perhaps derived from environmental sources—and this is obviously true for modern products made from sterilized (pasteurized) milk—it is clear that these cultures (aka bacteria) can also come intrinsically from milk and may be important for imparting optimal fermentation, preservation, and hedonic characteristics. This has undoubtedly been the case for traditional cheese makers for centuries, and likely millennia.

2.2 MILK-DERIVED "STARTER" CULTURES

Traditional farmstead cheese and yogurt production methods have typically relied on the use of "mother cultures" developed from previously fermented milk products over generations. However, because of a reasonable fear about pathogenic bacteria causing food-borne illness combined with a need for consistent results, most fermented dairy products in the United States are now made by adding commercial starter organisms to milk made mostly "sterile" via heat pasteurization. For instance, to meet the standard of identify in the United States, yogurt is produced using a commercially available coculture of *Lactobacillus delbrueckii* subsp. b*ulgaricus* and *Streptococcus thermophilus* bacteria (Shiby and Mishra, 2013; Tunick, 2009), although other *lactobacilli* and *bifidobacteria* are also sometimes added. Interestingly, however, these "starter" bacteria were invariably first isolated from dairy products, again providing additional evidence that milk intrinsically contains these microorganisms.

Moreover, aside from a variety of fermented fruits and vegetables that are common in some cultures around the world (e.g., Franz et al., 2014), it is interesting that many "probiotic" foods (e.g., yogurt, kefir, cheese) consumed globally are indeed made from milk. And even many such foods that are not dairy based are fermented using lactic acid bacteria initially isolated from dairy foods (e.g., Yu et al., 2015). This begs the question as to whether there is something particular about milk that lends itself to providing a successful growth medium for these bacteria. We speculate that the answer to this question is *yes*. As pointed out by Heller (2001), "There is the important technologic reason for the use of dairy products as carriers of probiotic bacteria: many of these products have already been optimized to some extent for survival of the fermentation organisms." This statement is interesting because it gives the impression that the consumer—in this case, humans—has over the millennia somehow optimized dairy products to support the growth of commonly used probiotic starter cultures. Alternatively, we posit that it is more likely that dairy products are inherently capable of supporting the growth of selected bacteria because milk is, by nature, a bacteria-containing fluid.

3. SPONTANEOUS GENERATION, GERM THEORY, AND FOOD-BORNE ILLNESS: OH MY!

Nonetheless, clinicians and researchers working in this area have—at least, in recent history—tended to consider the presence of bacteria in milk to reflect contamination or mammary infection. This viewpoint has been, for the most part, perpetuated by methodologic limitations allowing the identification and quantification of only those bacterial strains for which there existed an adequate culture medium coupled with a general belief that all fluids (e.g., blood, lymph, amniotic fluid) within the healthy body were microbe-free. In addition, food-borne illness (e.g., listeriosis, typhoid fever, tuberculosis, diphtheria, and brucellosis) sometimes caused by raw milk and other dairy products have been enduringly common and life-threatening—in part, spurring Louis Pasteur's seminal research and scientific career (Keim and Lumet, 2015). Indeed, Pasteur (1822–95; Fig. 10.2) revolutionized scientific thought in terms of shifting dogma away from a belief in "spontaneous generation" (Aristotle's conviction that life could come forth from inanimate objects; Brack, 1998), instead to an evidence-driven belief in Koch's "germ theory" (the belief that diseases can be caused by microorganisms). Of course, Pasteur's most publically recognized contribution to microbiology and human health is often said to be the development, understanding, and use of pasteurization, because it not only demonstrated that many common food-borne illnesses and food spoilage problems could be due to microbes but also that these offending organisms could be killed if the food was heated at a sufficient temperature for an ample amount of time.

3.1 DAIRY-RELATED FOOD-BORNE ILLNESS

Pasteur's work along with that of many others, including the likes of Alice Catherine Evans (1881–1975), a gifted American microbiologist with a keen interest in and

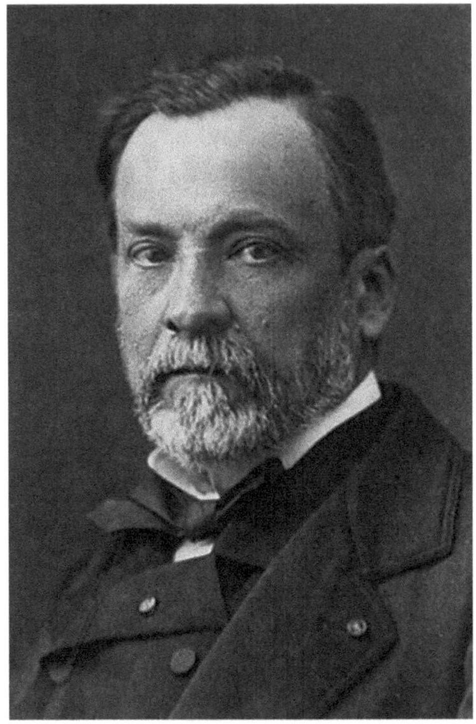

FIGURE 10.2

Louis Pasteur (1822–95) was responsible for disproving the doctrine of spontaneous generation.

Photograph by Pierre Lamy Petit.

understanding of dairy-related food-borne illness (Fig. 10.3), and Ilya Mechnikov (1845–1916), a Russian immunologist (Fig. 10.4) with profound observational and intuitive skills which he used in conjunction with scientific method, have undoubtedly saved the lives of countless people over the last two centuries. However, this period in history was clearly characterized by the general scientific thought that microbes (e.g., bacteria) are dangerous to human health.

Despite this generalized "microbes cause illness" thinking at the time, Mechnikov (who, along with Paul Ehrlich,[2] was awarded the Nobel Prize in Physiology or Medicine in 1908) made the important observation that peasants living in extremely poor, rural Bulgaria often survived to very old ages (Fig. 10.5). In fact, they lived much longer than many contemporary wealthy Europeans. Noting that their diets were rich in naturally fermented "soured milks," Mechnikov proposed that consumption of these foods could

[2] Coincidentally, Ehrlich was one of the first researchers actively interested in understanding the complex composition of human milk (especially immune components) and how it might confer health benefits to the infant.

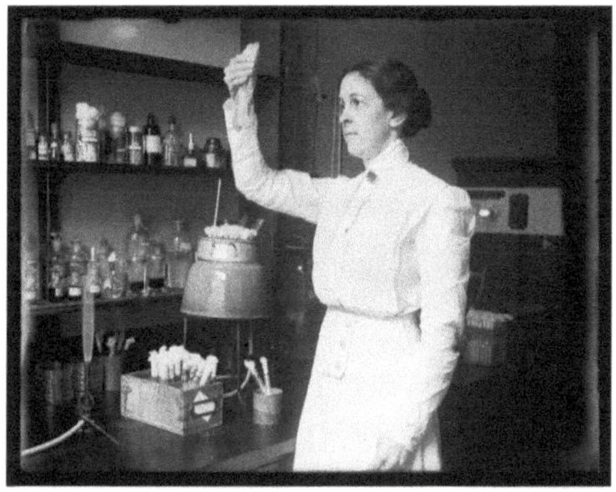

FIGURE 10.3

Alice Catherine Evans (1881–1975) in the Dairy Division of the Department of Agriculture. Evans was instrumental in demonstrating that milk-borne *Bacillus abortus* caused brucellosis in cows and humans.

Courtesy of the National Photo Company, Library of Congress.

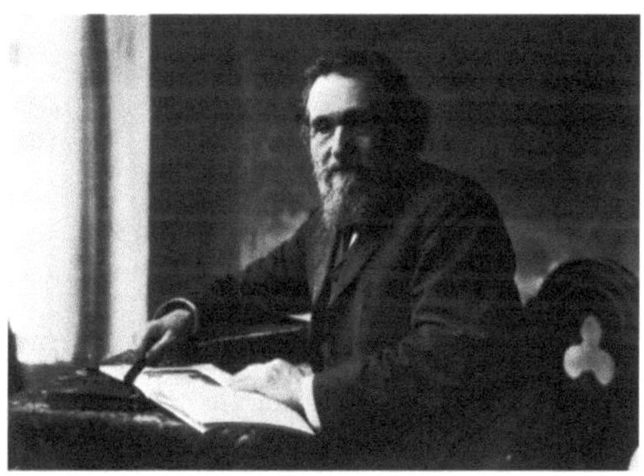

FIGURE 10.4

Ilya Ilyich Mechnikov (1845–1916), a Nobel laureate for his seminal research related to immunology was also known for his work related to the health benefits of lactic acid bacteria-fermented dairy products.

Obtained from Wikimedia.

result in a health-promoting shift in the bacteria present in the large intestine (reviewed by McGuire and McGuire, 2015). Of course, this line of thought contrasted starkly with the current dogma that intestinal bacteria generally promoted ill health.

3.2 MILK-BORNE BACTERIA AND HEALTH

Mechnikov's later work at the Pasteur Institute in Paris reinforced his theories on the benefits of the lactic acid bacteria so common in naturally fermented milk and earned

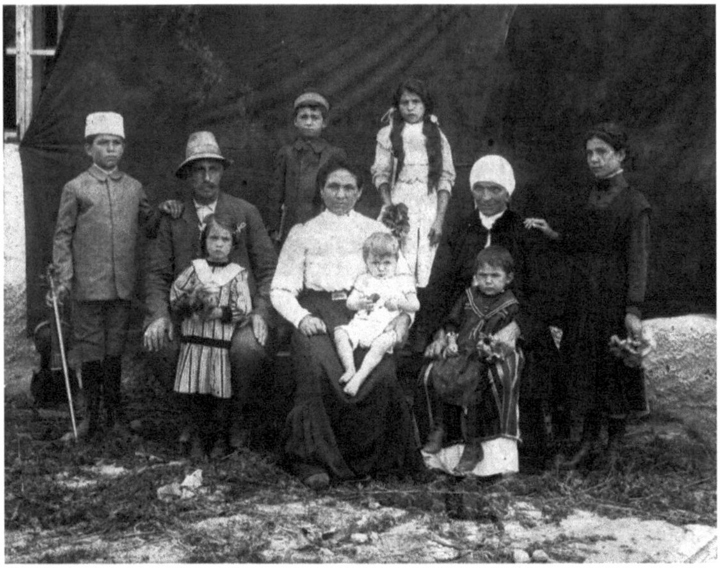

FIGURE 10.5

Mechnikov observed in the late 19th century that rural Bulgarian peasants like those shown here (Petar Konstantinov family, Mihajlovo, Vraca Province, Bulgaria, 1912) often lived very long lives. Mechnikov attributed this to their consumption of traditionally fermented milk products.

him the title of "father of probiotics," although he was never known to use this term. Mechnikov's work nonetheless formed the foundation for decades of research related to understanding how intestinal bacteria both positively and negatively impact human health, and how dietary manipulation via prebiotic and probiotic foods (mostly bacteria-containing dairy products) might moderate these effects.

3.3 MILK MICROBES: RISK VERSUS BENEFIT

Nevertheless, the tension between wanting foods to be sterile and acknowledging potential benefits of bacterially fermented foods has persisted. For instance, to minimize bacteria in raw milk with the goal of decreasing mastitis on the farm, lowering the chance of food-borne illness in the consumer, and maximizing dairy product acceptability on the table, the US National Mastitis Council currently declares bovine milk acceptable for sale only if its bacterial content does not exceed 100 CFU/mL (National Mastitis Council, 2001). This represents current policy even when the milk will be pasteurized prior to consumption and is understandable because bacterial content of milk often reflects animal health, and optimal animal husbandry techniques and approaches are desired to benefit livestock health. In addition, the threat of milk-derived food-borne illness to human health is real: between 1993 and 2006, more than 1500 people in the United States became sick from drinking raw milk or eating cheese made from raw milk (US Food and Drug Administration, 2012). Additionally, unpasteurized milk is 150 times more likely to cause illness than are pasteurized dairy products (US Food and Drug Administration, 2012).

Today, the US Food and Drug Administration (2012) recommends that all milk, cream, soft cheeses, processed cheeses, yogurt, puddings, and ice cream be made from pasteurized rather than raw milk. In this sense, and in this era of somewhat "black and white" thinking in terms of decreasing risk for food-borne illness by eliminating bacterial content, it seems reasonable to conclude that the fewer bacteria (preferably no bacteria) that are in raw milk the better. This idea, clearly stemming from as far back as Pasteur's era, is also often construed to suggest that milk produced by healthy cows should also ideally contain as few bacteria (preferably none) as possible. However, as previously discussed, a long-standing scientific body of literature coupled with current National Mastitis Council recommendations for acceptable bacterial counts based on culture-dependent methods (which undoubtedly underestimate the true bacterial content of milk) suggest otherwise.

3.4 USE OF MOLECULAR TECHNIQUES TO DETECT AND CHARACTERIZE BOVINE MILK MICROBES

Indeed, there are undoubtedly bacteria in bovine milk, even when it is produced by healthy cows and collected/processed using state-of-the-art, sanitary methods. Quigley et al. (2013) reviewed the bacterial composition of raw milk from several important species for human food including cows. The bacterial composition of raw milk from cows identified in both culture-dependent and -independent assessments are diverse with over 250 species detected in culture-independent studies (Masoud et al., 2012). The most abundant genera found in healthy bovine milk were *Ralstonia, Pseudomonas*, *Sphingomonas*, *Stenotrophomonas*, *Psychrobacter*, *Bradyrhizobium, Corynebacterium, Pelomonas, Staphylococcus, Faecalibacterium* spp., *Lachnospiraceae, Propionibacterium* spp., and *Aeribacillus* spp. (Kuehn et al., 2013; Oikonomou et al., 2014). Bovine milk contains a significant population of lactic acid bacteria, including *Lactococcus, Streptococcus, Lactobacillus, Leuconostoc*, and *Enterococcus* spp. Even anaerobic organisms such as *Bacteroides faecalibacterium*, and *Prevotella* are routinely detected. Unclassified and unknown bacteria found in culture-independent evaluations further suggest that the diversity and complexity of bovine milk are much greater than what is currently thought.

3.5 SUMMARY: COW'S MILK ISN'T STERILE

The presence of bacteria inherent to milk produced by healthy cows has been a part of cultural knowledge and has been used (knowingly and unknowingly) for millennia to produce fermented dairy products having both extended shelf lives and the ability to provide delicious, nutritious foods for human consumption. However, emerging knowledge garnered in the 19th century related to germ theory, infectious disease, and bacterially derived, food-borne illness shifted public perception such that the elimination of all (or most) bacteria from milk products seemed prudent. This, along with the fact that most bacteria (at least those which were not thought to harm health) could not be cultured in the laboratory, perpetuated the concept that milk produced by a healthy cow should be sterile. The advent of molecular techniques able to identify the presence of nonculturable microorganisms has now shown, beyond the shadow of a doubt, that this is assumption was incorrect.

4. HUMAN MILK STERILITY—GUILTY UNLESS PROVEN OTHERWISE

Like bovine milk, human milk has also historically been considered sterile unless produced by an infected breast or contaminated after being expressed. This belief was based in large part on the same assumptions applied to bovine milk coupled with methodologic limitations related to selective use of culture-dependent techniques to detect only bacteria known to be pathogenic.

4.1 INFECTIOUS VERSUS NONINFECTIOUS HUMAN MASTITIS

More specifically, results from many now-outdated studies using culture-dependent methods (e.g., Osterman and Rahm, 2000; Thomsen et al., 1983, 1984) suggested, although most human milk samples appeared to be sterile using methods available at the time, those produced by women suffering from mastitis contained cultivable bacteria: primarily *Staphylococcus aureus* and, to a lesser extent, streptococci. However, other studies have long provided evidence that some women with mastitis produce "sterile" milk, and cultivable bacteria can sometimes be detected in milk produced by healthy women (Kvist, 2010; Kvist et al., 2008). These seemingly disparate findings have, for some time, led human-milk experts to question the prevailing dogma related to "infectious" versus "noninfectious" mastitis (i.e., bacterial vs nonbacterial); the precise role of bacteria in the etiology of breast inflammation; and the implications this might have for or against antibiotic use in affected women (e.g., Kvist, 2010; Kvist et al., 2008; Fetherston, 2001).

4.2 ADVENT OF MOLECULAR METHODS

Indeed, as with studies related to microbial content (or lack thereof) of bovine milk, recent use of culture-independent techniques that do not rely on taxa-specific growth media but instead identify bacterial groups based on variation in specific DNA segments, has led to a paradigm shift in this regard (e.g., Hunt et al., 2011; Martín et al., 2003; Fernández et al., 2013). These studies using molecular techniques often coupled with more classic culture-dependent approaches, now overwhelmingly support the existence of a rich and diverse community of bacteria in human milk, regardless of whether it is produced by healthy or mastitic women. Details concerning the origins of and variability in these bacteria as well as their potential benefits to mothers and infants are provided in the following chapters.

4.3 REVOLVING DOOR OF CHALLENGING SCIENTIFIC DOGMA

It is worthwhile to point out, though, that this paradigm shift has not occurred without considerable hesitation and critical evaluation amongst lactation researchers—an important safeguard in any scientific discipline. Indeed, our experience as well as that of others (e.g., Dr. Juan Miguel Rodriguez, personal communications) has been that allied scientists rightly and severely have questioned whether the presence of bacteria in human milk might be attributed to inadequate milk collection techniques. Although this is clearly a reasonable concern, the ability for multiple groups around the world to identify bacteria in carefully collected milk produced by women residing in the United States (Hunt et al., 2011), Spain (Khodayar-Pardo et al., 2014), Canada (Urbaniak et al., 2016), Mexico (Davé et al., 2016), Finland (Cabrera-Rubio et al., 2012), and Mozambique (Gonzáez et al., 2013) coupled with associated studies in production animals (e.g., Callon et al., 2007; Liu et al., 2015) and rigorous evidence that live bacteria are present in the human breast even when it is not producing milk (Urbaniak et al., 2014a,b) collectively provide growing evidence that human milk inherently contains live bacteria.

Of course, scientific hesitation to adopt game-changing paradigm shifts such as this related to human physiology are expected, desirable, and historically common. Illustrating this reality as it relates to another seminal finding connected with the topic of microbes in milk is the fact that van Leeuwenhoek's initial proposition that living microscopic organisms even existed was certainly not immediately accepted by scientists, and there is considerable evidence that he was internationally mocked for his proposition (Moll, 2006). And to be fair, it is understandable why thoughtful scientists at the time might consider the following passage from van Leeuwenhoek's description of his own oral plaque too fanciful to be true (Snyde, 2015; Fig. 10.6).

> *"I then most always saw, with great wonder, that in the said matter there were many very little living animalcules, very prettily a-moving. The biggest sort … had a very strong and swift motion, and shot through the water (or spittle) like a pike does through the water. The second sort … oft-times spun round like a top … and these were far more in number." In the mouth of one of the old men, Leeuwenhoek found "an unbelievably great company of living animalcules, a-swimming more nimbly than any I had ever seen up to this time. The biggest sort … bent their body into curves in going forwards … Moreover, the other animalcules were in such enormous numbers, that all the water … seemed to be alive."*

4.4 SEEING IS BELIEVING

Despite the overwhelming initial disbelief in van Leeuwenhoek's theories, his descriptions turned out to be among the first observations of living bacteria ever recorded. Clearly, despite the fact that (by definition), microorganisms cannot be seen by the naked eye, van Leeuwenhoek's seemingly "naïve" suggestion that extremely small living organisms could be inherently found in biological and environmental fluids formed the underlying paradigm shift shaping modern microbiology. In this case, the creative use of new technology (in this case a simple microscope) to find answers

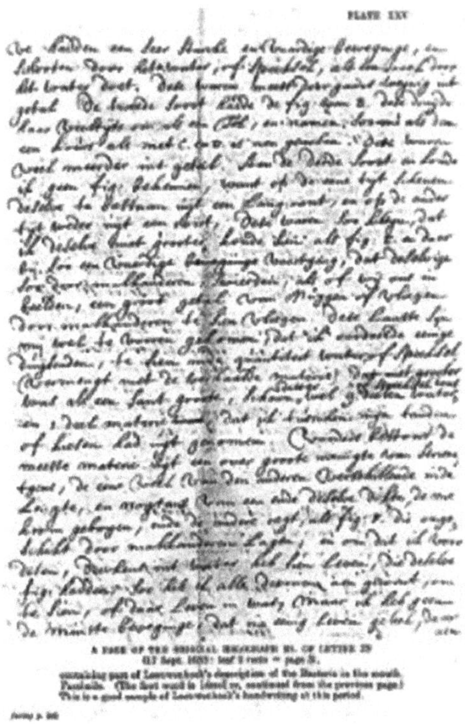

FIGURE 10.6

A page of the original holograph manuscript of letter 39 dated September 17, 1683 (leaf 2 recto, page 3) containing part of van Leeuwenhoek's description of the bacteria in the mouth.

to questions that may have not even been previously asked illuminated seemingly implausible facts about the world in which we live. As the idiom suggests: *Seeing is believing*. Being able to see microscopic bacteria opened the door to a new biological discipline: microbiology.

But then again, convincing the scientific community that microscopic organisms existed marked only the first phase of microbiology. Understanding how these minute organisms live and impact health and disease was the critical next step, and assigning microbial causality to disease was not universally accepted by the scientific community until the work of Heinrich Hermann Robert Koch (1843–1910) who distilled this causal relationship down to four repeatable, experimental steps. Indeed, Koch's "postulates" were essential in proving the germ theory of disease which was, in turn, essential in providing evidence that such diseases were infectious in nature (Brock, 1999). For his discoveries, Koch was awarded the Nobel Prize for Physiology or Medicine in 1905 (Nobel Media AB). It is noteworthy, however, that like those of van Leeuwenhoek, Koch's discoveries relied fundamentally upon *seeing* bacteria and/or describing their growth. Selective growth media developed by Koch made possible the detection and

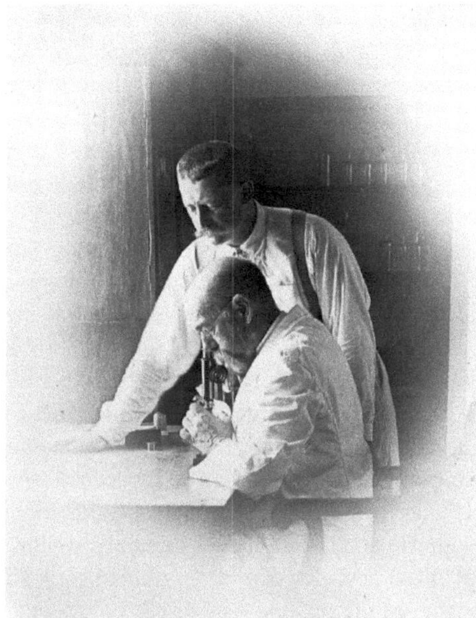

FIGURE 10.7

Robert Koch (seated) and Richard Friedrich Johannes Pfeiffer investigating the plague in Bombay, India, using a microscope.

Photograph attributed to Captain C. Moss, 1897.

characterization of bacteria; for instance, he used the aqueous humor of the ox's eye to culture and study *Bacillus anthracis*, the causative agent for anthrax. To aid in his work, Koch also developed new methods of staining bacteria, making them more easily visible and allowing them to be identified—again illustrating the "seeing-is-believing" phase of microbiology originating from van Leeuwenhoek's earlier work (Fig. 10.7).

This phase of microbiology, relying primarily on the visual identification and enumeration of bacteria, was and continues to be critical to understanding how microbes interact with each other, the environment (including foods), and human health. However, the advent of molecular techniques has now unmistakably augmented and enhanced the breadth and scope of microbes that can be detected and studied such that we now know that almost nothing, including bovine and human milks, is bacteria free.

5. SUMMARY: BELIEVING DOESN'T NECESSARILY REQUIRE SEEING

The presence of microorganisms in dairy products has long conferred nutritional significance to humans, in that they allowed natural fermentation and subsequent lower lactose concentrations and availability of nutrient-dense dairy products year-round.

Nonetheless, beginning in the 19th century, researchers have generally considered milk produced by healthy animals to be sterile—largely because of the prevailing dogma that bodily fluids were sterile combined with the low abundance of microbes in "healthy" milk and the fact that most inherent bacteria in milk are not typically grown on standard pathology-based media. These findings coupled with continued and understandable concern about dairy-related, food-borne illnesses have perpetuated the general concept that milk should be sterile.

However, many carefully conducted studies have long suggested that neither bovine nor human milk is sterile—instead containing low levels of bacteria and other microorganisms. Indeed, culture-dependent microbiological methods coupled with microscopy are still critically important to the field of microbiology and will continue to be fundamental in terms of understanding the role that bacteria play in the mammary gland, milk, and recipient infant's gastrointestinal tract. These methods, along with more recent advances in molecular methods that can detect the presence of DNA from uncultivable (and often undescribed) bacteria, are paving the way to a newly accepted reality that, in fact, many biological fluids thought previously to be sterile are, in fact, not sterile at all. This reality certainly applies to milk.

The application of these new discoveries to human milk has opened up a new frontier—in fact, a game-changing one—in terms of understanding human milk composition and how variation, therein, might impact both maternal and infant health. We have long known that milk supplies all of the essential and conditionally essential nutrients to infants and that it is also a rich source of immune cells and other bioactive compounds (e.g., hormones, immunoglobulins). We can now add living microbes to this long and impressive list of milk constituents. It is essential to remember that, although seeing sometimes facilitates believing, believing does not always require seeing. Sometimes discovery simply requires a curious mind, fearless use of ever-evolving methods and techniques, rigorous application of scientific method, and resolute persistence.

REFERENCES

Astrup, A., 2014. Yogurt and dairy product consumption to prevent cardiometabolic diseases: epidemiologic and experimental studies. The American Journal of Clinical Nutrition 99, 1235S–1242S.

Brack, A., 1998. The Molecular Origins of Life. Cambridge University Press, New York.

Brock, T.D., 1999. Robert Koch: A Life in Medicine and Bacteriology. American Society for Microbiology, Washington, DC.

Cabrera-Rubio, R., Collado, M.C., Laitinen, K., Salminen, S., Isolauri, E., Mira, A., 2012. The human milk microbiome changes over lactation and is shaped by maternal weight and mode of delivery. The American Journal of Clinical Nutrition 96, 544–551.

Callon, C., Duthoit, F., Delbès, C., Ferrand, M., Le Frileux, Y., De Crémoux, R., Montel, M.-C., 2007. Stability of microbial communities in goat milk during a lactation year: molecular approaches. Systematic and Applied Microbiology 30, 547–560.

Copley, M.S., Berstan, R., Dudd, S.N., Docherty, G., Mukherjee, A.J., Straker, V., Payne, S., Evershed, R.P., 2003. Direct chemical evidence for widespread dairying in prehistoric Britain. Proceeding of the National Academy of Sciences of the United States of America 100, 1524–1529.

Curry, A., 2013. Archaeology: the milk revolution. Nature 500, 20–22.

Davé, V., Street, K., Francis, S., Bradman, A., Riley, L., Eskenazi, B., Holland, N., 2016. Bacterial microbiome of breast milk and child saliva from low-income Mexican-American women and children. Pediatric Research. http://dx.doi.org/10.1038/pr.2016.9 (Epub ahead of print).

Dunne, J., Evershed, R.P., Salque, M., Cramp, L., Bruni, S., Ryan, K., Biagetti, S., di Lernia, S., 2012. First dairying in green Saharan Africa in the fifth millennium BC. Nature 486, 390–394.

Evershed, R.P., Payne, S., Sherratt, A.G., Copley, M.S., Coolidge, J., Urem-Kotsu, D., Kotsakis, K., Ozdoğan, M., Ozdoğan, A.E., Nieuwenhuyse, O., Akkermans, P.M., Bailey, D., Andeescu, R.R., Campbell, S., Farid, S., Hodder, I., Yalman, N., Ozbaşaran, M., Biçakci, E., Garfinkel, Y., Levy, T., Burton, M.M., 2008. Earliest date for milk use in the near East and Southeastern Europe linked to cattle herding. Nature 455, 528–531.

Fernández, L., Langa, S., Martín, V., Jiménez, E., Martín, R., Rodríguez, J.M., 2013. The microbiota of human milk in healthy women. Cellular and Molecular Biology (Noisy-le-Grand, France) 59, 31–42.

Fetherston, C., 2001. Mastitis in lactating women: physiology or pathology? Breastfeeding Review 9, 5–12.

Food and Agriculture/World Health Organization Working Group on Drafting Guidelines for the Evaluation of Probiotics in Food. Guidelines for the Evaluation of Probiotics in Food: Report of a Joint FAO/WHO Working Group on Drafting Guidelines for the Evaluation of Probiotics in Food, London, Ontario, Canada, April 30 and May 1, 2002. Available at: http://www.who.int/foodsafety/publications/fs_management/probiotics2/en/index.html.

Franz, C.M., Huch, M., Mathara, J.M., Abriouel, H., Benomar, N., Reid, G., Galvez, A., Holzapfel, W.H., 2014. African fermented foods and probiotics. International Journal of Food Microbiology 190, 84–96.

Gayne, R.P., 2011. Germ Theory: Medical Pioneers in Infectious Diseases. American Society of Microbiology Press, Washington, DC.

Gonzáez, R., Maldonado, A., Martín, V., Mandomando, I., Fumadó, V., Metzner, K.J., Sacoor, C., Fernández, L., Macete, E., Alonso, P.L., Rodríguez, J.M., Menendez, C., 2013. Breast milk and gut microbiota in African mothers and infants from an area of high HIV prevalence. PLoS ONE 8, e80299. http://dx.doi.org/10.1371/journal.pone.0080299.

Han, X.Y., Silva, F.J., 2014. On the age of leprosy. PLoS Neglected Tropical Diseases 8, e2544. http://dx.doi.org/10.1371/journal.pntd.0002544.

Heller, K.J., 2001. Probiotic bacteria in fermented foods: product characteristics and starter organisms. The American Journal of Clinical Nutrition 73 (Suppl.), 374S–379S.

Hunt, K.M., Foster, J.A., Forney, L.J., Schutte, U.M.E., Beck, D.L., Abdo, Z., Fox, L.K., Williams, J.E., McGuire, M.K., McGuire, M.A., 2011. Characterization of the diversity and temporal stability of bacterial communities in human milk. PLoS ONE 6, e21313. http://dx.doi.org/10.1371/journal.pone.0021313.

Itan, Y., Powell, A., Beaumont, M.A., Burger, J., Thomas, M.G., 2009. The origins of lactase persistence in Europe. PLoS Computational Biology 5 (8), e1000491. http://dx.doi.org/10.1371/journal.pcbi.100049.

Keim, A., Lumet, L., 2015. Louis Pasteur. Waxkeep Publishing.
Khodayar-Pardo, P., Mira-Pascual, L., Collado, M.C., Martínez-Costa, C., 2014. Impact of lactation stage, gestational age and mode of delivery on breast milk microbiota. Journal of Perinatology 34, 599–605.
Kuehn, J.S., Gorden, P.J., Munro, D., Rong, R., Dong, Q., Plummer, P.J., Wang, C., Phillips, G.J., 2013. Bacterial community profiling of milk samples as a means to understand culture-negative bovine clinical mastitis. PLoS ONE 8, e61959. http://dx.doi.org/10.1371/journal.pone.0061959.
Kvist, J., 2010. Toward a clarification of the concept of mastitis as used in empirical studies of breast inflammation during lactation. Journal of Human Lactation 26, 53–59.
Kvist, J., Wilde Larsson, B., Hall-Lord, M.L., Steen, A., Schalén, C., 2008. The role of bacteria in lactational mastitis and some considerations of the use of antibiotic treatment. International Breastfeeding Journal 3, 6. http://dx.doi.org/10.1186/1746-4358-3-6.
Le Bar, M., Anhê, F.F., Varin, T.V., Desjardins, Y., Levy, E., Roy, D., Urdaci, M.C., Marette, A., 2015. Probiotics as complementary treatment for metabolic disorders. Diabetes and Metabolism Journal 39, 291–303.
Liu, W., Zheng, Y., Kwok, L.Y., Sun, Z., Zhang, J., Guo, Z., Hou, Q., Menhe, B., Zhang, H., 2015. High-throughput sequencing for the detection of the bacterial and fungal diversity in Mongolian naturally fermented cow's milk in Russia. BMC Microbiology 22, 15–45.
Martín, R., Langa, S., Reviriego, C., Jimínez, E., Marín, M.L., Xaus, J., Fernández, L., Rodríguez, J.M., 2003. Human milk is a source of lactic acid bacteria for the infant gut. Journal of Pediatrics 143, 754–758.
Masoud, W., Vogensen, F.K., Lillevang, S., Abu Al-Soud, W., Sorensen, S.J., Jakobsen, M., 2012. The fate of indigenous microbiota, starter cultures, *Escherichia coli*, *Listeria innocua* and *Staphylococcus aureus* in Danish raw milk and cheeses determined by pyrosequencing and quantitative real time (qRT)-PCR. International Journal of Food and Microbiology 153, 192–202.
McGuire, M.K., McGuire, M.A., 2015. Human milk: mother nature's prototypical probiotic food? Advances in Nutrition 6, 112–123.
Mendelson, A., 2013. Milk. The Surprising Story of Milk Through the Ages. Knopf, New York.
Moll, W., 2006. Antonie Va Leeuwenhoek. Available on-line at: http://www.faculty.umb.edu/gary_zabel/Courses/Spinoza/Texts/WAW%20Moll%20Antonie%20van%20Leeuwenhoek.htm.
Montel, M.C., Buchin, S., Mallet, A., Delbes-Paus, C., Vuitton, D.A., Desmasures, N., Berthier, F., 2014. Traditional cheeses: rich and diverse microbiota with associated benefits. Journal of Food Microbiology 177, 136–154.
National Mastitis Council, 2001. Guidelines on Normal and Abnormal Raw Milk Based on Somatic Cell Counts and Signs of Clinical Mastitis. Available at: http://nmconline.org/docs/abnmilk.pdf.
Nobel Media AB. Robert Koch—Biographical. Available at: http://www.nobelprize.org/nobel_prizes/medicine/laureates/1905/koch-bio.html.
Nobel Media AB. Ilya Mechnikov—Biographical. Available at: http://www.nobelprize.org/nobel_prizes/medicine/laureates/1908/mechnikov-bio.html.
Oikonomou, G., Bicalho, M.L., Meira, E., Rossi, R.E., Foditsch, C., Machado, V.S., Teixeira, A.G.V., Santisteban, C., Schukken, Y.H., Bicalho, R.C., 2014. Microbiota of cow's milk; distinguishing healthy sub-clinically and clinically diseased quarters. PLoS One 9, e85904. http://dx.doi.org/10.1371/journal.pone.0085904.

Osterman, K.L., Rahm, V.-A., 2000. Lactation mastitis: bacterial cultivation of breast milk, symptoms, treatment, and outcomes. Journal of Human Lactation 16, 297–302.

Quigley, L., O'Sullivan, O., Stanton, C., Beresford, T.P., Ross, R.P., Fitzgerald, G.F., Cotter, P.D., 2013. The complex microbiota of raw milk. FEMS Microbiology Review 37, 664–698.

Rasinperä, H., Kuokkanen, M., Kolho, K.L., Lindahl, H., Enattah, N.S., Savilahti, E., Orpana, A., Järvelä, I., 2005. Transcriptional downregulation of the lactase (LCT) gene during childhood. Gut 54, 1660–1661.

Salque, M., Bogucki, P.I., Pyzel, J., Sobkowiak-Tabaka, I., Grygiel, R., Szmyt, M., Evershed, R.P., 2013. Earliest evidence for cheese making in the sixth millennium BC in northern Europe. Nature 493, 522–525.

Schmalstieg Jr., F.C., Goldman, A.S., 2008. Ilya Ilich Metchnikoff (1845–1915) and Paul Ehrlich (1854–1915): the centennial of the 1908 Nobel Prize in Physiology or Medicine. Journal of Medical Biography 16, 96–103.

Shiby, K., Mishra, H.N., 2013. Fermented milks and milk products as functional foods: a review. Critical Reviews in Food Science and Nutrition 53, 482–496.

Snyde, L.J., 2015. Eye of the Beholder: Johannes Vermeer, Antoni Van Leeuwenhoek, and the Reinvention of Seeing. WW Norton & Company, New York.

Tapsell, L.C., 2015. Fermented dairy food and CVD risk. British Journal of Nutrition 113 (Suppl. 2), S131–S135.

Thomsen, A.C., Hansen, K.B., Moller, B.R., 1983. Leukocyte counts and microbiological cultivation in the diagnosis of puerperal mastitis. American Journal of Obstetrics and Gynecology 146, 938–941.

Thomsen, A.C., Espersen, T., Maigaard, S., 1984. Course and treatment of milk stasis, noninfectious inflammation of the breast, and infectious mastitis in nursing women. American Journal of Obstetrics and Gynecology 149, 492–495.

Tunick, M.H., 2009. Dairy innovations in the past 100 Years. Journal of Agricultural and Food Chemistry 57, 8093–8097.

Urbaniak, C., McMillan, A., Angelini, M., Gloor, G.B., Sumarah, M., Burton, J.P., Reid, G., 2014a. Effect of chemotherapy on the microbiota and metabolome of human milk, a case report. Microbiome 2, 24. http://dx.doi.org/10.1186/2049-2618-2-24.

Urbaniak, C., Cummins, J., Brackstone, M., Macklaim, J.M., Gloor, G.B., Baban, C.K., Scott, L., O'Hanlon, D.M., Burton, J.P., Francis, K.P., Tangney, M., Reid, G., 2014b. Microbiota of human breast tissue. Applied Environmental Microbiology 80, 3007–3014.

Urbaniak, C., Angelini, M., Gloor, G.B., Reid, G., 2016. Human milk microbiota profiles in relation to birthing method, gestation and infant gender. Microbiome 4, 1. http://dx.doi.org/10.1186/s40168-015-0145-y.

US Food and Drug Administration, 2012. The Dangers of Raw Milk: Unpasteurized Milk Can Pose a Serious Health Risk. Available at: http://www.fda.gov/downloads/Food/FoodborneIllnessContaminants/UCM239493.pdf.

Wang, Y., Harvey, C.B., Hollox, E.J., Phillips, A.D., Poulter, M., Clay, P., Walker-Smith, J.A., Swallow, D.M., 1998. The genetically programmed down-regulation of lactase in children. Gastroenterology 114, 1230–1236.

Yu, J., Sun, Z., Liu, W., Xi, X., Song, Y., Xu, H., Lv, Q., Bao, Q., Menghe, B., Sun, T., 2015. Multilocus sequence typing of *Streptococcus thermophilus* from naturally fermented dairy foods in China and Mongolia. BMC Microbiology 15, 236.

CHAPTER

11 From the Human Milk Microbiota to the Human Milk Metagenome: Evolution of Methods to Study Human Milk Microbial Communities

Esther Jimenez[1,2]

[1]ProbiSearch, SL. Tres cantos, Madrid, Spain; [2]Universidad Complutense de Madrid, Madrid, Spain

Knowledge about the presence of bacteria in human milk has evolved in the past 40 years from studies on the microbiology of human milk in the 1970–1980s restricted to the identification of potential pathogenic bacteria in stored milk of milk banks and in clinical cases of mastitis or infant's infection (Eidelman and Szilagyi, 1979; Law et al., 1989; Lucas and Roberts, 1979; West et al., 1979) to the correlation between the human milk microbiota composition and woman's health status today (Fernández et al., 2013). The application of numerous laboratory culture-dependent and -independent techniques (Fig. 11.1) has contributed to this evolution.

1. CULTURE TECHNIQUES

Bacterial content of human milk has been one of the main concerns of human milk banks throughout history. Freshly collected human milk was considered contaminated with microbiota from the skin and nipples (Björkstén et al., 1980). Culture media normally used in milk banks were nutrient agar, blood agar, and MacConkey agar. These laboratory procedures led to the isolation of coagulase-negative and -positive staphylococci, streptococci, enterococci, and enterobacteria; all considered as potential pathogens.

In 2003, the inclusion of MRS (de Man, Rogosa, and Sharpe) medium and anaerobic incubation conditions allowed the isolation of lactic acid bacteria like *Lactobacillus gasseri*, *Lactobacillus fermentum*, *Lactobacillus crispatus*, *Lactobacillus rhamnosus*, *Lactococcus lactis*, and *Leuconostoc mesenteroides* (Heikkila and Saris, 2003; Martín et al., 2003). This fact changed the perception of human milk from a microbiological point of view as a source of potentially probiotic bacteria instead of potential pathogens.

Prebiotics and Probiotics in Human Milk. http://dx.doi.org/10.1016/B978-0-12-802725-7.00011-7

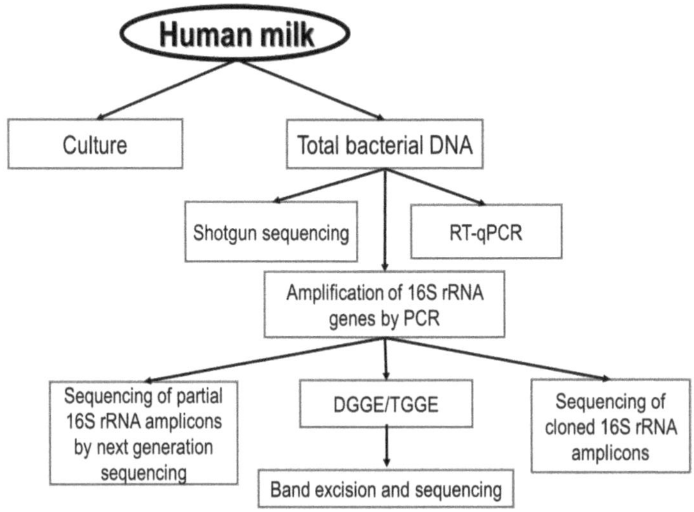

FIGURE 11.1

Summary of techniques used to characterize human milk microbiota.

Later, the use of a higher diversity of culture media allowed a deeper examination of the microbiota present in colostrum (Table 11.1) and human milk (Table 11.2). Predominance of staphylococci and streptococci was shown, while other bacteria such as lactic acid bacteria, propionibacteria, and occasionally gram-negative bacteria were present at subdominant levels (Albesharat et al., 2011; Jiménez et al., 2008a, b; Martín et al., 2012). Furthermore, new bacterial species, such as *Streptococcus lactarius* (Martín et al., 2011), were isolated and described.

The isolation of viable bifidobacteria required special effort. Two different research groups (Gueimonde et al., 2007; Perez et al., 2007) detected the presence of bifidobacterial DNA in human milk, but attempts to isolate bifidobacteria from human milk were not successful until later. Martín et al. (2009) cultured 20 human milk samples in MRS (de Man, Rogosa, Sharpe) supplemented with cysteine inside an anaerobic workstation (85% nitrogen, 10% hydrogen, 5% carbon dioxide). The authors were able to isolate and identify bifidobacteria from eight milk samples belonging to three species: *Bifidobacterium breve* (in four milk samples), *Bifidobacterium adolescentis* (in two samples), and *Bifidobacterium bifidum* (in two samples). Later, Jost et al. (2013) were able to isolate viable obligate anaerobes including not only bifidobacteria but also *Veillonella* for the first time. Bifidobacteria are important members of the human gastrointestinal (GI) microbiota that belong to a strictly anaerobic genus and, therefore, skin is a very unlikely source of these bacteria. This suggests that at least some of the bacteria present in the maternal GI tract could reach the mammary gland through an endogenous route (Martín et al., 2004; Pérez et al., 2007; Rodríguez et al., 2014).

One of the main advantages of culture-dependent techniques is that they allow further studies of bacterial isolates. Several research projects have submitted human milk isolates for in-depth characterization including detection of possible virulence

Table 11.1 Prevalence of Bacterial Species Isolated From Colostrum Samples ($n=35$)

Genus	Species	Number of Positive Samples (%)	Total Number of Isolates
Staphylococcus	*S. epidermidis*	30 (83.33)	284
	S. lugdunensis	8 (22.22)	23
	S. hominis	4 (11.11)	6
	S. pasteuri	3 (8.33)	3
	S. capitis	1 (2.77)	1
	S. haemolyticus	1 (2.77)	1
	S. aureus	2 (5.55)	3
Enterococcus	*E. faecalis*	15 (41.66)	35
	E. faecium	2 (5.55)	2
	E. durans	2 (5.55)	2
Streptococcus	*S. mitis*	9 (25.00)	27
	S. oralis	3 (8.33)	6
	S. parasanguinis	2 (5.55)	6
	S. pneumoniae	1 (2.77)	1
	S. anginosus	1 (2.77)	1
	S. salivarius	1 (2.77)	1
Propionibacterium	*P. acnes*	8 (22.22)	11
	P. avidum	1 (2.77)	2
	P. granulosum	2 (5.55)	4
Leuconostoc	*L. mesenteroides*	4 (11.11)	4
Lactobacillus	*Lb. paracasei*	1 (2.77)	2
Bifidobacterium	*B. breve*	1 (2.77)	1
Actinomyces	*A. neuii*	3 (8.33)	4
Arthrobacter	spp.	1 (2.77)	1
Corynebacterium	*C. amicolatum*	1 (2.77)	2
Finegoldia	*F. magna*	1 (2.77)	1
Gemella	*G. haemolysans*	2 (5.55)	2
Rothia	*R. mucilaginosa*	4 (11.11)	5
Enterobacter	spp.	2 (5.55)	4
Escherichia	*E. coli*	2 (5.55)	2
Klebsiella	spp.	1 (2.77)	2

Reproduced from Jiménez, E., Fernández, L., Delgado, S., García, N., Albújar, M., Gómez, A., Rodríguez J.M., 2008. Assessment of the bacterial diversity of human colostrum by cultural-based techniques. Analysis of the staphylococcal and enterococcal populations. Research in Microbiology 159, 595–601.

attributes, sensitivity to antibiotics (Jiménez et al., 2008a,b), or potential probiotic traits (Martín et al., 2005). In fact, some of the lactic acid bacteria strains isolated from human milk have been shown to possess probiotic properties, including the inhibition of a wide spectrum of infant pathogenic bacteria by competitive exclusion and/or through the

Table 11.2 Main Bacterial Groups Detected Using Culture-Dependent and Culture-Independent Techniques in Human Milk Manually Expressed By Healthy Women

Method	Main Bacterial Groups[a]	References
Culture	*En. faecium, L. fermentum, L. gasseri*	Martín et al. (2003)
	A. odontolyticus, En. faecalis, L. crispatus, L. rhamnosus, Lc. lactis, Leuc. mesenteroides, R. mucilaginosa, S. aureus, S. capitis, S. epidermidis, S. hominis, Str. Agalactiae, Str. mitis, Str. oralis, Str. parasanguis, Str. Peroris, Str. salivarius	Heikkila and Saris (2003)
	L. salivarius	Martín et al. (2006)
	Corynebacterium spp., *Enterococcus* spp., *Escherichia* spp., *Lactobacillus* spp., *Peptostreptococcus* spp.,*Staphylococcus* spp., *Streptococcus* spp.	Pérez et al. (2007)
	L. reuteri	Sinkiewicz and Ljunggren (2008)[b]
	A. johnsonii, Bifidobacterium spp., *Burkholderia* spp., *Citrobacter* spp., *Enterococcus* spp., *En. faecalis, E. coli, Klebsiella* spp. *Lactobacillus* spp., *Propionibacterium* spp., *Pseudomonas* spp., *Staphylococcus* spp. *S. epidermidis, Streptococcus* spp.	Jiménez et al. (2008a)
	A. neuii, Arthrobacter spp., *B. breve, C. amicolatum, E. coli, Enterobacter spp., En. faecalis, En. faecium, En. durans, F. magna, G. haemolysans, Klebsiella spp., L. paracasei, Leuc. mesenteroides, R. mucilaginosa, S. epidermidis, S. lugdunensis, S. hominis, S. pasteuri, S. capitis, S. haemolyticus, S. aureus, Str. mitis, Str. oralis, Str. parasanguinis, Str. pneumonia, Str. anginosus, Str. salivarius, Prop. acnes, Prop. avidum, Prop. granulosum*	Jiménez et al. (2008b)
	B. adolescentis, B. bifidum, B. breve	Martín et al. (2009)
	Str. lactarius	Martín et al. (2011)
	B. breve, B. longum, L. casei, L. gasseri, L. gastricus, L. fermentum, L. plantarum, L. reuteri, L. salivarius, L.vaginalis, S. epidermidis, S. hominis,	Martín et al. (2012)
	En. durans, En. faecalis, En. faecium, En. hirae, En. mundtii, L. animalis, L. brevis, L. fermentum, L. gasseri, L. helveticus, L. oris, L. plantarum, P. pentosaceous, Str. australis, Str. gallolyticus, Str. Vestibularis	Albesharat et al. (2011)
	B. longum	Makino et al. (2011)[c]

DGGE/TGGE	*B. longum, S. epidermidis, Str. thermophilus/salivarius*	Pérez et al. (2007)
	E. coli, En. faecalis, En. faecium, L. fermentum, L. gasseri, L. jensenii, L. rhamnosus, L. plantarum, Lc. lactis, Leuc. citreum, Leuc. fallax, Ps. synxantha, Prop. acnes, S. epidermidis, S. hominis, Str. mitis, Str. parasanguis, Str. salivarius, W. cibaria, W. confuse.	Martín et al. (2007a,b)
	B. adolescentis B. animalis, B. bifidum, B. breve, B. catenolatum, B. longum	Gueimonde et al. (2007)
	B. adolescentis B. animalis, B. bifidum, B. breve, B. catenolatum, B. longum	Martín et al. (2009)
RT-qPCR	*Bacteroides,* spp., *Bifidobacterium* spp., *Clostridium* spp., *Enterococcus* spp., *Lactobacillus* spp., *Staphylococcus* spp., *Streptococcus* spp.	Collado et al. (2009)
	Bifidobacterium spp., *B. fragilis*, *Enterobacteriaceae*, *Lactobacillus* spp., *C. coccoides*, *Streptococcus* spp., *Enterococcus* spp.	Olivares et al. (2015)
Pyrosequencing	*Actinomyces* spp., *Bradyrhizobium* spp., *Corynebacterium* spp., *Gemella* spp., *Granulicatella* spp., *Prevotella* spp., *Propionibacterium* spp., *Pseudomonas* spp., *Ralstonia* spp., *Rothia* spp., *Serratia* spp., *Sphingomonas* spp., *Staphylococcus* spp., *Streptococcus* spp, Veionella spp.	Hunt et al. (2011)
	Bifidobacterium spp., *Blautia* spp., *Brevundimonas* spp., *Burkholderia* spp., *Corynebacterium* spp., *Flavobacterium* spp., *Propionibacterium* spp., *Pseudomonas* spp., *Ralstonia* spp., *Rothia* spp., *Staphylococcus* spp., *Streptococcus* spp.,	Jost et al. (2013)
Illumina®	*Edwardsiella* spp., *Campylobacter* spp., *Corynebacterium* spp., *Lactobacillus* spp., *Mycoplasma* spp., *Pantoea* spp., *Pseudomonas* spp., *Staphylococcus* spp., *Streptococcus* spp., *Treponema* spp.	Ward et al. (2013)

[a]*Abbreviations: A.,* Actinomyces*; B.,* Bifidobacterium*; E.,* Escherichia*; En.,* Enterococcus*; F.,* Finegoldia*; G.,* Gemella*; K.,* Kocuria*; L.,* Lactobacillus*; Lc.,* Lactococcus*; Leuc.,* Leuconostoc*; P.,* Pediococcus*; Prop.,* Propionibacterium*; Ps.,* Pseudomonas*; R.,* Rothia*; S.,* Staphylococcus*; Str.,* Streptococcus*; W.,* Weissella.

[b]Sinkiewicz, G., Ljunggren, L., 2008. Occurrence of *Lactobacillus reuteri* in human breast milk. Microbial Ecology in Health and Disease 20, 122–126.

[c]Makino, H., Kushiro, A., Ishikawa, E., Muylaert, D., Kubota, H., Sakai, T., Oishi, K., Martin, R., Ben Amor, K., Oozeer, R., Knol, J., Tanaka, R., 2011. Transmission of intestinal *Bifidobacterium longum* subsp. *longum* strains from mother to infant, determined by multilocus sequencing typing and amplified fragment length polymorphism. Applied and Environmental Microbiology 77, 6788–6793.

production of antimicrobial compounds, such as bacteriocins, organic acids, reuterin, or hydrogen peroxide (Beasley and Saris, 2004; Heikkilä and Saris, 2003; Martín et al., 2005; Olivares et al., 2006).

The efficacy of oral administration of either *L. salivarius* CECT5713 or *L. gasseri.* CECT5714 in a pilot trial with 20 women was an effective alternative for treating staphylococcal mastitis in cases in which previous antibiotic therapy had been unsuccessful (Jiménez et al., 2008c). Later, a larger trial with 352 participants found that oral administration of each of two lactobacilli strains isolated from human milk, *L. fermentum* CECT5716 and *L. salivarius* CECT5713, were more effective than antibiotic therapy usually prescribed to treat lactational mastitis (Arroyo et al., 2010). Both studies showed not only the transfer of such strains from the maternal GI tract to the mammary gland and milk but, also, a notable or total improvement of the condition.

The main disadvantage of culture-dependent techniques seems to be the low number of cultivable species within any given ecological niche. Lack of knowledge of the real conditions under which most of the bacteria are growing in their natural environment may be one of the main factors affecting bacterial isolation. Therefore, the new cultivation techniques developed recently, or "culturomics" (Lagier et al., 2012; Singh et al., 2013), undoubtedly will contribute to increase the number of different bacterial species isolated from this source.

2. CULTURE-INDEPENDENT MOLECULAR TECHNIQUES

The cultivable microorganisms represent only a small fraction of natural microbial communities. Therefore, the application of culture-independent molecular techniques, and particularly those based on sequence divergences of the small subunit ribosomal RNA (16S rRNA) genes, has provided complementary biodiversity assessment of the human milk microbiome (Table 11.2).

However, each physical, chemical, and biological step involved in the molecular analysis of a microbial community represents a potential source of bias (von Wintzingerode et al., 1997). This molecular approach involves extraction of the DNA from the biological samples and polymerase chain reaction (PCR) amplification of 16S rRNA gene fragments with universal or group-specific bacterial primers. Regarding bacterial DNA extraction, insufficient or preferential lysis of cells will most likely result in bacterial composition bias. Gram-positive organisms typically require harsh conditions to disrupt the bacterial cell wall (which is thicker than in gram-negative bacteria), while the same conditions may cause excessive fragmentation of gram-negative chromosomal DNA affecting subsequent PCR amplification (Fraher et al., 2012). Another crucial point in the molecular analysis of a microbial community is PCR. Several factors can diminish the efficiency and accuracy of PCR, including primer-template mismatches, reactant concentrations, number of PCR cycles, annealing temperature, and complexity of the DNA template, among others (Mao et al., 2012). All of these factors should be taken in consideration when performing this type of analysis.

Various techniques, such as denaturing gradient gel electrophoresis (DGGE), temperature gradient gel electrophoresis (TGGE), real-time quantitative polymerase chain reaction (RT-qPCR), and next-generation sequencing of the 16S rRNA gene have been used to characterize the bacterial composition of human milk.

2.1 DENATURING GRADIENT GEL ELECTROPHORESIS AND TEMPERATURE GRADIENT GEL ELECTROPHORESIS

DGGE/TGGE are genetic fingerprinting techniques suitable for studies in microbial ecology. They were applied in microbial ecology in the 1990s (Muyzer et al., 1993) and had been widely used for human and environmental samples.

DGGE/TGGE separates complex mixtures of 16S rRNA gene amplicons, which are the same length but have different DNA sequences (Fig. 11.2). Separation is based on the decreased electrophoretic mobility of a partially melted double-stranded DNA molecule in a polyacrylamide gel that contains a linearly increasing gradient of denaturant (formamide and/or urea) (DGGE) or a linear temperature gradient (TGGE). Variations in DNA sequence result in different melting temperatures;

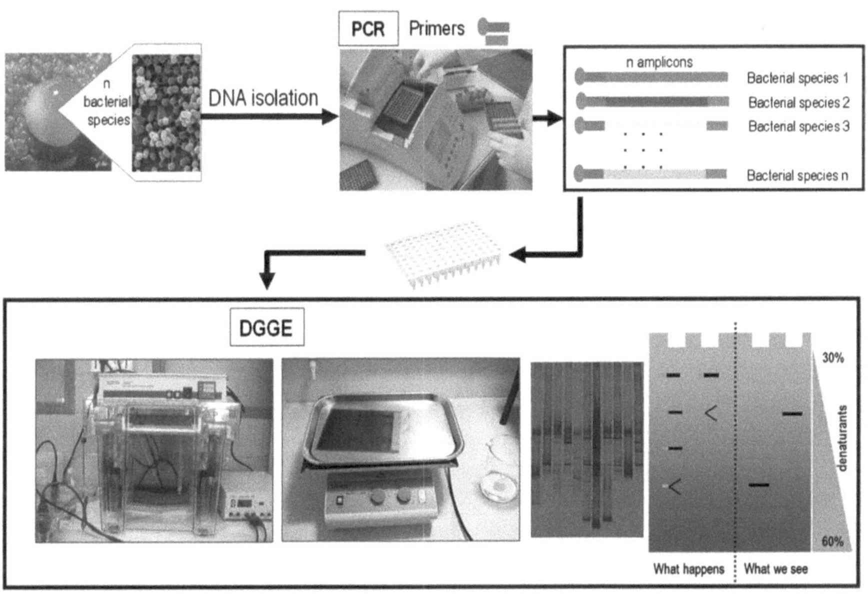

FIGURE 11.2

Schematic representation of the DGGE technique.

migration through the denaturant agent or temperature gradient gel halts at different positions, resulting in the separation of the amplicons that belong to different species.

TGGE has been used to examine the bacterial ribosomal DNA content in milk cells, maternal peripheral blood mononuclear cells, and feces obtained from mothers and their corresponding infants (Perez et al., 2007). Although milk cells had a less complex microbiota than maternal feces, TTGE revealed a greater biodiversity than observed previously when using classic plating methods. Some of the bands were identified after excision from the gel and sequencing. One band was particularly intense in infant fecal samples and comigrated with bands from maternal fecal and blood samples; this band was identified as *B. longum*. The presence of *B. longum* was also confirmed in the milk and infant feces obtained from four mother–infant dyads. This observation supports the hypothesis that bacteria found in human milk migrate within intestinally-derived cells from the maternal GI tract to the breast (Perez et al., 2007).

DGGE has extended the knowledge of the diversity and dominant bacteria existing in human milk of healthy women by using universal primers (Martin et al., 2007a) and primers initially targeting the *Lactobacillus* group, which included the genera *Leuconostoc, Pediococcus,* and *Weissella* (Martin et al., 2007b). In addition, the influence of the delivery method (vaginal delivery or cesarean section) in the acquisition of human milk bacteria has been investigated (Martín et al., 2007a,b). Samples of fresh human milk, vaginal swabs, and infant feces were collected from five mother–infant pairs and analyzed by DGGE. Cluster analysis of the DGGE profiles indicated that delivery-specific clustering could not be observed. In fact, unweighted pair group method with arithmetic mean (UPGMA) analysis revealed that sample profiles from the different mothers clustered together independently of the delivery mode (Martin et al., 2007a,b). On the other hand, none of the *Lactobacillus* phylotypes detected in the vaginal samples (*L. crispatus*, *Lactobacillus jensenii,* and *Lactobacillus inners*) were present in milk produced by the women whose neonates were born by vaginal delivery. This fact suggests that transit through the vagina does not play a determinant role in the establishment of lactobacilli found in human milk (Martin et al., 2007a,b).

Regarding the bacterial composition of milk from women with mastitis, DGGE had shown that infectious mastitis may be the consequence of a dysbiotic process leading to an overgrowth of certain bacterial species (Delgado et al., 2008). In this study where the milk samples of 20 women were analyzed, staphylococci were the dominant bacterial group and *Staphylococcus epidermidis* was the dominant species. Other bacteria (mainly streptococci and a few gram-negative species) were also identified in fewer samples. Globally, PCR-DGGE results were correlated with those obtained by culture-based methods (Delgado et al., 2008).

2.2 REAL-TIME QUANTITATIVE POLYMERASE CHAIN REACTION

The RT-qPCR technique is similar to the standard PCR except that the reaction mixture contains a DNA-binding dye that fluoresces when it binds to double-stranded

DNA, that is, the PCR product. The amount of DNA present in a sample can be quantified by comparison with DNA standards using a calibration curve.

RT-qPCR has been used to study the bacterial composition of human milk from healthy women (Collado et al., 2009; Gueimonde et al., 2007; Martin et al., 2009). The first studies focused on the detection of bifidobacteria (Gueimonde et al., 2007; Martin et al., 2009). This genus has been considered to represent the dominant component of the neonatal GI microbiota and consequently, human milk, which has been described as a source of bacteria influencing the development of the infant GI microbiota, should contain bifidobacterial DNA. Both studies, performed independently, reported that all the analyzed human milk samples contained bifidobacterial DNA confirming that this biological fluid is a source of bifidobacteria for the infant GI tract.

In order to detect and quantify several relevant bacterial groups that had never been found in human milk before, such as *Clostridium leptum–Faecalibacterium prausnitzii* subgroup (*Clostridium* cluster IV), *Clostridium coccoides–Eubacterium rectale* subgroup (*Clostridium* clusters XIVa and XIVb), and *Bacteroidetes* group (including *Prevotella* and *Porphyromonas*), another research group analyzed 50 human milk samples (Collado et al., 2009). Their results indicated that *Clostridium* XIVa–XIVb and *Enterococcus* were detected in most (>76%) of the samples in contrast to the *Bacteroides* and *Clostridium* cluster IV groups that were only found in 20 and two samples, respectively.

RT-qPCR has also been used to differentiate Raynaud's syndrome from infectious mastitis during lactation (Delgado et al., 2009). Milk samples from 10 lactating women, five with mastitis and the other five with Raynaud's syndrome, were analyzed with RT-qPCR. The concentration of total bacterial and staphylococcal DNA in mastitic milk were between 2 and 3 log units greater than those obtained from women with Raynaud's phenomenon symptoms.

More recently, bacterial composition of human milk from mothers with celiac disease has been assessed by RT-qPCR and compared with those from healthy women (Olivares et al., 2015). In this study, mothers with celiac disease had a reduction in the gene copy numbers of *Bifidobacterium* spp. and *B. fragilis* group in their milk compared with milk from healthy mothers. These results, together with the reduced abundance of immunoprotective compounds in human milk from women with celiac disease, could theoretically diminish the protective effect of breastfeeding on the child's future risk of developing celiac disease, although further prospective studies are needed (Olivares et al., 2015).

2.3 NEXT-GENERATION SEQUENCING

Genomic science has expanded considerably and the rate of genomic discovery has grown exponentially thanks to the innovations in high-throughput DNA sequencing, high-performance computing, and bioinformatics. Nowadays, there are several sequencing technologies that can be used for microbiome studies based on 16S rRNA taxonomic profiling, and shotgun metagenomics studies. Commercially available technologies include pyrosequencing (e.g., the Roche 454 Genome Sequencer

GS, FLX and FLX Titanium), Illumina's clonal arrays (e.g., the Illumina MiSeq and HiSeq2000), or parallel semiconductor-sensing device or ion chip of IonTorrent (e.g., the Ion S5 and Ion S5 XL).

The first research work that used next-generation sequencing to study the human milk microbiome was published in 2011 (Hunt et al., 2011). The authors performed pyrosequencing of the V1–V2 hypervariable regions of the 16S rRNA gene to characterize the bacterial communities present in milk samples from 16 healthy women at three time-points over 4 weeks. Results indicated a high interindividual variability but stability of the milk microbiome over time within an individual. The genera *Streptococcus, Staphylococcus,* and *Serratia* each represented more than 5% of the total DNA sequences of each sample. A core microbiome formed by nine genera (*Streptococcus, Staphylococcus, Serratia, Pseudomonas, Corynebacterium, Ralstonia, Propionibacterium, Sphingomonas*, and *Bradyrhizobium)* was present in every sample from every woman despite interindividual variability.

In a different pyrosequencing study in human milk samples, the presence of DNA of several major gut-associated obligate anaerobes such as *Bacteroides* and *Clostridia*, including butyrate producers, such as *Faecalibacterium* and *Roseburia*, which are important for colonic health was revealed (Jost et al., 2013). Several studies had shown that human milk provided a wealth of aerobic bacteria, which played a role in the colonization of the infant GI tract. However, anaerobic bacteria, which are very important in breastfeeding neonates, have been more difficult to detect in human milk.

Regarding the functional capability of the human milk microbiome, a metagenomic analysis of a pooled milk sample from 10 healthy donors was performed using an Illumina GAIIx Genome Analyzer (Ward et al., 2013). The objective of this study was not only to characterize the bacterial community but also to determine the types of bacterial open reading frames that may influence bacterial establishment and stability in this biological fluid. The results obtained in the analyzed pool sample showed over 360 prokaryotic genera, with sequences aligning predominantly to the genera *Pseudomonas*, *Staphylococcus*, and *Streptococcus*. The discovery of immunomodulatory motifs in this study indicates that more exhaustive analyses of the functionality of the human milk microbiome should be performed (Ward et al., 2013).

The use of 16S rRNA technology has greatly advanced our understanding of the bacterial composition of the human milk microbiota of healthy women. Identifying prenatal and postnatal factors or diseases that influence the composition of the bacterial communities in human milk is also a matter of utmost importance.

Milk samples from mothers who had elective but not from nonelective cesarean delivery contained a different bacterial community than milk samples from individuals who gave birth by vaginal delivery (Cabrera-Rubio et al., 2012). This finding suggests that it is not the surgery per se but rather the absence of physiological stress or hormonal signals that could influence the microbial transmission process from the gastrointestinal tract to the mammary gland (Cabrera-Rubio et al., 2012). On the other hand, milk samples from obese mothers contained a different and less diverse bacterial community compared with those from healthy-weight mothers (Cabrera-Rubio et al., 2012).

The metagenome of human milk samples obtained from healthy women and women with mastitis has revealed that the milk microbiome reflects a loss of bacterial diversity and a high increase in number of the sequences related to the presumptive etiological agents in mastitis cases (Jiménez et al., 2015). In fact, the results of this study clearly showed the strong effect of the pathogen responsible for acute mastitis (*S. aureus*) whose presence was associated with a drastic reduction of the microbial diversity in the samples; the Shannon-Weaver diversity index for these samples was lowest among all the samples included in this work. A less intense, but still noticeable, effect was demonstrated in the samples provided by the women who had subacute mastitis that showed a higher concentration of the genus *Staphylococcus* and the species *S. epidermidis* than healthy women (Jiménez et al., 2015).

Recently, the first report was published on the effects of chemotherapy on microbial and metabolomic profiles in human milk over a 4-month period in a breastfeeding woman undergoing treatment for Hodgkin's lymphoma (Urbaniak et al., 2014). The authors analyzed the bacterial composition of human milk samples by sequencing the V6 16S rRNA gene using the Ion Torrent platform. Results showed a decrease of *Bifidobacterium*, *Eubacterium*, *Staphylococcus,* and *Cloacibacterium* and an increase in *Acinetobacter*, *Xanthomonadaceae,* and *Stenotrophomonas* in human milk samples during chemotherapy. On the other hand, the metabolic profile, assessed by gas chromatography–mass spectrometry, also changed as a result of chemotherapy; the metabolites docosahexaenoic acid and inositol were decreased. These findings suggest that bacterial and metabolic composition of human milk, so critical for immunity and infant development, can change significantly after maternal exposure to chemotherapeutic agents (Urbaniak et al., 2014).

In summary, culture-dependent and -independent techniques have described in the past decade that human milk has its own complex microbiota (Table 11.2) affected by woman's health and physiology as well as predelivery and postdelivery factors. Differences observed in bacterial diversity among studies may result from different methodologies including selection of appropriate culture media, DNA isolation, PCR primers, etc. More studies focusing on the standardization of methodologic procedures are needed; likewise, characterization of similarities and differences in bacterial composition of human milk produced by women from different countries and lifestyles should be performed.

REFERENCES

Albesharat, R., Ehrmann, M.A., Korakli, M., Yazaji, S., Vogel, R.F., 2011. Phenotypic and genotypic analyses of lactic acid bacteria in local fermented food, breast milk and faeces of mothers and their babies. Systematic and Applied Microbiology 34, 148–155.

Arroyo, R., Martín, V., Maldonado, A., Jiménez, E., Fernández, L., Rodríguez, J.M., 2010. Treatment of infectious mastitis during lactation: antibiotics versus oral administration of lactobacilli isolated from breast milk. Clinical Infectious Diseases 50, 1551–1558.

Beasley, S.S., Saris, P.E.J., 2004. Nisin-producing *Lactococcus lactis* strains isolated from human milk. Applied and Environment Microbiology 70, 5051–5053.

Björkstén, B., Burman, L.G., De Chateau, P., Fredrikzon, B., Gothefors, L., Hernell, O., 1980. Collecting and banking human milk: to heat or not to heat? British Medical Journal 281, 765–769.

Cabrera-Rubio, R., Collado, M.C., Laitinen, K., Salminen, S., Isolauri, E., Mira, A., 2012. The human milk microbiome changes over lactation and is shaped by maternal weight and mode of delivery. American Journal of Clinical Nutrition 96, 544–551.

Collado, M.C., Delgado, S., Maldonado, A., Rodríguez, J.M., 2009. Assessment of the bacterial diversity of breast milk of healthy women by quantitative real time PCR. Letters in Applied Microbiology 48, 523–528.

Delgado, S., Collado, M.C., Fernández, L., Rodríguez, J.M., 2009. Bacterial analysis of breast milk: a tool to differentiate Raynaud's phenomenon from infectious mastitis during lactation. Current Microbiology 59, 59–64.

Delgado, S., Arroyo, R., Martín, R., Rodríguez, J.M., 2008. PCR-DGGE assessment of the bacterial diversity of breast milk in women with lactational infectious mastitis. BMC Infectious Diseases 8, 51.

Eidelman, A.I., Szilagyi, G., 1979. Patterns of bacterial colonization of human milk. Obstetrics & Gynecology 53, 550–552.

Fernández, L., Langa, S., Martín, V., Maldonado, A., Jiménez, E., Martín, R., Rodríguez, J.M., 2013. The human milk microbiota: origin and potential roles in health and disease. Pharmacology Research 69, 1–10.

Fraher, M.H., O'Toole, P.W., Quigley, E.M.M., 2012. Techniques used to characterize the gut microbiota: a guide for the clinician. Nature Reviews Gastroenterology & Hepatology 9, 312–322.

Gueimonde, M., Laitinen, K., Salminen, S., Isolauri, E., 2007. Breastmilk: a source ofbifidobacteria for infant gut development and maturation? Neonatology 92, 64–66.

Heikkilä, M.P., Saris, P.E.J., 2003. Inhibition of *Staphylococcus aureus* by the commensal bacteria of human milk. Journal of Applied Microbiology 95, 471–478.

Hunt, K.M., Foster, J.A., Forney, L.J., Schütte, U.M.E., Beck, D.L., Abdo, Z., Fox, L.K., Williams, J.E., McGuire, M.K., McGuire, M.A., 2011. Characterization of the diversity and temporal stability of bacterial communities in human milk. PLoS ONE 6, e21313.

Jiménez, E., Delgado, S., Maldonado, A., Arroyo, R., Albújar, M., García, N., Jariod, M., Fernández, L., Gómez, A., Rodríguez, J.M., 2008a. *Staphylococcus epidermidis*: a differential trait of the fecal microbiota of breast-fed infants. BMC Microbiology 8, 143.

Jiménez, E., Fernández, L., Delgado, S., García, N., Albújar, M., Gómez, A., Rodríguez, J.M., 2008b. Assessment of the bacterial diversity of human colostrum by cultural-based techniques. Analysis of the staphylococcal and enterococcal populations. Research in Microbiology 159, 595–601.

Jiménez, E., Fernández, L., Maldonado, A., Martín, R., Olivares, M., Xaus, J., Rodríguez, J.M., 2008c. Oral administration of lactobacilli strains isolated from breast milk as an alternative for the treatment of infectious mastitis during lactation. Applied and Environment Microbiology 74, 4650–4655.

Jiménez, E., de Andrés, J., Manrique, M., Pareja-Tobes, P., Tobes, R., Martínez-Blanch, J.F., Codoñer, F.M., Ramón, D., Fernández, L., Rodríguez, J.M., 2015. Metagenomic analysis of milk of healthy and mastitis-suffering women. Journal of Human Lactation 31, 406–415.

Jost, T., Lacroix, C., Braegger, C., Chassard, C., 2013. Assessment of bacterial diversity in breast milk using culture-dependent and culture-independent approaches. British Journal of Nutrition 110, 1253–1262.

Lagier, J.C., Armougom, F., Million, M., Hugon, P., Pagnier, I., Robert, C., Bittar, F., Fournous, G., Gimenez, G., Maraninchi, M., Trape, J.F., Koonin, E.V., La Scola, B., Raoult, D., 2012. Microbial culturomics: paradigm shift in the human gut microbiome study. Clinical Microbiology and Infection 18, 1185–1193.

Law, B.J., Urias, B.A., Lertzman, J., Robson, D., Romance, L., 1989. Is ingestion of milk-associated bacteria by premature infants fed raw human milk controlled by routine bacteriologic screening? Journal of Clinical Microbiology 1560–1566.

Lucas, A., Roberts, C.D., 1979. Bacteriological quality control in human milk-banking. British Medical Journal 1, 80–82.

Mao, D.P., Zhou, Q., Chen, C.Y., Quan, Z.X., 2012. Coverage evaluation of universal bacterial primers using the metagenomic datasets. BMC Microbiology 12, 66.

Martín, R., Langa, S., Reviriego, C., Jiménez, E., Marín, M.L., Xaus, J., Fernández, L., Rodríguez, J.M., 2003. Human milk is a source of lactic acid bacteria for the infant gut. Journal of Pediatrics 143, 754–758.

Martín, R., Langa, S., Reviriego, C., Jiménez, E., Marín, M.L., Olivares, M., Boza, J., Jiménez, J., Fernández, L., Xaus, J., Rodríguez, J.M., 2004. The commensal microflora of human milk: new perspectives for food bacteriotherapy and probiotics. Trends in Food Science and Technology 15, 121–127.

Martín, R., Olivares, M., Marín, M.L., Xaus, J., Rodriguez, J.M., 2005. Probiotic potential of 3 *Lactobacilli* strains isolated from breast milk. Journal of Human Lactation 21, 18–21.

Martín, R., Heilig, H.G., Zoetendal, E.G., Jiménez, E., Fernández, L., Smidt, H., Rodríguez, J.M., 2007a. Cultivation-independent assessment of the bacterial diversity of breast milk among healthy women. Research in Microbiology 158, 31–37.

Martín, R., Heilig, H.G., Zoetendal, E.G., Smidt, H., Rodríguez, J.M., 2007b. Diversity of the *Lactobacillus* group in breast milk and vagina of healthy women and potential role in the colonization of the infant gut. Journal of Applied Microbiology 103, 2638–2644.

Martín, R., Jiménez, E., Heilig, H.G., Fernández, L., Marín, M.L., Zoetendal, E.G., Rodríguez, J.M., 2009. Isolation of bifidobacteria from breast milk and assessment of the bifidobacterial population by PCR-denaturing gradient gel electrophoresis and quantitative real-time PCR. Applied and Environment Microbiology 75, 965–969.

Martín, R., Jiménez, E., Olivares, M., Marín, M.L., Fernández, L., Xaus, J., Rodríguez, J.M., 2006. Lactobacillus salivarius CECT 5713, a potential probiotic strain isolated from infant feces and breast milk of a mother-child pair. International Journal of Food Microbiology 112, 35–43.

Martín, V., Mañés-Lázaro, R., Rodríguez, J.M., Maldonado, A., 2011. *Streptococcus lactarius* sp. nov., isolated from breast milk of healthy women. International Journal of Systematic and Evolutionary Microbiology 61, 1048–1052.

Martín, V., Maldonado, A., Moles, L., Rodríguez-Baños, M., Del Campo, R., Fernández, L., Rodríguez, J.M., Jiménez, E., 2012. Sharing of bacterial strains between breast milk and infant feces. Journal of Human Lactation 28, 36–44.

Muyzer, G., de Waal, E.C., Uitterlinden, A.G., 1993. Profiling of complex microbial populations by denaturing gradient gel electrophoresis analysis of polymerase chain reaction-amplified genes coding for 16S rRNA. Applied and Environmental Microbiology 59, 695–700.

Olivares, M., Díaz-Ropero, M.P., Martín, R., Rodríguez, J.M., Xaus, J., 2006. Antimicrobial potential of four *Lactobacillus* strains isolated from breast milk. Journal of Applied Microbiology 101, 72–79.

Olivares, M., Albrecht, S., De Palma, G., Ferrer, M.D., Castillejo, G., Schols, H.A., Sanz, Y., 2015. Human milk composition differs in healthy mothers and mothers with celiac disease. European Journal of Nutrition 54, 119–128.

Perez, P.F., Doré, J., Leclerc, M., Levenez, F., Benyacoub, J., Serrant, P., Segura-Roggero, I., Schiffrin, E.J., Donnet-Hughes, A., 2007. Bacterial imprinting of the neonatal immune system: lessons from maternal cells? Pediatrics 119, e724–e732.

Rodríguez, J.M., 2014. The origin of human milk bacteria: is there a bacterial entero-mammary pathway during late pregnancy and lactation? Advances in Nutrition 5, 779–784.

Singh, S., Eldin, C., Kowalczewska, M., Raoult, D., 2013. Axenic culture of fastidious and intracellular bacteria. Trends in Microbiology 21, 92–99.

Urbaniak, C., McMillan, A., Angelini, M., Gloor, G.B., Sumarah, M., Burton, J.P., Reid, G., 2014. Effect of chemotherapy on the microbiota and metabolome of human milk, a case report. Microbiome 2, 24.

von Wintzingerode, F., Gobel, U.B., Stackebrandt, E., 1997. Determination of microbial diversity in environmental samples: pitfalls of PCR-based rRNA analysis. FEMS Microbiology Reviews 21, 213–229.

Ward, T.L., Hosid, S., Ioshikhes, I., Altosaar, I., 2013. Human milk metagenome: a functional capacity analysis. BMC Microbiology 13, 116.

West, P.A., Hewitt, J.H., Murphy, O.M., 1979. The influence of methods of collection and storage on the bacteriology of human milk. Journal of Applied Bacteriology 46, 269–277.

CHAPTER

Maternal Factors Related to Variability in the Human Milk Microbiome

12

Izaskun Garcia-Mantrana[1,a], Carlos Gómez-Gallego[2,3,a], Raul Cabrera-Rubio[1,4], Maria Carmen Collado[1]

[1]Institute of Agrochemistry and Food Technology-National Research Council (IATA-CSIC), Valencia, Spain; [2]University of Murcia, Murcia, Spain; [3]University of Turku, Turku, Finland; [4]TEAGASC Food Research Centre, Cork, Ireland

1. INTRODUCTION

Infant contact with microbes is initially provided by the maternal microbial communities. The microbial colonization process in infants affects metabolic and immunological development (Hooper and Macpherson, 2010; Hooper et al., 2012). The microbiota that colonize a healthy, breastfed, vaginally-delivered, full-term baby who remains healthy for a long follow-up period are considered the gold standard. Any alterations in this process may be associated with aberrancies leading to a higher risk of developing non-communicable diseases (NCDs) (Collado et al., 2015a; Rodriguez et al., 2015). The development of the human gastrointestinal (GI) microbiome is a complex and stepwise process that is thought to be initiated at birth when maternal microbes come in contact with the infant through delivery and then is supported by breastfeeding. Continual exposure to new microbes throughout life may alter the human microbiome. However, this understanding is currently changing as microorganisms have been found in the maternal-neonatal interfaces such as placenta, amniotic fluid, fetal membranes, umbilical cord, and also, in meconium, and colostrum (Jiménez et al., 2008; Domínguez-Bello et al., 2010; Vaishampayan et al., 2010; Aagaard et al., 2014; Hansen et al., 2015). At birth, the mode of delivery and other perinatal factors, such as gestational age, antibiotic treatment, and instrumentation, may also influence the establishment of the first microbiota (Dominguez-Bello et al., 2010).

Microbial alterations depending related to mode of delivery have been described to be associated with infant microbial colonization and differ in infants born by cesarean section (C-section) compared with infants born vaginally (Dominguez-Bello et al., 2010; Valles et al., 2014; Azad et al., 2015; Bäckhed et al., 2015). Modern society is experiencing a progressive increase in immunological and metabolic

[a]Both authors contributed equally to this work.

Prebiotics and Probiotics in Human Milk. http://dx.doi.org/10.1016/B978-0-12-802725-7.00012-9

diseases, and the increase is particularly alarming in infants. This situation could be linked to the increase in C-section births, which have exponentially increased beyond the 15% recommended by the World Health Organization (WHO, 2015), and with the decrease in exclusive breastfeeding practices (Victora et al., 2016). An increased risk for specific diseases such as asthma, allergic diseases, celiac disease, and obesity has been described for C-section infants (Decker et al., 2010; Kulas et al., 2013; Dogra et al., 2015) and for infants who are not breastfed in early life (Horta et al., 2013; Minnitti et al., 2014; Li et al., 2014; Stuebe, 2015; Lodge et al., 2015).

Breastfeeding represents the main postnatal link between mother and infant. It is considered protective and stimulates innate immunity (Petherick, 2010; Walker, 2010). Human milk (HM) is unique in its ability to fulfill infant nutritional requirements, and its composition "constantly" adapts to neonatal requirements. Human milk contains bioactive components that directly influence and shape the intestinal microbiota colonization. Beyond its nutritional characteristics, HM contains many immuno-modulatory substances, such as hormones, cytokines, growth factors, antibodies, and microRNA. In addition, HM contains compounds, such as lysozyme, proteins and peptides, oligosaccharides, and bacteria, which may also reinforce the immuno-modulatory and protective properties (Petherick, 2010; Walker, 2010; Lawrence and Lawrence, 2011). A delicate and complex balance of these components in conjunction with other as-of-yet uncharacterized components in milk are transferred from mother to infant via breastfeeding.

It has been suggested that perinatal factors may affect the mother-infant transfer of microbial and bioactive compounds during breastfeeding. Perinatal microbial transfer would provide novel targets for developing nutritional and dietary tools to reduce the risk of diseases in the infant population. Likewise, these potential data may drive the identification of new targets to support an adequate microbial contact mainly in those cases where the microbial contact will be not adequate (C-section, antibiotic use, etc).

HM is the key postnatal element for the metabolic, microbial and immunological programming of an infant's health (Aaltonen et al., 2011). Right after birth, the microbial transfer is supported by breastfeeding, (Roger et al., 2010; Jost et al., 2014, 2015; Vallés et al., 2014; Azad et al., 2015). *Bifidobacterium* spp. are more common in feces from breastfed infants than in formula-fed infants, and it was recently reported that specific intestinal *Bifidobacterium* strains are transmitted from mothers to breastfed infants (Makino et al., 2011, 2013; Takanashi et al., 2010). Human milk contains a high diversity of microbes that may drive microbial colonization in infants (Cabrera-Rubio et al., 2012; Hunt et al., 2011; Jost et al., 2013, 2014). HM also contains complex carbohydrates, oligosaccharides with prebiotic characteristics and activity that favor the growth of specific GI bacterial groups such as *Staphylococcus* and *Bifidobacterium* spp. (Zivkovic et al., 2011; Hunt et al., 2012). In addition, the maternal transmission of specific intestinal microbes, such as *Bifidobacterium* and *Staphylococcus* spp., to infants has been described (Makino et al., 2011, 2013; Benito et al., 2015). Those results suggest that each mother-infant dyads share specific microbes and suggest the potential biological role of maternal microbes to infant's health.

2. HUMAN MILK MICROBIOME

Historically, HM was considered sterile fluid, but this idea has changed in recent years. Accumulating evidence has shown the presence of microbes in milk with culture-dependent techniques, and most are *Staphylococcus*, *Streptococcus*, *Lactobacillus,* and *Bifidobacterium* spp. The development and application of culture-independent techniques confirmed the presence of microbial DNA and the existence of a rich and diverse HM microbial community (Gueimonde et al., 2007; Hunt et al., 2011; Jost et al., 2013; Martin et al., 2003; McGuire and McGuire, 2015). Despite the evidence, the scientific community is concerned that microbes in HM are from cross-contamination of maternal skin and infant oral cavity. However, the detection of live bacteria and the presence of strictly anaerobic species such as *Bifidobacterium*, *Clostridium*, and *Bacteroides* (Jost et al., 2013) that are usually related to GI environments and that cannot survive in aerobic environments have sustained the discussion about the origin of HM bacteria. More recently, high throughput sequencing showed the presence of anaerobic gut-associated strictly anaerobic microbes in the *Clostridia* family (*Blautia*, *Clostridium*, *Collinsella*, and *Veillonella*) in HM, and they are shared among the maternal intestinal microbiota, milk, and the infant intestinal microbiota (Jost et al., 2014, 2015). Furthermore, butyrate-producing bacteria, such as *Coprococcus*, *Faecalibacterium*, and *Roseburia*, are also present and shared in maternal feces and HM. The origin of the bacteria in HM is currently not known, but recent findings suggest a connection between the maternal GI microbiota and mammary tissue through an enteromammary pathway (Rodriguez et al., 2014; Fernandez et al., 2013; Rautava et al., 2015).

Studies have shown that HM harbors a unique microbial ecosystem that differs from other human niches. The milk microbiota are not linked to mucosal or fecal samples and do not seem to be a subset of any specific human niche (Cabrera-Rubio et al., 2012). The diversity of the microbiota in HM has been studied by different research groups (Cabrera-Rubio et al., 2012; Hunt et al., 2011; Jost et al., 2014; Fernandez et al., 2013), suggesting that *Staphylococcus* spp., *Enterococcus* spp., *Streptococcus* spp., and other lactic acid bacteria are the most common groups. The first study on the milk microbiome using pyrosequencing showed that milk bacterial communities are generally complex (Hunt et al., 2011). Among the microbial diversity present in each breast milk sample, specific bacteria such as *Streptococcus*, *Staphylococcus*, *Serratia*, *Pseudomonas*, *Corynebacterium*, *Ralstonia*, *Propionibacterium*, *Sphingomonas*, and *Bradyrhizobiaceae* were detected in all samples (Hunt et al., 2011). The bacterial complexity of human breast milk was later confirmed although differences were reported due to different sampling and process protocols, DNA extraction, and sequencing platforms (Cabrera-Rubio et al., 2012; Jost et al., 2014; McGuire and McGuire, 2015).

Microbes have been also detected in human mammary tissue (Urbaniak et al., 2014a; Xuan et al., 2014), suggesting that specific microbes inhabit the mammary epithelia, and likely milk ducts. The milk microbiota have also been described in the rhesus monkey (O'Sullivan et al., 2013) and in other mammals such as the cow

(Quigley et al., 2013). However, the biological influence of those milk microbes on infant health has not been resolved (Cabrera-Rubio et al., 2012), although it has been a key challenge in research during the last decade.

3. POTENTIAL FACTORS INFLUENCING THE HUMAN MILK MICROBIOME

Although in the past HM was considered homogeneous, variations in its composition have recently received more research attention, and considerable individual variation has been documented (Quinn et al., 2012). The composition of HM is influenced by genetic factors, mode of delivery, and maternal nutrition, and differs among feeds, time of day, and lactation stage and between mothers and populations. However, scarce data are available on the relationship between perinatal factors on maternal microbiota including HM microbes and other bioactive compouunds. The potential modifications and shifts in the composition of the HM microbiota may have biological implications for infant microbial colonization and for the development and maturation of the infant immune system, rendering infants more susceptible to specific diseases and disorders later in life.

3.1 LACTATION PERIOD

Human milk is a dynamic, complex fluid that changes in composition from colostrum to mature milk according to an infant's nutritional requirements. Colostrum contains higher amounts of immunological compounds, including cytokines, secretory immunoglobulin A (IgA), lactoferrin, as well as epidermal growth factor (EGF) and transforming growth factor-beta (TGF-β), suggesting that colostrum has primary immunological and trophic targets instead of nutritional function. Transitional milk is similar to colostrum and this transition period represents a critical milk production period during which nutritional and developmental needs increase. After this period, milk is considered more stable and mature.

It has been reported that the milk bacterial community is generally stable over time within an individual (Hunt et al., 2011), but specific shifts in microbial compositions in HM during lactation have been observed. The use of 454 pyrosequencing demonstrated large microbial biodiversity in colostrum samples and then mild temporal variations in the milk microbiome during first 6 months of breastfeeding (Cabrera-Rubio et al., 2012). The initial microbial community of colostrum in a study of Finnish mothers was dominated by *Weissella*, *Leuconostoc*, *Staphylococcus*, *Streptococcus*, and *Lactococcus* spp., whereas in mature milk, a significant increase in *Veillonella*, *Prevotella*, and *Leptotrichia* took place. In another study, while *Lactobacillus, Streptococcus*, and *Enterococcus* spp. were predominant, the *Bifidobacterium* and *Enterococcus* spp. in particular increased throughout the lactation period (Khodayar-Pardo et al., 2014).

3.2 MATERNAL DIET/NUTRITION

Studies on how the maternal diet modulates HM microbiota are scarce. Most studies find weak or modest associations between maternal diet and the macronutrient composition of the mother's milk (Chang et al., 2015; Quinn et al., 2012; Yang et al., 2014), although maternal nutrition may be compromised. However, other nutrients, such as vitamins A and D, several water-soluble vitamins (including vitamin B_6, vitamin B_{12}, and folate), iodine and selenium, and certain fatty acids, quickly respond to changes in the mother's diet (Harzer et al., 1984; Innis, 2014; Ares Segura et al., 2015). The relationship between dietary constituents and the composition of the intestinal microbiota from lactating mothers has been reported (Carrothers et al., 2015). The main finding was a positive relationship between vitamin B_{12} intake and Proteobacteria. However, other studies on populations with religious fasting showed that this practice affects some of the micronutrients of HM such as zinc, magnesium, and potassium (Rakicioğlu et al., 2006). Moreover, studies have reported that cyclical changes in the GI microbiota from feeding/fasting rhythms may alter the microbial diversity and likely represent a potential host–microbiota mechanism by which the bacteria may affect human metabolism (Zarrinpar et al., 2014). Although more studies are needed, if feeding patterns and time of harvest modulate the intestinal microbiota and HM micronutrients, changes in the HM microbiota might also be expected. Shared microbial features between bacteria present in local foods and traditional vegetable-, dairy-, and meat-based probiotic foods (e.g., Siria hand-made products such as *kishk*, *shanklish*, and *makdous*) and mother–infant microbial GI tract and HM have been reported (Albesharat et al., 2011). In summary, there is some (albeit weak) data suggesting a role for maternal diet in modulating microbial transfer from mother to infants.

However, HM contains substantial amounts of lipids, which are present as globules composed of nonpolar lipids, including triglycerides, cholesterol esters, retinyl esters, and other lipophilic nutrients, surrounded by the milk fat globule membrane. HM lipid concentrations vary widely between individuals, but this variability appears to be largely independent of maternal nutrition (Innis, 2014). However, HM fatty acids are derived from endogenous synthesis in the mammary gland and uptake from the maternal plasma, and both sources are influenced by maternal nutrition (Innis, 2014). The long-chain polyunsaturated fatty acid content in HM, especially linoleic acid (LA), arachidonic acid (AA), docosahexaenoic acid (DHA), and eicosapentaenoic acid (EPA), and the ω-3 to ω-6 ratio vary widely as a result of diverse food consumption (Nishimura et al., 2014; Peng et al., 2009), without changes in total fatty acids. This variation could be explained by differences in maternal fish and/or fish oil supplement intake (Harris et al., 1984; Lauritzen et al., 2002). Human milk fatty acids possess immunomodulatory properties, and the presence of fatty acids in milk could be modulated by probiotic intake (Hoppu et al., 2012), but no information about whether dietary fatty acids modulate the milk microbiota has been published. However, an assay with atopic mothers showed that ω-3 polyunsaturated fatty acid supplementation increases IgA and the soluble form of CD14 (sCD14) levels in HM

(Dunstan et al., 2004), which may affect the milk microbiota. Moreover, maternal consumption of high-fat dairy products increased milk lipid content and expression of genes related to the biosynthesis of milk lipids, which may also have an effect on the milk microbiota (Yahvah et al., 2015).

Other compounds that could be present in HM are volatile compounds. Volatile compounds related to the flavor from vegetables and foods, such as garlic, beer, eucalyptus, tea, several spices, or carrots, are present in HM and can be perceived by breastfed children (Mennella and Beauchamp, 1991, 1993, 1999; Denzer et al., 2015). Some of these volatile compounds exert antioxidant and antibacterial activities (Lu et al., 2011; Bugarin et al., 2014), and the presence of these volatile compounds in HM may affect the microbiota due to these activities.

The growth factors naturally present in HM polyamines might affect the milk microbiome. A correlation between dietary polyamine intake and polyamine concentration in HM has been demonstrated (Atiya Ali et al., 2014). Animal studies have shown that polyamines play an important role modulating the microbiota along the GI tract during lactation (Gómez-Gallego et al., 2014). Due to their effect on cell proliferation, different levels of polyamines in HM probably modulate the microbiota, but data are not available to test this hypothesis. Future studies should investigate the interactions among nutrients in the maternal diet and the HM microbiota and their health effects on infants.

3.3 MODE OF DELIVERY

The mode of delivery is also associated with variation in the macronutrient composition of HM (Dizdar et al., 2014). Vaginal births are associated with higher protein content in colostrum samples compared to colostrum produced by women who underwent C-section births. These results suggest that hormonal activity during labor might affect the protein composition of milk to facilitate optimal development of important physiologic functions in newborns.

The mode of delivery is also related to variation in the composition of the neonatal GI microbiota. Several studies have shown differences in the composition of the intestinal microbiota among infants depending on the mode of delivery (Dominguez-Bello et al., 2010). In addition, the GI microbiota of infants delivered by C-section were different than their mothers' GI microbiota (Backed et al., 2015), but only a few studies examined if delivery mode is associated with variation in the composition of the HM microbiota. HM from vaginal deliveries show higher microbial diversity and distinct microbial composition compared to that produced by women who delivered by C-section (Cabrera-Rubio et al., 2012, 2015; Khodayar-Pardo et al., 2014) although other studies did not report differences in microbial profiles based on gestation, mode of delivery, or infant gender (Urbaniak et al., 2016). Higher bacterial concentrations in colostrum and transitional milk have been reported in C-section deliveries (Cabrera-Rubio et al., 2012). Nevertheless, *Bifidobacterium* spp. was detected more frequently in HM from mothers with vaginal deliveries than in mothers with C-secton deliveries (Khodayar-Pardo et al., 2014).

Another study (Cabrera-Rubio et al., 2012) showed that milk from mothers who gave birth by elective C-section delivery but not from mothers with nonelective C-section deliveries contained a different bacterial composition than milk samples from mothers who gave birth vaginally. The mothers with elective C-section deliveries showed a significant compositional shift compared with the other two groups of mothers. The composition of the HM microbiota of the mothers with nonelective C-sections was more similar to that of mothers who gave birth vaginally, reinforcing the hypothesis of the role of physiological stress or hormonal signals could contribute to the microbial transmission process to milk (Cabrera-Rubio et al., 2012). Furthermore, decreased bacterial diversity has been reported in C-section samples compared with vaginal samples. Milk from women undergoing C-section deliveries and/or who received anesthesia or antibiotics during delivery tended to be less likely to contain lactobacilli (Soto et al., 2014). Decreased bacterial diversity has been associated with children developing various allergic conditions (Wang et al., 2008; Forno et al., 2008); infants delivered by C-section have different and less diverse GI microbial composition (Jakobsson et al., 2014) and are more prone to developing NCDs such as allergies, asthma, type 1 diabetes, and also, obesity (Barros et al., 2012; Cardwell et al., 2008). More studies are needed to understand the perinatal factors influencing milk bacterial communities and how they have an impact on neonatal and maternal health.

3.4 GESTATIONAL AGE

The composition of the HM microbiota is influenced by gestational age, according to a study that collected milk samples from prematurely ended pregnancies from 24 weeks onward (Khodayar-Pardo et al., 2014). Significant differences in HM microbiota were found between term and preterm groups and throughout the different stages of lactation. Lower counts of *Enterococcus* spp. in colostrum and higher presence of *Bifidobacterium* spp. were detected in milk samples from term deliveries. Taking into consideration that the milk of the mothers in the preterm delivery group presents specific microbiota characteristics, suggests that those differences may have an potential biological role in preterm infants. Human milk from preterm deliveries showed slightly different compositions, at least for the first several weeks, and this difference may be further studied as those changed would fit to meet the infant's particular needs as happen with nutritional compounds as proteins and fat in milk. Necrotizing enterocolitis (NEC) is one of the most common diseases in preterm babies, and HM helps in the prevention of this disease (Good et al., 2014; Collado et al., 2015b). Sometimes infants with NEC cannot breastfeed from their mothers, but specifically in this group, it is important to emphasize and promote HM consumption and/or to promote donor breast milk. Usually, donor milk is pasteurized (processed) to avoid potential contaminations to be transferred to the neonates. This thermal processing affects not only nutritional but also immunological quality (Espinosa-Martos et al., 2013; Garcia-Lara et al., 2013; Sousa et al., 2014). Therefore, further investigation is required to determine the impact of pasteurization and storage of HM and how they impact on infant health.

3.5 MATERNAL HEALTH

Specific microbial shifts in human milk have been associated with health status such as obesity, allergy, celiac disease, and HIV (Cabrera-Rubio et al., 2012; Collado et al., 2012; Olivares et al., 2015 and Gonzalez et al., 2013). In a recent study, HM from HIV-positive African women had more bacterial diversity and frequency of *Lactobacillus* spp. and lower frequency of *Staphylococcus* spp., including *S. hominis* and *S. aureus,* than non–HIV-positive women (González et al., 2013). Human milk from mothers with celiac disease is characterized by a reduced concentration of immunoprotective compounds (TGF-β1 and sIgA) and relative abundance of *Bifidobacterium* spp. and *Bacteroides fragilis* groups compared with that from healthy mothers (Olivares et al., 2015). Obesity and allergies are also related to the *Bifidobacterium* spp. levels present in HM (Gronlund et al., 2007; Collado et al., 2012). In addition, a study reported that maternal obesity and excessive weight gain during pregnancy was associated with the concentrations of specific immune factors in milk; TGF-β2, sCD14, and cytokines were lower in milk produced by obese mothers compared with milk produced by non-obese mothers (Collado et al., 2012). Reduction in bacterial diversity is also related to obesity (Cabrera-Rubio et al., 2012). Lower abundance of *Bifidobacterium* group bacteria and higher relative abundance of *Staphylococcus* group numbers were reported in milk produced by obese women (Collado et al., 2012). The greater concentrations or abundance of *Bifidobacterium* spp. in healthy infants would suggest the beneficial and protective role against the risk of diseases attributed to HM (Le Huërou-Luron et al., 2010), and also, the higher abundance of this bacterial group in exclusively breastfed infant microbiota (Gueimonde et al., 2007; Jost et al., 2015). The results indicate a relationship between obesity, microbiota, and breastfeeding. In this scenario, the biological impact of milk microbes on infant health is unknown and remains a key question in scientific research.

A better understanding about the role of maternal health in mediating maternal microbes including milk microbiota is needed (Fig. 12. 1).

3.6 GEOGRAPHIC LOCATION

Due to the strong geographic influence on the composition of GI microbial populations (Yatsunenko et al., 2012), geographic influences on pathways related to vitamin biosynthesis and carbohydrate metabolism has been observed. Yatsunenko et al. (2012) examined how GI microbes differ between human populations and compared 531 healthy Amerindian, Malawian, and American metropolitan inhabitants. Aside from less diversity among inhabitants in developed communities in the United States, the researchers observed differences in the metabolic profiles. As expected, compared with adults, infant microbiomes were enriched in genes involved in the forage of glycans present in HM and the intestinal mucosa. Several bacterial genes involved in using these host glycans were overrepresented in the Amerindian and Malawian compared with the US infant microbiomes. These population-specific biomarkers may reflect differences

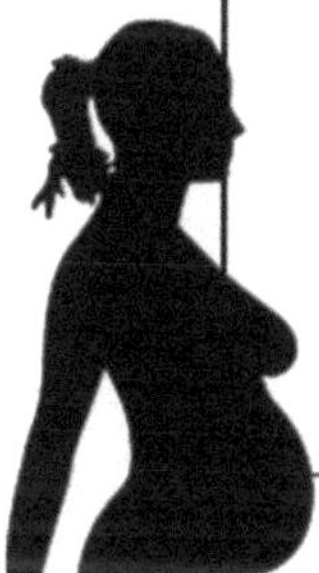
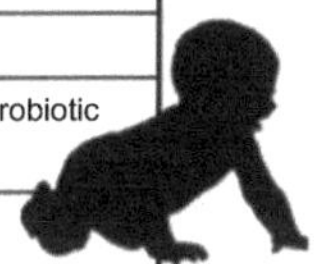

Factor		Changes in milk microbiota and immune factors
Lactation period	Calostrum	*Weisella, Leuconostoc, Staphylococcus, Streptococcus* and *Lactococcus*
	Mature Milk	*Veillonella, Prevotella , Leptotricia Lactobacillus, Streptococcus and Enterococcus, Bifidobacterium* and *Enterococcus*
Delivery	C-section	↑Bacterial concentrations ↓ *Bifidobacterium* ↓Bacterial diversity
Diet	Feeding/fasting rhythms	Changes in diversity
	ω-3 polyunsaturated fatty acids	Changes in IgA and sCD14 levels on breast milk
	Volatile compounds related with flavor from vegetables	Antibacterial activities
	Polyamines	
	Probiotics	Effect dependent of the probiotic strains
Gestational age	Term	↓*Enterococcus* ↑ *Bifidobacterium*
	Preterm	↑*Enterococcus* ↓ *Bifidobacterium*
Maternal health	Obesity Allergy Celiac disease	Changes in *Bifidobacterium*
	HIV	↑*Lactobacillus* ↓*Staphylococcus*
Geographical location		
Antibiotics, chemotherapy, medicines and others	Antibiotics Chemotherapy	↓bacterial diversity

FIGURE 12.1

Summary of the main factors that may modulate human milk microbiota and immune factors. Changes in human milk microbiota may lead to alterations in the infant GI microbiome with implications for infant health.

in the glycan content of HM. The presence of glycoside hydrolases decreased as the Malawian and Amerindian infants matured and transitioned to a diet dominated by vegetables including maize, cassava, and other plant-derived polysaccharides. In contrast, α-L-fucosidase gene representation in the US infants showed an increased trend (Rho = 0.29 and p value = .09) with age (Yatsunenko et al., 2012).

Differences in HM composition have been reported in mothers under different environmental exposures such as living in rural areas and being exposed to farm animals (Tomicic et al., 2010; Holmlund et al., 2010). Country of birth (Africa, Swedish immigrants, and native Swedish) was associated with variation in the immunological profiles (cytokine/chemokines) in HM, and how HM produced by women from different countries was associated with the host response (cord blood mononuclear cells (CBMCs) and intestinal epithelial cells) was investigated (Holmlund et al., 2010). Nonlactating mammary tissue microbiomes from women living in Canada and Ireland were different (Urnaniak et al., 2014a). The most abundant taxa in the Canadian samples were *Bacillus, Acinetobacter,* Enterobacteriaceae, and *Staphylococcus* spp. while in the Irish samples, the most abundant taxa were Enterobacteriaceae and *Staphylococcus*, followed by *Listeria* spp. Differences in microbiomes between women with breast cancer and healthy women were detected in both locations, Canada and Ireland. In HM from African mothers, *Staphylococcus* spp., *Streptococcus* spp., and lactic acid bacteria species were the main bacterial groups present according to traditional culture-dependent methods, while according to molecular techniques, the most predominant groups were *Streptococcus* followed by *Staphylococcus*, *Enterococcus*, *Bifidobacterium*, and lactic acid bacteria groups in African mothers (Gonzalez et al., 2013). These results showed similar bacterial profiles than those studies conducted with European women in whom *Staphylococcus* and lactic acid bacteria such as *Enterococcus* and *Lactococcus* were the most common microbes isolated from HM (Jost et al., 2014; Cabrera-Rubio et al., 2012, 2015). These data suggest the presence of a microbial core in HM formed by *Staphylococcus*, *Streptococcus*, and lactic acid bacteria. However, large-scale studies with samples from different geographic locations are needed.

3.7 ANTIBIOTICS, CHEMOTHERAPY, MEDICATIONS, AND OTHERS

Recently, Soto et al. (2014) demonstrated a lower occurrence of lactobacilli and bifidobacteria in milk produced by 160 women who received antibiotics during pregnancy or lactation. Lactobacilli were also less frequently detected in the milk from mothers with C-section deliveries likely due to the antibiotic treatment related to the surgery (Soto et al., 2014). The effects of antibiotics on the microbiome, leading to antibiotic-associated diarrhea and related problems such as gastroenteritis, and infections, have long been known (Willing et al., 2011). It is becoming evident that perinatal antibiotherapy has an impact on maternal microbiota, which may have negative consequences for infant health (Arboleya et al., 2015; Cox et al., 2015; Blaser & Bello, 2014).

Chemotherapy has also been associated with microbial shifts and with a reduction in bacterial diversity in HM (Urbaniak et al., 2014b). The same study reported that chemotherapy treatment increased the presence of *Acinetobacter* and Xanthomonadaceae and decreased the abundance of specific bacteria, such as *Bifidobacterium*, *Staphylococcus*, and *Eubacterium* spp., in milk samples.

4. STRATEGIES FOR MODULATING THE MATERNAL MICROBIOTA

Diet is probably one of the most important factors in determining and shaping the GI microbiota composition. Consequently, the development of dietary interventions inducing microbiota modifications may have a key impact on human physiology and metabolism. Recent evidence suggests that maternal consumption of a high-fat diet during pregnancy can influence the infant's GI microbiome (Ma et al., 2014). Thus, the contribution of specific microbes, diet,nutrition, and lifestyle may create a specific beneficial environment with impact on health and may reduce the incidence of specific disorders related alterations in the composition of the GI microbiota. Accumulating evidence suggests that early dietary interventions may result in programming effects on adult health.

Maternal probiotic interventions would have an impact on both maternal metabolic status and also, fetal physiology (Rautava et al., 2012a). Furthermore, nutrition counseling and probiotic intervention have been described to impact on gestational diabetes (GD) on differential way; probiotic intervention would reduce the risk of the GD while nutritional counseling was able to reduce the risk of associated fetal overgrowth (Luoto et al., 2010a). Different studies and some meta-analysis showed a significant reduction in the incidence of atopic eczema and allergies in children whose mothers consumed perinatal probiotics (Doege et al., 2012; Rautava et al., 2002), however no evidence has been shown regarding the perinatal use of probiotics and asthma or childhood wheeze (Azad et al., 2013). A recent study reported that perinatal probiotic intervention was able to stabilize weight gain during early infancy, the impact was most pronounced at the age of 4 years (Rautava et al., 2012b). Extended follow-up studies are needed to define the potential effect of perinatal probiotics in prevention and treatment of specific diseases as asthma, allergy, and obesity.

Moreover, the potential modulation of HM would open new research possibilities to manage and reduce the risk of disease (Munblit and Boyle, 2012; Munblit et al., 2015). There is evidence that probiotic consumption can modulate the composition of HM immunological compounds such as TGF-β2 (Prescott et al., 2008; Munblit and Boyle, 2012; Rautava et al., 2002; Kuitunen et al., 2012). In addition, specific probiotics consumed during lactation were detected in HM and in the infant GI tract (Abrahamsson et al., 2009). A recent study including 37 prenatal probiotic trials showed that probiotics prenatally were able to modulate immunological profile in the serum and HM; modulate maternal glucose response, and also, reduce the prevalence of GD and preeclampsia (Vandevusse et al., 2013).

Prenatal and postnatal probiotics consumption have been reported to induce specific changes in infant bifidobacteria colonization and to modulate HM microbiota compared to those observed in placebo group (Gueimonde et al., 2006). Recently, the effects of perinatal probiotic supplementation on milk bioactive composition, such as microbes (including *Bifidobacterium* and *Lactobacillus* spp.) and also, human milk oligosaccharides and lactoferrin, were reported (Mastroimarino et al., 2015).

The same study found a beneficial effect only for mothers with vaginal deliveries but no differences in those delivering via C-section suggesting a specific milk microbiota moculation and also, specific-probiotic effect dependent in vaginal deliveries.

In brief, there may be a "window of opportunity" during early life in which maternal microbial exposition and diet would have a key role in short and long-term health benefits in mother-infant dyad, and some of this effect may be due to modulation of the HM microbiome.

5. CONCLUSIONS

Alterations in the maternal environment (including diet, nutrition, hygiene, and microbes) has been related to high risk of childhood diseases that may persist during adulthood and later in life. For instance, maternal obesity may impact maternal microbes during pregnancy and lactation affecting microbial composition and diversity and activity. Those shifts may be transferred to offspring during delivery and during lactation, providing the neonate an atypical and abnormal environment that may drive infant microbial colonization and immune system development. Increasing our understanding of the role of maternal bacteria in the colonization of the infant would aid in the development of new strategies based on microbial modulation and focused at the beneficial metabolic, microbiological and immunological programming of health.

Based on the accumulating data, perinatal factors likely influence mother-to-infant microbial transfer. The lactation period may provide a new target for developing novel maternal dietary tools to modulate the HM microbiome and reduce the risk of both acute and chronic disease risk for the breastfed infant. Our knowledge of the HM microbiota is increasing, although further studies in different geographic locations and with larger sample sizes are required to explain the biological role of microbes for infant health.

REFERENCES

Aagaard, K., Ma, J., Antony, K.M., Ganu, R., Petrosino, J., Versalovic, J., 2014. The placenta harbors a unique microbiome. Science Translational Medicine 6 (237), 237ra65.

Aaltonen, J., Ojala, T., Laitinen, K., Poussa, T., Ozanne, S., Isolauri, E., 2011. Impact of maternal diet during pregnancy and breastfeeding on infant metabolic programming: a prospective randomized controlled study. European Journal of Clinical Nutrition 65 (1), 10–19.

Abrahamsson, T.R., Sinkiewicz, G., Jakobsson, T., Fredrikson, M., Björkstén, B., 2009. Probiotic lactobacilli in breast milk and infant stool in relation to oral intake during the first year of life. Journal of Pediatric Gastroenterology and Nutrition 49 (3), 349–355.Albesharat, R., Ehrmann, M.A., Korakli, M., Yazaji, S., Vogel, R.F., 2011. Phenotypic and genotypic analyses of lactic acid bacteria in local fermented food, breast milk and faeces of mothers and their babies. Systematic and Applied Microbiology 34, 148–155.

Arboleya, S., Sánchez, B., Milani, C., Duranti, S., Solís, G., Fernández, N., de los Reyes-Gavilán, C.G., Ventura, M., Margolles, A., Gueimonde, M., 2015. Intestinal microbiota development in preterm neonates and effect of perinatal antibiotics. Journal of Pediatrics 166 (3), 538–544.

Ares Segura, S., Arena Ansótegui, J., Díaz-Gómez, N.M., 2015. La importancia de la nutrición materna durante la lactancia, ¿necesitan las madres lactantes suplementos nutricionales? Anales de Pediatría. http://dx.doi.org/10.1016/j.anpedi.2015.07.024.

Atiya Ali, M., Strandvik, B., Sabel, K.G., Palme Kilander, C., Strömberg, R., Yngve, A., 2014. Polyamine levels in breast milk are associated with mothers' dietary intake and are higher in preterm than full-term human milk and formulas. Journal of Human Nutrition and Dietetics 27 (5), 459–467.

Azad, M.B., Coneys, J.G., Kozyrskyj, A.L., Field, C.J., Ramsey, C.D., Becker, A.B., Friesen, C., Abou-Setta, A.M., Zarychanski, R., 2013. Probiotic supplementation during pregnancy or infancy for the prevention of asthma and wheeze: systematic review and meta-analysis. BMJ 347, f6471.

Azad, M.B., Konya, T., Persaud, R.R., Guttman, D.S., Chari, R.S., Field, C.J., Sears, M.R., Mandhane, P.J., Turvey, S.E., Subbarao, P., Becker, A.B., Scott, J.A., Kozyrskyj, A.L., Child study investigators, 2015. Impact of maternal intrapartum antibiotics, method of birth and breastfeeding on gut microbiota during the first year of life: a prospective cohort study. BJOG: An International Journal of Obstetrics & Gynaecology. http://dx.doi.org/10.1111/1471-0528.13601.

Bäckhed, F., Roswall, J., Peng, Y., Feng, Q., Jia, H., Kovatcheva-Datchary, P., Li, Y., Xia, Y., Xie, H., Zhong, H., Khan, M.T., Zhang, J., Li, J., Xiao, L., Al-Aama, J., Zhang, D., Lee, Y.S., Kotowska, D., Colding, C., Tremaroli, V., Yin, Y., Bergman, S., Xu, X., Madsen, L., Kristiansen, K., Dahlgren, J., Wang, J., 2015. Dynamics and stabilization of the human gut microbiome during the first year of life. Cell Host & Microbe 17 (6), 852.

Barros, F.C., Matijasevich, A., Hallal, P.C., Horta, B.L., Barros, A.J., Menezes, A.B., Santos, I.S., Gigante, D.P., Victora, C.G., 2012. Cesarean section and risk of obesity in childhood, adolescence, and early adulthood: evidence from 3 Brazilian birth cohorts. American Journal of Clinical Nutrition 95 (2), 465–470.

Benito, D., Lozano, C., Jiménez, E., Albújar, M., Gómez, A., Rodríguez, J.M., Torres, C., 2015. Characterization of *Staphylococcus aureus* strains isolated from faeces of healthy neonates and potential mother-to-infant microbial transmission through breastfeeding. FEMS Microbiology Ecology 91 (3) pii: fiv007.

Blaser, M.J., Bello, M.G., 2014. Maternal antibiotic use and risk of asthma in offspring. Lancet Respiratory Medicine 2 (10), e16.

Bugarin, D., Grbović, S., Orčič, D., Mitić-Ćulafić, D., Knežević-Vukčević, J., Mimica-Dukić, N., 2014. Essential oil of *Eucalyptus gunnii* hook. As a novel source of antioxidant, antimutagenic and antibacterial agents. Molecules 19 (11), 19007–19020.

Cabrera-Rubio, R., Collado, M.C., Laitinen, K., Salminen, S., Isolauri, E., Mira, A., 2012. The human milk microbiome changes over lactation and is shaped by maternal weight and mode of delivery. American Journal of Clinical Nutrition 96 (3), 544–551.

Cabrera-Rubio, R., Mira-Pascual, L., Mira, A., Collado, M.C., 2015. Impact of mode of delivery on the milk microbiota composition of healthy women. Journal of Developmental Origins of Health and Disease 19, 1–7.

Cardwell, C.R., Stene, L.C., Joner, G., Cinek, O., Svensson, J., Goldacre, M.J., Parslow, R.C., Pozzilli, P., Brigis, G., Stoyanov, D., Urbonaite, B., Sipetić, S., Schober, E., Ionescu-Tirgoviste, C., Devoti, G., de Beaufort, C.E., Buschard, K., Patterson, C.C., 2008. Caesarean section is associated with an increased risk of childhood-onset type 1 diabetes mellitus: a meta-analysis of observational studies. Diabetologia 51 (5), 726–735.

Carrothers, J.M., York, M.A., Brooker, S.L., Lackey, K.A., Williams, J.E., Shafii, B., Price, W.J., Settles, M.L., McGuire, M.A., McGuire, M.K., 2015. Fecal microbial community structure is stable over time and related to variation in macronutrient and micronutrient intakes in lactating women. Journal of Nutrition 145 (10), 2379–2388.

Chang, N., Jung, J.A., Kim, H., Jo, A., Kang, S., Lee, S.W., Yi, H., Kim, J., Yim, J.G., Jung, B.M., 2015. Macronutrient composition of human milk from Korean mothers of full term infants born at 37–42 gestational weeks. Nutrition Research and Practice 9 (4), 433–438.

Collado, M.C., Cernada, M., Neu, J., Pérez-Martínez, G., Gormaz, M., Vento, M., 2015b. Factors influencing gastrointestinal tract and microbiota immune interaction in preterm infants. Pediatric Research 77 (6), 726–731.

Collado, M.C., Laitinen, K., Salminen, S., Isolauri, E., 2012. Maternal weight and excessive weight gain during pregnancy modify the immunomodulatory potential of breast milk. Pediatric Research 72, 77–85.

Collado, M.C., Rautava, S., Isolauri, E., Salminen, S., 2015a. Gut microbiota: a source of novel tools to reduce the risk of human disease? Pediatric Research 77 (1–2), 182–188.

Cox, L.M., Blaser, M.J., 2015. Antibiotics in early life and obesity. Nature Reviews Endocrinology 11 (3), 182–1890.

Decker, E., Engelmann, G., Findeisen, A., Gerner, P., Laass, M., Ney, D., Posovszky, C., Hoy, L., Hornef, M.W., 2010. Cesarean delivery is associated with celiac disease but not inflammatory bowel disease in children. Pediatrics 125 (6), e1433–40.

Denzer, M.Y., Kirsch, F., Buettner, A., 2015. Are odorant constituents of herbal tea transferred into human milk? Journal of Agricultural and Food Chemistry 63 (1), 104–111.

Dizdar, E.A., Sari, F.N., Degirmencioglu, H., Canpolat, F.E., Oguz, S.S., Uras, N., Dilmen, U., 2014. Effect of mode of delivery on macronutrient content of breast milk. Journal of Maternal-Fetal & Neonatal Medicine 27 (11), 1099–1102.

Doege, K., Grajecki, D., Zyriax, B.C., Detinkina, E., Zu Eulenburg, C., Buhling, K.J., 2012. Impact of maternal supplementation with probiotics during pregnancy on atopic eczema in childhood–a meta-analysis. British Journal of Nutrition 107 (1), 1–6.

Dogra, S., Sakwinska, O., Soh, S.E., Ngom-Bru, C., Brück, W.M., Berger, B., Brüssow, H., Lee, Y.S, Yap, F., Chong, Y.S., Godfrey, K.M., Holbrook, J.D., 2015. Dynamics of infant gut microbiota are influenced by delivery mode and gestational duration and are associated with subsequent adiposity. GUSTO Study Group. MBio 6 (1), e02419–14.

Dominguez-Bello, M.G., Costello, E.K., Contreras, M., Magris, M., Hidalgo, G., Fierer, N., Knight, R., 2010. Delivery mode shapes the acquisition and structure of the initial microbiota across multiple body habitats in newborns. Proceedings of the National Academy of Sciences of the United States of America 107 (26), 11971–11975.

Dunstan, J.A., Roper, J., Mitoulas, L., Hartmann, P.E., Simmer, K., Prescott, S.L., 2004. The effect of supplementation with fish oil during pregnancy on breast milk immunoglobulin A, soluble CD14, cytokine levels and fatty acid composition. Clinical & Experimental Allergy 34 (8), 1237–1242.

Espinosa-Martos, I., Montilla, A., de Segura, A.G., Escuder, D., Bustos, G., Pallás, C., Rodríguez, J.M., Corzo, N., Fernández, L., 2013. Bacteriological, biochemical, and immunological modifications in human colostrum after Holder pasteurisation. Journal of Pediatric Gastroenterology and Nutrition 56 (5), 560–568.

Fernández, L., Langa, S., Martín, V., Maldonado, A., Jiménez, E., Martín, R., Rodríguez, J.M., 2013. The human milk microbiota: origin and potential roles in health and disease. Pharmacological Research 69, 1–10.

Forno, E., Onderdonk, A.B., McCracken, J., Litonjua, A.A., Laskey, D., Delaney, M.L., Dubois, A.M., Gold, D.R., Ryan, L.M., Weiss, S.T., Celedón, J.C., 2008. Diversity of the gut microbiota and eczema in early life. Clinical & Experimental Allergy 6, 11.

García-Lara, N.R., Vieco, D.E., De la Cruz-Bértolo, J., Lora-Pablos, D., Velasco, N.U., Pallás-Alonso, C.R., 2013. Effect of Holder pasteurization and frozen storage on macronutrients and energy content of breast milk. Journal of Pediatric Gastroenterology and Nutrition 57 (3), 377–382.

Gómez-Gallego, C., Collado, M.C., Pérez, G., Ilo, T., Jaakkola, U.M., Bernal, M.J., Periago, M.J., Frias, R., Ros, G., Salminen, S., 2014. Resembling breast milk: influence of polyamine-supplemented formula on neonatal BALB/cOlaHsd mouse microbiota. Brithis Journal of Nutrition 111 (6), 1050–1058.

González, R., Maldonado, A., Martín, V., Mandomando, I., Fumadó, V., Metzner, K.J., Sacoor, C., Fernández, L., Macete, E., Alonso, P.L., Rodríguez, J.M., Menendez, C., 2013. Breast milk and gut microbiota in African mothers and infants from an area of high HIV prevalence. PLoS One 8, e80299.

Good, M., Sodhi, C.P., Hackam, D.J., 2014. Evidence-based feeding strategies before and after the development of necrotizing enterocolitis. Expert Review of Clinical Immunology 10 (7), 875–884.

Grönlund, M.M., Gueimonde, M., Laitinen, K., Kociubinski, G., Grönroos, T., Salminen, S., Isolauri, E., 2007. Maternal breast-milk and intestinal *bifidobacteria* guide the compositional development of the *Bifidobacterium* microbiota in infants at risk of allergic disease. Clinical Experimental Allergy 37, 1764–1772.

Gueimonde, M., Laitinen, K., Salminen, S., Isolauri, E., 2007. Breast milk: a source of Bifidobacteria for infant gut development and maturation? Neonatology 92 (1), 64–66.

Gueimonde, M., Sakata, S., Kalliomäki, M., Isolauri, E., Benno, Y., Salminen, S., 2006. Effect of maternal consumption of lactobacillus GG on transfer and establishment of fecal Bifidobacterial microbiota in neonates. Journal of Pediatric Gastroenterology and Nutrition 42 (2), 166–1670.

Hansen, R., Scott, K.P., Khan, S., Martin, J.C., Berry, S.H., Stevenson, M., Okpapi, A., Munro, M.J., Hold, G.L., 2015. First-pass meconium samples from healthy term vaginally-delivered neonates: an analysis of the microbiota. PLoS One 10 (7), e0133320.

Harris, W.S., Connor, W.E., Lindsey, S., 1984. Will dietary omega-3 fatty acids change the composition of human milk? American Journal of Clinical Nutrition 40 (4), 780–785.

Harzer, G., Dieterich, I., Haug, M., 1984. Effects of the diet on the composition of human milk. Annals of Nutrition and Metabolism 28 (4), 231–239.

Holmlund, U., Amoudruz, P., Johansson, M.A., Haileselassie, Y., Ongoiba, A., Kayentao, K., Traoré, B., Doumbo, S., Schollin, J., Doumbo, O., Montgomery, S.M., Sverremark-Ekström, E., 2010. Maternal country of origin, breast milk characteristics and potential influences on immunity in offspring. Clinical Experimental Immunolpgy 162, 500–509.

Hooper, L.V., Littman, D.R., Macpherson, A.J., 2012. Interactions between the microbiota and the immune system. Science 336, 1268–1273.

Hooper, L.V., Macpherson, A.J., 2010. Immune adaptations that maintain homeostasis with the intestinal microbiota. Nature Reviews Immunology 10, 159–169.

Hoppu, U., Isolauri, E., Laakso, P., Matomäki, J., Laitinen, K., 2012. Probiotics and dietary counselling targeting maternal dietary fat intake modifies breast milk fatty acids and cytokines. European Journal of Nutrition 51, 211–219.

Horta, B.L., Gigante, D.P., Lima, R.C., Barros, F.C., Victora, C.G., 2013. Birth by caesarean section and prevalence of risk factors for non-communicable diseases in young adults: a birth cohort study. PLoS One 8 (9), e74301.

Hunt, K.M., Foster, J.A., Forney, L.J., Schütte, U.M., Beck, D.L., Abdo, Z., Fox, L.K., Williams, J.E., McGuire, M.K., McGuire, M.A., 2011. Characterization of the diversity and temporal stability of bacterial communities in human milk. PLoS One 6, e21313.

Hunt, K.M., Preuss, J., Nissan, C., Davlin, C.A., Williams, J.E., Shafii, B., Richardson, A.D., McGuire, M.K., Bode, L., McGuire, M.A., 2012. Human milk oligosaccharides promote the growth of staphylococci. Applied and Environmental Microbiology 78 (14), 4763–4770.

Innis, S.M., 2014. Impact of maternal diet on human milk composition and neurological development of infants. American Journal of Clinical Nutrition 99, 734S–741S.

Jakobsson, H.E., Abrahamsson, T.R., Jenmalm, M.C., Harris, K., Quince, C., Jernberg, C., Björkstén, B., Engstrand, L., Andersson, A.F., 2014. Decreased gut microbiota diversity, delayed Bacteroidetes colonisation and reduced Th1 responses in infants delivered by caesarean section. Gut 63 (4), 559–566.

Jiménez, E., Marín, M.L., Martín, R., Odriozola, J.M., Olivares, M., Xaus, J., Fernández, L., Rodríguez, J.M., 2008. Is meconium from healthy newborns actually sterile? Research in Microbiology 159 (3), 187–193.

Jost, T., Lacroix, C., Braegger, C., Chassard, C., 2013. Assessment of bacterial diversity in breast milk using culture-dependent and culture-independent approaches. British Journal of Nutrition 110 (7), 1253–1262.

Jost, T., Lacroix, C., Braegger, C., Chassard, C., 2015. Impact of human milk bacteria and oligosaccharides on neonatal gut microbiota establishment and gut health. Nutrition Reviews 73 (7), 426–437.

Jost, T., Lacroix, C., Braegger, C., Rochat, F., Chassard, C., 2014. Vertical mother-neonate transfer of maternal gut bacteria via breastfeeding. Environmental Microbiology 16 (9), 2891–2904.

Khodayar-Pardo, P., Mira-Pascual, L., Collado, M.C., Martínez-Costa, C., 2014. Impact of lactation stage, gestational age and mode of delivery on breast milk microbiota. Journal of Perinatology 34, 599–605.

Kuitunen, M., Kukkonen, A.K., Savilahti, E., 2012. Impact of maternal allergy and use of probiotics during pregnancy on breast milk cytokines and food antibodies and development of allergy in children until 5 years. International Archives of Allergy and Immunology 159, 162–170.

Kulas, T., Bursac, D., Zegarac, Z., Planinic-Rados, G., Hrgovic, Z., 2013. New views on cesarean section, its possible complications and long-term consequences for children's health. Medical Archives 67 (6), 460–463.

Lauritzen, L., Jørgensen, M.H., Hansen, H.S., Michaelsen, K.F., 2002. Fluctuations in human milk long-chain PUFA levels in relation to dietary fish intake. Lipids 37 (3), 237–244.

Lawrence, R.A., Lawrence, R.M., 2011. Breastfeeding: A Guide for the Medical Profession, seventh ed. Elsevier Mosby, Maryland Hts, Missouri.

Le Huërou-Luron, I., Blat, S., Boudry, G., 2010. Breast- v. formula-feeding: impacts on the digestive tract and immediate and long-term health effects. Nutrition Research Reviews 23 (1), 23–36.

Li, R., Dee, D., Li, C.M., Hoffman, H.J., Grummer-Strawn, L.M., 2014. Breastfeeding and risk of infections at 6 years. Pediatrics 134 (1), S13–S20.

Lodge, C.J., Tan, D.J., Lau, M., Dai, X., Tham, R., Lowe, A.J., Bowatte, G., Allen, K.J., Dharmage, S.C., 2015. Breastfeeding and asthma and allergies: a systematic review and meta-analysis. Acta Paediatrica Supplement 104 (467), 38–53.

Lu, X., Rasco, B.A., Jabal, J.M., Aston, D.E., Lin, M., Konkel, M.E., 2011. Investigating antibacterial effects of garlic (*Allium sativum*) concentrate and garlic-derived organosulfur compounds on Campylobacter jejuni by using Fourier transform infrared spectroscopy, Raman spectroscopy, and electron microscopy. Applied and Environmental Microbiology 77 (15), 5257–5269.

Luoto, R., Laitinen, K., Nermes, M., Isolauri, E., 2010. Impact of maternal probiotic-supplemented dietary counselling on pregnancy outcome and prenatal and postnatal growth: a double-blind, placebo-controlled study. British Journal of Nutrition 103 (12), 1792–1799.

Ma, J., Prince, A.L., Bader, D., Hu, M., Ganu, R., Baquero, K., Blundell, P., Alan Harris, R., Frias, A.E., Grove, K.L., Aagaard, K.M., 2014. High-fat maternal diet during pregnancy persistently alters the offspring microbiome in a primate model. Nature Communications 5, 3889.

Makino, H., Kushiro, A., Ishikawa, E., Kubota, H., Gawad, A., Sakai, T., Oishi, K., Martin, R., Ben-Amor, K., Knol, J., Tanaka, R., 2013. Mother-to-infant transmission of intestinal Bifidobacterial strains has an impact on the early development of vaginally delivered infant's microbiota. PLoS One 8 (11), e7833.

Makino, H., Kushiro, A., Ishikawa, E., Muylaert, D., Kubota, H., Sakai, T., Oishi, K., Martin, R., Ben Amor, K., Oozeer, R., Knol, J., Tanaka, R., 2011. Transmission of intestinal *Bifidobacterium longum* subsp. *longum* strains from mother to infant, determined by multilocus sequencing typing and amplified fragment length polymorphism. Applied and Environmental Microbiology 77 (19), 6788–6793.

Martin, R., Langa, S., Reviriego, C., Jimínez, E., Marín, M.L., Xaus, J., Fernández, L., Rodríguez, J.M., 2003. Human milk is a source of lactic acid bacteria for the infant gut. Journal of Pediatrics 143, 754–758.

Mastroimarino, P., Capobianco, D., Miccheli, A., Praticò, G., Campagna, G., Laforgia, N., Capursi, T., Baldassarre, M.E., 2015. Administration of a multistrain probiotic product (VSL#3) to women in the perinatal period differentially affects breast milk beneficial microbiota in relation to mode of delivery. Pharmacology Research 95–96, 63–70.

McGuire, M.K., McGuire, M.A., 2015. Human milk: mother nature's prototypical probiotic food? Advances in Nutrition 6 (1), 112–123.

Mennella, J.A., Beauchamp, G.K., 1991. Maternal diet alters the sensory qualities of human milk and the nursling's behavior. Pediatrics 88, 737–744.

Mennella, J.A., Beauchamp, G.K., 1993. Beer breast feeding and folklore. Developmental Psychobiology 26, 459–466.

Mennella, J.A., Beauchamp, G.K., 1999. Experience with a flavor in mother's milk modifies the infant's acceptance of flavored cereal. Developmental Psychobiology 35, 197–203.

Minniti, F., Comberiati, P., Munblit, D., Piacentini, G.L., Antoniazzi, E., Zanoni, L., Boner, A.L., Peroni, D.G., 2014. Breast-milk characteristics protecting against allergy. Endocrine, Metabolic & Immune Disorders - Drug Targets 14 (1), 9–15.

Munblit, D., Boyle, R.J., 2012. Modulating breast milk composition – the key to allergy prevention? International Archives of Allergy and Immunology 159 (2), 107–108.

Munblit, D., Boyle, R.J., Warner, J.O., 2015. Factors affecting breast milk composition and potential consequences for development of the allergic phenotype. Clinical Experimental Allergy 45 (3), 583–601.

Nishimura, R.Y., Barbieiri, P., Castro, G.S., Jordão Jr., A.A., Perdoná, Gda, S., Sartorelli, D.S., 2014. Dietary polyunsaturated fatty acid intake during late pregnancy affects fatty acid composition of mature breast milk. Nutrition 30 (6), 685–689.

Olivares, M., Albrecht, S., De Palma, G., Ferrer, M.D., Castillejo, G., Schols, H.A., Sanz, Y., 2015. Human milk composition differs in healthy mothers and mothers with celiac disease. European Journal of Nutrition 54, 119–128.

O'Sullivan, A., He, X., McNiven, E.M., Hinde, K., Haggarty, N.W., Lönnerdal, B., Slupsky, C.M., 2013. Metabolomic phenotyping validates the infant rhesus monkey as a model of human infant metabolism. Journal of Pediatric Gastroenterology and Nutrition 56 (4), 355–363.

Peng, Y., Zhou, T., Wang, Q., Liu, P., Zhang, T., Zetterström, R., Strandvik, B., 2009. Fatty acid composition of diet, cord blood and breast milk in Chinese mothers with different dietary habits. Prostaglandins, Leukotrienes and Essential Fatty Acids 81 (5–6), 325–330.

Petherick, A., 2010. Development Mother's milk: a rich opportunity. Nature 468 (7327), S5–S7.

Prescott, S.L., Wickens, K., Westcott, L., Jung, W., Currie, H., Black, P.N., Stanley, T.V., Mitchell, E.A., Fitzharris, P., Siebers, R., Wu, L., Crane, J., 2008. Supplementation with *Lactobacillus rhamnosus* or *Bifidobacterium lactis* probiotics in pregnancy increases cord blood interferon-gamma and breast milk transforming growth factor-beta and immunoglobin A detection. Clinical Experimenal Allergy 38, 1606–1614.

Quigley, L., O'Sullivan, O., Stanton, C., Beresford, T.P., Ross, R.P., Fitzgerald, G.F., Cotter, P.D., 2013. The complex microbiota of raw milk. FEMS Microbiology Reviews 37 (5), 664–698.

Quinn, E.A., Largado, F., Power, M., Kuzawa, C.W., 2012. Predictors of breast milk macronutrient composition in Filipino mothers. American Journal of Human Biology 24 (4), 533–540.

Rakicioğlu, N., Samur, G., Topçu, A., Topçu, A.A., 2006. The effect of Ramadan on maternal nutrition and composition of breast milk. Pediatric International 48 (3), 278–283.

Rautava, S., 2015. Early microbial contact, the breast milk microbiome and child health. Journal of Developmental Origins of Health and Disease 8, 1–10.

Rautava, S., Collado, M.C., Salminen, S., Isolauri, E., 2012a. Probiotics modulate host-microbe interaction in the placenta and fetal gut: a randomized, double-blind, placebo-controlled trial. Neonatology 102 (3), 178–184.

Rautava, S., Kainonen, E., Salminen, S., Isolauri, E., 2012b. Maternal probiotic supplementation during pregnancy and breast-feeding reduces the risk of eczema in the infant. Journal of Allergy and Clinical Immunology 130 (6), 1355–1360.

Rautava, S., Kalliomäki, M., Isolauri, E., 2002. Probiotics during pregnancy and breast-feeding might confer immunomodulatory protection against atopic disease in the infant. Journal of Allergy and Clinical Immunology 109 (1), 119–121.

Rodríguez, J.M., 2014. The origin of human milk bacteria: is there a bacterial entero-mammary pathway during late pregnancy and lactation? Advances in Nutrition 5 (6), 779–784.

Rodríguez, J.M., Murphy, K., Stanton, C., Ross, R.P., Kober, O.I., Juge, N., Avershina, E., Rudi, K., Narbad, A., Jenmalm, M.C., Marchesi, J.R., Collado, M.C., 2015. The composition of the gut microbiota throughout life, with an emphasis on early life. Microbial Ecology in Health and Disease 26, 26050.

Roger, L.C., Costabile, A., Holland, D.T., Hoyles, L., McCartney, A.L., 2010. Examination of faecal *Bifidobacterium* populations in breast- and formula-fed infants during the first 18 months of life. Microbiology 156 (Pt 11), 3329–3341.

Soto, A., Martín, V., Jiménez, E., Mader, I., Rodríguez, J.M., Fernández, L., 2014. Lactobacilli and *Bifidobacteria* in human breast milk: influence of antibiotherapy and other host and clinical factors. Journal of Pediatric Gastroenterology and Nutrition 59, 78–88.

Sousa, S.G., Delgadillo, I., Saraiva, J.A., 2014. Effect of thermal pasteurisation and high-pressure processing on immunoglobulin content and lysozyme and lactoperoxidase activity in human colostrum. Food Chemistry 151, 79–85.

Stuebe, A.M., 2015. Does breastfeeding prevent the metabolic syndrome, or does the metabolic syndrome prevent breastfeeding? Seminars in Perinatology 39 (4), 290–295.

Takahashi, H., Mikami, K., Nishino, R., Matsuoka, T., Kimura, M., Koga, Y., 2010. Comparative analysis of the properties of bifidobacterial isolates from fecal samples of mother-infant pairs. Journal of Pediatric Gastroenterology and Nutrition 51 (5), 653–660.

Tomicic, S., Johansson, G., Voor, T., Björkstén, B., Böttcher, M.F., Jenmalm, M.C., 2010. Breast milk cytokine and IgA composition differ in Estonian and Swedish mothers – relationship to microbial pressure and infant allergy. Pediatric Research 68, 330–334.

Urbaniak, C., Angelini, M., Gloor, G.B., Reid, G., 2016. Human milk microbiota profiles in relation to birthing method, gestation and infant gender. Microbiome 4 (1), 1.

Urbaniak, C., Cummins, J., Brackstone, M., Macklaim, J.M., Gloor, G.B., Baban, C.K., Scott, L., O'Hanlon, D.M., Burton, J.P., Francis, K.P., Tangney, M., Reid, G., 2014a. Microbiota of human breast tissue. Applied and Environmental Microbiology 80 (10), 3007–3014.

Urbaniak, C., McMillan, A., Angelini, M., Gloor, G.B., Sumarah, M., Burton, J.P., Reid, G., 2014b. Effect of chemotherapy on the microbiota and metabolome of human milk, a case report. Microbiome 2, 24.

Vaishampayan, P.A., Kuehl, J.V., Froula, J.L., Morgan, J.L., Ochman, H., Francino, M.P., 2010. Comparative metagenomics and population dynamics of the gut microbiota in mother and infant. Genome Biology and Evolution 2, 53–66.

Vallés, Y., Artacho, A., Pascual-García, A., Ferrús, M.L., Gosalbes, M.J., Abellán, J.J., Francino, M.P., 2014. Microbial succession in the gut: directional trends of taxonomic and functional change in a birth cohort of Spanish infants. PLoS Genetics 10 (6), e1004406.

VandeVusse, L., Hanson, L., Safdar, N., 2013. Perinatal outcomes of prenatal probiotic and prebiotic administration: an integrative review. The Journal of Perinatal & Neonatal Nursing 27 (4), 288–301.

Victora, C.G., Bahl, R., Barros, A.J.D., França, G.V.A., Horton, S., Krasevec, J., Murch, S., Sankar, M.J., Walker, N., Rollins, N.G., 2016. Breastfeeding in the 21st century: epidemiology, mechanisms, and lifelong effect. The Lancet Breastfeeding Series Group Breastfeeding. The Lancet. www.thelancet.com/series/breastfeeding.

Walker, A., 2010. Breast milk as the gold standard for protective nutrients. Journal of Pediatrics 156 (2), S3–S7.

Wang, M., Karlsson, C., Olsson, C., Adlerberth, I., Wold, A.E., Strachan, D.P., Martricardi, P.M., Aberg, N., Perkin, M.R., Tripodi, S., Coates, A.R., Hesselmar, B., Saalman, R., Molin, G., Ahrné, S., 2008. Reduced diversity in the early fecal microbiota of infants with atopic eczema. Journal of Allergy and Clinical Immunology 121 (1), 129–134.

WHO, 2015. Statement on Caesarean Section Rates. WHO/RHR/15.02 http://www.who.int/reproductivehealth/publications/maternal_perinatal_health/cs-statement/en/.

Willing, B.P., Russell, S.L., Finlay, B.B., 2011. Shifting the balance: antibiotic effects on host-microbiota mutualism. Nature Reviews Microbiology 9, 233–243.

Xuan, C., Shamonki, J.M., Chung, A., Dinome, M.L., Chung, M., Sieling, P.A., Lee, D.J., 2014. Microbial dysbiosis is associated with human breast cancer. PLoS One 9 (1), e83744.

Yahvah, K.M., Brooker, S.L., Williams, J.E., Settles, M., McGuire, M.A., McGuire, M.K., 2015. Elevated dairy fat intake in lactating women alters milk lipid and fatty acids without detectible changes in expression of genes related to lipid uptake or synthesis. Nutrition Research 35 (3), 221–228.

Yang, T., Zhang, Y., Ning, Y., You, L., Ma, D., Zheng, Y., Yang, X., Li, W., Wang, J., Wang, P., 2014. Breast milk macronutrient composition and the associated factors in urban Chinese mothers. Chinese Medical Journal 127 (9), 1721–1725.

Yatsunenko, T., Rey, F.E., Manary, M.J., Trehan, I., Dominguez-Bello, M.G., Contreras, M., Magris, M., Hidalgo, G., Baldassano, R.N., Anokhin, A.P., Heath, A.C., Warner, B., Reeder, J., Kuczynski, J., Caporaso, J.G., Lozupone, C.A., Lauber, C., Clemente, J.C., Knights, D., Knight, R., Gordon, J.I., 2012. Human gut microbiome viewed across age and geography. Nature 486, 222–227.

Zarrinpar, A., Chaix, A., Yooseph, S., Panda, S., 2014. Diet and feeding pattern affect the diurnal dynamics of the gut microbiome. Cell Metabolism 20 (6), 1006–1017.

Zivkovic, A.M., German, J.B., Lebrilla, C.B., Mills, D.A., 2011. Human milk glycobiome and its impact on the infant gastrointestinal microbiota. Proceedings of the National Academy of Sciences USA 108, 4653–4658.

CHAPTER

The Origin of Human Milk Bacteria

13

Álex Mira[1], Juan M. Rodríguez[1,2]

[1]Complutense University of Madrid, Madrid, Spain; [2]Center for Advanced Research in Public Health (CSISP), Valencia, Spain

1. INTRODUCTION

In the past few years, culture-dependent studies have revealed that colostrum and milk from healthy women contain bacteria, including staphylococci, streptococci, corynebacteria, lactic acid bacteria, propionibacteria, and bifidobacteria (Fernández et al., 2013). More recently, the application of culture-independent techniques, including microbiomic and metagenomic approaches, confirmed the presence of DNA from these and other bacterial genera (Hunt et al., 2011; Cabrera-Rubio et al., 2012; Fernández et al., 2013; Jost et al., 2013, 2014; Ward et al., 2013; Jiménez et al., 2015). Therefore, such biological fluids are continuous sources of live bacteria to the infant gastrointestinal (GI) (McGuire and McGuire, 2015) tract and, in fact, other studies have shown that there is mother-to-infant transfer of bacterial strains through breastfeeding (Albesharat et al., 2011; Martín et al., 2012; Jost et al., 2014).

Traditionally, any bacterial cell present in human milk was considered the result of contamination arising from the infant's oral cavity or the mother's skin (West et al., 1979). However, the detection of live bacterial cells and/or DNA from anaerobic species that are generally related to gut environments and that cannot survive in aerobic locations has fueled a scientific debate on the origin of milk-associated bacteria. The microbiome of different human body locations constitutes a dynamic network of interrelated communities (Costello et al., 2009). Therefore, the fact that the infant's mouth or the maternal skin may provide some bacteria to milk is compatible with the potential interconnections between milk and other sites in mothers, especially during the last stages of pregnancy (Fig. 13.1).

2. POTENTIAL SOURCES OF BACTERIA TO MAMMARY STRUCTURES AND MILK

2.1 INFANT'S MOUTH

Some bacteria from the infant's oral cavity may contaminate milk during suckling due to milk flow back into mammary ducts (Ramsey et al., 2004); however, presence

Prebiotics and Probiotics in Human Milk. http://dx.doi.org/10.1016/B978-0-12-802725-7.00013-0

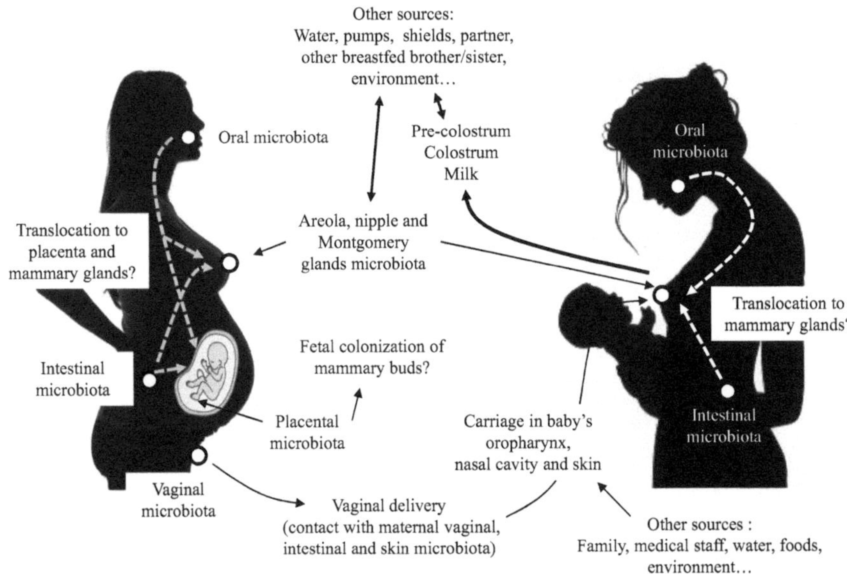

FIGURE 13.1

Potential sources of microbes to human colostrum and milk.

of oral-related bacteria in milk may precede the first feeding since colostrum collected within 24h after birth has been found to contain typical oral bacteria like *Veillonella*, *Leptotrichia*, and *Prevotella* (Cabrera-Rubio et al., 2012). In addition, contamination from the breastfed baby's oral cavity does not explain why precolostrum secreted by some women before delivery (and, obviously, before any contact with the baby's mouth) already contains the microbiota that characterizes human milk (Martín et al., 2004).

Although the origin of the human salivary microbiome is still widely unknown (Zaura et al., 2014), *Streptococcus* spp. seem to be one of the dominant microorganisms both in adults (Aas et al., 2005; Nasidze et al., 2009; Yang et al., 2012) and in edentulous infants (Li et al., 1997; Caufield et al., 2000; Bearfield et al., 2002; Cephas et al., 2011). Streptococci are also among the dominant phylotypes in human milk (Jiménez et al., 2008a,b; Hunt et al., 2011; Martín et al., 2015), suggesting a potential role in the shaping of the salivary microbiota. Although no longitudinal studies have been performed to characterize oral microbiota development during infancy and childhood, it is thought that facultative anaerobes such as streptococci and staphylococci initially colonize oral mucosal surfaces, followed by the settlement of anaerobic colonizers due to environmental modifications and species–species interactions (Sampaio-Maia and Monteiro-Silva, 2014). Similarly to the milk microbiome (Cabrera-Rubio et al., 2015), the infant oral microbiota seems to be affected by birth mode, as shown by reduced bacterial diversity at 3 months in infants born by cesarean section (Lif Holgerson et al., 2011).

Although oral colonization by bacteria causing dental caries was initially thought to happen during tooth eruption, it has later been demonstrated that the cariogenic organism *Streptococcus mutans* can be present in the infant before the appearance of hard tissues (Law et al., 2007); interestingly, this species has already been isolated from human milk (Martín et al., 2015). Given that the mother's oral health has been correlated with dental caries in the child and that the main source of oral bacteria for the infant has been shown to be the mother, the potential role of milk in the acquisition and development of oral bacteria deserves future research attention (Zaura et al., 2014).

The origin of the oral microbiota has relevant implications for human health, including the development of the immune system and the risk for tooth decay in the child. It is also interesting to note that some human milk compounds (e.g., human milk oligosaccharides, proteins) can influence the settlement of oral bacteria indirectly. For instance, milk proteins, such as caseins and lactoferrin, have been found to inhibit the attachment of cariogenic mutans streptococci to hydroxyapatite and to promote the attachment of commensal bacteria in vitro, while phosphorylated milk-derived peptides promote maintenance of tooth minerals, thereby contributing to the infant's oral health (Johansson and Lif Holgerson, 2011).

Finally, it should be noted that, as a result of sexual activity, the oral microbiota of the partner might provide microorganisms to human milk.

2.2 MATERNAL SKIN

Although it has long been known that bacteria, viruses, fungi, and arthropods inhabit the skin, recent studies have shown that the community of microorganisms on human skin is more complex than once thought (Schommer and Gallo, 2013). However, our knowledge of the skin microbiota pales in comparison with that of our GI microbiota despite the fact that the vast majority of our resident skin microorganisms are non-pathogenic, and many of these probably contribute to maintaining health. Microbes inhabiting maternal skin and, particularly, the external surfaces closer to milk exits (nipples, mammary areolas, Montgomery glands) can be transferred to this biological fluid during milk ejection (Fig. 13.1). The skin of the infant, partner, and/or other people (members of the family, friends, medical staff, etc.) can also be a source of microorganisms to the maternal skin (Fig. 13.1).

The skin is a variable ecosystem, providing many niches in which microbes are subjected to myriad ecological pressures including humidity, temperature, pH, and the composition of antimicrobial peptides and lipids. In addition, skin structures such as hair follicles and sebaceous, eccrine, and apocrine glands constitute discrete niches that harbor unique microbiota (Grice et al., 2008). Physiologically comparable body sites harbor similar microbial communities in healthy individuals (Grice et al., 2009; Findley et al., 2013), and shifts in skin communities are associated with development and immune status (Oh et al., 2012, 2013). Instead of merely sampling the random bacteria in our environment with which our bodies interact, skin can differentially select for specific populations. Therefore, scientists have now moved beyond the question of which microbes are present on the skin to assessing what they might be doing. Among the most abundant bacterial populations, Oh et al. (2014) identified numerous strains of some species and genera that are common in human milk: *Propionibacterium acnes*, *Corynebacterium* spp., and, particularly, *Staphylococcus epidermidis*. Investigating the spatial and personal distribution, they observed that the distribution of *P. acnes* strains was more individual specific than site specific, whereas *S. epidermidis* strains were more site specific than individual specific. On the other hand, the presence of lipophilic *Corynebacterium* populations in healthy people suggests that moisturizing creams (which are widely used) could be acting as a prebiotic to feed these organisms.

Mammary external surfaces (nipple, mammary areola, Montgomery glands) are very peculiar in relation to the skin structures found in other body sites, undergoing relevant anatomic and physiological changes throughout pregnancy. Future investigations will need to focus on how the distribution of these strains in mammary structures (and, also, in colostrum and milk) varies over time (from early pregnancy to weaning), and with changes in health, including the development of mastitis. Antibiotic-resistance genes seem to be specific to individuals and body sites, and knowing the diversity and distribution of such genes across mammary structures could prove crucial in customizing therapies for the treatment of nipple and breast infections during lactation.

It must be highlighted that although staphylococci, corynebacteria, and propionibacteria have been traditionally associated to the skin, they are widespread in most, if not all, human mucosal surfaces; in fact, the populations of such bacterial groups reach their highest concentrations in the mucosal layers of the digestive and genitourinary tracts. In addition, these bacteria have been detected in samples of chorioamnion and amniotic fluid from pregnant women and in umbilical cord blood obtained from healthy neonates born via either labor or cesarean section (Bearfield et al., 2002; Jiménez et al., 2005; Aagaard et al., 2014). This suggests that staphylococci, corynebacteria, and propionibacteria may colonize fetal skin and the digestive tract in utero and raises the possibility that the presence of bacteria in chorioamnion, amniotic fluid, colostrum, and milk may share a common or similar mechanism in healthy hosts (Fig. 13.1). This is supported by the overlapping bacterial composition between milk and aseptically collected meconium samples from newly born infants, which also contain a high frequency of lactic acid bacteria as determined by high-throughput sequencing of the 16S rRNA gene (Gosalbes et al., 2013).

2.3 MATERNAL GASTROINTESTINAL TRACT

Despite sharing of some phylotypes, the comparison between the bacterial communities detected in milk and those found on breast skin or in the infant's mouth reveals major differences between them (Hunt et al., 2011; Cabrera-Rubio et al., 2012; Jost et al., 2013; Jiménez et al., 2015). As an example, *Bifidobacterium* is a strictly anaerobic genus and, therefore, skin is a highly improbable source of such microorganisms to milk (Gueimonde et al., 2007). *Bifidobacterium longum* DNA in maternal feces, human milk, and neonatal feces within the same mother–neonate pair was clearly shared (Perez et al., 2007). More recently, pyrosequencing allowed identifying gut-associated obligate anaerobic genera, like *Bifidobacterium*, *Bacteroides*, *Parabacteroides*, and members of the Clostridia class (*Blautia*, *Clostridium*, *Collinsella*, and *Veillonella*), within maternal feces, milk, and neonatal feces (Jost et al., 2014). Furthermore, several butyrate-producing members of Clostridia (*Coprococcus*, *Faecalibacterium*, *Roseburia*, and *Subdoligranulum*) were shared between maternal feces and human milk. A recent metagenome analysis of human milk has also revealed the presence of DNA belonging to such anaerobes (Jiménez et al., 2015).

A major drawback of culture-independent studies is the lack of information about the viability of the detected populations and the lack of possibility for strain-level discrimination, which is necessary for demonstrating that the same bacterial strain was shared between mother and neonate. A second caveat of molecular methods is the low amount of DNA typically extracted from milk samples, making the relative proportion of contaminant DNA from sample manipulation and from DNA extraction reagents more important than when analyzing other biological samples (Salter et al., 2014; Jiménez et al., 2015). Thus, without confirming the presence of these populations by culture, isolation, and strain-level discrimination, it remains unclear whether human milk is a source of viable gut-associated obligate anaerobes or if dead cells or parts thereof are transferred to the breastfed neonate (Jost et al., 2014). However, transfer of bifidobacteria, lactobacilli, and/or other bacteria, at the strain level, from the maternal GI tract to the neonatal GI tract (Kulagina et al., 2010; Takahashi et al., 2010; Makino et al., 2011), from maternal GI tract to human milk (Martín et al., 2006; Jiménez et al., 2008c; Abrahamsson et al., 2009; Arroyo et al., 2010; Fernández et al., 2015), from milk to the neonatal GI tract (Martín et al., 2003, 2009, 2012; Jiménez et al., 2008a), and from the maternal GI tract to milk and infant GI tract (Albesharat et al., 2011; Jost et al., 2014) has also been demonstrated using culture- and strain-level discrimination. Such studies reinforce the hypothesis that at least some bacteria, including obligate anaerobes, may be vertically transferred from mother to neonate via breastfeeding.

3. ORAL AND GASTROINTESTINAL BACTERIAL TRANSLOCATION DURING LATE PREGNANCY AND LACTATION

Oral health is highly affected during pregnancy, with a high proportion of women undergoing inflammatory processes in gums leading to bleeding and gingivitis. Overproduction of some female hormones during pregnancy affects vascular permeability (Straka, 2011) facilitating the translocation of bacterial cells to the bloodstream. The use of molecular techniques has allowed the detection of DNA belonging to oral bacteria, such as *Fusobacterium nucleatum*, in placental tissue (Blanc et al., 2015) and, in fact, the composition of the oral microbiota may be a key player in the pregnancy outcome. As stated, bacteria present in placental or amniotic environment may colonize fetal skin, including the mammary buds (Fig. 13.1).

Recent findings suggest that selected bacteria of the maternal GI microbiota can access the mammary glands through oromammary and enteromammary pathways

(Martín et al., 2004; Rodríguez et al., 2014). Previous studies have indicated that certain bacteria from the maternal GI tract may spread to extraintestinal locations in healthy hosts (Ouwehand et al., 2001; Vankerckhoven et al., 2004; Begier et al., 2005; Jiménez et al., 2005; Dasanayake et al., 2005). Although this constitutes a controversial issue, some studies have offered a scientific basis for such physiological translocation (Rodríguez et al., 2014). The mechanism would involve dendritic cells (DCs) and CD18$^+$ cells (Vazquez-Torres et al., 1999; Rescigno et al., 2001; Macpherson and Uhr, 2004), which would be able to take up nonpathogenic bacteria from the GI lumen and, subsequently, to carry them to other locations, including the lactating mammary gland (Roitt, 2001) (Fig. 13.2). There is an intense efflux of intestinal immune cells to mammary glands during late pregnancy and lactation (Bertotto et al., 1991) and that, in fact, the existence of an enteromammary circulation of IgA-producing cells is long known (Newburg, 2005).

Two independent groups obtained in vitro and in vivo data reinforcing the hypothesis that at least some human milk bacteria may reach the mammary glands through an internal route, involving maternal DCs and macrophages (Langa, 2006; Perez et al., 2007; Langa et al., 2012). Two lactobacilli strains isolated from human milk (*Lactobacillus salivarius* CECT 5713 and *Lactobacillus gasseri* CECT 5713) translocated across a Caco-2 cell monolayer through a DC-mediated mechanism (Langa, 2006) (Fig. 13.3). In addition, oral inoculation of pregnant mice with a genetically labeled *E. faecium* M1a strain led to the isolation and polymerase chain reaction (PCR) detection of the labeled strain in amniotic fluid (Jiménez et al., 2005) and milk (unpublished results) of the inoculated animals. In contrast, the strain could not be detected in the respective samples obtained from a noninoculated control group. Similarly, oral administration of lactobacilli strains isolated from human milk led to their presence in the milk of more than 50% of the recruited women (Jiménez et al., 2008c; Arroyo et al., 2010; Fernández et al., 2015).

An increased bacterial translocation from the GI tract to mesenteric lymph nodes and mammary glands in pregnant and lactating mice was observed in another study (Perez et al., 2007). Bacteria could be observed histologically in the subepithelial dome and interfollicular regions of Peyer's patches, in the *lamina propria* of the small bowel, and associated with cells in the glandular tissue of the mammary gland. The Peyer's patches of pregnant and lactating mice were macroscopically larger than those of control animals and had a more prominent subepithelial dome and more dilated draining lymphatic vessels, containing mononuclear cells. The same study showed that human milk contains viable bacteria, including *Streptococcus*, *Lactobacillus*, and *Bifidobacterium*, while acridine orange staining of milk and blood cytopreparations identified bacterial cells in association with maternal mononuclear cells. Globally, these results strongly suggest the involvement of mononuclear cells in the transport of GI bacteria to mammary glands in late pregnancy.

The passage of viable bacteria through the intact intestinal mucosa is known as bacterial translocation. This phenomenon was postulated more than 60 years ago (Schweinburg et al., 1950), although the term "translocation" was first used to describe the passage of *Serratia marcescens* from the duodenum of rats, where it

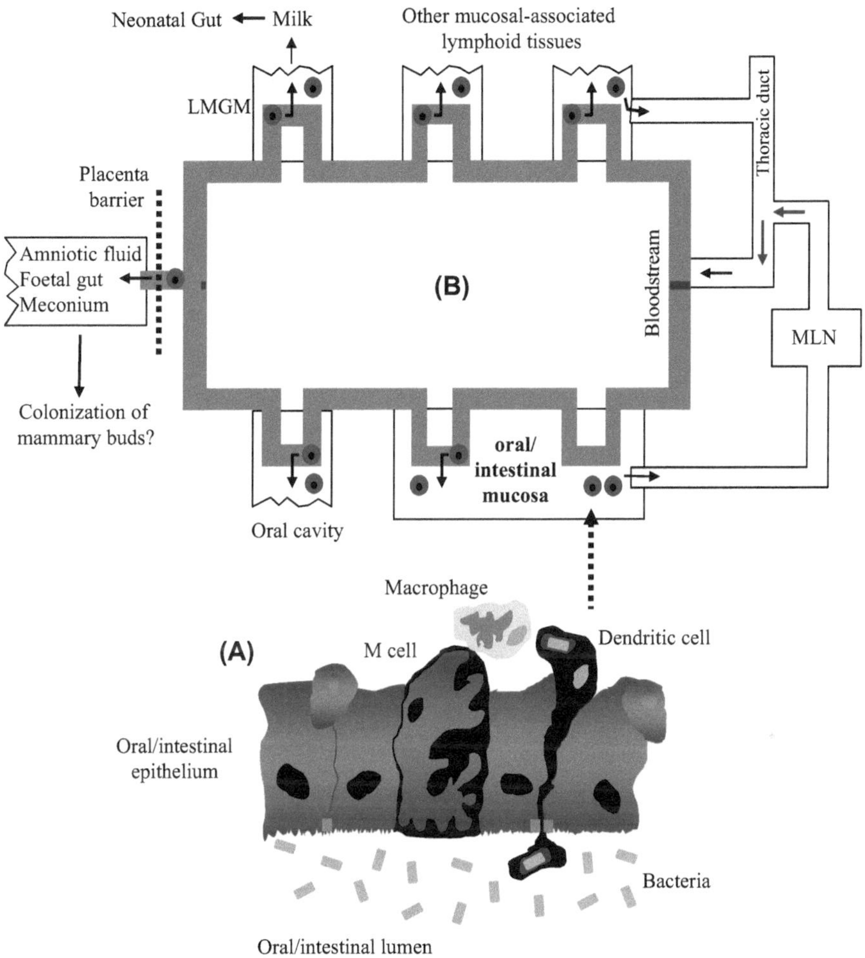

FIGURE 13.2

A hypothetical model to explain how some maternal bacterial strains could be transferred from the gastrointestinal tract (including the oral cavity) to the placenta and mammary glands during pregnancy and/or lactation. (A) Dendritic cells and/or other monocytes could penetrate the oral or intestinal epithelium to take up bacteria directly from lumen. (B) Once inside antigen-stimulated cells, bacteria could move from the digestive mucosa to colonize distant mucosal surfaces, since there is a circulation of lymphocytes within the mucosal associated lymphoid tissues, including those found in the genitourinary tracts, and, most significantly, that of the lactating mammary gland. *LMGM*, mucosa of the lactating mammary gland; *MLN*, mesenteric lymph node.

Adapted from Martín, R., Langa, S., Reviriego, C., Jiménez, E., Marín, M.L., Olivares, M., Boza, J., Jiménez, J., Fernández, L., Xaus, J., Rodríguez, J.M., 2004. The commensal microflora of human milk: new perspectives for food bacteriotherapy and probiotics. Trends in Food Science and Technology 15, 121–127.

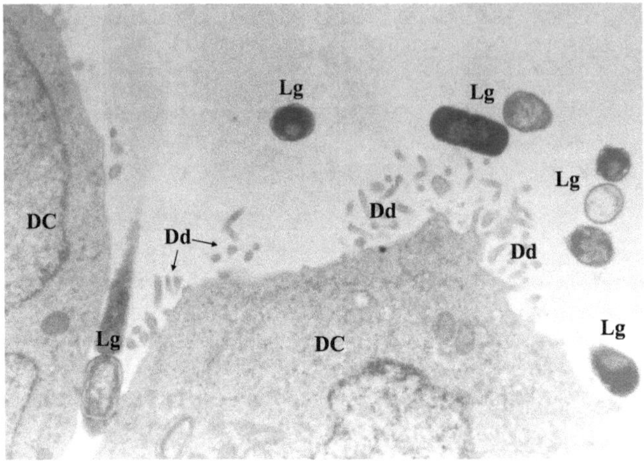

FIGURE 13.3

Specific interactions between cells of a *Lactobacillus gasseri* strain isolated from human milk (Lg) and dendritic cells (DCs), as assessed by transmission electron microscopy (Langa, 2006). The interactions were studied using transwell bicompartmental assays in which bacterial cells and immature DCs were initially separated by a monolayer of Caco-2 cells. *Dd*, DC dendrites.

had been inoculated, to the lymph (Wolochow et al., 1966). Later, the term "bacterial translocation" was defined as the passage of viable bacteria from the GI tract into the lamina propria and, then, to the mesenteric lymph nodes and other extraintestinal organs such as spleen, liver, kidneys, peritoneal cavity, or bloodstream (Berg and Garlington, 1979). Traditionally, GI bacteria translocation has been associated with pathogenic conditions and, therefore, it has been mainly studied in patients (e.g., severe burns, transplants, pancreatitis, cardiopulmonary diseases, AIDS) in whom pathogenic bacteria spread throughout the body causing sepsis, multiorgan failure, and, sometimes, death (Lichtman, 2001). However, it is known that a low-rate bacterial translocation also occurs in healthy individuals without causing detrimental effects on the host (Berg, 1995; Lichtman, 2001; Rodriguez et al., 2001). In a study involving 132 patients who underwent laparotomy, five showed positive culture results in their blood samples but the isolated bacteria lacked pathogenic traits and were not related to the patient morbidity (Moore et al., 1992). Langa (2006) reported that the rate of translocation of some lactic acid bacteria (0.002–0.009% after 2h) through a transwell system, involving interactions between immune cells and Caco-2 cells, were notably lower than those (>20%) reported for *Vibrio cholerae* (Kerneis et al., 2000) and invasive *Salmonella* (Jepson and Clark, 2001). In fact, it has been suggested that bacterial translocation to extraintestinal tissues is a beneficial physiological event in healthy hosts since it may be associated with immunomodulation, including the initial maturation of the neonatal immune system (Bengmark and Jeppsson, 1995; MacFie et al., 2004; Perez et al., 2007).

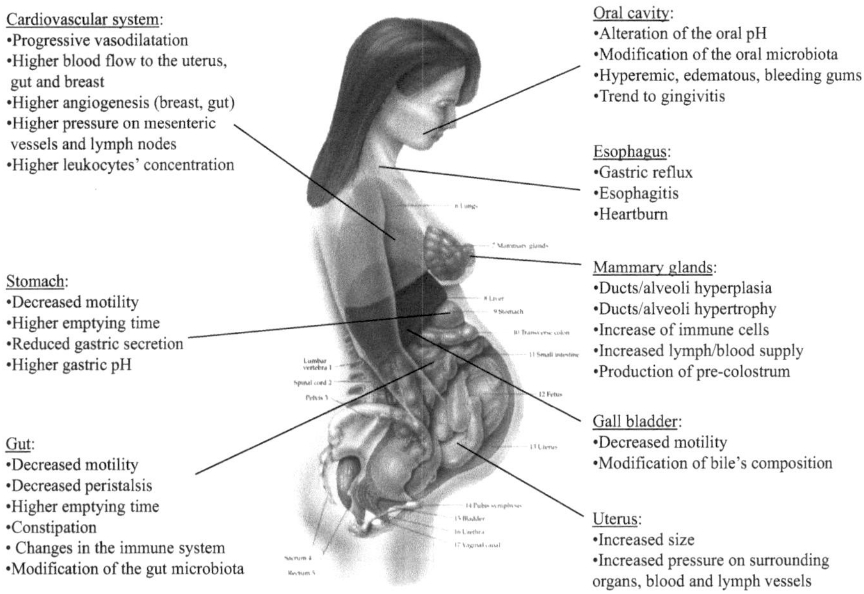

FIGURE 13.4

Physiological adaptations of the body during pregnancy predispose a mother to increased bacterial translocation.

Many transient anatomical and physiological changes occur during pregnancy and lactation to provide a suitable framework for the development of the fetus, first, and the neonate, later. These changes affect virtually all systems, including cardiovascular, respiratory, genitourinary, and digestive systems. Interestingly, such adaptations may favor an increased bacterial translocation during late pregnancy and early lactation (Fig. 13.4). Adequate cardiovascular adaptations must secure good placental development and appropriate fetal growth. Therefore, changes in the cardiovascular system are characterized by a progressive and generalized state of vasodilatation and an increase in several parameters or processes, including blood volume, stroke volume, cardiac output, heart rate, regional blood flow to various organs (uterus, kidneys, GI tract, skin, breasts), angiogenesis, and concentrations of coagulation factors and leukocytes in the blood.

As stated, the hormonal action induces relevant oral changes during pregnancy, affecting its pH and microbiota; the gums become hyperemic and edematous and tend to bleed, and the transfer of some bacterial species and inflammatory compounds to the bloodstream have been associated with the onset of premature birth (Straka, 2011). The main effects of gestation on the GI system are associated to the displacement of the abdominal organs by the progressive growth of the uterus and, also, to a decreased motility, presumably due to the effect of progesterone on smooth muscle contractility. This causes an increase in the gastric emptying time, while decreased gastric secretion results in a more basic gastric pH. The decreased GI motility and peristalsis, particularly in the last third of pregnancy, along with the increased pressure of the uterus, can cause problems of constipation and hemorrhoids. In addition, the maternal mesenteric blood vessels are exposed to estrogens and to increasing fetal pressure, leading to transient vascular engorgements and blood stasis. Additionally, one of the body's most dramatic adaptations to late pregnancy and lactation is a large increase in the size and complexity of the maternal intestine (Hammond, 1997). Globally, the digestive tract is characterized by weakened barriers against bacterial growth, increased permeability, and reduced peristalsis, three factors that are closely associated to bacterial translocation (Berg, 1995). Finally, several anatomical and physiological changes of the mammary system, including ducts, areola, and nipples (Beischer et al., 1997), during pregnancy facilitate the formation of a specific mammary microbiota (Fernández et al., 2013). Interestingly, there is a functional relationship between the GI tract and mammary glands during late pregnancy and lactation (Hammond, 1997).

The potential translocation process to the mammary gland may take place not only from the colon but also from other mucosal tissues. In this context, a study comparing different body locations found that the milk microbiome was most similar to that in the vaginal and oral niches (Cabrera-Rubio et al., 2012). Interestingly, it has been found that the placental microbiome is also most similar to that of the oral cavity (Aagaard et al., 2014). As a consequence, it is tempting to hypothesize that some bacteria make use of a similar mechanism to endogenously reach either the placenta or mammary glands during pregnancy. It is also important to note that fecal samples are the biological material routinely used to describe the GI microbiome and that the presence of lactic acid bacteria and typical oral inhabitants is limited in such samples. In contrast, the still scarce studies dealing with the microbial composition of the small intestine indicate a high presence of lactobacilli as well as oral microorganisms, including *Streptococcus* spp. or *Veillonella* spp. (Hayashi et al., 2005; de Meij et al., 2013; Leimena et al., 2013), which are also frequently present in milk under physiological conditions. Globally, this suggests that the oropharyngeal tract and the small intestine may be important and underestimated sources of bacteria to human milk (Fig. 13.1). The existence of such bacterial oromammary and enteromammary pathways would provide new opportunities for manipulating an altered maternal–fetal microbiota, reducing the risk of preterm birth and infant diseases (Martín et al., 2004; Rautava et al., 2012).

4. OTHER SOURCES OF BACTERIA TO HUMAN MILK: PUMPS AND OTHER BREASTFEEDING ACCESSORIES

The use of pumps to collect milk samples is associated with a high concentration of bacteria in milk, and particularly enterobacteria, which are not related to the usual human milk microbiota (Marín et al., 2009). Contamination of milk during pumping has been reported previously and seems to be of particular concern for premature infants or ill infants in neonatal intensive care units (Boo et al., 2001; Brown et al., 2005).

Pumps and other breastfeeding accessories such as nipple shields are frequently rinsed at home with tap water, and it must be highlighted that drinkable water is not sterile but contains microorganisms, including enterobacteria, *Pseudomonas*, *Stenotrophomonas*, and related gram-negative bacteria. Even hospital pumps and/or their accessories may not be properly sanitized and/or sterilized. Bacteria and yeasts usually persist after application of current cleaning protocols due to the formation of biofilms in the inner surfaces of such devices. Therefore, the design of new pumping devices that can be sterilized and subjected to more efficient cleaning and disinfection procedures is highly desirable.

REFERENCES

Aagaard, K., Ma, J., Antony, K.M., Ganu, R., Petrosino, J., Versalovic, J., 2014. The placenta harbors a unique microbiome. Science Translational Medicine 6, 237ra65.

Aas, J.A., Paster, B.J., Stokes, L.N., Olsen, I., Dewhirst, F.E., 2005. Defining the normal bacterial flora of the oral cavity. Journal of Clinical Microbiology 43, 5721–5732.

Abrahamsson, T.R., Sinkiewicz, G., Jakobsson, T., Fredrikson, M., Björkstén, B., 2009. Probiotic lactobacilli in breast milk and infant stool in relation to oral intake during the first year of life. Journal of Pediatric Gastroenterology and Nutrition 49, 349–354.

Albesharat, R., Ehrmann, M.A., Korakli, M., Yazaji, S., Vogel, R.F., 2011. Phenotypic and genotypic analyses of lactic acid bacteria in local fermented food, breast milk and faeces of mothers and their babies. Systematic and Applied Microbiology 34, 148–155.

Arroyo, R., Martin, V., Maldonado, A., Jimenez, E., Fernandez, L., Rodriguez, J.M., 2010. Treatment of infectious mastitis during lactation: antibiotics versus oral administration of lactobacilli isolated from breast milk. Clinical Infectious Diseases 50, 1551–1558.

Bearfield, C., Davenport, E.S., Sivapathasundaram, V., Allaker, R.P., 2002. Possible association between amniotic fluid micro-organism infection and microflora in the mouth. British Journal of Obstetrics and Gynaecology 109, 527–533.

Begier, E.M., Barrett, N.L., Mshar, P.A., Johnson, D.G., Hadler, J.L., Connecticut Bioterrorism Field Epidemiology Response Team, 2005. Gram-positive rod surveillance for early anthrax detection. Emerging Infectious Diseases 11, 1483–1486.

Beischer, N.A., Mackay, E.V., Colditz, P.B., 1997. Obstetrics and the Newborn. W.B. Saunders Company, Philadelphia.

Bengmark, S., Jeppsson, B., 1995. Gastrointestinal surface protection and mucosa reconditioning. Journal of Parenteral and Enteral Nutrition 19, 410–415.

Berg, R.D., 1995. Bacterial translocation from the gastrointestinal tract. Trends Microbiology 3, 149–154.

Berg, R.D., Garlington, A.W., 1979. Translocation of certain indigenous bacteria from the gastrointestinal tract to the mesenteric lymph nodes and other organs in a gnotobiotic mouse model. Infection and Immunology 23, 403–411.

Bertotto, A., Gerli, R., Castellucci, G., Scalise, F., Vaccaro, R., 1991. Human milk lymphocytes bearing the gamma/delta T-cell receptor are mostly delta TCS1-positive cells. Immunology 74, 360–361.

Blanc, V., O'Valle, F., Pozo, E., Puertas, A., León, R., Mesa, F., 2015. Oral bacteria in placental tissues: increased molecular detection in pregnant periodontitis patients. Oral Diseases 21, 905–912.

Boo, N.Y., Nordiah, A.J., Alfizah, H., Nor-Rohaini, A.H., Lim, V.K., 2001. Contamination of breast milk obtained by manual expression and breast pumps in mothers of very low birthweight infants. Journal of Hospital Infection 49, 274–281.

Brown, S.L., Bright, R.S., Dwyer, D.E., Forman, B., 2005. Breast pump adverse events: reports to the food and drug administration. Journal of Human Lactation 21, 169–174.

Cabrera-Rubio, R., Collado, M.C., Laitinen, K., Salminen, S., Isolauri, E., Mira, A., 2012. The human milk microbiome changes over lactation and is shaped by maternal weight and mode of delivery. American Journal of Clinical Nutrition 96, 544–551.

Cabrera-Rubio, R., Mira-Pascual, L., Mira, A., Collado, M.C., 2015. Impact of mode of delivery on the milk microbiota composition of healthy women. Journal of Developmental Origins of Health and Disease 19, 1–7.

Caufield, P.W., Dasanayake, A.P., Li, Y., Pan, Y., Hsu, J., Hardin, J.M., 2000. Natural history of *Streptococcus sanguinis* in the oral cavity of infants: evidence for a discrete window of infectivity. Infection and Immunity 68, 4018–4023.

Cephas, K.D., Kim, J., Mathai, R.A., Barry, K.A., Dowd, S.E., Meline, B.S., Swanson, K.S., 2011. Comparative analysis of salivary bacterial microbiome diversity in edentulous infants and their mothers or primary care givers using pyrosequencing. PLoS ONE 6, e23503.

Costello, E.K., Lauber, C.L., Hamady, M., Fierer, N., Gordon, J., Knight, R., 2009. Bacterial community variation in human body habitats across space and time. Science 326, 1694–1697.

Dasanayake, A.P., Li, Y., Wiener, H., Ruby, J.D., Lee, M.J., 2005. Salivary *Actinomyces naeslundii* genospecies 2 and *Lactobacillus casei* levels predict pregnancy outcomes. Journal of Periodontology 76, 171–177.

De Meij, T.G., Budding, A.E., Grasman, M.E., Kneepkens, C.M., Savelkoul, P.H., Mearin, M.L., 2013. Composition and diversity of the duodenal mucosa-associated microbiome in children with untreated coeliac disease. Scandinavian Journal of Gastroenterology 48, 530–536.

Fernández, L., Langa, S., Martín, V., Maldonado, A., Jiménez, E., Martín, R., Rodríguez, J.M., 2013. The human milk microbiota: origin and potential roles in health and disease. Pharmacological Research 69, 1–10.

Fernández, L., Cárdenas, N., Arroyo, R., Manzano, S., Jiménez, E., Martín, V., Rodríguez, J.M., 2015. Prevention of infectious mastitis by oral administration of *Lactobacillus salivarius* PS2 during late pregnancy. Clinical Infectious Diseases pii: civ974. PMID: 26611780.

Findley, K., Oh, J., Yang, J., Conlan, S., Deming, C., Meyer, J.A., Schoenfeld, D., Nomicos, E., Park, M., NIH Intramural Sequencing Center Comparative Sequencing Program, Kong, H.H., Segre, J.A., 2013. Topographic diversity of fungal and bacterial communities in human skin. Nature 498, 367–370.

Gosalbes, M.J., Llop, S., Vallès, Y., Moya, A., Ballester, F., Francino, M.P., 2013. Meconium microbiota types dominated by lactic acid or enteric bacteria are differentially associated with maternal eczema and respiratory problems in infants. Clinical & Experimental Allergy 43, 198–211.

Grice, E.A., Kong, H.H., Renaud, G., Young, A.C., NISC Comparative Sequencing Program, Bouffard, G.G., Blakesley, R.W., Wolfsberg, T.G., Turner, M.L., Segre, J.A., 2008. A diversity profile of the human skin microbiota. Genome Research 18, 1043–1050.

Grice, E.A., Kong, H.H., Conlan, S., Deming, C.B., Davis, J., Young, A.C., NISC Comparative Sequencing Program, Bouffard, G.G., Blakesley, R.W., Murray, P.R., Green, E.D., Turner, M.L., Segre, J.A., 2009. Topographical and temporal diversity of the human skin microbiome. Science 324, 1190–1192.

Gueimonde, M., Laitinen, K., Salminen, S., Isolauri, E., 2007. Breast milk: a source of bifidobacteria for infant gut development and maturation? Neonatology 92, 64–66.

Hammond, K.A., 1997. Adaptation of the maternal intestine during lactation. Journal of Mammary Gland Biology and Neoplasia 2, 243–252.

Hayashi, H., Takahashi, R., Nishi, T., Sakamoto, M., Benno, Y., 2005. Molecular analysis of jejunal, ileal, caecal and recto-sigmoidal human colonic microbiota using 16S rRNA gene libraries and terminal restriction fragment length polymorphism. Journal of Medical Microbiology 54, 1093–1101.

Hunt, K.M., Foster, J.A., Forney, L.J., Schütte, U.M.E., Beck, D.L., Abdo, Z., Fox, L.K., Williams, J.E., McGuire, M.K., McGuire, M.A., 2011. Characterization of the diversity and temporal stability of bacterial communities in human milk. PLoS ONE 6, e21313.

Jepson, M.A., Clark, M.A., 2001. The role of M cells in *Salmonella* infection. Microbes and Infection 3, 1183–1190.

Jiménez, E., Fernández, L., Marín, M.L., Martín, R., Odriozola, J.M., Nueno-Palop, C., Narrad, A., Olivares, M., Xaus, J., Rodríguez, J.M., 2005. Isolation of commensal bacteria from umbilical cord blood of healthy neonates born by caesarean section. Current Microbiology 51, 270–274.

Jimenez, E., Delgado, S., Maldonado, A., Arroyo, R., Albujar, M., Garcia, N., Jariod, M., Fernandez, L., Gomez, A., Rodriguez, J.M., 2008a. *Staphylococcus epidermidis*: a differential trait of the fecal microbiota of breast-fed infants. BMC Microbiology 8, 143.

Jiménez, E., Fernández, L., Delgado, S., García, N., Albújar, M., Gómez, A., Rodríguez, J.M., 2008b. Assessment of the bacterial diversity of human colostrum by cultural-based techniques. Analysis of the staphylococcal and enterococcal populations. Research in Microbiology 159, 595–601.

Jimenez, E., Fernandez, L., Maldonado, A., Martin, R., Olivares, M., Xaus, J., Rodriguez, J.M., 2008c. Oral administration of *Lactobacillus* strains isolated from breast milk as an alternative for the treatment of infectious mastitis during lactation. Applied and Environmental Microbiology 74, 4650–4655.

Jiménez, E., de Andrés, J., Manrique, M., Pareja-Tobes, P., Tobes, R., Martínez-Blanch, J.F., Codoñer, F.M., Ramón, D., Fernández, L., Rodríguez, J.M., 2015. Metagenomic analysis of milk of healthy and mastitis-suffering women. Journal of Human Lactation 31, 406–415.

Johansson, I., Lif Holgerson, P., 2011. Milk and oral health. Nestle Nutrition Workshop Series 67, 55–66.

Jost, T., Lacroix, C., Braegger, C., Chassard, C., 2013. Assessment of bacterial diversity in breast milk using culture-dependent and culture-independent approaches. British Journal of Nutrition 14, 1–10.

Jost, T., Lacroix, C., Braegger, C., Rochat, F., Chassard, C., 2014. Vertical mother-neonate transfer of maternal gut bacteria via breastfeeding. Environmental Microbiology 16, 2891–2904.

Kerneis, S., Caliot, E., Stubbe, H., Bogdanova, A., Kraehenbuhl, J., Pringault, E., 2000. Molecular studies of the intestinal mucosal barrier physiopathology using cocultures of epithelial and immune cells: a technical update. Microbes and Infection 2, 1119–1124.

Kulagina, E.V., Shkoporov, A.N., Kafarskaia, L.I., Khokhlova, E.V., Volodin, N.N., Donskikh, E.E., Korshunova, O.V., Efimov, B.A., 2010. Molecular genetic study of species and strain variability in bifidobacteria population in intestinal microflora of breastfed infants and their mothers. Bulletin of Experimental Biology and Medicine 150, 61–64.

Langa, S., 2006. Interactions Between Lactic Acid Bacteria, Intestinal Epithelial Cells and Immune Cells. Development of *In Vitro* Models (Ph.D. thesis). Complutense University of Madrid, Madrid.

Langa, S., Maldonado, A., Delgado, S., Martín, R., Martín, V., Jiménez, E., Ruíz-Barba, J.L., Mayo, B., Connor, R.I., Suárez, E., Rodríguez, J.M., 2012. Characterization of *Lactobacillus salivarius* CECT 5713, a strain isolated from human milk: from genotype to phenotype. Applied Microbiology and Biotechnology 94, 1279–1287.

Law, V., Seow, W.K., Townsend, G., 2007. Factors influencing oral colonization of mutans streptococci in young children. Australian Dental Journal 52, 93–100.

Leimena, M.M., Ramiro-Garcia, J., Davids, M., van den Bogert, B., Smidt, H., Smid, E.J., Boekhorst, J., Zoetendal, E.G., Schaap, P.J., Kleerebezem, M., 2013. A comprehensive metatranscriptome analysis pipeline and its validation using human small intestine microbiota datasets. BMC Genomics 14, 530.

Li, Y., Teague, E., Zhuang, Z., Caufield, P.W., 1997. Screening for the *spaP* gene of *Streptococcus mutans* in predentate infants. Journal of Dental Research 76, 102.

Lichtman, S.M., 2001. Bacterial translocation in humans. Journal of Pediatric Gastroenterology and Nutrition 33, 1–10.

Lif Holgerson, P., Harnevik, L., Hernell, O., Tanner, A.C., Johansson, I., 2011. Mode of birth delivery affects oral microbiota in infants. Journal of Dental Research 90, 1183–1188.

MacFie, J., 2004. Current status of bacterial translocation as a cause of surgical sepsis. British Medical Bulletin 71, 1–11.

Macpherson, A.J., Uhr, T., 2004. Induction of protective IgA by intestinal dendritic cells carrying commensal bacteria. Science 303, 1662–1665.

Makino, H., Kushiro, A., Ishikawa, E., Muylaert, D., Kubota, H., Sakai, T., Oishi, K., Martin, R., Ben Amor, K., Oozeer, R., Knol, J., Tanaka, R., 2011. Transmission of intestinal *Bifidobacterium longum* subsp. longum strains from mother to infant, determined by multilocus sequencing typing and amplified fragment length polymorphism. Applied and Environmental Microbiology 77, 6788–6793.

Marín, M.L., Arroyo, R., Jiménez, E., Gómez, A., Fernández, L., Rodríguez, J.M., 2009. Cold storage of human milk: effect on its bacterial composition. Journal of Pediatric Gastroenterology and Nutrition 49, 343–348.

Martín, R., Jiménez, E., Heilig, H.G., Fernández, L., Marín, M.L., Zoetendal, E.G., Rodríguez, J.M., 2009. Isolation of bifidobacteria from breast milk and assessment of the bifidobacterial population by PCR-denaturing gradient gel electrophoresis and quantitative real-time PCR. Applied and Environmental Microbiology 75, 965–969.

Martín, R., Jiménez, E., Olivares, M., Marín, M.L., Fernández, L., Xaus, J., Rodríguez, J.M., 2006. *Lactobacillus salivarius* CECT 5713, a potential probiotic strain isolated from infant feces and breast milk of a mother-child pair. International Journal of Food Microbiology 112, 35–43.

Martín, R., Langa, S., Reviriego, C., Jiménez, E., Marín, M.L., Olivares, M., Boza, J., Jiménez, J., Fernández, L., Xaus, J., Rodríguez, J.M., 2004. The commensal microflora of human milk: new perspectives for food bacteriotherapy and probiotics. Trends in Food Science and Technology 15, 121–127.

Martín, R., Langa, S., Reviriego, C., Jiménez, E., Marín, M.L., Xaus, J., Fernández, L., Rodríguez, J.M., 2003. Human milk is a source of lactic acid bacteria for the infant gut. Journal of Pediatrics 143, 754–758.

Martín, V., Maldonado, A., Moles, L., Rodríguez-Baños, M., Del Campo, R., Fernández, L., Rodríguez, J.M., Jiménez, E., 2012. Sharing of bacterial strains between breast milk and infant feces. Journal of Human Lactation 28, 36–44.

Martín, V., Mediano, P., Del Campo, R., Rodríguez, J.M., Marín, M., 2015. Streptococcal diversity of human milk and comparison of different methods for the taxonomic identification of streptococci. Journal of Human Lactation pii: 0890334415597901.

McGuire, M.K., McGuire, M.A., 2015. Human milk: mother nature's prototypical probiotic food? Advances in Nutrition 6, 112–123.

Moore, F.A., Moore, E.E., Poggetti, R.S., Read, R.A., 1992. Postinjury shock and early bacteremia: a lethal combination. Archives in Surgery 127, 893–898.

Nasidze, I., Li, J., Quinque, D., Tang, K., Stoneking, M., 2009. Global diversity in the human salivary microbiome. Genome Research 19, 636–643.

Newburg, D.S., 2005. Innate immunity and human milk. Journal of Nutrition 135, 1308–1312.

Oh, J., Byrd, A.L., Deming, C., Conlan, S., NISC Comparative Sequencing Program, Kong, H.H., Segre, J.A., 2014. Biogeography and individuality shape function in the human skin metagenome. Nature 514, 59–64.

Oh, J., Conlan, S., Polley, E.C., Segre, J.A., Kong, H.H., 2012. Shifts in human skin and nares microbiota of healthy children and adults. Genome Medicine 4, 77.

Oh, J., Freeman, A.F., NISC Comparative Sequencing Program, Park, M., Sokolic, R., Candotti, F., Holland, S.M., Segre, J.A., Kong, H.H., 2013. The altered landscape of the human skin microbiome in patients with primary immunodeficiencies. Genome Research 23, 2103–2114.

Ouwehand, A.C., Isolauri, E., He, F., Hashimoto, H., Benno, Y., Salminen, S., 2001. Differences in *Bifidobacterium flora* composition in allergic and healthy infants. Journal of Allergy and Clinical Immunology 108 144–145.

Perez, P.F., Doré, J., Leclerc, M., Lévense, F., Benyacoub, J., Serrant, P., Segura-Roggero, I., Schiffrin, E.J., Donnet-Hughes, A., 2007. Bacterial imprinting of the neonatal immune system: lessons from maternal cells? Pediatrics 119, 724–732.

Ramsey, D.T., Kent, J.C., Owens, R.A., Hartmann, P.E., 2004. Ultrasound imaging of milk ejection in the breast of lactating women. Pediatrics 113, 361–367.

Rautava, S., Luoto, R., Salminen, S., Isolauri, E., 2012. Microbial contact during pregnancy, intestinal colonization and human disease. Nature Reviews in Gastroenterology and Hepatology 9, 565–576.

Rescigno, M., Urbano, M., Valzasina, B., Francolín, M., Rotta, G., Bonasio, R., Granucci, F., Kraehenbuhl, J., Ricciardi-Castagnoli, P., 2001. Dendritic cells express tight junction proteins and penetrate gut epithelial monolayers to sample bacteria. Nature Immunology 2, 361–367.

Rodriguez, A.V., Baigorí, M.D., Alvarez, S., Castro, G.R., Oliver, G., 2001. Phosphatidylinositol-specific phospholipase C activity in *Lactobacillus rhamnosus* with capacity to translocate. FEMS Microbiology Letters 204, 33–38.

Rodríguez, J.M., 2014. The origin of human milk bacteria: is there a bacterial entero-mammary pathway during late pregnancy and lactation? Advances in Nutrition 2014 (5), 779–784.

Roitt, I., 2001. Essential Immunology. Blackwell Scientific Publications, Oxford.

Salter, S.J., Cox, M.J., Turek, E.M., Calus, S.T., Cookson, W.O., Moffatt, M.F., Turner, P., Parkhill, J., Loman, N.J., Walker, A.W., 2014. Reagent and laboratory contamination can critically impact sequence-based microbiome analyses. BMC Biology 12, 87.

Sampaio-Maia, B., Monteiro-Silva, F., 2014. Acquisition and maturation of oral microbiome throughout childhood: an update. Dental Research Journal 11, 291–301.

Schommer, N., Gallo, R.L., 2013. Structure and function of the human skin microbiome. Trends in Microbiology 21, 660–668.

Schweinburg, F.B., Seligman, A.M., Fine, J., 1950. Transmural migration of intestinal bacteria. Study based on use of radioactive *Escherichia coli*. New England Journal of Medicine 242, 747–751.

Straka, M., 2011. Pregnancy and periodontal tissues. Neuroendocrinology Letters 32, 34–38.

Takahashi, H., Mikami, K., Nishino, R., Matsuoka, T., Kimura, M., Koga, Y., 2010. Comparative analysis of the properties of bifidobacterial isolates from fecal samples of mother-infant pairs. Journal of Pediatric Gastroenterology and Nutrition 51, 653–660.

Vankerckhoven, V.V., Autgaerden, T.A., Huys, G., Vancanneyt, M., Swings, J., Goossens, H., 2004. Establishment of the PROSAFE collection of probiotic and human lactic acid bacteria. Microbial Ecology in Health and Disease 16, 131–136.

Vazquez-Torres, A., Jones-Carson, J., Baumler, A.J., Falkow, S., Valdivia, R., Brown, W., Le, M., Berggren, R., Parks, W.T., Fang, F.C., 1999. Extraintestinal dissemination of *Salmonella* by CD18-expressing phagocytes. Nature 401, 804–808.

Ward, T.L., Hosid, S., Ioshikhes, I., Altosaar, I., 2013. Human milk metagenome: a functional capacity analysis. BMC Microbiology 13, 116.

West, P.A., Hewitt, J.H., Murphy, O.M., 1979. The influence of methods of collection and storage on the bacteriology of human milk. Journal of Applied Bacteriology 46, 269–277.

Wolochow, H., Hildebrand, G.J., Lammanna, C., 1966. Translocation of microorganism across the intestinal wall in rats: effect of microbial size and concentration. Journal of Infectious Diseases 116, 523–528.

Yang, F., Zeng, X., Ning, K., Liu, K.L., Lo, C.C., Wang, W., Chen, J., Wang, D., Huang, R., Chang, X., Chain, P.S., Xie, G., Ling, J., Xu, J., 2012. Saliva microbiomes distinguish caries-active from healthy human populations. ISME Journal 6, 1–10.

Zaura, E., Nicu, E.A., Krom, B.P., Keijser, B.J., 2014. Acquiring and maintaining a normal oral microbiome: current perspective. Frontiers in Cell Infection and Microbiology 24, 85.

SECTION

E

Human Milk Microbes and Health

CHAPTER

An Evolutionary, Biosocial Perspective on Variation in Human Milk Microbes and Oligosaccharides: An Example of Eco-Homeorhesis?

14

Michelle K. McGuire[1], Courtney L. Meehan[1], Sarah Brooker[2], Janet E. Williams[2], James A. Foster[2], Mark A. McGuire[2]

[1]Washington State University, Pullman, WA, United States; [2]University of Idaho, Moscow, ID, United States

1. INTRODUCTION

Evolutionary processes have been critically important in shaping mammary gland structure and function as well as the process of lactation (a distinguishing characteristic of members of the class Mammalia) and its life-supporting product: milk (Capuco and Akers, 2009; Lemay et al., 2009; Oftedal, 2002). Indeed, given that milk is critical to the growth and development of mammalian neonates, evolutionary processes have surely played important roles in shaping both milk production and its composition. We posit that environmental microbes have likely also played an important role in this regard, but note that this is not a novel hypothesis.

Hayssen and Blackburn (1985) suggested more than three decades ago that lactation, itself, evolved due to selective pressures from microbial predation and that perhaps one of the important original roles of lactation was to provide the neonate with protection from microbes. Several decades later, Rosenberg and Rosenberg (2008), although not discussing lactation specifically, proposed that microbes and animals have coevolved in such a way that during periods of rapid environmental change, the diverse microbial community aided the combined human/microbe entity (referred to as the "holobiont") in surviving, multiplying, and "buying the time necessary for the host genome to evolve." Others (e.g., Dethlefsen et al., 2007) have also suggested a coevolution of microbes and humans, such that rapid shifts in ecological and behavioral factors (e.g., diet) influencing the delicate balance between the two taxa might result in disease.

Here, we review evidence that milk composition evolved via environmental and selective pressures across mammalian taxa and, more importantly, we argue that milk composition has likely evolved across *Homo sapiens* subgroups, to support neonatal

Prebiotics and Probiotics in Human Milk. http://dx.doi.org/10.1016/B978-0-12-802725-7.00014-2

survival within specific eco-cultural settings. Although our focus is on milk microbes and complex carbohydrates, we also briefly discuss other milk constituents such as lipids. In addition, we discuss selected sociocultural, behavioral, and environmental variables that may be important in shaping milk microbial communities worldwide and next steps as they relate to the use of population genetics approaches to investigate global milk composition variation.

2. MILK COMPOSITION: ONE-SIZE-FITS-ALL?

Milk composition varies among phylogenetic taxa. These compositional differences are thought to be a result of both genetic and environmental variation that respond to different selective pressures. Several examples of this "one-size-*does-not*-fit-all" construct are provided here.

2.1 INTERGENUS VARIATION IN MILK COMPOSITION

Although the etiological basis (including selective factors, if they exist) for evolutionary changes that have clearly taken place in terms of milk production and composition are not well understood, examples of variation in the evolution of lactation have been well described and explored across mammalian genera, particularly for total lipid content, the primary source of energy during early life. For instance, Oftedal has published several articles related to milk lipids in bears, true seals, and whales: large mammals that fast during much or all of their lactation (e.g., Oftedal, 1993, 1997). These mammals produce milk with exceptionally high lipid content (200–500 g/L) while fasting by mobilizing up to 40% of their body weight. These species have greater adipose and protein stores relative to rates of milk production, so that this intensive lactation period can occur without jeopardizing maternal health and subsequent reproductive efforts. This is not the case for other taxa, for example, *H. sapiens*; human milk typically contains 30–50 g/L lipids (Jensen, 1995). As described by Capuco and Akers (2009), these and other differences in lactation strategy and milk production are thought to have evolved to meet the diverse reproductive strategies and environmental demands of different mammals.

Concentrations and profiles of milk carbohydrates also vastly differ among genera. For instance, whereas primates and some ruminants produce milk with relatively high levels of lactose (~50–70 g/L), rodent milk has less (~30–50 g/L), and that of pinnipeds, cetaceans, bears, and marsupials often even less (~5–20 g/L, as reviewed by Jensen, 1995). Total complex carbohydrate (oligosaccharide) content and composition also vary among genera. For instance, bovine milk typically has a much lower oligosaccharide concentration and diversity than human milk (0.05 and 5–15 g/L, respectively), and the majority of the bovine oligosaccharides are more simplistic in their chemical structure than are those found in human milk. To date, only 40 different bovine milk oligosaccharides have been identified in the colostrum of Holstein-Friesian cows (Barile et al., 2010), whereas there are reportedly at least 100 human milk oligosaccharides (HMOs) (reviewed by Bode, 2012). Lactose concentration and oligosaccharide content and diversity also differ greatly among New and Old World monkeys (Goto et al., 2010), and between humans and apes (Urashima et al., 2009). As proposed by Urashima et al. (2012), it is possible that these vast differences in lactose and oligosaccharide profiles in milk are a result of gradual and bifurcated shifts in the function of the evolving mammary gland—first acting primarily as an innate immune tissue with high expression of lysozyme (an enzyme that helps destroy bacterial cell walls) and eventually, as the DNA encoding for α-lactalbumin evolved from DNA encoding for lysozyme, to a nutritive organ. Indeed, milk oligosaccharides predominate over lactose in monotremes and marsupials (more primitive mammals, Messer and Kerry, 1973), whereas milk produced by most of Eutherian taxa contains lactose as the dominant carbohydrate (Urashima et al., 2009). Urashima et al. (2012) have speculated that the high oligosaccharide concentration and somewhat unique oligosaccharide profile of human milk (compared with closely related apes) is an evolutionary consequence of human neonates being relatively more altricial and needing additional milk-borne protection from pathogenic organisms. How this likely relates to environmental microbial exposures is discussed later in this chapter.

Milk also differs in micronutrient concentrations. For instance, iron concentrations are low in human and bovine milk (0.3–0.9 and 0.2–0.6 μg/mL, respectively) relative to that produced by dogs (6.5–7.6 μg/mL) (Jensen, 1995). Iron, although essential for growth and development throughout the human lifecycle and still a major public health concern globally, is also necessary for the growth and replication of many bacteria. Iron's role in infectious disease (e.g., malaria) etiology is well known (e.g., Bullen et al., 1991; Gera and Sachdev, 2002; Murray et al., 1978; Ward et al., 1996). As such, the maintenance of very low iron levels in human milk has been hypothesized by some to represent an important evolutionary tradeoff favoring reduced risk of infectious disease during infancy over increased risk for mild iron deficiency (Quinn, 2014). This begs the questions of whether all human infants (regardless of their infectious disease risk) benefit from similar iron intake levels and if current practices related to iron supplementation during infancy and fortification of infant formulas with relatively high levels of iron are wise across the board.

In summary, there exist ample data suggesting that milk composition, at both macronutrient and micronutrient levels, varies among genera and that these differences may have evolved to maintain health across various environmental constraints (e.g., microbial exposures and risks) and behavioral contexts.

2.2 INTRASPECIES VARIATION IN MILK COMPOSITION

Certain milk components can also vary greatly even *within* a species. Take, for example, human milk lipids (including their fatty acid profiles), which are affected by maternal diet and maternal body composition. One of the first studies to provide evidence of this was conducted by Insull et al. (1959), who reported rapid, reversible shifts in milk fat in response to dietary macronutrient manipulation in a single, hospitalized breastfeeding woman. Karmarkar et al. (1963) also observed a 25% increase in milk fat content with dietary lipid supplementation. Similarly, Park et al. (1999) showed that milk fat was 18% higher when subjects consumed a high–dairy fat diet, and Mohammad et al. (2009) reported 12% greater milk fat when women consumed a high-lipid diet compared with an isocaloric, low-fat diet. Martín et al. (2012) provide similar data for forager-horticulturalists in Bolivia.

In addition to acute (proximal) effects of diet, long-term energy balance is also associated with total milk fat content: women with higher maternal body mass or body mass index (BMI) tend to produce higher-fat milk than those with lower BMI (Anderson et al., 2005; Quinn et al., 2016). This difference may both protect women living in regions with chronic malnutrition from mobilizing excess body weight during lactation and result in smaller offspring who will, across their entire lifespan, require fewer calories—an example of the "small but healthy" hypothesis (Messer, 1986; Pelto and Pelto, 1989). However, as discussed by Prendergast and Humphrey (2014), the tradeoff for stunted growth and decreased caloric requirements across the lifespan is likely increased morbidity and mortality in early life.

It is noteworthy that whereas lipids and selected other components (e.g., B vitamins) tend to be variable in milk produced by different women, concentrations of other components (e.g., iron) appear to be more conserved. As described previously for differences in milk iron concentrations among genera, it is thought that there may exist adaptive advantages to maintaining low iron content in human milk. This low level of variation for certain milk constituents, such as iron, may indicate a protective advantage that is not modified by other more fluid factors such as maternal nutritional status, environmental microbial exposures, and feeding practices. Conversely, greater plasticity in some components (e.g., lipids) might represent an important ability to adjust milk production and/or composition to adapt to more acute environmental conditions.

In addition to the essential and energy-yielding nutrients that are in milk, such as iron and lipids, there is also an impressive host of other biologically active components whose concentrations vary (or are conserved) among women. Of particular interest to us in this regard is the relatively high abundance and variability in complex carbohydrates and microbial taxa in milk, which are discussed in detail in the next section.

3. VARIABILITY IN HUMAN MILK OLIGOSACCHARIDES AND MICROBES: ECO-HOMEORHESIS?

As described briefly earlier and throughout this book, the overall concentration and profile of milk-borne complex carbohydrates differ among both genera and species. Furthermore, although an individual woman appears to have a somewhat consistent HMO profile over lactation, there exists significant variation among women (reviewed by Kobata, 2010). In addition to their importance for nourishing health-promoting bacteria in the breastfed infant's gastrointestinal (GI) tract, emerging research also shows that HMOs act as antiadhesive antimicrobials that serve as soluble decoy receptors as well as modulate epithelial and immune cell responses; many of these effects are thought to be HMO isoform specific. To date, however, there has been almost no parallel research documenting and understanding milk microbe variation among and within mammalian taxa. Neither has there been much work describing the relationship between HMO profiles and milk microbial community structure, a connection that makes as much intuitive and scientific sense as that of the importance of HMOs on the recipient infant's GI microbiome.

Here, we explore the possibility that differences in longstanding microbial exposures due to a combination of environmental and sociocultural factors may have resulted in milk microbe variability among human populations. In addition, optimal milk microbial community structures in a particular location and culture may have been, at least in part, shaped by selective pressures resulting in the evolution of genes responsible for HMO synthesis. If true, this would represent an example of host–microbe coevolution, as described previously. Indeed, what is "normal" milk composition in terms of milk microbes and HMOs in one population may not be optimal in another. We refer to this overarching concept as an example of "*eco-homeorhesis*," which we define here as a shift in what would be considered a "normal" homeostatic range or profile *to support health in a particular ecological/behavioral niche*. The term *eco-homeorhesis* represents a modification of the term "homeorhesis," the orchestrated or coordinated shift in what would be considered a "normal" homeostatic range *to support a physiological state*, such as pregnancy or lactation (Bauman and Curie, 1980). We recognize that substantial interdisciplinary work, including focused research from a population genetics viewpoint, will be required to provide "hard" evidence for our theory of eco-homeorhesis as it might relate to variation in milk composition. Nonetheless, to our knowledge, the possibility that normal milk composition may vary across human populations to specifically support health, therein, has not been seriously considered by others in the field and, if true, may have important implications for infant feeding in various environments and cultures.

3.1 GENOMIC VARIATION AND HUMAN MILK OLIGOSACCHARIDE SYNTHESIS

Because relatively little is known about the complex and diverse metabolic pathways underlying the synthesis of the known 100-plus complex carbohydrates moieties present in human milk, almost nothing is known about whether variation in HMO profiles among women is evolutionarily derived via natural selection, genetic drift, or some other factor(s) influencing genetic variation. Nonetheless, some inferential evidence can be gleaned from basic observational data related to phenotypic differences in HMOs as well as genomic variation in *FUT2* and *FUT3*, two relatively well characterized genes encoding for α1,2-fucosyltransferase (FUT2) and α1,3/4-fucosyltransferase (FUT3), respectively. As described in more detail elsewhere in this book, FUT2 transfers a fucose residue to a Gal*β*(1→3)GlcNAc unit (type 1 chain), and its presence characterizes positive "secretor" (Se) status and forms the basis of the ABO blood-typing system. FUT3 transfers a fucose in an α(1-4)-linkage to a subterminal *N*-acetylglucosamine residue of a type 1 chain to produce the Lewis B antigen in secretors and the Lewis A antigen in nonsecretors. Because of the intimate associations of FUT2 and FUT3 activities with these commonly used blood typing schemes, their distributions, evolution, and potential health outcomes have been relatively well studied.

In this section, we will first briefly describe what is known about phenotypic differences in HMO profiles, particularly as they relate to FUT2 and FUT3 patterns, among women and populations around the globe. Then, we will draw on the blood group literature to infer the possibility that this variation is or is not driven by selection and, if so, briefly review contemporary thought related to potential fitness benefits derived from this selection.

3.1.1 Global Variation in Human Milk Oligosaccharide Profiles

Oligosaccharide profiles vary among populations and women, although the relative proportions of the HMOs present tend to be more consistent within an individual woman than between women. For instance, in a study designed to examine the complex human milk metabolome, Smilowitz et al. (2013) found that in a largely Caucasian sample of American women, although total HMO concentration was relatively conserved across women, several of the most variable metabolites were HMO (e.g., 2′-FL) or their constituents (e.g., fucose). Currently, almost nothing is known about the etiology of this variability aside from activity of FUT2 and FUT3, which not only influence the presence or absence of α1-2-fucosylated and α1-4-fucosylated HMO (respectively) but also many other HMO varieties because their precursors compete with those of FUT2 and/or FUT3 (Kumazaki and Yoshida, 1984; Xu et al., 1996). In addition, it is clear that other fucosyltransferases are also involved (Newburg et al., 2005), complicating the predictability of HMO profiles purely from genetics. Indeed, aside from genetic predisposition, it is also theoretically possible that other factors such as acute and chronic maternal nutritional status and environmental variables might impact HMO profiles via either acute effects or more long-term programming (potentially via epigenetic modification), but there exist no data to support or refute this possibility.

Although published nearly two decades ago, perhaps the most relevant study conducted to date in which interpopulation variation in HMO profiles was investigated was conducted by Erney (2000), who compared neutral oligosaccharides in milk collected from 435 women living in 10 countries. Consistency in milk collection and analysis methods makes the results of this study powerful in terms of population comparisons. Although the authors recognize that in some cases small sample sizes within countries make comparisons and generalizations difficult, several findings were of significance. For instance, 2′-FL was found in every milk sample collected in Mexico ($n = 156$) and Sweden ($n = 7$) but in only 46% of samples collected in the Philippines ($n = 22$). Sweden, although composing the smallest sample size, presented a particularly interesting picture; with all samples containing eight of the nine HMOs studied, and none of the samples containing the other (3-FL). In all, 85%

and 86% of the women tested could be classified as secretors and Lewis positive, respectively, based on their HMO profile. When locations were grouped into region (Asia, Europe, Latin America, and United States), the authors concluded that 3-FL showed the most interregional variability, with an average of 1.87 g/L in the United States compared with 0.76 g/L in Latin American counties combined. Although these data are observational in nature and it is clear that environmental and behavioral confounders might help explain population differences, they provide some evidence that group differences exist in the presence and/or activity of both FUT2 and FUT3 as they relate to HMO synthesis in the human mammary gland. Future studies of this type should also strive to use consistent sample collection, storage, and analysis procedures to be able to make cross-population comparisons. In addition, collecting information about genetic ethnicity or race, relating genotypes to phenotypes, and including African populations that might be expected to present the greatest diversity in terms of genetics would lend important information related to evolutionary theory in this regard.

In one of the few studies to focus on milk produced by any African population, Totten et al. (2012) evaluated HMO profiles in 60 Gambian women with various Lewis and secretor blood groups: as expected, there was a relatively high proportion of women (27%) who were nonsecretors in terms of blood group type. Milk from secretor mothers had higher total oligosaccharide concentrations and fucosylated HMOs than that produced by nonsecretors. Based on previous reports of higher levels of nonsecretor phenotypes occurring in other African locations, Central Asia and Pacific regions, and Far East populations, the authors posit that this may be related to providing protection against viral infections common to those locals (e.g., certain strains of norovirus, influenza, rhinovirus, and HIV) as hypothesized by Anstee (2010). They also note that, in order to investigate whether various HMOs might foster growth of locally adapted microbial communities in the recipient infant, future studies should aim to relate variation in HMO profiles to infant GI microbial community structures.

3.1.2 Human Milk Oligosaccharide Profiles and Infectious Disease Risk

HMO profiles were also assessed in 187 HIV-infected and 36 uninfected women living in or around Lusaka, Zambia, to determine if risk for vertical transmission of the virus from mother to infant was related to abundance (or presence/absence) of a particular carbohydrate moiety or profile (Bode et al., 2012). Mothers and infants were studied from birth to 2 years postpartum, largely during the time prior to wide availability of antiretroviral therapy. Although blood group (secretor and Lewis status) was not associated with risk for transmission, lower total HMO level and higher proportion of 3′-SL (alternatively lower proportions of non–3′-SL HMOs) were related to greater rates of transmission. Although it is possible that HIV infection might induce greater synthesis of 3′-SL via epigenetic reprogramming (a host response; Giordanengo et al., 2004), it is also possible that increased presence of 3′-SL in the mammary gland or infant GI tract might directly or indirectly promote HIV infection in the infant. If the latter is true, one would expect that in regions of the world with high prevalence of poorly controlled HIV infection, genetic variation responsible for lower 3′-SL levels in milk might be selected for and future generations of women would, on average, produce milk with lower average 3′-SL concentrations.

Using this logic, it would be interesting and informative to test findings from animal and in vitro work showing that particular oligosaccharides commonly found in milk differentially influence growth and/or virulence of potential pathogens in populations where that particular pathogen commonly causes or does not cause childhood mortality. In addition, because these complex carbohydrates are thought to act as important prebiotics influencing microbial community patterns in the neonatal GI tract, understanding whether there exist relationships among endemic environmental pathogen burden, milk HMO profile, infant GI microbiome, and neonatal disease incidence and severity would lend insight into possible evolutionary shifts that have either coincidentally or selectively shaped human milk composition to best suit various socioecological contexts.

For instance, in locations where clean water is available at the turn of a spigot, excellent medical care widely accessible, and adequate nutrition the norm, neither HMO consumption nor GI microbiota might greatly impact diarrhea risk due to *Campylobacter pylori* infection. However, in a setting where infants live in proximity to domestic fowl (a common carrier of *C. pylori*) and do not have access to clean water and optimal nutrition, higher consumption of certain HMOs, like 2′-FL, known to impact infection (Ruiz-Palacios et al., 2003) might have fitness benefits. Indeed, incidence of *Campylobacter*-associated diarrhea was found to be substantially reduced in infants living in San Pedro Martir (a transitional neighborhood of Mexico City) consuming medium– to high–2′-FL milk compared with those consuming low amounts (Morrow et al., 2004). Similar associative findings were reported for lacto-*N*-difucohexaose (LDFH-1) content in milk and norovirus diarrhea. Of interest is the fact that, like Erney et al. (2000), Morrow et al. (2004) reported that 100% of the milk samples they collected from Mexican women contained 2′-FL.

A similar story can be told involving rotovirus diarrhea—common in both human infants and farm animals—but in this instance, lactadherin (a milk fat membrane–bound sialylated glycoprotein) appears to act as a decoy for rotovirus binding to intestinal cells (Yolken et al., 1992). Extending these findings are those of Newberg et al. (1998) showing that, in breastfed infants who present with rotovirus in their stools, those who exhibited symptoms of diarrhea were consuming milk with reduced levels of lactadherin. Again, it is possible that—particularly in populations with endemic livestock-related rotovirus burden combined with the enhanced potential for zoonotic transmission due to close contact of animals with infants—evolutionary pressures have favored increased acidic (sialylated) oligosaccharide content of human milk.

Clearly, environmental pathogen exposure and relationship with early life disease vary among populations and contexts worldwide. Importantly, whether these exposures lead to disease is confounded by a host of environmental, ecological, and sociocultural factors—for instance, availability of clean water and overall hygiene behaviors, general nutritional status and food intake patterns, customary childcare and parenting patterns, and availability of medical care. Untangling this complicated web of factors, including how breastfeeding and milk composition may mediate its various components and the possibility that milk composition (particularly HMO profiles) has been selectively shaped over time by culture- and location-specific variables, will necessitate careful data collection and collaborations among seasoned researchers in a multitude of disciplines.

3.1.3 Blood Group Type and Infectious Disease Risk

Although beyond the scope of this book, it is relevant to note that there is an extensive literature outlining the potential relationship between blood groups and host susceptibility to various infectious diseases (as reviewed by Cooling, 2015). In addition, there appears to be a somewhat coordinated relationship between blood group expression and maturation of the infant's GI microbiome; for instance, commensal bacteria that use fucose as a nutrient appear to be able to upregulate expression of *FUT2* (Meng et al., 2007; Nanthakumar et al., 2003). Various microbes can also induce the synthesis of ABO antibodies (Galili et al., 1988; Springer, 1971; Springer et al., 1959). As such, there appears to be a bidirectional and intimate physiological relationship between bacteria and blood group antigens that is likely important in disease modulation.

Examples of this relationship are two studies suggesting a possible role for FUT2 in influencing risk of cholera infection. Chaudhuri and DasAdhikary (1978) documented that nonsecretor status was twofold higher than expected (from population statistics) in cholera patients. Arifuzzaman et al. (2011) also found that the prevalence of a nonsecretor, Lewis(a^+b^-) phenotype was significantly increased in cholera patients compared with household contacts and healthy controls. Similarly, a nonsecretor blood group phenotype has been associated with greater likelihood of *H. pylori* disease (Heneghan et al., 2000; Rothenbacher et al., 2004), although this relationship has not been consistently found (DeMattos et al., 2002; Martins et al., 2006). Secretor status has also been identified as a biomarker for necrotizing enterocolitis risk in premature infants; those who were either nonsecretors or heterozygous for *FUT2* were at greater risk than secretors (Morrow et al., 2011). Of course, infant secretor status is a factor of parental secretor status and related to milk HMO content, making assessment of causality particularly complicated. Nonsecretor blood type is also related to lower HIV transmission, especially among heterosexuals (Ali et al., 2000; Kindberg et al., 2006). In conclusion, there are ample examples of relationships between various FUT2 (secretor)- and FUT3 (Lewis)-dependent blood groups and disease risk. Whether the well-documented population differences in these blood groups were the result of random genetic drift and/or founder effect or were the result of natural selection arising from differences in fitness within a sociocultural/environmental milieu remains a matter of debate (Anstee, 2010; Cooling, 2015). We posit that the same can be said for HMOs, their variation among populations, and their genomic basis.

3.2 VARIATION IN HUMAN MILK MICROBES

As previously noted, it has been suggested that the human–microbiome complex can be treated as a combined organism, a holobiont, with the genetic material composing a hologenome. We propose that this construct could be extended one step further: treating the mother and child along with their collective microbial communities as a larger holobiont or an "*epi-holobiont*" during the period of breastfeeding and consistent intimate contact between mothers and their infants. Here, we define an *epi-holobiont* as a collective comprising more than one individual (e.g., mother–infant dyad) and their associated microbiota. Consequently, the combined genetic material within an epi-holobiont would be its *epi-holobiome*. Furthermore, if microbe–host coevolution has indeed occurred across human populations to improve fitness, then perhaps instead of considering an individual and his/her microbes as the unit of measure of interest (i.e., the holobiont), we might instead consider the maternal–infant dyad along with their combined interacting microbes (i.e., the epi-holobiont).

The presence of bacteria in many human niches such as the GI tract and skin has been recognized for decades. More recently, emerging data convincingly show that the mammary gland itself contains a resident network of living bacteria that become milk constituents during the period of lactation. These microbes are thought to originate from several sources, including the infant's mouth, areola, and surrounding skin and the mother's own circulatory system (Fernández et al., 2013). As such, their composition is likely influenced directly by environmental microbial exposure and, indirectly, by factors that influence this exposure. As described previously in this and other chapters, HMO concentrations and profiles, via their prebiotic properties, have long been thought to impact early colonization of the *infant's* GI microbial communities. It is equally as likely, however, that oligosaccharide profiles in the mammary gland and milk impact growth and community structure of *milk-borne* microbes. If, as argued previously, maternal genomic variation (and perhaps evolutionary pressures that have shaped it) impacts milk carbohydrate profiles in ways that we are just beginning to understand, this logic would also support the concept that a woman's particular genetic makeup might, at least in part, also indirectly influence the microbial communities in the milk she produces.

Not much is known about variation in the human milk microbiome among women and populations, but limited data suggest variation among populations, and there is some (but conflicting) evidence that demographic, environmental, and physiological variables might be related to this variation. These variables include geographic location (which encompasses myriad variables including genetics and dietary patterns Cabrera-Rubio et al., 2012), time postpartum (Cabrera-Rubio et al., 2012; Urbaniak et al., 2016), reproductive variables (e.g., delivery mode; Cabrera-Rubio et al., 2012, 2016; Hoashi et al., 2015; Khodayar-Pardo et al., 2014; Urbaniak et al., 2016), and maternal health (e.g., obesity and disease, Cabrera-Rubio et al., 2012; Olivares et al., 2015). Of particular interest to this chapter is the potential interactive impact of chronic microbial exposures, disease risk, culturally relevant dietary patterns (e.g., probiotic foods), reproductive variables (e.g., delivery mode and location), and child-rearing practices (e.g., feeding colostrum, introduction of supplementary foods) as these might work together to shape the milk microbiome to support optimal child health.

3.2.1 Milk Microbes, Infection, and Maternal Health

Several research groups have reported differences in milk microbial communities based on maternal health status. For example, González et al. (2013) found higher bacterial diversity and frequency of *Lactobacillus* spp. in HIV-positive, Mozambique women and lower frequency of *Staphylococcus hominis* and *S. aureus* than in their HIV-counterparts. These differences are likely not related to sampling or methodological issues because all samples were collected and analyzed in a similar manner. However, one cannot infer causality (or directionality) from these differences. It is possible that factors associated with different microbial ecologies in milk might influence susceptibility to HIV, but equally possible that HIV infection triggers microbial community shifts. Unfortunately, because HMO were not reported, it is not possible to assess the more complex multivariate relationships among HMO profiles, milk microbes, and HIV susceptibility. In addition, breastfeeding characteristics and other sociocultural factors, such as probiotic and other dietary intake, were not reported in detail, although milk produced by exclusively breastfeeding women was found to have higher proportions of *Streptococcus parasanguis* than that of women who had already introduced supplementary foods; presence of *S. parasanguis* in milk also decreased with time postpartum. As such, and although these findings represent an important observation relating differences in milk microbial communities with maternal health, it is not possible to draw any causal conclusions.

Similarly, Olivares et al. (2015) reported in a cross-sectional study that concentrations (number of gene copies/mL) of *Bifidobacterium* spp. and *Bacteroides fragilis* group were higher in milk produced by 12 self-reported healthy, Spanish mothers than that collected from 12 lactating, Spanish women with celiac disease. Whether these differences are due strictly to the disease or other confounding factors, such as gluten or other components of the diet, are not known. Again, HMOs were not reported.

Although a connection between HMOs and milk microbe variability is intriguing and biologically plausible, currently almost nothing is known about the relationship between HMO content and profile and variation of microbes in milk. However, Hunt et al. (2012) have provided in vitro evidence that HMOs can interact with the bacterial communities present in milk—specifically with regard to enhancing growth of *Staphylococcus* spp. Whether this effect occurs within a woman's mammary gland is unknown.

In conclusion, there is limited evidence that demographic, physiological, and environmental factors are associated with variation in the microbes present in a woman's milk. Please refer to Chapter 12 in this book for more detail about what is known in this regard. As such, it will likely be impossible to describe a single "normal" milk microbiome, as its membership and distribution probably are dependent on other important factors such as environment, dietary habits, delivery mode, and other birth attributes, time postpartum, breastfeeding behaviors, and even genetics.

Some of these factors are described next. In particular, they are examined using an anthropological, rather than a purely biological, viewpoint.

4. SOCIOCULTURAL FACTORS AND MATERNAL–INFANT MICROBIAL EXPOSURES

Here we examine cross-cultural variation in maternal and early infant physical, social, and cultural environments that might lead to differential microbial exposure for mothers and infants and argue that such factors may be possible candidates for driving variation in milk components—particularly microbes. The major factors suggested to influence infant microbial colonization, although their effects are variable, include birth mode, feeding pattern, neonatal intensive care practices, antibiotic usage, sanitary conditions, family composition, and physical location (e.g., country of birth) (Adlerberth and Wold, 2009; Fallani et al., 2010; Penders et al., 2006). Additional inquiry including whether presence of animals and maternal diet are factors in early microbial colonization, to date, have indicated no or minimal influence (Adlerberth and Wold, 2009; Penders et al., 2006; Song et al., 2013). However, in a study conducted by Albesharat et al. (2011) in Syria, genotypic and phenotypic analyses of lactic acid bacteria in locally produced fermented foods were compared with that of human milk and fecal samples collected from mother–infant dyads. The results revealed striking similarities among sample types, prompting the researchers to conclude that there may be vertical transfer of bacteria ingested by the mother to her infant via an enteromammary route. In other words, these results provide evidence that environmental bacteria (in this case from foods) directly influences milk composition and, in turn, infant GI microbiota.

Given the relative newness of these lines of investigation, it is perhaps not surprising that much of the research has been done in Western populations, although there are notable exceptions (e.g., Adlerberth et al., 1991; Bennet et al., 1991). Yet, the vast variability in maternal and early infant environments and experiences around the world makes it essential for future research to remain vigilant to cross-cultural variation. Attention to the diversity of infants' environments and experiences will help elucidate factors related to bacteria–host coevolution, particularly as it relates to the maternal/infant epi-holobiont, and help us identify factors that may influence variation in milk composition and its influence on infant health and development (Benezra et al., 2012). Attention to such diversity is particularly important for the most at-risk infants around the world.

In the majority of the world, infants are born into and mother–infant dyads reside in environments that do not resemble Western physical or social environments. Thus, it is perhaps best to consider infants' early microbial exposure through a biosocial lens. We use the term "*biosocial*" because early life experiences are simultaneously biological and universal but mediated by the range of social and cultural options available. For instance, the biosocial nature of birth (see Jordan, 1992) has universal components to it which every neonate and mother experience, but the location, interventions, presence or absence of particular individuals, and procedures during and following birth [such as treatment of the vernix caseosa, a substance containing antimicrobial agents (Tollin et al., 2005; Yoshio et al., 2003)] alter the pathways as well as the type and level of microbial exposure the mother-infant dyad experiences. Thus, we consider and explore the current state-of-knowledge related to mother–infant microbial exposure through this biosocial lens. A holistic perspective is essential for us to not only understand factors that affect mother–infant microbial exposure and the development of complex epi-holobiont's microbiological communities, but it will also enhance our understanding regarding the scope and extent of such variation at the species level (see Fortenberry, 2013).

4.1 BIRTH MODE

One of the most recognized sources of microbial exposure and subsequent influences on the infant microbiome is birth mode. Exposure to the maternal vaginal, fecal, and perineal microbes during birth begins the process of microbial colonization in neonates (Dominguez-Bello et al., 2010; Fallani et al., 2010; Koenig et al., 2011; Madan et al., 2016; Penders et al., 2006). Yet, location and hospital practice may be equally important in terms of exposure and early colonization. Pakistani infants delivered via cesarean acquire *E. coli* (most frequently via mothers during birth) almost as early as do infants delivered vaginally, suggesting substantial environmental exposure to *E. coli* in Pakistani hospitals (Adlerberth et al., 1991). Additionally, Ethiopian newborn infants showed no consistent change in GI microbes attributable to antibiotic treatment (Bennet et al., 1991), a finding in opposition to multiple studies on the effects of antibiotics on the infant gut microbiome in Western cultures (e.g., Penders et al., 2006). Bennet et al. (1991) hypothesize that one reason for the difference may lie in Ethiopians' overall greater exposure to bacteria in their environment. Last, changes in the development of the infant GI microbiome over the last 30 years in Sweden, as outlined by Adlerberth et al. (2006), suggest that even in the short term, evolving hospital hygienic practices in this country are significantly altering early infant GI colonization. In this case, changes in infant GI microbiota indicate a reduction in gram-negative bacteria over the last several decades. As a whole, such studies suggest differential environmental exposure and GI colonization are heavily influenced by infants' immediate physical environment following birth.

For the millions of infants around the world who are not born in Western-style hospitals, but rather in clinics, homes, or even nearby fields, environmental exposure and local practice may be of particular relevance for maternal and infant microbial colonization and their collective epi-holobiome. For instance, although data do not exist to examine this directly, it has been suggested that the position of the mother during birth may influence an infant's exposure to fecal bacteria (Adlerberth and Wold, 2009). A nonsupine position, cross-culturally common (Trevathan, 2011) may increase maternal to infant fecal bacterial transfer during parturition (Adlerberth and Wold, 2009). If the infant is then put directly to the breast and concomitant transfer occurs from the infant's mouth to the mother's breast, this may theoretically affect the milk microbiome.

4.2 FEEDING PATTERN

The composition of infants' diets is also one of the earliest factors affecting early microbial exposure and colonization of the infant GI tract (Edwards and Parrett, 2002; Penders et al., 2006; Thompson, 2012). For most infants, it is thought that the early influence of breastfeeding (or not) has the most lasting influence. For instance, bacteria in human milk (Jeurink et al., 2013; Hunt et al., 2011; Martín et al., 2012) likely contribute directly to the colonization of the neonatal GI microbes, leading to significant differences in infant fecal microbiota between breastfed and formula-fed infants (Fanaro et al., 2003; Madan et al., 2016; Penders et al., 2006). Of course, other factors in human milk such as its oligosaccharides (described earlier) also influence the infant's GI microbiome. Although the source of the human milk microbiome is still debated (Cabrera-Rubio et al., 2012; Jeurink et al., 2013; Hunt et al., 2011), maternal microbial exposure through biosocial and environmental exposures may prime infants for their specific ecological niche. Future research is needed to tease apart the biosocial and environmental factors driving variation in the milk microbiome. But, since human milk is one of the earliest influences on the development on infant GI tract, and variation in milk microbiome has been posited to be responsive to genetic, cultural, environmental, or dietary influences (Hunt et al., 2011), this line of inquiry may illuminate yet another pathway by which milk constituents have evolved to protect infants in environments they would be otherwise immunologically ill prepared with meet.

Cross-cultural differences in microbial exposure continue to increase as infants' diets expand. Even in the United States, where early supplementation is generally more limited than what is seen cross-culturally, the influence of a mixed diet (breastmilk and formula) is still substantial. Maden et al. (2016), in a study of 6-week-old infants living in New Hampshire, found that the microbial community composition of infants fed a mixed diet resembled that of formula-fed infants more than exclusively breastfed infants. Moreover, GI microbiota appear to diversify with the introduction of solid foods, pointing to weaning as a later (albeit currently argued to be less influential) factor influencing infants' microbiome maturation process (Fallani et al., 2011). Yet, cross-culturally, breastfeeding practices are fluid and, in many regions of the world, early supplementation goes beyond formula-derived from clean water sources. In many small-scale societies, women breastfeed on average for more than 2 years (Sellen and Smay 2001), far exceeding the average in the United States where only 27% of infants are still breastfed at 12 months of age (National Center for Chronic Disease Prevention and Health Promotion, 2014). Moreover, late initiation of breastfeeding, colostrum taboos, and the early introduction of non–breast milk substances are common in non-Western societies (Sellen and Smay, 2001).

Some of the best examples of maladaptive feeding behaviors are the cultural taboos surrounding colostrum that abound around the world (Morse et al., 1990). UNICEF (2008) reports that among the 47 priority countries (those with the highest burden of child and maternal mortality) with available data, median prevalence for early initiation of breastfeeding was only 43%, indicating that many infants do not receive colostrum: one of evolution's most protective inocula. For instance, Aka hunter-gatherer mothers in the Central African Republic expel colostrum into the fire, believing it dangerous to their infants (Hewlett, 2012; Meehan and Roulette, 2013), and colostrum is reported to evoke "disgust" in Nepalese mothers, a response that delays initiation of breastfeeding for several days (Reissland and Bhurghart, 1989).

Cultural taboos surrounding colostrum result in one of two alternatives: early supplementation or allomaternal nursing, both of which open distinct avenues of differential microbial exposure and likely represent important factors influencing early infant GI colonization under these circumstances. To our knowledge, these impacts have not been studied. Frequently when denying colostrum, mothers supplement with water, broth, or other soft foods. The Aka newborns, mentioned, are provided water from nearby streams almost immediately following birth (Meehan and Roulette, 2013), and Nepalese neonates receive sweetened water, as well as goat and cow milk until mothers commence breastfeeding (Reissland and Bhurghart, 1989). Thus, early supplementation exposes infants to a host of bacteria not commonly assumed to be influential in colonization in the West. How this affects both the infant's GI and mother's milk microbiota is not known.

Alternatively, or in addition to supplementation, cross-culturally infants frequently receive human milk through wet nurses or lactating allomothers (nonmaternal caregivers, Hewlett and Winn, 2014). Hewlett and Winn report that this most frequently occurs upon maternal death or when a mother is unable to breastfeed, but the belief that colostrum is dangerous prompts allomaternal nursing practice in approximately 10% of cultures surveyed with data on nonmaternal breastfeeding. Among the Efe foragers in the Ituri forest (Democratic Republic of the Congo), where mothers deny colostrum, infants suckle on the breasts of multiple women immediately following birth "whether or not [the women] are lactating" (Tronick et al., 1987). Following the initial reception of the infant, a lactating woman will be found to nurse the infant until the mother's lactation is fully established (Tronick et al., 1987). The practice results in infants having direct contact with skin and milk microbiota from multiple individuals within their first days of life. Allomaternal nursing has been suggested to improve immunocompetence (Roulin and Heeb, 1999; Roulin, 2002), but future studies will need to explore whether and how allomaternal nursing effects colonization and diversity of microbiota in infants and/or their mother's milk. In addition to the potential for allomaternal milk to expose infants to a more diverse microbiota, there is a likely feedback loop through retrograde backflow (Ramsey et al., 2004), wherein the infant affects the microbial community structure of the lactating allomother and his or her own mother. It would be interesting to determine whether infant GI microbiomes and milk microbial communities are less individualized among infants and women living in these cultures than in those living in societies where allomaternal breastfeeding is not practiced.

Beyond circumstances influencing supplementation from delayed breastfeeding initiation, infants around the world are frequently fed a diet of human milk and non–breast milk liquids and semisolid foods, essentially beginning the weaning process during early infancy. Yet, weaning has not been considered overwhelmingly influential on infant GI colonization. UNICEF (2008) reports the median rate of exclusive breastfeeding in priority countries is only 28%, although few studies exist that examine microbial colonization in infants who are both breastfed and supplemented (Edwards and Parrett, 2002; Madan et al., 2016; Thompson, 2012). Fallani and colleagues found that, while weaning promotes increased microbial diversity, the age when weaning commences does not appear to influence GI microbial composition—instead, other early life factors (country of birth, feeding method, and mode of delivery) have more lasting influences (Fallani et al., 2011). While these results are likely true in the West, we must consider the age at which exposure to non–breast milk liquids and foods begin to occur around the world. As noted, even in the United States, infants with a mixed diet of formula and breast milk have markedly different microbial communities than do breastfed infants (Madan et al., 2016). Cross-culturally, low rates early initiation combined with low rates of exclusive breastfeeding (UNICEF, 2008) almost guarantee early exposure to local pathogens, making cross-cultural patterns of infant feeding ripe for investigation. In many instances, cross-cultural patterns of early supplementation present an interesting dichotomy in regard to microbial exposure. Populations that supplement earliest also tend to breastfeed the longest (Sellen and Smay, 2001; Meehan and Roulette, 2013). Thus, infants who are exposed to potentially pathogenic bacteria in early infancy are also most likely to receive the benefits of breastfeeding the longest.

4.3 PHYSICAL AND SOCIAL ENVIRONMENTS

Throughout the world mothers are primary caregivers (Konner, 2016), and their contact with their infants arguably makes them one of the most influential individuals in terms of the development of their infants' microbiomes (Matamoros et al., 2013). Yet, child-rearing patterns differ dramatically across cultures. Due to cultural expectations and practice, including the lack of co-sleeping in American society, American mothers are estimated to hold or touch their infants only 18% of a 24-h day (Hewlett and Lamb, 2002). When compared with mothers living in a non-Western horticultural population who hold their infants 79% of the day and hunter-gatherers, who hold their infants over average 99% of the day, the difference is dramatic (Hewlett and Lamb, 2002). Moreover, the majority of mother–infant interactions in Western societies are not skin-to-skin in their nature. In much of the world, depending of course on environmental conditions, infant clothing is not as common, and maternal–infant skin-to-skin contact is greater. Unknown is whether the level of contact between mothers and infants, particularly in regions where individual and household hygiene varies from Western patterns, results in different levels and diversity of microbial exposure and colonization patterns. It is possible that where mother–infant contact is greatest, variation in microbial communities across the myriad of niches making up the mother–infant epi-holobiont might be the least pronounced. However, as with so many other related aspects, there exist data to neither support nor refute this possibility.

Moreover, to-date we know little about the role of others (cohabitants of the mother–infant dyad) on microbial exposure and its effect on mother's milk or the infant's GI tract. Extended contact among individuals, however, had been attributed to lower within-group taxonomic diversity in adult GI microbiota (Schnorr et al., 2014). However, we do not know whether such contact alters the human milk microbiome or exposes the infant to greater microbial diversity through breastfeeding and/or contact with others. In a study of three European birth cohorts, singleton infants were found to have different colonization patterns than infants with siblings—singleton children's GI microbiota showed some resemblance to those of infants born via cesarean section (i.e., a less mature pattern) (Adlerberth et al., 2007). An additional study in the Netherlands indicates that singleton infants have lower counts of bifidobacteria at 1 month of age than infants with siblings (Penders et al., 2006). These results are telling as they both indicate a possible role of others and because they suggest this line of inquiry may be particularly important when investigating the role of family environments in the majority world.

Throughout human evolutionary history, infants have been reared in dense social units, and care by allomothers was essential to successful maternal reproduction and infant survivorship (Hardy, 2009). In much of the world today, human allomaternal investment remains ubiquitous and is most notable in the non-Western world (Meehan, 2014). The West is anomalous in its emphasis on the mother–infant dyad, and although siblings are noted to have an effect in the studies given, sibling interactions with infants is likely much less frequent in the West than throughout the rest of the world. Indeed, in over 90% of the world's cultures, mothers are not the first to hold their infants (Hewlett, 1996). Efe forager mothers only receive their infant several hours after birth (Tronick et al., 1987). In this culture, at 3, 7, and 18 weeks of age, infants are transferred to caregiver on average 3.7, 5.6, and 8.3 times/h, respectively. Infants are in contact with nonmaternal caregivers almost 40% of the time at 3 weeks and time in contact with others increases as children age (Tronick et al., 1987). Among the Aka, discussed earlier, infants are in proximity (within a forearm's distance) to 20 individuals on a daily basis and are intimately cared for (e.g., held, fed, touched, etc.) by an average of 10 individuals each day (Meehan, 2009). Allomothers among the Ngandu (a Central African horticultural population) provide approximately half of the holding infants receive (Meehan, 2005). Similarly, in periurban and rural Argentinean Toba populations, allomothers are in charge of infants 23–50% of the time (Valeggia, 2009). Such contact clearly opens new avenues for microbial exposure in early infancy and may serve to prime infants for their environments.

In addition to the role of caregivers, interesting inquiries into the role of pets or human–animal cohabitation on microbial communities are beginning to emerge. It would not be surprising given our 15,000-year history of domestication (Shannon et al., 2015) that our cohabitation with animals might influence our microbiomes. However, to date, there is minimal evidence that animals have a strong influence on the development of the GI or skin microbiota *of infants* (see Adlerberth et al., 2007; Penders et al., 2006; Song et al., 2013). Yet this is not the case *for adults*. In the United States, dog ownership is associated with increased similarities in skin microbiota in cohabiting adults, and adult dog owners share more skin microbiota with their own dogs than with other dogs (Song et al., 2013)—making a human, his or her dog, and their combined microbiota another possible example of an epi-holobiont. Song and colleagues attributed the lack of associations between microbes of infants and their family dogs to be due to behavioral differences—US adults have more contact with dogs than do infants. If true, it is possible that pet ownership or animal husbandry will have a larger influence on infant microbial communities in cultures where the physical distance between humans and animals is reduced. Moreover, it is possible that, in regions where there is minimal distance separating humans and animals, animals may influence infants indirectly, through maternal exposure and the human milk microbiome. For instance, in pastoral communities in Ethiopia, families reside in the same structure as their cattle and livestock, resulting in minimal distance between family members, animals, and animal waste (Quinlan et al., 2015). Moreover, women and young girls, responsible for most of the infant care, are in charge of removing the animal waste, by hand, from the home and yard. The influence of such intimate contact with animals, whether such exposure affects infants through indirect transfer, and its effects on maternal and infant microbiota and health remain open questions.

4.4 CONCLUSIONS

There exist myriad potential biosocial variables that may influence maternal and infant microbial exposures and thus may affect the combined mother–infant epi-holobiont microbiome. These include a complex web of reproductive and childcare practices (e.g., birth mode, communal childcare, and allomaternal breastfeeding) combined with environmental and social environments (e.g., presence and care of animals) that impact overall microbial exposures. Whether these and other long-held practices and living conditions have resulted in population differences in maternal and infant microbial communities, particularly in terms of human milk and infant GI tract, is a research area that has not been previously considered in an adequate interdisciplinary approach, though we are currently pursuing this line of investigation.

Moreover, whether these potential population differences in long-term microbial exposures may be related to evolution of and/or variation in other milk constituents to result in an eco-homeorhesis, therein, will require collaboration among human milk researchers, anthropologists, evolutionary biologists, and population geneticists. A targeted discussion as to how this approach might be applied to variation in HMO profile (particularly FUT2 and FUT3) is provided next.

5. USING POPULATION GENETICS TO EXAMINE ECO-HOMEORHESIS OF MILK COMPOSITION

Here, we discuss scientific approaches that might be taken to identify and distinguish among potential types of selection (such as purifying, positive, or diversifying) that may have affected genes associated with HMO production. To accomplish this, we first briefly discuss several basic concepts related to population-level genetics. Then we apply these concepts to how one might test whether milk composition, in particular HMO profiles, might have evolved to support infant health in divergent locations and populations. It is noteworthy that substantial data have already been published suggesting that genes encoding the casein proteins, which modulate the delivery of calcium in milk, show strong positive selection, since their variation is deeply conserved in the mammalian phylogeny (Khaldi et al., 2011; Lefevre et al., 2010; Ward et al., 1997). Here, we focus on using similar and expanded methods to evaluate evolution of HMO production, in part because HMOs are a main focus of this monograph, but moreover because of their putative importance in determining milk microbial community structure and, in turn, that of the recipient infant's GI tract.

5.1 POPULATION GENETICS OVERVIEW

The basis of genetic variation is carried in alleles: genetic variants passed from parent to offspring. The specific variants of an allele (or combination of alleles) determines the genotype of an individual. Given the most basic scenario of diploid genetics—that one locus contains two alleles (A and a)—we can begin to discuss the framework for determining genetic variation. The most basic analysis of population genetics considers allele frequency and genotype frequency, where allele frequency is the number of alleles (N_A or N_a) divided by the total population (designated as 2N, the population size). Expanding this to genotypic frequency adds a letter to the subscript, with N_{AA} denoting the genotype of the individual (Nielsen and Slatkin, 2013). For instance, *FUT3* has been studied in several populations and several single nucleotide polymorphisms (SNPs), or different alleles, have been detected (reviewed by Soejima and Koda, 2005). Many of these SNPs show population-specific polymorphic patterns leading to different genotypic frequencies across populations. For example, the *Le/Le* genotype has a genotypic frequency of 15.3% in an Amazonian population (Corvelo et al., 2013), whereas in a Korean population, the genotypic frequency for *Le/Le* was found to be 49.2% (Park et al., 2010). Population-specific mutations that are enzyme-inactivating mutations or that alter substrate activity of FUT3 also exist leading to many different haplotypes (sets of DNA variations or polymorphisms) that tend to be inherited together. Soejima and Koda (2005) have postulated that, because the various secretor and Lewis phenotypes exhibit different susceptibility to microbes and diseases, local adaptation to region-specific microbes may be one of the selective forces that have led to the population-specific, polymorphic patterns of these genes.

One of the fundamental assumptions of population genetics is that under no selection (or genetic drift) the above frequencies will be maintained in equilibrium, commonly referred to as Hardy–Weinberg equilibrium. The assumption that allele frequencies follow this equilibrium allows us to test for signatures of selection by finding allele frequencies that deviate from equilibrium. The assumption that allele frequencies follow this equilibrium is based in the "neutral theory" of genetic evolution, which in its most-simple form proposes that random genetic drift is the primary driver of genetic variation and that all differences between populations are derived from random mutation or nearly neutral mutations, which can occur in many ways, rather than Darwinian selection (Kimura, 1968; King and Jukes, 1969).

5.2 TYPES OF SELECTION

If neutral theory proposes that genetic variation is only caused by genetic drift or random mutations accumulated over many generations, how are deviations from this assumption tested? Some of the popular tests for neutrality include Tajima's D (Tajima, 1989), Fay and Wu's H (Fay et al., 2002), the McDonald–Kreitman test (McDonald and Kreitman, 1991), and the Hudson–Kreitman–Aguadé test (Hudson et al., 1987). The basic principles for these tests are to determine if the genetic variation seen in a set of sequences is different than what would be expected under neutral theory. These tests take into consideration different types of mutations (point, polymorphic, and fixed mutations) and the population allele frequencies to help determine the type of selective forces that might be in play. There are many types of selection, with "directional selection" (the favor of one allele over another) being one of the most traditionally considered forms of Darwinian selection. However, other types of selection include "distributive selection" (which removes low-frequency polymorphisms while keeping extreme traits) and "purifying selection" (purging genomes of deleterious mutations and overall decreasing the genetic variation at that locus). Alternatively, "balancing selection" refers to a force of selection that maintains genetic variation in a population. Balancing selection has been suggested to have driven worldwide variation in several genes, many of which have immune-related functions (Akey et al., 2004; Andrés et al., 2009; Ferrer-Admetlla et al., 2008). For instance, there is mounting evidence that balancing selection has acted on *FUT2* (Fumagalli et al., 2009; Ferrer-Admetlla et al., 2009; Silva et al., 2010). Koda and coworkers have conducted several studies that provide support for this scenario (Koda et al., 2000, 2001a,b; Soejima et al., 2007; Soejima and Koda, 2008). Although Gagneux and Varki (1999) have explored the biological repercussions of genetic polymorphisms on oligosaccharide diversity in a general fashion, the effects of balancing selection (i.e., increased genetic variation of *FUT2*, *FUT3*, and possibly other genes involved in oligosaccharide synthesis) on HMO isoform presence and concentrations have not been thoroughly investigated.

5.3 MODELS FOR POPULATION GENETICS

Another approach to studying dynamics of allele frequencies is the utilization of models such as the Wright–Fisher model (Wakeley, 2008). This is one of the basic and most referenced models for population genetics. This model uses a series of assumptions to compare real data (i.e., population allele frequencies) to the neutral theory. The Wright–Fisher model can be summarized as follows: the expected allele frequency in the next generation ($t+1$) is equal to the allele frequency in the current generation (t). Deviations from this are due to genetic drift and after many generations, these deviations can add up to large population differences in allele frequency.

The assumptions that go with the Wright–Fisher model approach are that there exists a fixed (unchanging) populations size; there are discrete (nonoverlapping) generations; and gene copies are transmitted randomly to the next generation. In general, the time it takes for any allele frequency to change depends on the population size; this reality, consequently, blurs the line between signatures of selection and population structure changes, such as a bottleneck (defined as a sudden, significant decrease in population size). Thus, despite the fact that we can test for evidence of selection by comparing the sequences of genes (such as *FUT2* and *FUT3*), the variation can be caused by selection or by alterations to the population, and these differences can be difficult to differentiate.

Alternatively, another approach to modeling evolutionary dynamics is to use "coalescent theory" (Wakeley, 2008). Coalescent theory works backward in time to track the changes in population allele frequency. It, too, is widely used to estimate population genetic parameters such as population size and migration and is concerned with the states that the population can exist in and defined by the number of separate lineages that have descendants in the current population. For example, imagine two individuals who have the same parent (like in a pedigree); their gene copies would converge or coalesce in the previous generation. The ancestry of these alleles is most often visualized as a tree showing the coalescent events leading back to a "most recent common ancestor" and calculates the time to each coalescent event as the length of the branch between the points. One important concept of coalescence theory is that the time between coalescent events decreases in length the closer one gets to the present. In general, one would expect more variants to arise as time progresses and thus for there to be more variants found in older populations (Botigue, 2013). Also, the structure of the branch lengths can tell researchers something about the population structure, such as whether the population size stayed constant, increased, or decreased with respect to the alleles being analyzed. Additionally, by applying coalescent theory to haplotype data for genes, the ages of SNP as well as the time to the most recent common ancestor (T_{MRCA}) can be estimated. For example, Soejima et al. (2007) estimated T_{MRCA} for *FUT2* to be $3{,}630{,}000 \pm 1{,}220{,}000$ years ago in a Ghanaian population. In fact, most of the variability in the *FUT2* haplotypes is thought to have developed over the last 730,000 years (Soejima et al., 2007). Work by Silva et al. (2010) has also estimated global genetic variation of *FUT2* to be over 3 million years old. Results of both of these studies support a role for balancing selection on the *FUT2* gene. How this genetic variation in *FUT2* across time and populations has impacted the global variation of milk oligosaccharides has yet to be determined.

5.4 POPULATION SUBDIVISION AND STRUCTURE

As noted here, most of the models discussed so far assume a single, well-mixed population within which there is random mating. In reality, populations are often structured into sets of subpopulations due to geographical distance and culture, resulting in a larger probability of mating within subpopulations than across subpopulations. If we begin from an "out-of-Africa" human migration assumption (see Botigue, 2013; Prezeworski,

2005), we make the assumption that isolation by distance happened over a long period of time in human history creating subdivision within the global human population. Consequently, population geneticists often look for historical patterns of population subdivision. Populations that are independently assumed to be in Hardy–Weinberg equilibrium will show this equilibrium independently as well as when the allele frequencies are pooled. However, if there is deviation from Hardy–Weinberg equilibrium, there will be a decrease in heterozygosity among the pooled population; this represents a signature of selection in one or both populations. The metric by which researchers determine this difference in allele frequencies is referred to as F_{ST}, which distinguishes between subpopulations and is calculated as the difference between heterozygosity of the subpopulation and the total (pooled) population divided by the total population heterozygosity. F_{ST} is one of the F statistics, or fixation indexes, introduced by Wright (1951) and the estimate varies between 0 and 1, where 0 indicates no population subdivision and 1 indicates that the differences between the populations are fixed (Weir and Cockerham, 1984; Holsinger and Weir, 2009). Generally, F_{ST} values are calculated for species that are completely diverged or split apart far back in history. However, humans have a relatively short divergence time, and thus have a subset of normal F_{ST} values. The general outline for interpreting F_{ST} values in humans looks more akin to 0–0.025 for populations on the same continent and 0.05–0.2 for populations on different continents, showing a much smaller range of values than 0 to 1 used in taxa with longer divergence times. In terms of HMO variability, we know that populations have polymorphic alleles in some of the genes responsible for HMO isoforms. Therefore, we would expect to look for these smaller variations in F_{ST}, and signatures of selection will be stronger comparing populations that live on different continents.

Migration also complicates interpretation of Hardy–Weinberg equilibrium and is often seen within population subdivisions. Changes in expected allele frequency will change depending on migration rate. Migration and isolation by distance (defined as the divergence of two populations due to inability to randomly mate) can be confounding events when looking for signatures of selection. Because these events will change the allele frequencies to something unexpected, they can look like selection when in reality, there is no selection at work. However, with regard to F_{ST} and migration, a general rule-of-thumb is that F_{ST} should increase as the distance between populations increases. Again, this would lead one to expect F_{ST} to be higher for populations on different continents. However, due to recent admixtures of all populations due to globalized travel, there may be random mutations and alleles shared with recent populations that are unexpected.

5.5 NEXT STEPS: TESTING FOR HUMAN MILK OLIGOSACCHARIDE SELECTION

Here, we briefly present a hypothetical experiment designed to determine if human genes related to HMO production (e.g., *FUT2* or *FUT3*) have signatures of selection. Przeworski et al. (2005) have previously stated that the advances in sequencing technology have allowed researchers to “analyze genetic variation within and between species, with the goal of identifying genomic regions that appear to have evolved under natural selection rather than by drift alone." In order to achieve this, the first step would be to collect human DNA and milk samples from populations of interest. Whereas the DNA would be sequenced to determine each woman's genotype at specific loci related to FUT2 or FUT3 synthesis, milk samples would be analyzed for their HMO profiles. Statistical tests, such as those described previously would then be applied to assess genomic variation. These approaches might be simple, such as sequencing a known gene such as *FUT2*, or more complex such as sequencing whole genomes or using multiethnic genotyping arrays, to look at variation across over a million markers in the human genome. Once the genetic information is processed and sequenced, allele frequencies could be calculated. To determine a signature of selection, the type of selection, or the population demographics at play, neutrality tests could be applied.

Examples of some of these approaches have been used for FUT2 and FUT3 (Soejima et al., 2007, 2009) as it relates to *FUT2* and *FUT3* expression and blood groups. If there are identifiable signatures of selection, where certain alleles are favored in a population, this information can be used to develop hypotheses linking evolutionary shifts to environmental and sociocultural variables that also differ between these populations. For example, if a population is particularly homogeneous for the secretor allele (a functional *FUT2*) involved in synthesis of fucosylated HMOs, this may be indicative that these specific types of carbohydrates are supporting growth of an important microbe or set of microbes particularly important in the milk and/or GI tract in that population and location. In other words, exploratory analysis using population genetics approaches to evaluate variation in HMO-synthesis genes might serve as an important engine to generate hypotheses related to how milk composition may (or may not) have been selectively shaped by factors such as disease risk, microbial exposures, and biosocial, cultural attributes around the world.

6. SUMMARY

Although researchers have long known that milk composition varies among and within mammalian taxa, aside from a handful of factors such as time postpartum, time since last breastfeeding bout, maternal health, and maternal nutritional status, very little is known about the cause of this variation in human milk. However, because of the importance of milk to the survival of humans, it is likely that at least some of this variation may be due to selective evolutionary pressures. In particular, milk composition has likely evolved in such a way to provide context-specific protection from environmental pathogens and to reflect local variations in ecosystem services, which vary among cultures and locations around the world. We propose, herein, that variability in milk composition is (at least in part) an example of eco-homeorhesis resulting in the existence of different "normal" milk compositions around the globe, and that at least a portion of this variation is due to evolutionary selection. To our knowledge, this overarching paradigm (particularly as it relates to HMO and milk microbes) has not been rigorously tested.

However, development of high-throughput sequencing techniques and population genetics methodologies coupled with advances in compositional analyses used with milk have collectively made it possible to obtain genetic sequence information on many individuals and then use these data to test various theories of evolution using milk composition as the phenotypic outcome. Although the study of molecular genetic variation is not new (e.g., Hirszfeld and Hirszfeld, 1919), the use of these techniques to study genes involved in human milk composition is very limited. Milk component genes that have been examined include the molecular divergence of α-lactalbumin from lysozyme (Urashima et al., 2012) and the evolution of casein genes (Ward et al., 1997). Two other genes, *FUT2* and *FUT3*, which we have discussed earlier because of their role in HMO synthesis, have also been described in detail (Koda et al., 2001a,b). But investigation into the molecular evolution of these genes has been driven by their involvement in blood group types, not their importance to milk carbohydrate synthesis and milk or infant GI microbiome profiles—relationships that probably impact short- and long-term disease risk in infants—and how these are related to variation in maternal and/or infant microbial exposures.

As such, we urge interdisciplinary researchers interested in exploring this complex web of biosocial, environmental, and genetic factors to ask questions, propose hypotheses, and carry out future studies in such a way that eco-homeorhetic shifts in milk composition to support optimal health in diverse cultures and locations can be holistically investigated. If evidence is obtained to support this paradigm, these analyses can then be used to generate follow-up hypotheses proposing biosocial factors which may have driven these evolutionary shifts as well as specific health and/or disease outcomes that they may potentially modify. As human milk is inarguably the only food ever "designed" to be consumed specifically and exclusively by humans (albeit only during early life), examining variation in its composition using an evolutionarily informed, biosocial lens may provide important insight as to the relationship between diet and health, not only during the neonatal period but also across the lifespan and around the world.

ACKNOWLEDGMENTS

We would like to sincerely thank Dr. Edward Hagen (Department of Anthropology, Washington State University) for his careful reading of and insightful comments on this manuscript. We are also grateful to Abby Biedenbach for her help in preparing this manuscript.

REFERENCES

Adlerberth, I., Wold, A., 2009. Establishment of the gut microbiota in Western infants. Acta Pædiatrica 98, 229–238.

Adlerberth, I., Carlsson, B., Man, P.D., Jalil, F., Khan, S.R., Larsson, P., Mellander, L., Svanborg, C., Wold, A.E., Hanson, L.Å., 1991. Intestinal colonization with enterobacteriaceae in Pakistani and Swedish hospital-delivered infants. Acta Pædiatrica 80, 602–610.

Adlerberth, I., Lindberg, E., Åberg, N., Hesselmar, B., Saalman, R., Strannegård, I.-L., Wold, A.E., 2006. Reduced enterobacterial and increased staphylococcal colonization of the infantile bowel: an effect of hygienic lifestyle? Pediatric Research 59, 96–101.

Adlerberth, I., Strachan, D.P., Matricardi, P.M., Ahrné, S., Orfei, L., Åberg, N., Perkin, M.R., Tripodi, S., Hesselmar, B., Saalman, R., Coates, A.R., Bonanno, C.L., Panetta, V., Wold, A.E., 2007. Gut microbiota and development of atopic eczema in 3 European birth cohorts. Journal of Allergy and Clinical Immunology 120, 343–350.

Akey, J.M., Eberle, M.A., Rieder, M.J., Carlson, C.S., Shriver, M.D., Nickerson, D.A., Kruglyak, L., 2004. Population history and natural selection shape patterns of genetic variation in 132 genes. PLoS Biology 2, e286.

Albesharat, R., Ehrmann, M.A., Korakli, M., Yazaji, S., Vogel, R.F., 2011. Phenotypic and genotypic analyses of lactic acid bacteria in local fermented food, breast milk and faeces of mothers and their babies. Systematic and Applied Microbiology 34, 148–155.

Ali, S., Niang, M.A., N'doye, I., Critchlow, C.W., Hawes, S.E., Hill, A.V., Kiviat, N.B., 2000. Secretor polymorphism and human immunodeficiency virus infection in Senegalese women. Journal of Infectious Diseases 181, 737–739.

Anderson, N.K., Beerman, K.A., McGuire, M.A., Dasgupta, N., Griinari, J.M., Williams, J., McGuire, M.K., 2005. Dietary fat type influences total milk fat content in lean women. Journal of Nutrition 135, 416–421.

Andrés, A.M., Hubisz, M.J., Indap, A., Torgerson, D.G., Degenhardt, J.D., Boyko, A.R., Gutenknunst, R.N., White, T.J., Green, E.D., Bustamante, C.D., Clark, A.G., Nielsen, R., 2009. Targets of balancing selection in the human genome. Molecular Biology and Evolution 26, 2755–2764.

Anstee, D.J., 2010. The relationship between blood groups and disease. Blood 115, 4635–4643.

Arifuzzaman, M., Ahmed, T., Rahman, M.A., Chowdhury, F., Rashu, R., Khan, A.I., LaRocque, R.C., Harris, J.B., Bhuiyan, T.R., Ryan, E.T., Calderwood, S.B., Qadri, F., 2011. Individuals with Le(a+b–) blood group have increased susceptibility to symptomatic vibrio cholerae O1 infection. PLoS Neglected Tropical Diseases 5, e1413. http://dx.doi.org/10.1371/journal.pntd.0001413.

Barile, D., Marotta, M., Chu, C., Mehra, R., Grimm, R., Lebrilla, C.B., German, J.B., 2010. Neutral and acidic oligosaccharides in Holstein-Friesian colostrum during the first 3 days of lactation measured by high performance liquid chromatography on a microfluidic chip and time-of-flight mass spectrometry. Journal of Dairy Science 93, 3940–3949.

Bauman, D.E., Currie, W.B., 1980. Partitioning of nutrients during pregnancy and lactation: a review of mechanisms involving homeostasis and homeorhesis. Journal of Dairy Science 63, 1514–1529.

Benezra, A., DeStefano, J., Gordon, J.I., 2012. Anthropology of microbes. Proceedings of the National Academy of Sciences 109, 6378–6381.

Bennet, R., Eriksson, M., Tafari, N., Nord, C.E., 1991. Intestinal bacteria of newborn Ethiopian infants in relation to antibiotic treatment and colonisation by potentially pathogenic gram-negative bacteria. Scandinavian Journal of Infectious Diseases 23, 63–69.

Bode, L., Kuhn, L., Kim, H.Y., Hsiao, L., Nissan, C., Sinkala, M., Kankasa, C., Mwiya, M., Thea, D.M., Aldrovandi, G.M., 2012. Human milk oligosaccharide concentration and risk of postnatal transmission of HIV through breastfeeding. The American Journal of Clinical Nutrition 96, 831–839.

Bode, L., 2012. Human milk oligosaccharides: every baby needs a sugar mama. Glycobiology 22, 1147–1162.

Botigue, L.R., Henn, B.M., Gravel, S., Maples, B.K., Gignoux, C.R., Corona, E., Atzmon, G., Burns, E., Ostrer, H., Flores, C., Bertranpetit, J., Comas, D., Bustamante, C.D., 2013. Gene flow from North Africa contributes to differential human genetic diversity in southern Europe. Proceedings of the National Academy of Sciences 110, 11791–11796.

Bullen, J.J., Ward, C.G., Rogers, H.J., 1991. The critical role of iron in some clinical infections. European Journal of Clinical Microbiology and Infectious Diseases 10, 613–617.

Cabrera-Rubio, R., Collado, M.C., Laitinen, K., Salminen, S., Isolauri, E., Mira, A., 2012. The human milk microbiome changes over lactation and is shaped by maternal weight and mode of delivery. American Journal of Clinical Nutrition 96, 544–551.

Cabrera-Rubio, R., Mira-Pascual, L., Mira, A., Collado, M.C., 2016. Impact of mode of delivery on the milk microbiota composition of healthy women. Journal of the Developmental Origins of Health and Disease 7, 54–60.

Capuco, A.V., Akers, R.M., 2009. The origin and evolution of lactation. Journal of Biology 8, 37.

Chaudhuri, A., DasAdhikary, C.R., 1978. Possible role of blood-group secretory substances in the aetiology of cholera. Transactions of the Royal Society of Tropical Medicine and Hygiene 172, 664–665.

Cooling, L., 2015. Blood groups in infection and host susceptibility. Clinical Microbiology Reviews 28, 801–871.

Corvelo, T.C., de Loiola, Rdo, S., Aguiar, D.C., Matos, G.C., de Brito, D.C., 2013. The Lewis histo-blood group system: molecular analysis of the 59→G, 508G→A, and 1067T→A polymorphisms in an Amazonian population. PLoS ONE 2, e69908.

de Mattos, L.C., Rodrigues, J.C., Sanches, F.E., Alves da Silva, R.C., Ruiz, M.A., Moreira, H.W., 2002. ABO, Lewis, secretor and non-secretor phenotypes in patients infected or uninfected by the *Helicobacter pylori* bacillus. Sao Paulo Medical Journal 120, 55–58.

Dethlefsen, L., McFall-Ngai, M., Relman, D.A., 2007. An ecological and evolutionary perspective on human-microbe mutualism and disease. Nature 449, 811–818.

Dominguez-Bello, M.G., Costello, E.K., Contreras, M., Magris, M., Hidalgo, G., Fierer, N., Knight, R., 2010. Delivery mode shapes the acquisition and structure of the initial microbiota across multiple body habitats in newborns. Proceedings of the National Academy of Sciences 107, 11971–11975.

Edwards, C.A., Parrett, A.M., 2002. Intestinal flora during the first months of life: new perspectives. British Journal of Nutrition 88, s11–s18.

Erney, R.M., Malone, W.T., Skelding, M.B., Marcon, A.A., Kleman-Leyer, K.M., O'Ryan, M.L., Ruiz-Palacios, G., Hilty, M.D., Pickering, L.K., Prieto, P.A., 2000. Variability of human milk neutral oligosaccharides in a diverse population. Journal of Pediatric Gastroenterology and Nutrition 30, 181–192.

Fallani, M., Young, D., Scott, J., Norin, E., Amarri, S., Adam, R., Aguilera, M., Khanna, S., Gil, A., Edwards, C.A., Doré, J., 2010. Intestinal microbiota of 6-week-old infants across Europe: geographic influence beyond delivery mode, breast-feeding, and antibiotics. Journal of Pediatric Gastroenterology and Nutrition 51, 77–84.

Fallani, M., Amarri, S., Uusijarvi, A., Adam, R., Khanna, S., Aguilera, M., Gil, A., Vieites, J.M., Norin, E., Young, D., Scott, J.A., Doré, J., Edwards, C.A., The INFABIO Team, 2011. Determinants of the human infant intestinal microbiota after the introduction of first complementary foods in infant samples from five European centres. Microbiology 157, 1385–1392.

Fanaro, S., Chierici, R., Guerrini, P., Vigi, V., 2003. Intestinal microflora in early infancy: composition and development. Acta Pædiatrica 92, 48–55.

Fay, J.C., Wyckoff, G.J., Wu, C.I., 2002. Testing the neutral theory of molecular evolution with genomic data from Drosophila. Nature 415, 1024–1026.

Fernández, L., Langa, S., Martín, V., Jiménez, E., Martín, R., Rodríguez, J.M., 2013. The microbiota of human milk in healthy women. Cellular and Molecular Biology (Noisy-le-grand, France) 59, 31–42.

Ferrer-Admetlla, A., Bosch, E., Sikora, M., Marqués-Bonet, T., Ramírez-Soriano, A., Muntasell, A., Navarro, A., Lazarus, R., Calafell, F., Bertranpetit, J., Casals, F., 2008. Balancing selection is the main force shaping the evolution of innate immunity genes. The Journal of Immunology 181, 1315–1322.

Ferrer-Admetlla, A., Sikora, M., Laayouni, H., Esteve, A., Roubinet, F., Blancher, A., Calafell, F., Bertranpetit, J., Casals, F., 2009. A natural history of FUT2 polymorphism in humans. Molecular Biology and Evolution 26, 1993–2003.

Fortenberry, J.D., 2013. The uses of race and ethnicity in human microbiome research. Trends in Microbiology 21, 165–166.

Fumagalli, M., Cagliani, R., Pozzoli, U., Riva, S., Comi, G.P., Menozzi, G., Bresolin, N., Sironi, M., 2009. Widespread balancing selection and pathogen-driven selection at blood group antigen genes. Genome Research 19, 199–212.

Gagneux, P., Varki, A., 1999. Evolutionary considerations in relating oligosaccharide diversity to biological function. Glycobiology 9, 747–755.

Galili, U., Mandrell, R.E., Hamadeh, R.M., Shohet, S.B., Griffiss, J.M., 1988. Interaction between human natural anti-alpha-galactosyl immunoglobulin G and bacteria of the human flora. Infection and Immunity 56, 1730–1737.

Gera, T., Sachdev, H.P., 2002. Effect of iron supplementation on incidence of infectious illness in children: systematic review. British Medical Journal 325, 1142.

Giordanengo, V., Ollier, L., Lanteri, M., Lesimple, J., March, D., Thyss, S., Lefebvre, J.C., 2004. Epigenetic reprogramming of UDP-N-acetylglucosamine 2-epimerase/N-acetylmannosamine kinase (GNE) in HIV-1-infected CEM T cells. The Federation of American Societies for Experimental Biology Journal 18, 1961–1963.

González, R., Maldonado, A., Martín, V., Mandomando, I., Fumadó, V., Metzner, K.J., Sacoor, C., Fernández, L., Macete, E., Alonso, P.L., Rodríguez, J.M., Menendez, C., 2013. Breast milk and gut microbiota in African mothers and infants from an area of high HIV prevalence. PLoS ONE 8, e80299.

Goto, K., Fukuda, K., Senda, A., Saito, T., Kimura, K., Glander, K.E., Hinde, K., Dittus, W., Milligan, L.A., Power, M.L., Oftedal, O.T., Urashima, T., 2010. Chemical characterization of oligosaccharides in the milk of six species of New and Old World monkeys. Glycoconjugate Journal 27, 703–715.

Hayssen, V., Blackburn, D.G., 1985. α-lactalbumin and the origins of lactation. Evolution 39, 1147–1149.

Heneghan, M.A., McCarthy, C.F., Moran, A.P., 2000. Relationship of blood group determinants on *Helicobacter pylori* lipopolysaccharide with host Lewis phenotype and inflammatory response. Infection and Immunity 68, 937–941.

Hewlett, B.S., Lamb, M.E., 2002. Integrating evolution, culture and developmental psychology: explaining caregiver-infant proximity and responsiveness in central Africa and the USA. In: Keller, H., Poortinga, Y.H. (Eds.), Between Culture and Biology: Perspectives on Ontogenetic Development. Cambridge University Press, pp. 241–269.

Hewlett, B.S., Winn, S., 2014. Allomaternal nursing in humans. Current Anthropology 55, 200–229.

Hewlett, B.S., 1996. Diverse contexts of human infancy. In: Ember, C.R., Ember, M. (Eds.), Cross-Cultural Research for Social Science. Prentice Hall, Upper Saddle River, NI, pp. 171–200.

Hewlett, B.L., 2012. Listen, Here Is a Story: Ethnographic Life Narratives from Aka and Ngandu Women of the Congo Basin. Oxford University Press, United Kingdom.

Hirszfeld, L., Hirszfeld, H., 1919. Serological differences between the blood of different races: the results of researches on the Macedonian front. Lancet 2, 675–679.

Hoashi, M., Meche, L., Mahal, L.K., Bakacs, E., Nardella, D., Naftolin, F., Bar-Yam, N., Dominguez-Bello, M.G., December 27, 2015. Human Milk Bacterial and Glycosylation Patterns Differ by Delivery Mode. Reproductive Sciences (Thousand Oaks, California) pii:1933719115623645. (Epub ahead of print).

Holsinger, K.E., Weir, B.S., 2009. Genetics in geographically structured populations: defining, estimating and interpreting FST. Nature Reviews Genetics 10, 639–650.

Hrdy, S.B., 2009. Mothers and Others: The Evolutionary Origins of Mutual Understanding. Harvard University Press, Cambridge, MA.

Hudson, R.R., Kreitman, M., Aguadé, M., 1987. A test of neutral molecular evolution based on nucleotide data. Genetics 116, 153–159.

Hunt, K.M., Foster, J.A., Forney, L.J., Schütte, U.M.E., Beck, D.L., Abdo, Z., Fox, L.K., Williams, J.E., McGuire, M.K., McGuire, M.A., 2011. Characterization of the diversity and temporal stability of bacterial communities in human milk. PLoS ONE 6, e21313.

Hunt, K.M., Preuss, J., Nissan, C., Davlin, C.A., Williams, J.E., Shafii, B., Richardson, A.D., McGuire, M.K., Bode, L., McGuire, M.A., 2012. Human milk oligosaccharides promote the growth of staphylococci. Applied Environmental Microbiology 78, 4763–4770.

Insull Jr., W., Hirsch, J., James, T., Ahrens Jr., E.H., 1959. The fatty acids of human milk. II. Alterations produced by manipulation of caloric balance and exchange of dietary fats. Journal of Clinical Investigations 38, 443–450.

Jensen, R.G., 1995. Handbook of Milk Composition. Academic Press, Inc., California.

Jeurink, P.V., van Bergenhenegouwen, J., Jiménez, E., Knippels, L.M., Fernández, L., Garssen, J., Knol, J., Rodríguez, J.M., Martín, R., 2013. Human milk: a source of more life than we imagine. Beneficial Microbes 4, 17–30.

Jordan, B., 1992. Birth in Four Cultures: A Crosscultural Investigation of Childbirth in Yucatan, Holland, Sweden, and the United States, fourth ed. Waveland Press, Illinois.

Karmarkar, M.G., Rajalakshmi, R., Ramakrishnan, C.V., 1963. Studies on human lactation. I. Effect on dietary protein and fat supplementation on protein, fat and essential amino acid contents of breast milk. Acta Paediatrica 52, 473–480.

Khaldi, N., Shields, D.C., 2011. Shift in the isoelectric-point of milk proteins as a consequence of adaptive divergence between the milks of mammalian species. Biology Direct 6, 40. http://dx.doi.org/10.1186/1745-6150-6-40.

Khodayar-Pardo, P., Mira-Pascual, L., Collado, M.C., Martínez-Costa, C., 2014. Impact of lactation stage, gestational age and mode of delivery on breast milk microbiota. Journal of Perinatology 34, 599–605.

Kimura, M., 1968. Evolutionary rate at the molecular level. Nature 217, 624–626.

Kindberg, E., Hejdeman, B., Bratt, G., Wahren, B., Lindblom, B., Hinkula, J., Svensson, L., 2006. A nonsense mutation (428G-->A) in the fucosyltransferase FUT2 gene affects the progression of HIV-1 infection. AIDS 20, 685–689.

King, J.L., Jukes, T.H., 1969. Non-Darwinian evolution. Science 164, 788–797.

Kobata, A., 2010. Structures and application of oligosaccharides in human milk. Proceedings of the Japan Academy, Series B Physical and Biological Sciences 86, 731–747.

Koda, Y., Tachida, H., Soejima, M., Takenaka, O., Kimura, H., 2000. Ancient origin of the null allele se(428) of the human ABO-secretor locus (FUT2). Journal of Molecular Evolution 50, 243–248.

Koda, Y., Soejima, M., Kimura, H., 2001a. The polymorphisms of fucosyltransferases. Legal Medicine 3, 2–14.

Koda, Y., Tachida, H., Pang, H., Liu, Y., Soejima, M., Ghaderi, A.A., Takenaka, O., Kimura, H., 2001b. Contrasting patterns of polymorphisms at the ABO-secretor gene (FUT2) and plasma alpha(1,3)fucosyltransferase gene (FUT6) in human populations. Genetics 158, 747–756.

Koenig, J.E., Spor, A., Scalfone, N., Fricker, A.D., Stombaugh, J., Knight, R., Angenent, L.T., Ley, R.E., 2011. Succession of microbial consortia in the developing infant gut microbiome. Proceedings of the National Academy of Sciences 108, 4578–4585.

Konner, M., 2016. Hunter-gatherer infancy and childhood in the context of human evolution. In: Meehan, C.L., Crittenden, A. (Eds.), Childhood: Origins, Implications, Evolution. School of Advanced Research Press, New Mexico, pp. 123–154.

Kumazaki, T., Yoshida, A., 1984. Biochemical evidence that secretor gene, Se, is a structural gene encoding a specific fucosyltransferase. Proceedings of the National Academy of Sciences 81, 4193–4197.

Lefèvre, C.M., Sharp, J.A., Nicholas, K.R., 2010. Evolution of lactation: ancient origin and extreme adaptations of the lactation system. Annual Review of Genomics and Human Genetics 11, 219–238.

Lemay, D.G., Lynn, D.J., Martin, W.F., Neville, M.C., Casey, T.M., Rincon, G., Kriventseva, E.V., Barris, W.C., Hinrichs, A.S., Molenaar, A.J., Pollard, K.S., Maqbool, N.J., Singh, K., Murney, R., Zdobnov, E.M., Tellam, R.L., Medrano, J.F., German, J.B., Rijnkels, M., 2009. The bovine lactation genome: insights into the evolution of mammalian milk. Genome Biology 10, R43.

Madan, J.C., Hoen, A.G., Lundgren, S.N., Farzan, S.F., Cottingham, K.L., Morrison, H.G., Sogin, M.L., Li, H., Moore, J.H., Karagas, M.R., 2016. Association of cesarean delivery and formula supplementation with the intestinal microbiome of 6-week-old infants. The Journal of the American Medical Association Pediatrics 11, 1–8.

Martín, V., Maldonado-Barragán, A., Moles, L., Rodriguez-Baños, M., del Campo, R., Fernández, L., Rodríguez, J.M., Jiménez, E., 2012. Sharing of bacterial strains between breast milk and infant feces. Journal of Human Lactation 28, 36–44.

Martins, L.C., de Oliveira Corvelo, T.C., Oti, H.T., do Socorro Pompeu Loiola, R., Aguiar, D.C., dos Santos Barile, K.A., do Amaral, R.K., Barbosa, H.P., Fecury, A.A., de Souza, J.T., 2006. ABH and Lewis antigen distributions in blood, saliva and gastric mucosa and *H. pylori* infection in gastric ulcer patients. World Journal of Gastroenterology 12, 1120–1124.

Matamoros, S., Gras-Leguen, C., Le Vacon, F., Potel, G., de La Cochetiere, M.F., 2013. Development of intestinal microbiota in infants and its impact on health. Trends in Microbiology 21, 167–173.

McDonald, J.H., Kreitman, M., 1991. Adaptive protein evolution at the Adh locus in Drosophila. Letters to Nature 351, 653–654.

Meehan, C.L., 2005. The effects of residential locality on parental and alloparental investment among the Aka foragers of the central African Republic. Hum. Nat. 16 (1), 58–80.

Meehan, C.L., 2014. Allomothers and child well-being. In: Ben-Arieh, B., Casas, F., Frones, I., Korbin, J.E. (Eds.), Handbook of Child Well-being: Theories, Methods, and Policies in Global Perspective, vol. 2. Springer, New York, pp. 1787–1816.

Meehan, C.L., 2009. Maternal time allocation in two cooperative childrearing societies. Human Nature 20, 375–393.

Meehan, C.L., Roulette, J.W., 2013. Early supplementary feeding among central African foragers and farmers: a biocultural approach. Social Science & Medicine 96, 112–120.

Meng, D., Newburg, D.S., Young, C., Baker, A., Tonkonogy, S.L., Sartor, R.B., Walker, W.A., Nanthakumar, N.N., 2007. Bacterial symbionts induce a FUT2-dependent fucosylated niche on colonic epithelium via ERK and JNK signaling. American Journal of Physiology Gastrointestinal and Liver Physiology 293, G780–G787.

Messer, E., 1986. The "small but healthy" hypothesis: historical, political, and ecological influences on nutritional standards. Human Ecology 14, 57–75.

Messer, M., Kerry, K.R., 1973. Milk carbohydrates of the echidna and the platypus. Science 180, 201–203.

Mohammad, M.A., Sunehag, A.L., Haymond, M.W., 2009. Effect of dietary macronutrient composition under moderate hypocaloric intake on maternal adaptation during lactation. The American Journal of Clinical Nutrition 89, 1821–1827.

Morrow, A.L., Ruiz-Palacios, G.M., Altaye, M., Jiang, X., Guerrero, M.L., Meinzen-Derr, J.K., Farkas, T., Chaturvedi, P., Pickering, L.K., Newburg, D.S., 2004. Human milk oligosaccharide blood group epitopes and innate immune protection against campylobacter and calicivirus diarrhea in breastfed infants. Advances in Experimental Medicine and Biology 554, 443–446.

Morrow, A.L., Meinzen-Derr, J., Huang, P., Schibler, K.R., Cahill, T., Keddache, M., Kallapur, S.G., Newburg, D.S., Tabangin, M., Warner, B.B., Jiang, X., 2011. Fucosyltransferase 2 non-secretor and low secretor status predicts severe outcomes in premature infants. Journal of Pediatrics 158, 745–751.

Morse, J.M., Jehle, C., Gamble, D., 1990. Initiating breastfeeding: a world survey of the timing of postpartum breastfeeding. International Journal of Nursing Studies 27, 303–313.

Murray, M.J., Murray, A.B., Murray, M.B., Murray, C.J., 1978. The adverse effect of iron repletion on the course of certain infections. British Medical Journal 2, 1113–1115.

Nanthakumar, N.N., Dai, D., Newburg, D.S., Walker, W.A., 2003. The role of indigenous microflora in the development of murine intestinal fucosyl- and sialyltransferases. The Federation of American Societies for Experimental Biology Journal 17, 44–46.

National Center for Chronic Disease Prevention and Health Promotion (CDC), 2014. Breastfeeding Report Card. United States/2014. Available at: https://www.cdc.gov/breastfeeding/pdf/2014breastfeedingreportcard.pdf.

Newburg, D.S., Peterson, J.A., Ruiz-Palacios, G.M., Matson, D.O., Morrow, A.L., Shults, J., Guerrero, M.L., Chaturvedi, P., Newburg, S.O., Scallan, C.D., Taylor, M.R., Ceriani, R.L., Pickering, L.K., 1998. Role of human-milk lactadherin in protection against symptomatic rotavirus infection. The Lancet 351, 1160–1164.

Newburg, D.S., Ruiz-Palacios, G.M., Morrow, A.L., 2005. Human milk glycans protect infants against enteric pathogens. Annual Review of Nutrition 25, 37–58.

Nielsen, R., Slatkin, M., 2013. An Introduction to Population Genetics: Theory and Applications. Sinauer Associates, Massachusetts.

Oftedal, O.T., 1993. The adaptation of milk secretion to the constraints of fasting in bears, seals, and baleen whales. Journal of Dairy Science 76, 3234–3246.

Oftedal, O.T., 1997. Lactation in whales and dolphins: evidence of divergence between baleen- and toothed-species. Journal of Mammary Gland Biology and Neoplasia 2, 205–230.

Oftedal, O.T., 2002. The mammary gland and its origin during synapsid evolution. Journal of Mammary Gland Biology and Neoplasia 7, 225–252.

Olivares, M., Albrecht, S., de Palma, G., Ferrer, M.D., Castillejo, G., Schols, H.A., Sanz, Y., 2015. Human milk composition differs in healthy mothers and mothers with celiac disease. Europe Journal of Nutrition 54, 119–128.

Park, H.-D., Park, K.U., Song, J., Ki, C.-S., Han, K.S., Kim, J.Q., 2010. The relationship between Lewis/Secretor genotypes and serum carbohydrate antigen 19-9 levels in a Korean population. The Korean Journal of Laboratory Medicine 30, 51–57.

Park, Y., McGuire, M.K., Behr, R., McGuire, M.A., Evans, M.A., Shultz, T.D., 1999. High-fat dairy product consumption increases delta 9c,11t-18:2 (rumenic acid) and total lipid concentrations of human milk. Lipids 34, 543–549.

Penders, J., Thijs, C., Vink, C., Stelma, F.F., Snijders, B., Kummeling, I., Van den Brandt, P.A., Stobberingh, E.E., 2006. Factors influencing the composition of the intestinal microbiota in early infancy. Pediatrics 118, 511–521.

Pelto, G., Pelto, P., 1989. Small but healthy? an anthropological perspective. Human Organization 48, 11–15.

Prendergast, A.J., Humphrey, J.H., 2014. The stunting syndrome in developing countries. Paediatrics and International Child Health 34, 250–265.

Przeworski, M., Coop, G., Wall, J.D., 2005. The signature of positive selection on standing genetic variation. Evolution 59, 2312–2323.

Quinlan, R.J., Quinlan, M.B., Dira, S., Caudell, M., Sooge, A., Assoma, A.A., 2015. Vulnerability and resilience of sidama enset and maize farms in Southwestern Ethiopia. Journal of Ethnobiology 35, 314–336.

Quinn, E.A., 2014. Too much of a good thing: evolutionary perspectives on infant formula fortification in the United States and its effects on infant health. American Journal of Human Biology 26, 10–17.

Quinn, E.A., Diki Bista, K., Childs, G., 2016. Milk at altitude: human milk macronutrient composition in a high-altitude adapted population of Tibetans. American Journal of Physical Anthropology 159, 233–243.

Ramsay, D.T., Kent, J.C., Owens, R.A., Hartmann, P.E., 2004. Ultrasound imaging of milk ejection in the breast of lactating women. Pediatrics 113, 361–367.

Reissland, N., Burghart, R., 1989. Active patients: the integration of modern and traditional obstetric practices in Nepal. Social Science & Medicine 29, 43–52.

Rothenbacher, D., Weyermann, M., Bode, G., Kulaksiz, M., Stahl, B., Brenner, H., 2004. Role of Lewis A and Lewis B blood group antigens in *Helicobacter pylori* infection. Helicobacter 9, 324–329.

Roulin, A., 2002. Why do lactating females nurse alien offspring? A review of hypotheses and empirical evidence. Animal Behaviour 63, 201–208.

Roulin, A., Heeb, P., 1999. The immunological function of allosuckling. Ecology Letters 2, 319–324.

Ruiz-Palacios, G.M., Cervantes, L.E., Ramos, P., Chavez-Munguia, B., Newburg, D.S., 2003. *Campylobacter jejuni* binds intestinal H(O) antigen (Fuc alpha 1, 2Gal beta 1, 4GlcNAc), and fucosyloligosaccharides of human milk inhibit its binding and infection. Journal of Biological Chemistry 278, 14112–14120.

Schnorr, S.L., Candela, M., Rampelli, S., Centanni, M., Consolandi, C., Basaglia, G., Turroni, S., Biagi, E., Peano, C., Severgnini, M., Fiori, J., Gotti, R., De Bellis, G., Luiselli, D., Brigidi, P., Mabulla, A., Marlowe, F., Henry, A.G., Crittenden, A.N., 2014. Gut microbiome of the Hadza hunter-gatherers. Nature Communications 5, 3654.

Sellen, D.W., Smay, D.B., 2001. Relationship between subsistence and age at weaning in "preindustrial" societies. Human Nature 12, 47–87.

Shannon, L.M., Boyko, R.H., Castelhano, M., Corey, E., Hayward, J.J., McLean, C., White, M.E., Said, M.A., Anita, B.A., Bondjengo, N.I., Calero, J., Galov, A., Hedimbi, M., Imam, B., Khalap, R., Lally, D., Masta, A., Oliveira, K.C., Pérez, L., Randall, J., Tam, N.M., Trujillo-Cornejo, F.J., Valeriano, C., Sutter, N.B., Todhunter, R.J., Bustamante, C.D., Boyko, A.R., 2015. Genetic structure in village dogs reveals a Central Asian domestication origin. Proceedings of the National Academy of Science 112, 13639–13644.

Silva, L.M., Carvalho, A.S., Guillon, P., Seixas, S., Azevedo, M., Almeida, R., Ruvoën-Clouet, N., Reis, C.A., Le Pendu, J., Rocha, J., David, L., 2010. Infection-associated FUT2 (Fucosyltransferase 2) genetic variation and impact on functionality assessed by in vivo studies. Glycoconjugate Journal 27, 61–68.

Smilowitz, J.T., O'Sullivan, A., Barile, D., German, J.B., Lönnerdal, B., Slupsky, C.M., 2013. The human milk metabolome reveals diverse oligosaccharide profiles. Journal of Nutrition 143, 1709–1718.

Soejima, M., Koda, Y., 2005. Molecular mechanisms of Lewis antigen expression. Legal Medicine 7, 266–269.

Soejima, M., Koda, Y., 2008. Distinct single nucleotide polymorphism patterns promoter among human populations. Annals of Hematology 87, 19–25.

Soejima, M., Pang, H., Koda, Y., 2007. Genetic variation of FUT2 in a Ghanaian population: identification of four novel mutations and inference of balancing selection. Annals of Hematology 86, 199–204.

Soejima, M., Munkhtulga, L., Iwamoto, S., Koda, Y., 2009. Genetic variation of FUT3 in Ghanaians, Caucasians, and Mongolians. Transfusion 49, 959–966.

Song, S.J., Lauber, C., Costello, E.K., Lozupone, C.A., Humphrey, G., Berg-Lyons, D., Caporaso, J.G., Knights, D., Clemente, J.C., Nakielny, S., Gordon, J.I., Fierer, N., Knight, R., 2013. Cohabiting family members share microbiota with one another and with their dogs. eLife Sciences 2, e00458.

Springer, G.F., 1971. Blood-group and Forssman antigenic determinants shared between microbes and mammalian cells. Progress of Allergy 15, 9–77.

Springer, G.F., Horton, R.E., Forbes, M., 1959. Origin of antihuman blood group B agglutinins in germfree chicks. Annals of New York Academy of Sciences 78, 272–275.

Tajima, F., 1989. Statistical method for testing the neutral mutation hypothesis by DNA polymorphism. Genetics 123, 585–595.

Thompson, A.L., 2012. Developmental origins of obesity: early feeding environments, infant growth, and the intestinal microbiome. American Journal of Human Biology 24, 350–360.

Tollin, M., Bergsson, G., Kai-Larsen, Y., Lengqvist, J., Sjövall, J., Griffiths, W., Skúladóttir, G.V., Haraldsson, Á., Jörnvall, H., Gudmundsson, G.H., Agerberth, B., 2005. Vernix caseosa as a multi-component defence system based on polypeptides, lipids and their interactions. Cellular and Molecular Life Sciences 62, 2390–2399.

Totten, S.M., Zivkovic, A.M., Wu, S., Ngyuen, U., Freeman, S.L., Ruhaak, L.R., Darboe, M.K., German, B.J., Prentice, A.M., Lebrilla, C.B., 2012. Comprehensive profiles of human milk oligosaccharides yield highly sensitive and specific markers for determining secretor status in lactating mothers. Journal of Proteome Research 11, 6124–6133.

Trevathan, W., 2011. Human Birth: An Evolutionary Perspective. Transaction Publishers, New Jersey.

Tronick, E.Z., Morelli, G.A., Winn, S., 1987. Multiple caretaking of Efe (pygmy) infants. American Anthropologist 89, 96–106.

Urbaniak, C., Angelini, M., Gloor, G.B., Reid, G., 2016. Human milk microbiota profiles in relation to birthing method, gestation and infant gender. Microbiome 4, 1. http://dx.doi.org/10.1186/s40168-015-0145-y.

Urashima, T., Odaka, G., Asakuma, S., Uemura, Y., Goto, K., Senda, A., Saito, T., Fukuda, K., Messer, M., Oftedal, O.T., 2009. Chemical characterization of oligosaccharides in chimpanzee, bonobo, gorilla, orangutan, and siamang milk or colostrum. Glycobiology 19, 499–508.

Urashima, T., Fukuda, K., Messer, M., 2012. Evolution of milk oligosaccharides and lactose: a hypothesis. Animal 6, 369–374.

UNICEF, 2008. Tracking Progress in Maternal, Newborn and Child Survival: the 2008 Report. UNICEF, New York.

Valeggia, C., 2009. Flexible caretakers: responses of Toba families in transition. In: Bentley, G., Mace, R. (Eds.), Substitute Parents: Biological and Social Perspectives on Alloparenting in Human SocietiesStudies in Biosocial Science Series, , pp. 100–115.

Wakeley, J., 2008. Coalescent Theory: An Introduction. Roberts & Co. Publishers, Texas.

Ward, C.G., Bullen, J.J., Rogers, H.J., 1996. Iron and infection: new developments and their implications. Journal of Trauma and Acute Care 41, 356–364.

Ward, T.J., Honeycutt, R.L., Derr, J.N., 1997. Nucleotide sequence evolution at the κ-casein locus: evidence for positive selection within the family Bovidae. Genetics 147, 1863–1872.

Weir, B.S., Cockerham, C.C., 1984. Estimating F-statistics for the analysis of population structure. Evolution 38, 1358–1370.

Wright, S., 1951. The genetical structure of populations. Annals of Eugenics 15, 323–354.

Xu, Y.H., Ponce, E., Sun, Y., Leonova, T., Bove, K., Witte, D., Grabowski, G.A., 1996. Turnover and distribution of intravenously administered mannose-terminated human acid beta-glucosidase in murine and human tissues. Pediatric Research 39, 313–322.

Yolken, R.H., Peterson, J.A., Vonderfecht, S.L., Fouts, E.T., Midthun, K., Newburg, D.S., 1992. Human milk mucin inhibits rotavirus replication and prevents experimental gastroenteritis. The Journal of Clinical Investigation 90, 1984–1991.

Yoshio, H., Tollin, M., Gudmundsson, G.H., Lagercrantz, H., Jörnvall, H., Marchini, G., Agerberth, B., 2003. Antimicrobial polypeptides of human vernix caseosa and amniotic fluid: implications for newborn innate defense. Pediatric Research 53, 211–216.

Zilber-Rosenberg, I., Rosenberg, E., 2008. Role of microorganisms in the evolution of animals. FEMS Microbiology Letters.

CHAPTER

Infectious Mastitis During Lactation: A Mammary Dysbiosis Model

15

Juan M. Rodríguez[1,2], Leonides Fernández[1]

[1]*Complutense University of Madrid, Madrid, Spain;* [2]*Center for Advanced Research in Public Health (CSISP), Valencia, Spain*

1. INTRODUCTION: LACTATIONAL MASTITIS IS A RELEVANT PUBLIC HEALTH ISSUE

In the past years, breastfeeding has received a renewed interest since its beneficial health, psychosocial, economic, and environmental effects are well recognized and apply to both developed and developing countries (Lawrence and Lawrence, 2010; US Department of Health and Human Services, 2011; Renfrew et al., 2012). Human milk is uniquely suited to the human infant's nutritional needs and is a living substance with unparalleled immunological, microbiological, and biochemical properties that protect against a host of illnesses and diseases for both mothers and children (Gartner et al., 2005). On this basis, international and national health organizations advise that infant feeding should not be considered as a lifestyle choice but rather as a basic public health issue, and strongly recommend exclusive breastfeeding for the first 6 months of life and, then, a gradual weaning process in which the infant receives human milk for 1 year or longer as mutually desired by mother and infant (WHO, 2001; American Academy of Pediatrics, 2012).

However, it is often difficult to cope with such recommendations due to several reasons (Li et al., 2008; US Department of Health and Human Services, 2011). From the medical point of view, mastitis represents the first cause of undesired precocious weaning (Walker, 2008), with an incidence among lactating women as high as 35% when any clinical mastitis case is considered (Michie et al., 2003; Delgado et al., 2009a; Jiménez et al., 2009; Schoenfeld and McKay, 2010). Taking into account that this condition may prevent many mother–infant pairs to receive the short- and long-term health benefits provided by breastfeeding, it seems logical that mastitis should be transformed from an underrated condition to a relevant public health issue, as soon as possible. The traditional lack of interest and knowledge about this disease in human medicine strongly contrasts with its huge relevance in veterinary medicine, due to the obvious animal welfare, economic, and sanitary impact for farmers and dairy companies.

Prebiotics and Probiotics in Human Milk. http://dx.doi.org/10.1016/B978-0-12-802725-7.00015-4

2. MASTITIS: DEFINITION AND CLASSIFICATION

Literally, "mastitis" means the inflammation of any part of a mammary gland, including not only intramammary tissues but also nipples and mammary areolas. However, in practice, this term is generally used to define an infectious process of the mammary gland, usually—but not always—occurring during the lactation or puerperal period, and characterized by a variety of local and, in some cases, systemic symptoms (Lawrence and Lawrence, 2010). The infectious nature of lactational mastitis usually serves to differentiate this condition from other inflammatory processes of the mammary gland, such as those associated with breast cancer and Raynaud's disease, a painful vasoconstriction of the nipple during breastfeeding.

Lactational mastitis has been often classified into subgroups depending on different and, sometimes, controversial criteria. One criterion is the presence of clinical manifestations (clinical vs subclinical mastitis). Clinical mastitis implies signs and symptoms of breast inflammation, which may or may not be accompanied by systemic signs and symptoms. The term "subclinical" is used to describe those cases characterized by reduced milk secretion and a high milk bacterial count in the absence of evident inflammatory changes, including pain (Contreras and Rodríguez, 2011). Milk somatic cell counts (SCCs) and microbial cultures are generally used to diagnose subclinical mastitis in veterinary medicine (National Mastitis Council, 2001) but, in contrast, there is no a routine scientific or medical approach to diagnose subclinical mastitis in humans. It has been suggested that the term "subclinical" should be used to describe those cases characterized by the absence of local and systemic inflammatory changes, a reduced milk secretion (usually falsely perceived by mothers/practitioners as "low production," "not having enough milk," or "not having enough nutritious milk"), and a high milk bacterial count (Willumsen et al., 2003; Fernández et al., 2014). Within clinical mastitis, the type of symptoms and course of the disease (acute, subacute, granulomatous, chronic, and/or recurrent) are useful criteria to subclassify the disease (see Section 3). These terms are suitable for the classification of human infectious and inflammatory diseases according to the US National Library of Medicine.

3. LACTATIONAL MASTITIS AS A DYSBIOSIS PROCESS

The process of lactation has been remarkably successful since the earliest mammals, allowing thousands of species to occupy a vast range of ecological niches. It has been stated that, shaped by millennia of (co)evolution, some host–bacterial associations have developed into beneficial relationships in the mammalian gastrointestinal (GI) tract, creating an environment for mutualism (Round and Mazmanian, 2009). It is highly probable that the same is applicable for the mammary gland and milk.

A healthy milk microbiota contains a balanced composition of many classes of bacteria. Some symbiotic bacterial strains isolated from human milk have the ability to prevent infectious and inflammatory disease. But, similar to other human sites, the "normal" milk microbiota may also contain microorganisms ("pathobionts") that have shown to induce inflammation under particular conditions, usually acting as opportunistic pathogens. Therefore, the human milk microbiota have the potential to exert both pro- and antiinflammatory responses, and the composition of the bacterial communities in the breast and milk may be intimately linked to the proper functioning of the mammary immune system and to the milk biochemical composition, which is very complex and shows a high degree of interindividual variability. This may help to explain why mastitis remains a common feeding complication among most, if not all, mammalian species (Michie et al., 2003).

The US National Library of Medicine defines "dysbiosis" as "changes in quantitative and qualitative composition of microbiota. The changes may lead to altered host microbial interaction or homeostatic imbalance that can contribute to a disease state often with inflammation" (MeSH Descriptor Data; ID: D064806). Globally, all the facts indicate that lactational mastitis may be the result of a process of dysbiosis in the mammary gland (Delgado et al., 2008, 2009a; Jiménez et al., 2009) (Fig. 15.1),

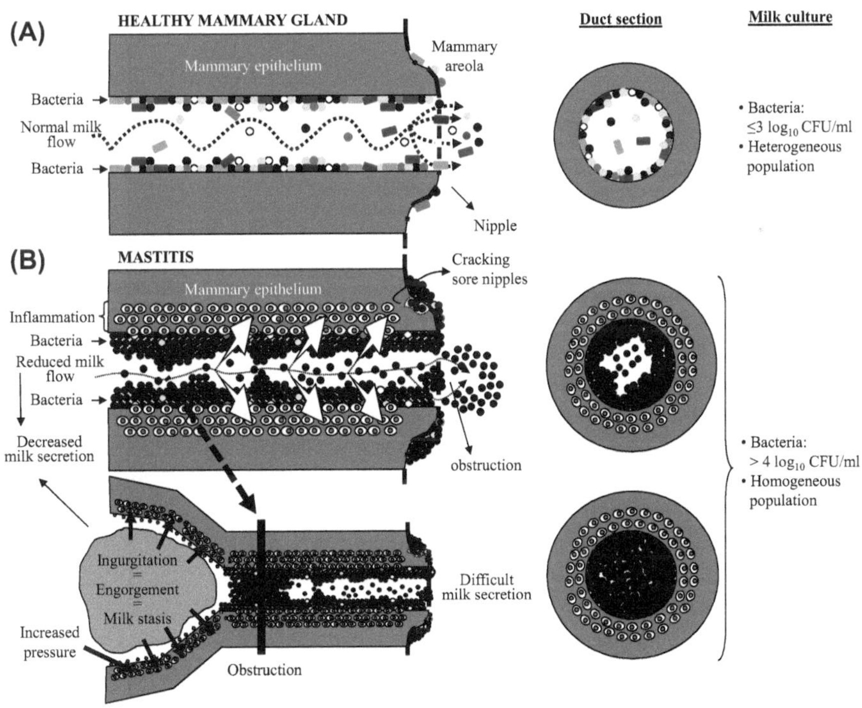

FIGURE 15.1

Schematic representation of the dysbiosis process leading to human mastitis. Mammary epithelium in physiological conditions (A) and during mastitis (B). *White arrows* indicate the excessive pressure of milk through an inflamed mammary epithelium, leading to cramps and typical burning and/or needle-like pain.

Adapted from Fernández, L., Arroyo, R., Espinosa, I., Marín, M., Jiménez, E., Rodríguez, J.M., 2014. Probiotics for human lactational mastitis. Beneficial Microbes 5, 169–183.

thus resembling the potential results of microbial dysbiosis in other locations, such as the GI tract (e.g., gastroenteritis, inflammatory bowel diseases) or in the vagina (vaginitis, vaginosis). In conditions of dysbiosis, there is a shift in the composition of the microbiota, which results in a loss of bacterial diversity, with a qualitative and quantitative reduction in the numbers of the symbionts and a usually sharp increase in the concentration of one or more pathobionts (Fig. 15.1). The causes for this shift are not entirely clear (see Section 5), but functional dysbiosis can affect host–microbe cross-talk interactions, resulting in disease. In general, more diversity seems to be more advantageous because it is thought that a diverse ecosystem is more resilient. Studies of the GI microbiome exemplify the enormous influence of a westernized lifestyle on microbial diversity and the pathophysiology of many diseases. Factors, such as the mode of birth delivery and feeding modality, improved sanitation, introduction of antibiotics and vaccines, a Western diet, and consumption of non-nutrients, greatly impact the GI microbiota. Since the GI microbiota seems to exert a strong influence on the human mammary microbiota, Western lifestyle may also have a similar impact on the milk microbiota.

4. ETIOPATHOGENESIS OF LACTATIONAL MASTITIS

It must be highlighted that microbiological analysis of milk is the only method that allows an etiological diagnosis of mastitis. As such, it would a very useful epidemiological tool if milk cultures became routine when mastitis is suspected. It may seem simple but it is not an easy issue, partly due to the absence of uniform or standard protocols for the collection of this biological fluid, the doubts that often arise for the interpretation of the results, and, in humans, the lack of tradition in milk microbiological analysis. The collection of a representative sample for microbial analysis is of utmost importance in order to get a correct diagnosis since there are many sampling-related factors that may affect the result (Arroyo et al., 2011). As an example, the use of nonsterile milk pumps and other devices to collect the samples is associated with a high concentration of some contaminant bacteria (particularly enterobacteria, *Pseudomonas* spp., *Stenotrophomonas* spp. and related gram-negative bacteria), and yeasts (*Candida* spp.) that arise from the rinsing water, manipulations, and other sources but are not related to the particular mastitis case (Brown et al., 2005; Marín et al., 2009). Other relevant factors that may be considered in making an etiological diagnosis include a reliable identification of the organism(s) detected on culture, its/their concentration(s), concurrent evidence of inflammation, and, if so, at what degree (Dohoo et al., 2011).

The introduction of molecular microbiology techniques to mastitis diagnosis has been extremely useful. Matrix-assisted laser desorption/ionization time-of-flight mass spectrometry (MALDI-TOF MS) is also spreading as a bacterial identification tool with high confidence and speed. In recent years, some identification schemes based on real-time polymerase chain reaction (RT-PCR) assays directly from milk have been proposed because of several benefits over conventional culture, including speed, automated interpretation of results, and increased sensitivity; however, the use of this technique must take into account that, in addition to live bacteria, milk contains a high quantity of dead bacteria and free bacterial DNA. There is no doubt that future improvements in the application of "-omics" to mastitic milk will provide more powerful tools for such a task but, at present, bacterial cultures are still required for routine etiological diagnosis of mastitis.

4.1 ACUTE MASTITIS

Staphylococcus aureus is the main etiological agent of acute mastitis (Reddy et al., 2007; Delgado et al., 2011; Jiménez et al., 2015). Once in the mammary gland, *S. aureus* can proliferate and produce toxins that lead to strong inflammation of the mammary tissue; as a consequence, intense local signs and symptoms (e.g., breast redness, heat, pain) usually arise (Fig. 15.2A). Since the mammary gland is highly vascularized throughout the lactation period, toxins are rapidly absorbed and reach the bloodstream causing an alteration in the host cytokine patterns and, eventually,

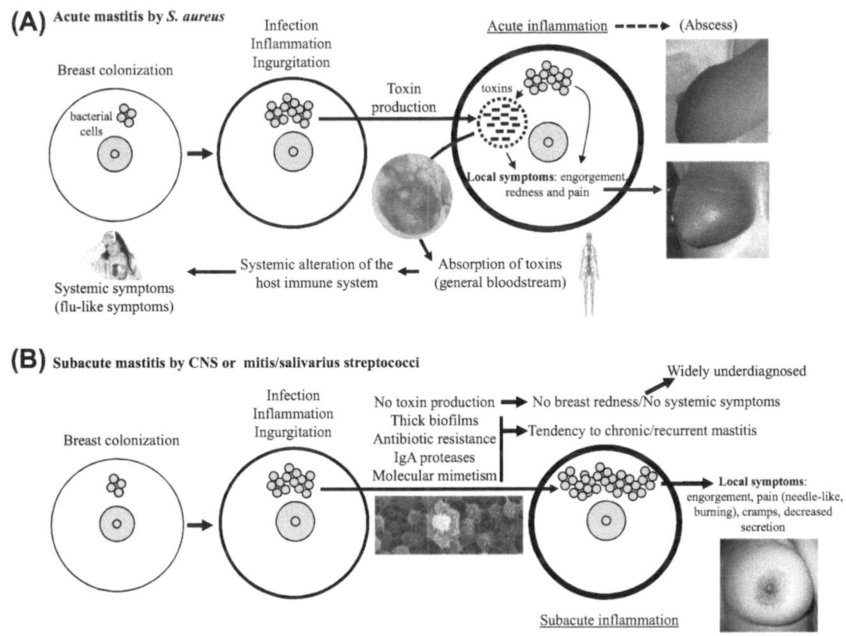

FIGURE 15.2

Schematic representation of the etiopathogenesis of acute (A) and subacute (B) mastitis. *CNS*, Coagulase-negative staphylococci; *IgA*, immunoglobulin A.

Adapted from Fernández, L., Arroyo, R., Espinosa, I., Marín, M., Jiménez, E., Rodríguez, J.M., 2014. Probiotics for human lactational mastitis. Beneficial Microbes 5, 169–183.

leading to systemic flu-like symptoms, which may include fever, muscular and joint pain, and general physical discomfort (Fig. 15.2A). Acute mastitis constitutes a relatively small fraction of human mastitis cases but due to the evident local and systemic signs, is the only type of mastitis correctly diagnosed.

4.2 SUBACUTE AND SUBCLINICAL MASTITIS

Coagulase-negative staphylococci (CNS) and *mitis* and *salivarius* streptococci are normal inhabitants of the mammary ecosystem during lactation. Under physiological conditions, they form thin biofilms that line the epithelium of the mammary ducts, allowing a normal milk flow (Fig. 15.2B). Pressure exerted by milk during its ejection sweeps along a relatively low number of bacteria, which are, subsequently, transferred to the infant (Fig. 15.2B). Different factors (discussed later) may favor an overgrowth of such bacterial species, leading to subacute or subclinical mastitis. Since CNS and *mitis/salivarius* streptococci do not produce the toxins responsible for acute mastitis, there are no systemic flu-like symptoms and, generally, local breast symptoms are milder and breast redness is absent. However, in some circumstances, these bacteria are able to form thick biofilms inside the ducts, inflaming the mammary epithelium and forcing milk to pass through an increasingly narrower lumen. The increasing milk pressure exerted on an inflamed epithelium results in a characteristic needle- or prick-like pain, often accompanied by breast cramps and a burning feeling. Eventually, bacterial biofilms may fill up some ducts, obstructing or blocking the milk flow and leading to a breast engorgement (Fig. 15.2B).

Unfortunately, in the few instances in which human milk culture examinations are performed, CNS are usually regarded as "commensal" or "saprophytic" bacteria, independent of their concentration. Therefore, if there is a high concentration (>3 $\log_{10}$CFU/mL) of CNS or streptococci in milk but, for example, *S. aureus* cannot be detected, then the case is usually wrongly reported as "noninfectious" mastitis. This means that subacute and subclinical mastitis are largely under-reported, despite being the most frequent cause of mastitis, painful breastfeeding, and precocious and undesired weaning (Delgado et al., 2009a; Jiménez et al., 2009).

Among CNS, *Streptococcus epidermidis* is the species most commonly associated with lactational mastitis in women (Thomsen et al., 1985; Delgado et al., 2008, 2009b; Jiménez et al., 2008a; Arroyo et al., 2010). Normally, it is a commensal inhabitant of healthy human skin and mucosal surfaces but, also, it is a common nosocomial pathogen (Otto, 2009). Living at the edge between commensalism and pathogenicity, *S. epidermidis* has developed interesting strategies to transform into a notorious pathogen (Schoenfelder et al., 2010). Similarly as in humans, CNS have become the most common mastitis-causing agents in ruminants and other mammals in many countries (Zhang and Maddox, 2000; Pyörälä and Taponen, 2009; Thorberg et al., 2009; Park et al., 2011a). Although CNS are not as pathogenic as *S. aureus* and infection mostly remains subacute or subclinical, CNS are relevant as they can cause persistent infections, which result in increased milk SCCs, tissue damage, and decreased milk quality and secretion.

Some species of the family Micrococcaceae (which is closely related, from a taxonomical point of view, to family Staphylococcaceae) may cause mastitis. They include *Rothia dentocariosa*, *Rothia mucilaginosa*, *Kocuria rosea,* and *Kocuria kristinae*, which are often involved in human opportunistic infections. In recent years, taxonomical rearrangements affecting these families may be responsible for a misidentification of isolates belonging to such species. More studies are required to clarify their role in this condition.

Streptococcus spp. associated with mastitis seem to be host specific. Group B streptococci such *Streptococcus uberis* or *Streptococcus dysgalactiae* are frequent agents of mastitis in cattle (Keefe, 1997) but are rarely, if ever, implicated in human mastitis. In contrast, the most common streptococcal species affecting humans include *Streptococcus mitis, Streptococcus salivarius,* and related species (Delgado et al., 2009a; Martín et al., 2015). It is important to note that streptococci have been subject to important taxonomical rearrangements and that many novel streptococcal species and closely related genera have been described in the last years; therefore, the implication of streptococci in mastitis should be carefully reevaluated.

4.3 GRANULOMATOUS MASTITIS

Some corynebacteria, including *Corynebacterium kroppenstedtii*, *Corynebacterium amycolatum,* and *Corynebacterium tuberculostearicum*, are involved in human granulomatous lobular mastitis, a chronic inflammatory disease that was previously considered of unknown etiology (Renshaw et al., 2011). Patients usually present an enlarged, mildly tender breast lump, which is sometimes associated with local inflammation, tenderness, and sinus formation and can become chronic and disfiguring in a large number of patients. Since corynebacteria stain poorly using the Gram stain technique, often fail to grow on routine media, and are found forming granulomatous structures deep in the breast tissue, it is probable that corynebacteria may have been overlooked as mastitis-causing agents (Paviour et al., 2002; Bercot et al., 2009). At present, *C. kroppenstedtii* is considered to be the main cause of granulomatous mastitis. It is a lipophilic species, and this feature seems particularly relevant in the pathogenesis of this condition. Such a property allows a firm attachment to fat globules, providing easy access to an abundant source of fatty acids. Therefore, it is not strange that histological preparations always show the bacterial cells within a central lipid-containing vacuole (Renshaw et al., 2011).

5. MASTITIS PROTECTING OR PREDISPOSING FACTORS

Similar to other body locations, breast health seems to depend on the balance between the state of the host and its microbiota, which may contain microorganisms ranging from symbionts or probiotic to pathobionts or potentially infectious agents. Therefore, there are many host, microbial, and medical factors that may play important roles in protection or predisposition to mastitis (Fig. 15.3).

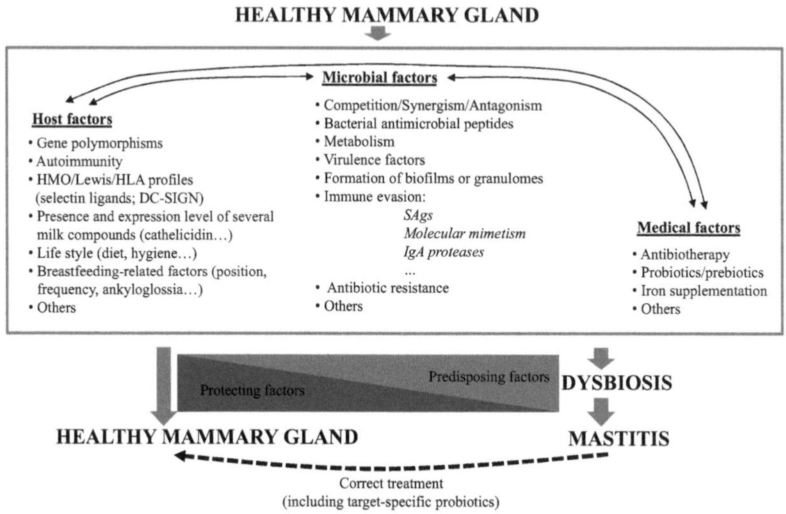

FIGURE 15.3

Several interrelated host-, microbial-, and medical-related factors may play a protecting or predisposing role concerning the development of mastitis.

5.1 HOST FACTORS

In order to ask why evolution has not managed to sort out the problem of mastitis or what mechanisms exist to prevent it developing, an insight into host differences is required. Although contemporary environmental factors such as a lower frequency of feeds, the wearing of a tight brassiere, or a higher perinatal use of antibiotics might increase this problem in humans, these seem irrelevant throughout mammalian evolutionary history (Michie et al., 2003). In contrast, the genetic background and the structure and immunology of the mammary gland differ notably among mammalian species, and individual differences are also observed within a given species. The interactions between the host immune system and the pathogen seem to be of particularly relevance in the etiopathogeny of mastitis (Burton and Erskine, 2003).

The existence of a genetic basis for host responses to bacterial intramammary infections has been widely documented in ruminants and, as an example, quantitative trait loci affecting the risk of *S. aureus* mastitis have been discovered (Sørensen et al., 2008). A few years ago, the first case of human granulomatous mastitis by a *C. kroppenstedtii* infection associated with a single nucleotide polymorphism (SNP) within the *NOD2* gene (SNP13 [Leu1007fsinsC]) was reported (Bercot et al., 2009). Such SNPs resulted in a strong impairment of the neutrophil responses to Nod2 agonists.

In addition, it has been suggested that some staphylococcal and streptococcal strains may use molecular mimetic mechanisms involving host-specific human leukocyte antigens (HLA) to evade the immune system response (Thibodeau et al., 1994; Giordano et al., 1996; Nooh et al., 2007). Toll-like receptor 2 (TLR2) signaling plays a key role in staphylococcal infections due to the interactions between this receptor and the major components (LTA and PGN) of the staphylococcal cell wall (Takeuchi et al., 1999, 2000; von Bernuth et al., 2008; Kawai and Akira, 2010). It has been observed that, after TLR2 signaling, *S. aureus* inhibits the interleukin (IL)-2 responses of T cells through the modulation of HLA-DR, the cluster of differentiation 86 (CD86 or B7.2), and the programmed cell death 1 ligand (PD-L1) (Wang et al., 2012).

Differences in selectin, Lewis antigens, and human milk oligosaccharide (HMO) gene determinants of the host may also predispose or protect against mastitis by altering neutrophils' activation and production of reactive oxygen species (Bode et al., 2004). Related to this, HMOs present in human milk are able to modulate the microbiota of breastfed infants (Bode, 2012). Therefore, it can be speculated that HMOs are also able to modulate the bacterial communities in the mammary gland. Interestingly, four different milk groups have been identified based on secretor and Lewis blood group systems (Albrecht et al., 2011; Thurl et al., 2010). While milk of "secretor" women is rich in 2′-fucosyllactose and other α1-2–fucosylated HMOs, "nonsecretor" women lack a functional FUT2 enzyme resulting in milk that does not contain α1-2–fucosylated HMOs. Interestingly, some strains of *Staphylococcus*, the major cause of mastitis, bind to 2′-fucosyllactose (Lane et al., 2011). Therefore, it is possible that susceptibility to suffer from mastitis is determined not only by the bacterial composition of the human milk but also by the blood group and corresponding type of HMOs in the milk.

Human milk contains a wide spectrum of other biologically active substances, and a higher or lower expression of the genes responsible for their biosynthesis may be related to a higher or lower risk of mastitis. In this context, polymorphisms or variations in the copy number of genes encoding eukaryotic antimicrobial peptides may be linked to mastitis susceptibility (Rivas-Santiago et al., 2009). As an example, cathelicidin LL-37, expressed in the mammary gland and secreted in milk, displays relevant antimicrobial activity against potential mastitis-causing agents (Murakami et al., 2005); interestingly, it has a strong antibiofilm effect even at subinhibitory concentrations (Jacobsen and Jenssen, 2012). Human alpha-lactalbumin made lethal to tumor cells (HAMLET) is another example. It is a protein–lipid complex from human milk with bactericidal activities. HAMLET exerts a rather specific bactericidal activity against some respiratory pathogens, with highest activity against *Streptococcus pneumoniae*. In addition, HAMLET acts as an antimicrobial adjuvant that can increase the activity of a broad spectrum of antibiotics (methicillin, vancomycin, gentamicin, and erythromycin) against multidrug-resistant *S. aureus* strains, to a degree where they become sensitive to those antibiotics, both in antimicrobial assays against planktonic and biofilm bacteria and in an in vivo model of nasopharyngeal colonization (Marks et al., 2013).

5.2 MICROBIAL FACTORS

The mammalian ecosystem is hospitable, or at least receptive, to many microorganisms, including the bacterial groups that have the potential to cause mastitis; this process of coevolution has led to a state of mutual acceptance or tolerance. However, on disturbance of this balanced state, localized or disseminated infection can occur. Unfortunately, the exact causal events leading to the transition from colonization to infection are still ill defined in vivo (van Belkum et al., 2009). The composition of the milk microbiome is host dependent (Martín et al., 2007; Hunt et al., 2011; Cabrera-Rubio et al., 2012; Jost et al., 2013; Jiménez et al., 2015). Therefore, this composition may be an important factor that determines whether a woman will have or will be protected against mastitis. Recently, Ma et al. (2015) reconstructed a milk bacterial community network based on the microbiome data obtained by Hunt et al. (2011). Their analysis revealed that the milk microbiome network consisted of two disconnected subnetworks. One subnetwork was a fully connected *complete graph* consisting of seven genera as nodes, and all of its pairwise interactions among the bacteria were facilitative or cooperative. In contrast, the interactions in the other subnetwork of eight nodes were mixed but dominantly cooperative. The only "non-cooperative" nodes in the second subnetwork were the mutually cooperative *Staphylococcus* and *Corynebacterium*, two genera that include some of the main mammary opportunistic pathogens. This potentially "evil" alliance between *Staphylococcus* and *Corynebacterium* could be inhibited by the remaining nodes that cooperate with one another in the second subnetwork. The authors postulated that the "confrontation" between the "evil" alliance and "benign" alliance and the shifting balance between them may be responsible for the dysbiosis of the milk microbiome that permits mastitis. Further research should focus on identifying the components of the milk microbiome associated with health benefits, and identify any other factor influencing these communities.

The ability to colonize and, eventually, infect a host depends not only on each bacterial species but also, most importantly, on each strain within a same species. It includes the expression of virulence factors, the resistance to antimicrobials, the formation of biofilms and the presence of other mechanisms to evade the immune response of the host.

At the species level, pathogen-specific local transcriptional disruptions in the mammary gland have been observed (Rinaldi et al., 2010). As an example, *S. aureus* elicits differential innate immune responses following intramammary infection in cows, which may determine the course and severity of the disease (Bannerman et al., 2004). The analysis of the genomes already available reveals that, globally, *S. aureus* is more suited to cause acute infections than CNS, which, in turn, have a higher propensity to cause subacute, subclinical or chronic infections (Gill et al., 2005). As an example, members of the enterotoxin and exotoxin families, which function as superantigens and inducers of a proinflammatory cytokine response, are usually associated with *S. aureus* (Larsen et al., 2002; Smyth et al., 2005; Hu et al., 2008). Seven pathogenicity genomic islands (νSas), carrying approximately one-half of the *S. aureus* toxins or virulence factors, have been identified in *S. aureus*. Variations in the pathogenic potential of strains belonging to this species depend largely on allelic variation of the virulence genes, on the presence or absence of individual νSas and on the presence of SNPs in key genes (Gill et al., 2005). Other studies, including genomic and proteomic approaches, have also found differences in genes and/or toxins related to virulence and antibiotic resistance among *S. aureus* strains involved in bovine and human mastitis (Barkema et al., 2006; Monecke et al., 2007; Delgado et al., 2011; Wolf et al., 2011).

As stated, the beneficial or detrimental effect of a mammary microorganism may depend not only on its relationships with other members of the microbiota but, also, on those established with the host. Some *S. epidermidis* strains constitute a good example of a beneficial relationship between bacteria and the mammary ecosystem through modulation of TLR3-dependent inflammation by initiating a TLR2-mediated cross-talk mechanism to suppress inflammation (Lai et al., 2009). In the skin, this bacterium also induces keratinocytes to express endogenous antimicrobial peptides through a TLR2-dependent mechanism (Lai et al., 2010), a property that has been unexplored in milk isolates so far. Furthermore, it has been reported that *S. epidermidis* has an autonomous function in controlling and tuning the functions of resident T lymphocytes in germ-free mice (Naik et al., 2012).

Commensal microorganisms can become pathogens, and thus no microbe can really be considered to be exclusively beneficial. Again, *S. epidermidis* is one of the most prominent and best-studied example although some questions are still to be answered such as the following. How does a commensal become a pathogen? Even more important, what are the unique factors that allow a commensal organism to be tolerated by a host? Among CNS, *S. epidermidis* causes the greatest number of infections. It is commonly regarded as the most frequent causative agent of infections of indwelling medical devices. Staphylococci are transferred into the patient's body from the skin of the patient or that of healthcare personnel during device insertion. Once the bacteria have entered the body, they use various virulence factors to facilitate interactions with host tissues and subvert the host's immune system. The most essential staphylococcal virulence factor is the characteristic biofilm formation on devices such as peripheral or central venous catheters. Interestingly, lactating mammary glands contain an extraordinary complex net of ducts during lactation that provides an excellent physical support to this microorganism (Fig. 15.4). In addition, its lactose and galactose metabolism is highly efficient through the D-tagatose-6-phosphate pathway (Schleifer et al., 1978). Finally, the growth of this bacterium is stimulated by HMOs (Hunt et al., 2012).

Biofilms are multicellular, surface-attached agglomerations of microorganisms (Fig. 15.4). Their regulation involves quorum-sensing systems and is not yet completely understood. Do all S. *epidermidis* species in the mammary environment have the potential to become a pathogen? Previous epidemiological and genetic studies suggest that *S. epidermidis* isolates in the hospital environment differ from those obtained outside of medical facilities in terms of biofilm formation, antibiotic resistance, and the presence of mobile DNA elements. For example, most disease-associated *S. epidermidis* biofilms are dependent on the expression of polysaccharide intercellular adhesin (PIA). However, the intercellular adhesion operon (*ica*) necessary for PIA production is rarely found in isolates obtained outside of hospital settings. To date, *icaA*, *mecA*, and *IS256* are used as markers for invasive nosocomial

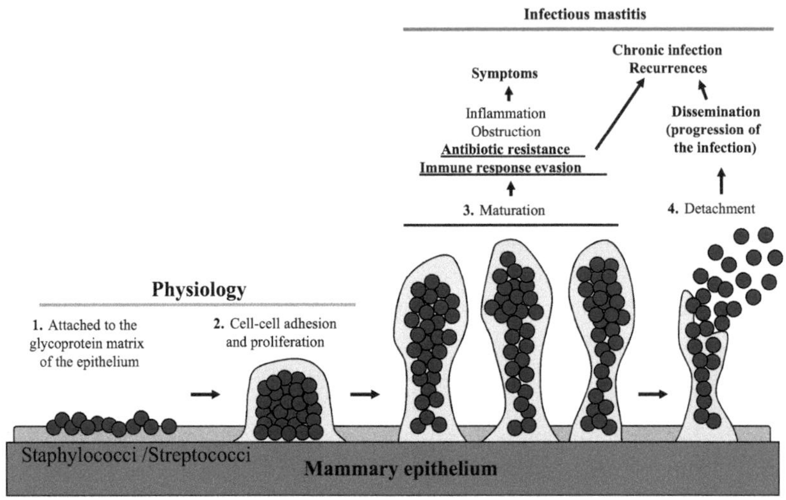

FIGURE 15.4

Stages of biofilm formation inside the mammary ducts, eventually leading to mastitis.

strains. Acquisition of these markers is associated with intra- and interspecific horizontal gene transfer. In this context, the comparison of several properties of 200 *S. epidermidis* strains isolated from women with mastitis with those displayed by 105 strains isolated from milk of healthy women revealed that the number of strains that contained biofilm-related genes and that showed resistance to oxacillin, erythromycin, clindamycin, and mupirocin was significantly higher among the strains isolated from mastitic milk (Delgado et al., 2009b). The authors suggested that resistance to diverse antibiotics and a greater ability to form biofilms found among the clinical strains may explain the chronic and recurrent nature of this infectious condition.

5.3 MEDICAL FACTORS

There are two common practices during late pregnancy, peripartum, and lactation that may have a profound impact on the mammary/milk microbiome: antibiotherapy and the use of iron. In a benefit–risk balance, both may be required to prevent or treat different conditions; however, their use should be avoided when there is not a clear medical indication.

Peripartum antibiotherapy, frequently related to cesarean section, premature or prolonged rupture of membranes, or group B streptococci intrapartum prophylaxis, has emerged as a strong risk factor for human mastitis because of the selection of antibiotic-resistant bacteria in the mammary environment and the elimination of potential natural competitors (Delgado et al., 2009a; Jiménez et al., 2009). Antibiotic resistance due to mechanisms both related and not related to biofilm formation seems to be a relatively widespread trait among mastitis-causing organisms (Delgado et al., 2009b; Begović et al., 2013).

In a recent study, the influence of several factors on the detection of lactobacilli and bifidobacterial DNA by PCR was assessed (Soto et al., 2014). The factor that exerted the strongest influence on the presence of lactobacilli or bifidobacteria was the administration of antibiotherapy to mothers during pregnancy or lactation. More specifically, detection of lactobacilli or bifidobacterial DNA in the milk samples was significantly lower in those women who had received antibiotherapy during such periods. Lactobacilli were also less frequently detected in milk of women who had been subjected to cesarean section, probably due to the antibiotherapy associated with such surgery.

It is widely accepted that antibiotics are responsible for dysbiosis processes in human microbiota leading to antibiotic-associated diarrhea and gastroenteritis and urogenital and oral infections. Host–microbiota interactions are dynamic and, therefore, changes in the microbiota as a consequence of antibiotic treatment can result in the dysregulation of host immune homeostasis and an increased susceptibility to infectious, allergic, and inflammatory diseases (Joffe and Simpson, 2009; Willing et al., 2011). In the past few years, it is becoming evident that antibiotherapy during pregnancy, intrapartum, or lactation alters the maternal (intestinal, vaginal, mammary) microbiota, a fact that may have negative consequences to infant health (Murk et al., 2011; Stensballe et al., 2013). The decrease in milk lactobacilli and bifidobacterial populations may have negative consequences for breastfed infants since they are important members of the human GI microbiota in early life and are believed to play a beneficial role in maintaining the health of the host. Some studies have suggested that infants with delayed colonization or decreased numbers of these bacteria may be more susceptible to a variety of GI or allergic conditions (Arvola et al., 2006). Recently, a comprehensive analysis of the fecal microbiota in infants with colic, compared with control infants, revealed that bifidobacteria and lactobacilli were reduced in infants with colic (de Weerth et al., 2013). Interestingly, several trials have shown that infants with colic benefit from the administration of a *Lactobacillus* strain, claimed to be of human milk origin (Savino et al., 2010; Sung et al., 2012; Szajewska et al., 2013). Finally, the antibiotic-associated loss of lactobacilli and bifidobacteria in milk may also have negative consequences for breast health because of the overgrowth of mastitis-causing agents (Contreras and Rodríguez, 2011).

The prescription of iron has become a routine practice during pregnancy and lactation, even for women whose iron-related hematological parameters are within physiological values and, therefore, do not need iron supplementation. The unique redox potential of iron makes it an ideal cofactor in diverse biochemical reactions. Iron is vital for the growth and proliferation of pathogenic bacteria. Vertebrates sequester excess iron within proteins in order to alleviate toxicity and restrict the amount of free iron available for invading pathogens (Hammer and Skaar, 2011). Restricting the growth of infectious microorganisms by sequestering essential nutrients is referred to as nutritional immunity. In order to circumvent nutritional immunity, bacterial pathogens have evolved elegant systems that allow for the acquisition of iron during infection. *S. aureus* is an organism that can cause severe disease when it gains access to underlying tissues. Iron acquisition, through the production of siderophores and the consumption of host heme, is required for *S. aureus* colonization, proliferation, and subsequent pathogenesis (Hammer and Skaar, 2012).

Similarly, the ability of *S. epidermidis* to withstand the high bactericidal activity of human blood is crucial for its systemic dissemination, including the colonization of the mammary gland during late pregnancy and lactation, periods in which it is highly vascularized. The study of the transcriptome of *S. epidermidis* biofilms, upon contact with human blood, showed an increased transcription of genes involved in biosynthesis and metabolism of amino acids, small molecules, carboxylic and organic acids, and cellular ketones (França et al., 2014). However, one of the most striking changes observed after 4 h of *S. epidermidis* exposure to human blood was an increased expression of genes involved in iron utilization. This finding suggests that iron acquisition is an important event for *S. epidermidis* survival in human blood (França et al., 2014). Therefore, intake of iron during late pregnancy and throughout the lactation period may favor the selective growth of mammary staphylococci, highly increasing the risk of mastitis and, as a consequence, it should be prescribed only when it is actually required but not in an indiscriminate manner during such life stages.

6. HUMAN MASTITIS: A TARGET FOR PROBIOTICS?

Potentially probiotic bacteria isolated from human milk seem to be particularly attractive organisms since they would fulfill some of the main criteria generally recommended for human probiotics, such as human origin, a history of safe prolonged intake by a particularly sensitive population (neonates, infants), and adaptation to mucosal and dairy substrates. Among the bacteria isolated from human milk, species like *Lactobacillus salivarius, L. reuteri, L. plantarum, L. paraplantarum, Lactobacillus gasseri, L. fermentum,* or *B. breve* are considered among those with probiotic potential and the *Qualified Presumption of Safety* status conceded by the European Food Safety Authority. In contrast to other bacteria, human milk strains seem to be uniquely adapted to reside in the human digestive tract and to interact in symbiosis from the time we are born (Jeurink et al., 2013).

As stated, multiresistance to antibiotics and the formation of biofilms and mechanisms for evasion of the host immune response are common features among clinical staphylococci involved in mastitis (Reddy et al., 2007; Delgado et al., 2011). In this context, the development of new strategies for mastitis management based on human milk probiotics, as an alternative or a complement to antibiotic therapy, is particularly appealing (Fernández et al., 2014).

For this purpose, our research group adopted the guidelines of the Food and Agriculture Organization/World Health Organization working groups on evaluation of the health and safety properties of probiotics in food (FAO/WHO, 2001, 2002) to select human milk lactobacilli strains with the ability for mastitis treatment. In parallel to the safety studies (including absence of antibiotic-resistance transmissible genes, deleterious metabolic activities, acute and repeated-dose toxicity in animal models, and adverse effects in human assays), the strains were selected on the basis of specific properties required for success in mastitis treatment after oral administration. Among the strains selected, we included a high survival rate during transit through the GI tract, specific interactions with dendritic cells, ability to colonize the mammary gland, and, once there, mechanisms for competitive exclusion of mastitis-causing staphylococci and streptococci.

Initially, a pilot trial highlighted the potential of *L. salivarius* CECT 5713 and *L. gasseri* CECT 5714, two strains isolated from milk, for the treatment of staphylococcal mastitis (Jiménez et al., 2008a). In the study, 20 women with staphylococcal mastitis were randomly divided in two groups. Those in the probiotic group daily ingested 10 $\log_{10}$ colony forming units (CFU) of *L. salivarius* CECT5713 and the same quantity of *L. gasseri* CECT5714 for 4 weeks while those in the placebo group only ingested the excipient. On day 0, the mean staphylococcal counts in the probiotic and placebo groups were similar (4.74 and 4.81 $\log_{10}$CFU/mL, respectively) but lactobacilli could not be detected. On day 30, the mean staphylococcal count in the probiotic group (2.96 $\log_{10}$CFU/mL) was significantly lower than that of the placebo group (4.79 $\log_{10}$CFU/mL). Colony hybridization and pulsed field gel electrophoresis profiling assays showed that *L. salivarius* CECT5713 and *L. gasseri* CECT5714 could be isolated from the milk samples of 6 of the 10 women in the probiotic group. On day 14, no clinical signs of mastitis were observed in the women assigned to this group but persisted throughout the study period in women given the placebo. These results revealed that *L. salivarius* CECT5713 and *L. gasseri* CECT5714 were an efficient alternative for the treatment of lactational mastitis.

Later, the efficacy of *L. fermentum* CECT 5716 or *L. salivarius* CECT 5713, two lactobacilli strains isolated from milk, to treat lactational mastitis when administered orally was evaluated and compared to antibiotic therapy (Arroyo et al., 2010). A total of 352 women with infectious mastitis were randomly divided in three groups. Those in groups A ($n=124$) and B ($n=127$) ingested daily 9 $\log_{10}$CFU of *L. fermentum* CECT 5716 or *L. salivarius* CECT 5713, respectively, for 3 weeks while those in group C ($n=101$) were submitted to antibiotic therapy prescribed in their respective primary care centers. On day 0, the mean staphylococcal and/or streptococcal counts in milk samples of the three groups were similar (4.35–4.47 $\log_{10}$CFU/mL) and lactobacilli could not be detected. On day 21, the mean staphylococcal and/or streptococcal counts in the probiotic groups (2.61 and 2.33 $\log_{10}$CFU/mL) were lower than that of the control group (3.28 $\log_{10}$CFU/mL). The probiotic treatment led to a significant reduction (1.7–2.1 $\log_{10}$CFU/mL) in the milk bacterial count and to a rapid improvement of the condition. The final staphylococcal and/or streptococcal count was approximately 2.5 $\log_{10}$CFU/mL, an acceptable bacterial load in milk of healthy women. After the probiotic treatment, *L. salivarius* CECT 5713 and *L. fermentum* CECT 5716 could be isolated from the milk samples of women of the probiotic groups A and B, respectively. On the basis of the bacterial counts, pain scores and clinical evolution, women in either of the probiotic groups improved significantly more than those assigned to the antibiotic group. However, the administration of

L. salivarius CECT 5713 was able to improve symptoms in 3–5 days while the effect of *L. fermentum* CECT 5716 was notably slower. In addition, the use of the probiotic strains prevented the mother from suffering side effects often associated with antibiotic treatment such as vaginal infections and recurrent mastitis episodes. Flatulence was the only adverse effect associated to probiotic treatment and was reported by a few percentage of the women receiving *L. fermentum* CECT5716.

Recently, another clinical assay was carried out to find microbiological, biochemical, and/or immunological biomarkers of the probiotic effect (Espinosa et al., 2015). Women with ($n=23$) and without ($n=8$) symptoms of mastitis received three daily doses (10^9 CFU) of *L. salivarius* PS2 for 21 days. Samples of milk, blood and urine were collected before and after the probiotic intervention, and screened for a wide spectrum of microbiological, biochemical, and immunological parameters. In the mastitis group, *L. salivarius* PS2 intake led to a decrease in the milk bacterial counts, milk and blood leukocyte counts and IL-8 milk concentration, to an increase in those of immunoglobulin (Ig)E, IgG3, epidermal growth factor, and IL-7, to a modification of the milk electrolyte profile, and to a reduction of some oxidative stress biomarkers. Such biomarkers will be useful in future clinical studies involving a larger cohort. In the same cohort, the characterization of the urine metabolic profile of the lactating women with mastitis at the beginning of a probiotic intervention with *L. salivarius* PS2 showed increased energy metabolism (lactate, citrate, formate, acetate, malonate) and decreased branched-chain amino acid catabolism (isocaproate and isovalerate) compared with that after probiotic intake (Vázquez-Fresno et al., 2014). Changes in the levels of acetate and 2-phenylpropionate after probiotic intake suggested an immunomodulatory role while increased level of malonate indicated an important antagonistic strategy of *L. salivarius* PS2 since this catabolite is a well-known repressor of the tricarboxylic acid cycle, which may alter staphylococcal and streptococcal metabolism and negatively affect their survival, virulence, and ability for biofilm formation (Gaupp et al., 2010; Leibig et al., 2010; Sun et al., 2012).

More recently, the potential of *L. salivarius* PS2 to prevent mastitis when orally administered during late pregnancy to women who had infectious mastitis after, at least, a previous pregnancy, was also investigated (Fernández et al., 2016). A total of 108 pregnant women were randomly divided in two groups. Those in the probiotic group ($n=55$) ingested daily 9 $\log_{10}$ CFU of *L. salivarius* PS2 from about week 30 of pregnancy until delivery while those in the control group ($n=53$) received a placebo. The occurrence of mastitis was evaluated during the first 3 months after delivery. Globally, 44 of 108 women (59.3%) had mastitis; however, the percentage of women with mastitis in the probiotic group (25.5%, $n=14$) was significantly lower than in the control group (56.6%, $n=30$). When mastitis occurred, the milk bacterial counts in the probiotic group were significantly lower than in the placebo one. Oral administration of *L. salivarius* PS2 during late pregnancy appears to be an efficient method to prevent infectious mastitis in a susceptible population.

It is important to note that efficacy of human milk lactobacilli in mastitis settings seems to be a strain-specific trait since only a few percentage of those isolated in our laboratory possess such ability (unpublished data). There may be different mechanisms by which some lactobacilli strains are able to control or, even to repress, mastitis-causing agents in the breast, including competitive exclusion for receptors or nutrients, or production of a variety of antimicrobials, including bacteriocins, organic acids, or hydrogen peroxide (Beasley and Saris, 2004; Martín et al., 2005; Olivares et al., 2006). After oral administration, a lactobacillus strain must be able to elicit potent responses from the mucosal immune system and/or to colonize the mammary gland in order to compete with the bacteria responsible for mastitis. The latter would imply that a lactobacillus strain must be able to reach the mammary gland upon ingestion, and, in fact, it has been suggested that the origin of, at least a part, of the live bacteria found in human milk could be the maternal GI tract through an enteromammary pathway, involving complex interactions with intestinal immune cells (Martín et al., 2004; Langa, 2006; Rodríguez, 2014). An increased bacterial translocation from the GI tract to mesenteric lymph nodes and mammary glands in pregnant and lactating mice has already been described (Perez et al., 2007). Bacteria could be observed histologically in the subepithelial dome and interfollicular regions of Peyer's patches, in the lamina propria of the small bowel, and associated with cells in the glandular tissue of the mammary gland. In the same study, acridine orange staining of human milk and blood cytopreparations allowed the detection of bacterial cells in association with maternal mononuclear cells.

A previous study showed that oral administration of a *Lactobacillus* strain to women during pregnancy resulted in colonization of their intestine and, subsequently, of their respective breastfed infant's GI tract (Schultz et al., 2004). Unfortunately, the role of milk bacteria as the potential source of the strain was not investigated. More recently, an *L. reuteri* strain could be detected in milk after oral supplementation to the mother (Abrahamsson et al., 2009). Therefore, it is not strange that oral administration of a few lactobacilli strains isolated from human milk, and specifically selected for the mastitis target, resulted not only in the transfer of such strains from the GI tract to the mammary gland and milk but, also, in a notable or total improvement of the condition (Jiménez et al., 2008b; Arroyo et al., 2010). Genome sequencing of some of these strains is providing some new clues to understand the relationship between phenotypic properties and their subjacent molecular basis (Langa et al., 2012).

At present, it is obvious that the interrelated nutritional, metabolic, microbiological, neurological, and immunological processes that take place in the GI tract have a direct impact in mammary gland and, as a consequence, in milk during late pregnancy and throughout lactation (Goldblum and Goldman, 1994; Fernández et al., 2013; Jeurink et al., 2013; Rodríguez, 2014). Therefore, manipulation of the maternal GI microbiota by probiotic supplementation has the potential to affect the immune composition of the mammary gland and milk and could be another mechanism explaining the antimastitis effect. It has been shown that administration of some probiotic strains belonging to different species, such as *Lactobacillus rhamnosus* or *Bifidobacterium animalis* subsp. *lactis*, during late pregnancy and/or breastfeeding increases IgA and transforming growth factor (TGF)-β2 levels in milk (Rautava et al., 2002; Prescott et al., 2008; Nikniaz et al., 2013). Increased IgA levels may help to limit the access of mastitis-causing bacteria to the mammary epithelium while TGF-β2 is a key mammary immunoregulatory factor, promoting local IgA production and inducing oral tolerance mechanisms in infants (Stavnezer, 1995; Oddy and Rosales, 2010). In contrast, oral supplementation with an *L. reuteri* strain to pregnant women resulted in a reduction of the TGF-β2 levels in colostrum and had no effect on milk IgA concentration (Böttcher et al., 2008). This contradictory result may be due to differential immune responses to different bacterial strains. Interestingly, none of the *L. reuteri* strains assayed by our group so far had a significant effect on human mastitis (unpublished data).

The potential of lactic acid bacteria to treat bovine mastitis has also been tested recently in two field trials and compared with conventional antibiotic therapy (Klostermann et al., 2008; Crispie et al., 2008). Results from both trials indicated that administration of *Lactococcus lactis* DPC3147 to the teat canal was, at least, as efficacious as common antibiotic treatments. Flow cytometry assays demonstrated that live *L. lactis* specifically triggered the mammary immune response to elicit neutrophil accumulation (Crispie et al., 2008). These results suggest that the mechanism responsible for this probiotic treatment of mastitis is associated with stimulation of the host intramammary immune system.

7. CNS AND VIRIDANS STREPTOCOCCI: POTENTIAL PROBIOTICS FOR MASTITIS?

Streptococci and staphylococci have received marginal attention regarding their role in the human mammary gland and in the early colonization of the infant GI tract despite being the dominant bacteria in human milk (Jiménez et al., 2008b; Martín et al., 2012; Hunt et al., 2012). Interestingly, an abundant presence of *S. epidermidis* in the infant GI tract seems to be a differential feature of the feces of breastfed infants compared with those of formula-fed infants (Sakata et al., 1985; Lundequist et al., 1985; Balmer and Wharton, 1989; Borderon et al., 1996; Adlerberth et al., 2006; Jiménez et al., 2008b).

Indeed, CNS and *mitis/salivarius* streptococci provided by milk can be particularly useful to reduce the acquisition of undesired pathogens by infants exposed to hospital environments. It has been proposed that *S. epidermidis* and other CNS may have a probiotic function by preventing colonization of the host by more severe pathogens, such as *S. aureus* (Otto, 2009). Quorum sensing interference favors at least one subtype of *S. epidermidis* over *S. aureus* in vitro (Otto et al., 1999; Carmody and Otto, 2004). A previous study showed that bovine mammary quarters infected with CNS were less susceptible to development of new mastitis after experimental challenge with *S. aureus* (Nickerson and Boddie, 1994). In fact, some *S. epidermidis* strains that inhibit in vivo colonization by *S. aureus* have been postulated as a future strategy to eradicate such a pathogen from the mucosal surfaces (Iwase et al., 2010; Park et al., 2011b). Similarly, it has been shown that *viridans* streptococci inhibit oral colonization by methicillin-resistant *S. aureus* in high-risk newborns exposed to hospital environments (Uehara et al., 2001). In addition, the presence of *viridans* streptococci seems to be a feature of the healthy infant GI tract in contrast with the atopic infant GI tract (Kirjavainen et al., 2001). Therefore, at least some staphylococcal and streptococcal strains present in human milk may play important empirical probiotic roles in the breast and in the breastfed infant. Obviously, a potential CNS probiotic approach should take into account that CNS provide a reservoir function for the transfer of genetic elements to enhance the pathogenic success and antibiotic resistance of *S. aureus* and, therefore, play an important role in human and animal disease (Gill et al., 2005). As a consequence, selection of potentially probiotic CNS should follow particularly strict safety criteria, including the lack of mechanisms to exchange genetic information with other bacteria.

8. BACTERIOCINS AND MASTITIS

Early attempts to find a practical application for nisin, a food-grade antimicrobial peptide produced by some strains of *L. lactis*, included the treatment of bovine mastitis (Taylor et al., 1949). However, such application was soon forgotten mainly due to the coming of the antibiotic age. In the past two decades, the increasing rate of antibiotic-resistant bacteria has led to a renewed interest in the use of nisin and other bacteriocins, such as lactacin 3147 and uberolysin, as therapeutic agents in bovine mastitis because of their activity against staphylococci and streptococci (Broadbent et al., 1989; Sears et al., 1992; Ryan et al., 1998; Wirawan et al., 2007; Klostermann et al., 2008; Crispie et al., 2008). *L. lactis* seems to be a common species in milk of healthy women (Heikkilä and Saris, 2003; Martín et al., 2007) and, approximately 30% of the isolates from this origin have the ability to produce nisin (Beasley and Saris, 2004). In fact, nisin-producing lactococci have shown potential to be used as biotherapeutic agents in preventing neonatal and maternal breast infections caused by *S. aureus* (Heikkilä and Saris, 2003). Obviously, application of bacteriocins for human mastitis faces the limitation that an intramammary application is not possible. However, topical application of nisin-containing preparations was efficient for treatment of the most painful manifestations of staphylococcal lactational mastitis: nipple and mammary areola fissures and wounds (Fernández et al., 2008). Its efficacy for such use is notably better than that of lanolin and other ointments frequently used for nipple and mammary areola cracking (unpublished results).

9. CONCLUSIONS

The composition of the human milk microbiota has implications not only for the infant but also for mammary health. Mammary microbial dysbiosis may lead to acute, subacute or subclinical mastitis, a frequently underrated and underdiagnosed condition that represents the first medical cause for undesired weaning. Since breastfeeding provides short- and long-term benefits to the mother–infant pair, lactational mastitis should be considered as a relevant public health issue. Many host, microbial, medical, and environmental factors may predispose a woman to or her protect against mastitis development. In the future, better knowledge on such factors could be used to design novel means of preventing bacterial colonization from proceeding into mastitis. Lactobacillus strains isolated from milk of healthy women, and specifically selected for the mastitis target, have shown a high efficacy as oral probiotics for the prevention and treatment of mastitis. Work is in progress to elucidate the local and systemic mechanisms responsible for such an effect by combining microbiological and immunological assays with "-omics" approaches.

ACKNOWLEDGMENTS

The work of our group in this field has been partly supported by the FUN-C-FOOD (Consolider-Ingenio, CSD2007-00063) and AGL2013-41980-P projects from the Ministerio de Economía y Competitividad (Spain).

REFERENCES

Abrahamsson, T.R., Sinkiewicz, G., Jakobsson, T., Fredrikson, M., Björkstén, B., 2009. Probiotic lactobacilli in breast milk and infant stool in relation to oral intake during the first year of life. Journal of Pediatric Gastroenterology and Nutrition 49, 349–354.

Adlerberth, I., Lindberg, E., Aberg, N., Hesselmar, B., Saalman, R., Strannegard, I.L., Wold, A.E., 2006. Reduced enterobacterial and increased staphylococcal colonization of the infantile bowel: an effect of hygienic lifestyle. Pediatric Research 59, 96–101.

Albrecht, S., Schols, H.A., van den Heuvel, E.G., Voragen, A.G., Gruppen, H., 2011. Occurrence of oligosaccharides in feces of breast-fed babies in their first six months of life an1d the corresponding breast milk. Carbohydrate Research 346, 2540–2550.

American Academy of Pediatrics, 2012. Breastfeeding and the use of human milk. Pediatrics 129, e827–41.

Arroyo, R., Martin, V., Maldonado, A., Jimenez, E., Fernandez, L., Rodriguez, J.M., 2010. Treatment of infectious mastitis during lactation: antibiotics versus oral administration of lactobacilli isolated from breast milk. Clinical Infectious Diseases 50, 1551–1558.

Arroyo, R., Mediano, P., Martín, V., Jiménez, E., Delgado, S., Fernández, L., Marín, M., Rodríguez, J.M., 2011. Etiological diagnosis of infectious mastitis: proposal of a protocol for the culture of human milk samples. Acta Pediatrica Española 69, 276–281.

Arvola, T., Ruuska, T., Keränen, J., Hyöty, H., Salminen, S., Isolauri, E., 2006. Rectal bleeding in infancy: clinical, allergological, and microbiological examination. Pediatrics 117, e760–768.

Balmer, S.E., Wharton, B.A., 1989. Diet and faecal flora in the newborn: breast milk and infant formula. Archives of Disease in Childhood 64, 1672–1681.

Bannerman, D.D., Paape, M.J., Lee, J.W., Zhao, X., Hope, J.C., Rainard, P., 2004. *Escherichia coli* and *Staphylococcus aureus* elicit differential innate immune responses following intramammary infection. Clinical and Diagnostic Laboratory Immunology 11, 463–472.

Barkema, H.W., Schukken, Y.H., Zadoks, R.N., 2006. The role of cow, pathogen, and treatment regimen in the therapeutic success of bovine *Staphylococcus aureus* mastitis. Journal of Dairy Science 89, 1877–1895.

Beasley, S.S., Saris, P.E., 2004. Nisin-producing *Lactococcus lactis* strains isolated from human milk. Applied and Environmental Microbiology 70, 5051–5053.

Begović, J., Jovčić, B., Papić-Obradović, M., Veljović, K., Lukić, J., Kojić, M., Topisirović, L., 2013. Genotypic diversity and virulent factors of *Staphylococcus epidermidis* isolated from human breast milk. Microbiology Research 168, 77–83.

Bercot, B., Kannengiesser, C., Oudin, C., Grandchamp, B., Sanson-le Pors, M.J., Mouly, S., Elbim, C., 2009. First description of NOD2 variant associated with defective neutrophil responses in a woman with granulomatous mastitis related to corynebacteria. Journal of Clinical Microbiology 47, 3034–3037.

Bode, L., 2012. Human milk oligosaccharides: every baby needs a sugar mama. Glycobiology 22, 1147–1162.

Bode, L., Rudloff, S., Kunz, C., Strobel, S., Klein, N., 2004. Human milk oligosaccharides reduce platelet-neutrophil complex formation leading to a decrease in neutrophil beta 2 integrin expression. Journal of Leukocyte Biology 76, 820–826.

Borderon, J.C., Lionnet, C., Rondeau, C., Suc, A.I., Laugier, J., Gold, F., 1996. Current aspects of fecal flora of the newborn without antibiotherapy during the first 7 days of life: *Enterobacteriaceae*, enterococci, staphylococci. Pathologie Biologie 44, 416–422.

Böttcher, M.F., Abrahamsson, T.R., Fredriksson, M., Jakobsson, T., Björkstén, B., 2008. Low breast milk TGF-beta2 is induced by *Lactobacillus reuteri* supplementation and associates with reduced risk of sensitization during infancy. Pediatric Allergy and Immunology 19, 497–504.

Broadbent, J.R., Chou, Y.C., Gillies, K., Kondo, J.K., 1989. Nisin inhibits several gram-positive, mastitis-causing pathogens. Journal of Dairy Science 72, 3342–3345.

Brown, S.L., Bright, R.S., Dwyer, D.E., Forman, B., 2005. Breast pump adverse events: reports to the Food and Drug Administration. Journal of Human Lactation 21, 169–174.

Burton, J.L., Erskine, R.J., 2003. Immunity and mastitis. Some new ideas for an old disease. Veterinary Clinics of North America: Food Animal Practice 19, 1–45.

Cabrera-Rubio, R., Collado, M.C., Laitinen, K., Salminen, S., Isolauri, E., Mira, A., 2012. The human milk microbiome changes over lactation and is shaped by maternal weight and mode of delivery. American Journal of Clinical Nutrition 96, 544–551.

Carmody, A.B., Otto, M., 2004. Specificity grouping of the accessory gene regulator quorum-sensing system of *Staphylococcus epidermidis* is linked to infection. Archives in Microbiology 181, 250–253.

Contreras, G.A., Rodriguez, J.M., 2011. Mastitis: comparative etiology and epidemiology. Journal of the Mammary Gland Biology and Neoplasia 16, 339–356.

Crispie, F., Alonso-Gómez, M., O'Loughlin, C., Klostermann, K., Flynn, J., Arkins, S., Meaney, W., Paul Ross, R., Hill, C., 2008. Intramammary infusion of a live culture for treatment of bovine mastitis: effect of live lactococci on the mammary immune response. Journal of Dairy Research 75, 374–384.

de Weerth, C., Fuentes, S., Puylaert, P., de Vos, W.M., 2013. Intestinal microbiota of infants with colic: development and specific signatures. Pediatrics 131, e550–e558.

Delgado, S., Arroyo, R., Martín, R., Rodríguez, J.M., 2008. PCR-DGGE assessment of the bacterial diversity of breast milk in women with lactational infectious mastitis. BMC Infectious Diseases 8, 51.

Delgado, S., Arroyo, R., Jiménez, E., Fernández, L., Rodríguez, J.M., 2009a. Infectious mastitis during lactation: an underrated condition (I). Acta Pediatrica Española 67, 77–84.

Delgado, S., Arroyo, R., Jiménez, E., Marin, M.L., del Campo, R., Fernandez, L., Rodriguez, J.M., 2009b. *Staphylococcus epidermidis* strains isolated from breast milk of women suffering infectious mastitis: potential virulence traits and resistance to antibiotics. BMC Microbiology 9, 82.

Delgado, S., García, P., Fernández, L., Jiménez, E., Rodríguez-Baños, M., del Campo, R., Rodríguez, J.M., 2011. Characterization of *Staphylococcus aureus* strains involved in human and bovine mastitis. FEMS Immunological and Medical Microbiology 62, 225–235.

Dohoo, I.R., Smith, J., Andersen, S., Kelton, D.F., Godden, S., 2011. Diagnosing intramammary infections: evaluation of definitions based on a single milk sample. Journal of Dairy Science 94, 250–261.

Espinosa-Martos, I., Jiménez, E., de Andrés, J., Rodríguez-Alcalá, L.M., Tavárez, S., Manzano, S., Fernández, L., Alonso, E., Fontecha, J., Rodríguez, J.M., 2015. Searching for milk and blood biomarkers associated to the clinical efficacy of a probiotic for the treatment of infectious mastitis. Beneficial Microbes (accepted).

FAO/WHO, 2001. Report on Joint FAO/WHO Expert Consultation on Evaluation of Health and Nutritional Properties of Probiotics in Food Including Powder Milk with Live Lactic Acid Bacteria.

FAO/WHO, 2002. Report of a Joint FAO/WHO Working Group on Drafting Guidelines for the Evaluation of Probiotics in Food.

Fernández, L., Delgado, S., Herrero, H., Maldonado, A., Rodríguez, J.M., 2008. The bacteriocin nisin, an effective agent for the treatment of staphylococcal mastitis during lactation. Journal of Human Lactation 24, 311–316.

Fernández, L., Langa, S., Martín, V., Maldonado, A., Jiménez, E., Martín, R., Rodríguez, J.M., 2013. The human milk microbiota: origin and potential roles in health and disease. Pharmacological Research 69, 1–10.

Fernández, L., Arroyo, R., Espinosa, I., Marín, M., Jiménez, E., Rodríguez, J.M., 2014. Probiotics for human lactational mastitis. Beneficial Microbes 5, 169–183.

Fernández, L., Cárdenas, N., Arroyo, R., Manzano, S., Jiménez, E., Martín, V., Rodríguez, J.M., 2016. Prevention of infectious mastitis by oral administration of *Lactobacillus salivarius* PS2 during late pregnancy. Clinical Infectious Disease 62, 568–573.

França, A., Carvalhais, V., Maira-Litrán, T., Vilanova, M., Cerca, N., Pier, G., 2014. Alterations in the *Staphylococcus epidermidis* biofilm transcriptome following interaction with whole human blood. Pathogens and Disease 70, 444–448.

Gartner, L.M., Morton, J., Lawrence, R.A., Naylor, A.J., O'Hare, D., Schanler, R.J., Eidelman, A.I., 2005. Breastfeeding and the use of human milk. Pediatrics 2005 (115), 496–506.

Gaupp, R., Schlag, S., Liebeke, M., Lalk, M., Gotz, F., 2010. Advantage of upregulation of succinate dehydrogenase in *Staphylococcus aureus* biofilms. Journal of Bacteriology 192, 2385–2394.

Gill, S.R., Fouts, D.E., Archer, G.L., Mongodin, E.F., Deboy, R.T., Ravel, J., Paulsen, I.T., Kolonay, J.F., Brinkac, L., Beanan, M., Dodson, R.J., Daugherty, S.C., Madupu, R., Angiuoli, S.V., Durkin, A.S., Haft, D.H., Vamathevan, J., Khouri, H., Utterback, T., Lee, C., Dimitrov, G., Jiang, L., Qin, H., Weidman, J., Tran, K., Kang, K., Hance, I.R., Nelson, K.E., Fraser, C.M., 2005. Insights on evolution of virulence and resistance from the complete genome analysis of an early methicillin-resistant *Staphylococcus aureus* strain and a biofilm-producing methicillin-resistant *Staphylococcus epidermidis* strain. Journal of Bacteriology 187, 2426–2438.

Giordano, N., Senesi, M., Battisti, E., Palumbo, F., Mondillo, S., Bargagli, G., Palazzuoli, V., Nardi, P., Gennari, C., 1996. Reactive arthritis by *Staphylococcus epidermidis*: report of an unusual case. Clinical Rheumatology 15, 59–61.

Goldblum, R.M., Goldman, A.S., 1994. Immunological components of milk: formation and function. In: Ogra, P.L., Strober, W., McGhee, G.R., Lamm, G.R., Bienenstock, J. (Eds.), Handbook of Mucosal Immunology. Academic Press, New York, pp. 643–652.

Hammer, N.D., Skaar, E.P., 2011. Molecular mechanisms of *Staphylococcus aureus* iron acquisition. Annual Review of Microbiology 65, 129–147.

Hammer, N.D., Skaar, E.P., 2012. A battle for iron: host sequestration and *Staphylococcus aureus* acquisition. Microbes and Infection 14, 217–227.

Heikkila, M.P., Saris, P.E., 2003. Inhibition of *Staphylococcus aureus* by the commensal bacteria of human milk. Journal of Applied Microbiology 95, 471–478.

Hu, D.L., Omoe, K., Inoue, F., Kasai, T., Yasujima, M., Shinagawa, K., Nekane, A., 2008. Comparative prevalence of superantigenic toxin genes in methicillin-resistant and meticillin-susceptible *Staphylococcus aureus* isolates. Journal of Medical Microbiology 57, 1106–1112.

Hunt, K.M., Foster, J.A., Forney, L.J., Schutte, U.M., Beck, D.L., Abdo, Z., Fox, L.K., Williams, J.E., McGuire, M.K., McGuire, M.A., 2011. Characterization of the diversity and temporal stability of bacterial communities in human milk. PLoS ONE 6, e21313.

Hunt, K.M., Preuss, J., Nissan, C., Davlin, C.A., Williams, J.E., Shafii, B., Richardson, A.D., McGuire, M.K., Bode, L., McGuire, M.A., 2012. Human milk oligosaccharides promote the growth of staphylococci. Applied and Environmental Microbiology 78, 4763–4770.

Iwase, T., Uehara, Y., Shinji, H., Tajima, A., Seo, H., Takada, K., Agata, T., Mizunoe, Y., 2010. *Staphylococcus epidermidis* Esp inhibits *Staphylococcus aureus* biofilm formation and nasal colonization. Nature 465, 346–349.

Jacobsen, A.S., Jenssen, H., 2012. Human cathelicidin LL-37 prevents bacterial biofilm formation. Future Medicine and Chemistry 4, 1587–1599.

Jeurink, P.V., van Bergenhenegouwen, J., Jimenez, E., Knippels, L.M., Fernandez, L., Garssen, J., Knol, J., Rodriguez, J.M., Martin, R., 2013. Human milk: a source of more life than we imagine. Beneficial Microbes 4, 17–30.

Jimenez, E., Fernandez, L., Maldonado, A., Martin, R., Olivares, M., Xaus, J., Rodriguez, J.M., 2008a. Oral administration of *Lactobacillus* strains isolated from breast milk as an alternative for the treatment of infectious mastitis during lactation. Applied and Environmental Microbiology 74, 4650–4655.

Jimenez, E., Delgado, S., Maldonado, A., Arroyo, R., Albujar, M., Garcia, N., Jariod, M., Fernandez, L., Gomez, A., Rodriguez, J.M., 2008b. *Staphylococcus epidermidis*: a differential trait of the fecal microbiota of breast-fed infants. BMC Microbiology 8, 143.

Jiménez, E., Delgado, S., Arroyo, R., Fernández, L., Rodríguez, J.M., 2009. Infectious mastitis during lactation: an underrated condition (II). Acta Pediatrica Española 67, 125–132.

Jiménez, E., de Andrés, J., Manrique, M., Pareja-Tobes, P., Tobes, R., Martínez-Blanch, J.F., Codoñer, F.M., Ramón, D., Fernández, L., Rodríguez, J.M., 2015. Metagenomic analysis of milk of healthy and mastitis-suffering women. Journal of Human Lactation 31, 406–415.

Joffe, T., Simpson, N., 2009. Cesarean section and risk of asthma. The role of intrapartum antibiotics: a missing piece? Journal of Pediatrics 154, 154.

Jost, T., Lacroix, C., Braegger, C., Chassard, C., 2013. Assessment of bacterial diversity in breast milk using culture-dependent and culture-independent approaches. British Journal of Nutrition 14, 1–10.

Kawai, T., Akira, S., 2010. The role of pattern-recognition receptors in innate immunity: update on Toll-like receptors. Nature Immunology 11, 373–384.

Keefe, K., 1997. *Streptococcus agalactiae* mastitis: a review. Canadian Veterinary Journal 38, 429–437.

Kirjavainen, P.V., Apostolou, E., Arvola, T., Salminen, S.J., Gibson, G.R., Isolauri, E., 2001. Characterizing the composition of intestinal microflora as a prospective treatment target in infant allergic disease. FEMS Immunological and Medical Microbiology 32, 1–7.

Klostermann, K., Crispie, F., Flynn, J., Ross, R.P., Hill, C., Meaney, W., 2008. Intramammary infusion of a live culture of *Lactococcus lactis* for treatment of bovine mastitis: comparison with antibiotic treatment in field trials. Journal of Dairy Research 75, 365–373.

Lai, Y., Di Nardo, A., Nakatsuji, T., Leichtle, A., Yang, Y., Cogen, A.L., Wu, Z.R., Hooper, L.V., Schmidt, R.R., von Aulock, S., Radek, K.A., Huang, C.M., Ryan, A.F., Gallo, R.L., 2009. Commensal bacteria regulate Toll-like receptor 3-dependent inflammation after skin injury. Nature Medicine 15, 1377–1382.

Lai, Y., Cogen, A.L., Radek, K.A., Park, H.J., Macleod, D.T., Leichtle, A., Ryan, A.F., Di Nardo, A., Gallo, R.L., 2010. Activation of TLR2 by a small molecule produced by *Staphylococcus epidermidis* increases antimicrobial defense against bacterial skin infections. Journal of Investigative Dermatology 130, 2211–2221.

Lane, J.A., Mehra, R.K., Carrington, S.D., Hickey, R.M., 2011. Development of biosensor-based assays to identify anti-infective oligosaccharides. Analytical Biochemistry 410, 200–205.

Langa, S., 2006. Interactions between Lactic Acid Bacteria, Intestinal Epithelial Cells and Immune Cells. Development of *In Vitro* Models (Ph.D. thesis). Complutense University of Madrid, Madrid.

Langa, S., Maldonado, A., Delgado, S., Martín, R., Martín, V., Jiménez, E., Ruíz-Barba, J.L., Mayo, B., Connor, R.I., Suárez, E., Rodríguez, J.M., 2012. Characterization of *Lactobacillus salivarius* CECT 5713, a strain isolated from human milk: from genotype to phenotype. Applied Microbiology and Biotechnology 94, 1279–1287.

Larsen, H.D., Aarestrup, F.M., Jensen, N.E., 2002. Geographical variation in the presence of genes encoding superantigenic exotoxins and ß-hemolysin among *Staphylococcus aureus* isolated from bovine mastitis in Europe and USA. Veterinary Microbiology 85, 61–67.

Lawrence, R.A., Lawrence, R.M., 2010. Breastfeeding. A Guide for the Medical Profession, seventh ed. Saunders, Philadelphia.

Leibig, M., Liebeke, M., Mader, D., Lalk, M., Peschel, A., Gotz, F., 2010. Pyruvate formate lyase acts as a formate supplier for metabolic processes during anaerobiosis in *Staphylococcus aureus*. Journal of Bacteriology 193, 952–962.

Li, R., Fein, S.B., Chen, J., Grummer-Strawn, L.M., 2008. Why mothers stop breastfeeding: mothers' self-reported reasons for stopping during the first year. Pediatrics 122 (Suppl. 2), S69–S76.

Lundequist, B., Nord, C.E., Winberg, J., 1985. The composition of the faecal microflora in breastfed and bottle-fed infants from birth to eight weeks. Acta Paediatrica Scandinavica 74, 45–51.

Ma, Z., Guan, Q., Ye, C., Zhang, C., Foster, J.A., Forney, L.J., 2015. Network analysis suggests a potentially "evil" alliance of opportunistic pathogens inhibited by a cooperative network in human milk bacterial communities. Scientific Reports 5, 8275.

Marín, M.L., Arroyo, R., Jiménez, E., Gómez, A., Fernández, L., Rodríguez, J.M., 2009. Cold storage of human milk: effect on its bacterial composition. Journal of Pediatric Gastroenterology and Nutrition 49, 343–348.

Marks, L.R., Clementi, E.A., Hakansson, A.P., 2013. Sensitization of *Staphylococcus aureus* to methicillin and other antibiotics *in vitro* and *in vivo* in the presence of HAMLET. PLoS ONE 8, e63158.

Martín, R., Langa, S., Reviriego, C., Jiménez, E., Marín, M.L., Olivares, M., Boza, J., Jiménez, J., Fernández, L., Xaus, J., Rodríguez, J.M., 2004. The commensal microflora of human milk: new perspectives for food bacteriotherapy and probiotics. Trends in Food Science and Technology 15, 121–127.

Martín, R., Heilig, H.G., Zoetendal, E.G., Jiménez, E., Fernández, L., Smidt, H., Rodríguez, J.M., 2007. Cultivation-independent assessment of the bacterial diversity of breast milk among healthy women. Research in Microbiology 158, 31–37.

Martín, R., Olivares, M., Marín, M.L., Fernández, L., Xaus, J., Rodríguez, J.M., 2005. Probiotic potential of 3 lactobacilli strains isolated from breast milk. Journal of Human Lactation 21, 8–17.

Martín, V., Maldonado, A., Moles, L., Rodríguez-Baños, M., Del Campo, R., Fernández, L., Rodríguez, J.M., Jiménez, E., 2012. Sharing of bacterial strains between breast milk and infant feces. Journal of Human Lactation 28, 36–44.

Martín, V., Mediano, P., Del Campo, R., Rodríguez, J.M., Marín, M., August 10, 2015. Streptococcal diversity of human milk and comparison of different methods for the taxonomic identification of streptococci. Journal of Human Lactation pii:0890334415597901.

Michie, C., Lockie, F., Lynn, W., 2003. The challenge of mastitis. Archives of Disease in Childhood 88, 818–821.

Monecke, S., Kuhnert, P., Hotzel, H., Slickers, P., Ehricht, R., 2007. Microarray based study on virulence-associated genes and resistance determinants of *Staphylococcus aureus* isolates from cattle. Veterinary Microbiology 125, 128–140.

Murakami, M., Dorschner, R.A., Stern, L.J., Lin, K.H., Gallo, R.L., 2005. Expression and secretion of cathelicidin antimicrobial peptides in murine mammary glands and human milk. Pediatric Research 57, 10–15.

Murk, W., Risnes, K.R., Bracken, M.B., 2011. Prenatal or early-life exposure to antibiotics and risk of childhood asthma: a systematic review. Pediatrics 127, 1125–1138.

Naik, S., Bouladoux, N., Wilhelm, C., Mohillo, M.J., Salcedo, R., Kastenmuller, W., Deming, C., Quiñónez, M., Koo, L., Conlan, S., Spencer, S., Hall, J.A., Dzutsev, A., Kong, H., Campbell, D.J., Trinchieri, G., Segre, J.A., Belkaid, Y., 2012. Compartmentalized control of skin immunity by resident commensals. Science 337, 1115–1119.

National Mastitis Council, 2001. Guidelines on Normal and Abnormal Raw Milk Based on Somatic Cell Counts and Signs of Clinical Mastitis. Madison.

Nickerson, S.C., Boddie, R.L., 1994. Effect of naturally occurring coagulase-negative staphylococcal infections on experimental challenge with major mastitis pathogens. Journal of Dairy Science 77, 2526–2536.

Nikniaz, L., Ostadrahimi, A., Mahdavi, R., Hejazi, M.A., Hosseini Salekdeh, G., 2013. Effects of synbiotic supplementation on breast milk levels of IgA, TGF-β1, and TGF-β2. Journal of Human Lactation 29, 591–596.

Nooh, M.M., El-Gengehi, N., Kansal, R., David, C.S., Kotb, M., 2007. HLA transgenic mice provide evidence for a direct and dominant role of HLA class II variation in modulating the severity of streptococcal sepsis. Journal of Immunology 178, 3076–3083.

Oddy, W.H., Rosales, F.A., 2010. Systematic review of the importance of milk TGF-beta on immunological outcomes in the infant and young child. Pediatric Allergy and Immunology 21, 47–59.

Olivares, M., Díaz-Ropero, M.P., Martín, R., Rodríguez, J.M., Xaus, J., 2006. Antimicrobial potential of four *Lactobacillus* strains isolated from breast milk. Journal of Applied Microbiology 101, 72–79.

Otto, M., 2009. Staphylococcus epidermidis; the 'accidental' pathogen. Nature Reviews Microbiology 7, 555–567.

Otto, M., Sussmuth, R., Vuong, C., Jung, G., Gotz, F., 1999. Inhibition of virulence factor expression in *Staphylococcus aureus* by the *Staphylococcus epidermidis agr* pheromone and derivatives. FEBS Letters 450, 257–262.

Park, B., Iwase, T., Liu, G.Y., 2011b. Intranasal application of *S. epidermidis* prevents colonization by methicillin-resistant *Staphylococcus aureus* in mice. PLoS ONE 6, e25880.

Park, J.Y., Fox, L.K., Seo, K.S., McGuire, M.A., Park, Y.H., Rurangirwa, F.R., Sischo, W.M., Bohach, G.A., 2011a. Detection of classical and newly described staphylococcal superantigen genes in coagulase-negative staphylococci isolated from bovine intramammary infections. Veterinary Microbiology 147, 149–154.

Paviour, S., Musaad, S., Roberts, S., Taylor, G., Taylor, S., Shore, K., Lang, S., Holland, D., 2002. *Corynebacterium* species isolated from patients with mastitis. Clinical Infectious Diseases 35, 1434–1440.

Perez, P.F., Doré, J., Leclerc, M., Lévense, F., Benyacoub, J., Serrant, P., Segura-Roggero, I., Schiffrin, E.J., Donnet-Hughes, A., 2007. Bacterial imprinting of the neonatal immune system: lessons from maternal cells? Pediatrics 119, 724–732.

Prescott, S.L., Wickens, K., Westcott, L., Jung, W., Currie, H., Black, P.N., Stanley, T.V., Mitchell, E.A., Fitzharris, P., Siebers, R., Wu, L., Crane, J., Probiotic Study Group, 2008. Supplementation with *Lactobacillus rhamnosus* or *Bifidobacterium lactis* probiotics in pregnancy increases cord blood interferon-gamma and breast milk transforming growth factor-beta and immunoglobin A detection. Clinical and Experimental Allergy 38, 1606–1614.

Pyörälä, S., Taponen, S., 2009. Coagulase-negative staphylococci-emerging mastitis pathogens. Veterinary Microbiology 134, 3–8.

Rautava, S., Kalliomäki, M., Isolauri, E., 2002. Probiotics during pregnancy and breast-feeding might confer immunomodulatory protection against atopic disease in the infant. Journal of Allergy and Clinical Immunology 109, 119–121.

Reddy, P., Qi, C., Zembower, T., Noskin, G.A., Bolon, M., 2007. Postpartum mastitis and community-acquired methicillin-resistant *Staphylococcus aureus*. Emerging Infectious Diseases 13, 298–301.

Renfrew, M.J., Pokhrel, S., Quigley, M., McCormick, F., Fox-Rushby, J., Dodds, R., Duffy, S., Trueman, P., Williams, A., 2012. Preventing disease and saving resources: the potential contribution of increasing breastfeeding rates in the UK. UNICEF, UK.

Renshaw, A.A., Derhagopian, R.P., Gould, E.W., 2011. Cystic neutrophilic granulomatous mastitis: an underappreciated pattern strongly associated with gram-positive bacilli. American Journal of Clinical Pathology 136, 424–427.

Rinaldi, M., Li, R.W., Capuco, A.V., 2010. Mastitis associated transcriptomic disruptions in cattle. Veterinary Immunology and Immunopathology 138, 267–279.

Rivas-Santiago, B., Serrano, C.J., Enciso-Moreno, J.A., 2009. Susceptibility to infectious diseases based on antimicrobial peptide production. Infection and Immunity 77, 4690–4695.

Rodríguez, J.M., 2014. The origin of human milk bacteria: is there a bacterial entero-mammary pathway during late pregnancy and lactation? Advances in Nutrition 5, 779–784.

Round, J.L., Mazmanian, S.K., 2009. The gut microbiota shapes intestinal immune responses during health and disease. Nature Reviews Immunology 9, 313–323.

Ryan, M.P., Meaney, W.J., Ross, R.P., Hill, C., 1998. Evaluation of lacticin. 3147 and teat seal containing this bacteriocin for inhibition of. mastitis pathogens. Applied and Environmental Microbiology 64, 2287–2290.

Sakata, H., Yoshioka, H., Fujita, K., 1985. Development of the intestinal flora in very low birth weight infants compared to normal full-term newborns. European Journal of Pediatrics 144, 186–190.

Savino, F., Cordisco, L., Tarasco, V., Palumeri, E., Calabrese, R., Oggero, R., Roos, S., Matteuzzi, D., 2010. *Lactobacillus reuteri* DSM 17938 in infantile colic: a randomized, double-blind, placebo-controlled trial. Pediatrics 126, e526–e533.

Schleifer, K.H., Hartinger, A., Götz, F., 1978. Occurrence of d-tagatose-6-phosphate pathway of d-galactose metabolism among staphylococci. FEMS Microbiology Letters 3, 9–11.

Schoenfeld, E.M., McKay, M.P., 2010. Mastitis and methicillin-resistant *Staphylococcus aureus* (MRSA): the calm before the storm? Journal of Emergency Medicine 38, 31–34.

Schoenfelder, S.M., Lange, C., Eckart, M., Hennig, S., Kozytska, S., Ziebuhr, W., 2010. Success through diversity – how *Staphylococcus epidermidis* establishes as a nosocomial pathogen. International Journal of Medical Microbiology 300, 380–386.

Schultz, M., Göttl, C., Young, R.J., Iwen, P., Vanderhoof, J.A., 2004. Administration of oral probiotic bacteria to pregnant women causes temporary infantile colonization. Journal of Pediatric Gastroenterology and Nutrition 38, 293–297.

Sears, P.M., Smith, B.S., Stewart, W.K., Gonzalez, R.N., 1992. Evaluation of a nisin based germicidal formulation on teat skin of live cows. Journal of Dairy Science 75, 3185–3190.

Smyth, D.S., Hartigan, P.J., Meaney, W.J., Fitzgerald, J.R., Deobald, C.F., Bohach, G.A., Smyth, C.J., 2005. Superantigen genes encoded by the *egc* cluster and SaPIbov are predominant among *Staphylococcus aureus* isolates from cows, goats, sheep, rabbits and poultry. Journal of Medical Microbiology 54, 401–411.

Sørensen, L.P., Guldbrandtsen, B., Thomasen, J.R., Lund, M.S., 2008. Pathogen-specific effects of quantitative trait loci affecting clinical mastitis and somatic cell count in Danish Holstein cattle. Journal of Dairy Science 91, 2493–2500.

Soto, A., Martín, V., Jiménez, E., Mader, I., Rodríguez, J.M., Fernández, L., 2014. *Lactobacilli* and bifidobacteria in human breast milk: influence of antibiotherapy and other host and clinical factors. Journal of Pediatric Gastroenterology and Nutrition 59, 78–88.

Stavnezer, J., 1995. Regulation of antibody production and class switching by TGF-beta. Journal of Immunology 155, 1647–1651.

Stensballe, L.G., Simonsen, J., Jensen, S.M., Bønnelykke, K., Bisgaard, H., 2013. Use of antibiotics during pregnancy increases the risk of asthma in early childhood. Journal of Pediatrics 162, 832–838.

Sun, J.L., Zhang, S.K., Chen, J.Y., Han, B.Z., 2012. Metabolic profiling of *Staphylococcus aureus* cultivated under aerobic and anaerobic conditions with (1)H NMR-based nontargeted analysis. Canadian Journal of Microbiology 58, 709–718.

Sung, V., Hiscock, H., Tang, M., Mensah, F.K., Heine, R.G., Stock, A., York, E., Barr, R.G., Wake, M., 2012. Probiotics to improve outcomes of colic in the community: protocol for the Baby Biotics randomised controlled trial. BMC Pediatrics 12, 135.

Szajewska, H., Gyrczuk, E., Horvath, A., 2013. *Lactobacillus reuteri* DSM 17938 for the management of infantile colic in breastfed infants: a randomized, double-blind, placebo-controlled trial. Journal of Pediatrics 162, 257–262.

Takeuchi, O., Hoshino, K., Kawai, T., Sanjo, H., Takada, H., Ogawa, T., Takeda, K., Akira, S., 1999. Differential roles of TLR2 and TLR4 in recognition of gram negative and gram-positive bacterial cell wall components. Immunity 11, 443–451.

Takeuchi, O., Hoshino, K., Akira, S., 2000. Cutting edge: TLR2-deficient and MyD88-deficient mice are highly susceptible to *Staphylococcus aureus* infection. Journal of Immunology 165, 5392–5396.

Taylor, J.I., Hirsch, A., Mattick, A.T.R., 1949. The treatment of bovine streptococcal and staphylococcal mastitis with nisin. Veterinary Record 61, 197–198.

Thibodeau, J., Cloutier, I., Lavoie, P., Labrecque, N., Mourad, W., Jardetzky, T., Sekaly, R., 1994. Subsets of HLA-DR1 molecules defined by SEB and TSST-1 binding. Science 266, 1874–1878.

Thomsen, A.C., Mogensen, S.C., Love Jepsen, F., 1985. Experimental mastitis in mice induced by coagulase-negative staphylococci isolated from cases of mastitis in nursing women. Acta Obstetricia et Gynecologica Scandinavica 64, 163–166.

Thorberg, B.M., Danielsson-Tham, M.L., Emanuelson, U., Persson Waller, K., 2009. Bovine subclinical mastitis caused by different types of coagulase-negative staphylococci. Journal of Dairy Science 92, 4962–4970.

Thurl, S., Munzert, M., Henker, J., Boehm, G., Muller-Werner, B., Jelinek, J., Stahl, B., 2010. Variation of human milk oligosaccharides in relation to milk groups and lactational periods. British Journal of Nutrition 104, 1261–1271.

Uehara, Y., Kikuchi, K., Nakamura, T., Nakama, H., Agematsu, K., Kawakami, Y., Maruchi, N., Totsuka, K., 2001. H_2O_2 produced by viridans group streptococci may contribute to inhibition of methicillin-resistant *Staphylococcus aureus* colonization of oral cavities in newborns. Clinical Infectious Diseases 32, 1408–1413.

US Department of Health and Human Services, 2011. The Surgeon General's Call to Action to Support Breastfeeding. US Department of Health and Human Services, Office of the Surgeon General, Washington, DC.

van Belkum, A., Melles, D.C., Nouwen, J., van Leeuwen, W.B., van Wamel, W., Vos, M.C., Wertheim, H.F., Verbrugh, H.A., 2009. Co-evolutionary aspects of human colonisation and infection by *Staphylococcus aureus*. Infection, Genetics and Evolution 9, 32–47.

Vázquez-Fresno, R., Llorach, R., Marinic, J., Tulipani, S., Garcia-Aloy, M., Espinosa-Martos, I., Jiménez, E., Rodríguez, J.M., Andres-Lacueva, C., 2014. Urinary metabolomic fingerprinting after consumption of a probiotic strain in women with mastitis. Pharmacology Research 87, 160–165.

von Bernuth, H., Picard, C., Jin, Z., Pankla, R., Xiao, H., Ku, C.L., Chrabieh, M., Mustapha, I.B., Ghandil, P., Camcioglu, Y., Vasconcelos, J., Sirvent, N., Guedes, M., Vitor, A.B., Herrero-Mata, M.J., Aróstegui, J.I., Rodrigo, C., Alsina, L., Ruiz-Ortiz, E., Juan, M., Fortuny, C., Yagüe, J., Antón, J., Pascal, M., Chang, H.H., Janniere, L., Rose, Y., Garty, B.Z., Chapel, H., Issekutz, A., Maródi, L., Rodriguez-Gallego, C., Banchereau, J., Abel, L., Li, X., Chaussabel, D., Puel, A., Casanova, J.L., 2008. Pyogenic bacterial infections in humans with MyD88 deficiency. Science 321, 691–696.

Walker, M., 2008. Conquering common breast-feeding problems. Journal of Perinatal and Neonatal Nursing 22, 267–274.

Wang, J., Roderiquez, G., Norcross, M.A., 2012. Control of adaptive immune responses by *Staphylococcus aureus* through IL-10, PD-L1, and TLR2. Science Reports 2, 606.

WHO, April 2, 2001. The Optimal Duration of Exclusive Breastfeeding. Results of a WHO Systematic Review. Note for the press n° 7 http://www.who.int/inf-pr-2001/en/note2001-07.html

Willing, B.P., Russell, S.L., Finlay, B.B., 2011. Shifting the balance: antibiotic effects on host-microbiota mutualism. Nature Reviews Microbiology 9, 233–243.

Willumsen, J.F., Filteau, S.M., Coutsoudis, A., Newell, M.-L., Rollins, N.C., Coovadia, H.M., Tomkins, A.M., 2003. Breastmilk RNA viral load in HIV-infected South African women: effects of subclinical mastitis and infant feeding. AIDS 17, 407–414.

Wirawan, R.E., Swanson, K.M., Kleffmann, T., Jack, R.W., Tagg, J.R., 2007. Uberolysin: a novel cyclic bacteriocin produced by *Streptococcus uberis*. Microbiology 153, 1619–1630.

Wolf, C., Kusch, H., Monecke, S., Albrecht, D., Holtfreter, S., von Eiff, C., Petzl, W., Rainard, P., Bröker, B.M., Engelmann, S., 2011. Genomic and proteomic characterization of *Staphylococcus aureus* mastitis isolates of bovine origin. Proteomics 11, 2491–2502.

Zhang, S., Maddox, C.W., 2000. Cytotoxic activity of coagulase-negative staphylococci in bovine mastitis. Infection and Immunity 68, 1102–1108.

CHAPTER

Probiotics During the Perinatal Period: Impact on the Health of Mothers and Infants

16

Elloise du Toit[1,a], Carlos Gómez-Gallego[2,3,a], Seppo Salminen[2]

[1]University of Cape Town, Cape Town, South Africa; [2]University of Turku, Turku, Finland; [3]University of Murcia, Murcia, Spain

1. DEFINITION OF "PROBIOTIC"

The definition of "probiotic" has gone through substantial development, and the widely accepted Food and Agriculture Organinzation/World Health Organization (2001) working group report has recently been grammatically corrected to the present form as follows: "Probiotics are live microorganisms that, when administered in adequate amounts, confer a health benefit to the host" (Hill et al., 2014). This definition has been construed by many to emphasize viability, strain identification, specificity of strains, and health benefits demonstrated in human studies. Consequently, foods and supplements labeled as probiotic have to be assessed for efficacy in strain-specific studies, and extrapolation of data from one strain to another is possible only if detailed knowledge of the strain genomes and practical knowledge on efficacy obtained in human intervention studies is available. The definition means that each probiotic strain and combination should be assessed separately and the properties of probiotics should include viability and defined dose of specific probiotic strains. In general, the term "probiotic" is a useful and accepted expression, and the definition has been widely adopted and has proved to be valuable to researchers, regulators, and consumers. However, in the European Union, the term is considered to bear a health message and thus can be used in foods only when regulatory authorities have approved a particular health claim for the probiotic. At the same time, the term "probiotic" is used in the recommendations of many medical societies including those of the European Society of Pediatric Gastroenterology, Hepatology and Nutrition (ESPGHAN). ESPGHAN recommends the use of specific well-studied probiotics to prevent and treat acute gastroenteritis in infants and children and to reduce antibiotic associated side effects (Szajewska et al., 2014). For a specific probiotic, for example, a meta-analysis concluded that the strain *Lactobacillus rhamnosus* GG (LGG) is effective in preventing antibiotic-associated diarrhea in

[a] Both authors contributed equally to this work.

Prebiotics and Probiotics in Human Milk. http://dx.doi.org/10.1016/B978-0-12-802725-7.00016-6

children and adults treated with antibiotics for any reason (Szajewska and Kołodziej, 2015). Probiotics are also mentioned and recommended in some European countries in nutrition guidelines and recommendations (Smug et al., 2014).

2. PROBIOTICS DURING THE PERINATAL PERIOD—SAFETY ASPECTS

Safety is a main concern in the perinatal use of probiotics. In theory, any microbe that is able to grow under conditions found in the human body might be able to cause an infection. In reality, infections are rare considering the widespread consumption of live microbes through probiotics and fermented foods and as incidental contaminants of foods. However, since reports of infections by common probiotic species are almost exclusively limited to people with seriously compromised health, serious underlying diseases, and several antibiotic treatments, their occurrence is relevant. Although infections by species used as probiotics have been documented, rarely have the microbes isolated from the infection been confirmed to be the same strain as a probiotic organism (Meini et al., 2015).

2.1 PREGNANT WOMEN AND PROBIOTICS

The hypertensive disorders of pregnancy remain the leading causes of maternal and perinatal morbidity and mortality (Center for Maternal and Child Enquiries, 2011). Approximately 1% of pregnancies are complicated by preexisting hypertension, 5–6% by gestational hypertension, and 1–2% by preeclampsia. Probiotics have been suggested to modify placental trophoblast inflammation, systemic inflammation, and blood pressure, all potential factors important to preeclampsia. In a Norwegian study of a prospective design in 33,399 primiparous women in 2002–2008 (Brantsaeter et al., 2011), consumption of probiotic milk products (estimated using validated self-reported food frequency questionnaires) was associated with reduced risk of pre-eclampsia, and this association was most prominent in cases of severe preeclampsia. No detrimental effects related to probiotics were observed; rather, the population presented with fewer problems during pregnancy and breastfeeding.

2.2 PRETERM INFANTS AND PROBIOTICS

Although there have been numerous studies assessing the effectiveness of probiotics for necrotizing enterocolitis (NEC) in preterm infants, prematurity has also been considered a risk factor for negative outcomes associated with probiotic use (Boyle and Tang, 2006). However, it is not clear if the risk is due to prematurity itself or other risk factors commonly associated with prematurity, such as the use of a central venous catheter, an immunocompromised state, an impaired intestinal barrier (which may increase the likelihood of bacterial translocation), or the use of broad-spectrum antibiotics. Furthermore, a review of 24 clinical trials assessing the effectiveness of probiotics for the prevention of NEC found no reports of systemic or other infection with the probiotic organism used (Robinson, 2014). However, like any population, premature infants are at risk from iatrogenic infection in any health care setting or infection secondary to a contaminated probiotic product (Vallabhaneni et al., 2014) or an inappropriately labeled product (Macrobal et al., 2008). A report from Finland suggests that postnatal use of LGG is safe for premature infants after 12 years of administration to all premature and very low birth weight infants born in one university hospital area (Luoto et al., 2010).

In a systematic review and meta-analysis (Dugoua et al., 2009), the evidence for safety of *Lactobacillus, Bifidobacterium,* and *Saccharomyces* probiotics during pregnancy was assessed. No malformations were reported in the probiotic group. No randomized control trials were available for *Saccharomyces* during pregnancy. *Lactobacillus* and *Bifidobacterium* probiotics had no effect on the incidence of caesarean section, birth weight, or gestational age.

3. IMPACT OF PROBIOTICS IN ANIMAL MODELS

3.1 TREATMENT OF RODENTS WITH PROBIOTICS

In rat and mouse models (Khailova et al., 2009; Liu et al., 2014), treatment of premature rodents with induced NEC with some strains of *Bifidobacterium bifidum* OLB6378 and *Lactobacillus reuteri* DSM 17,938 was protective with a reduction of inflammatory reaction in the ileum, regulation of main components of mucous layer, and improvement of intestinal integrity. Moreover, it has been shown that *Bifidobacterium infantis* KLDS2.0002 protected intestinal tissue from damage while decreasing inflammatory response (Wang et al., 2015). A similar protective effect has been reported for *L. rhamnosus* HN001 in mice and piglets (Good et al., 2014). Preinoculation of the murine gastrointestinal (GI) tract with probiotic *Lactobacillus acidophilus* early in life enhanced host defense against enteric bacterial infection and attenuated bacteria-mediated intestinal injury, which correlated with enhanced colonic gene expression of antiinflammatory cytokines (Foye et al., 2012).

Decreased environmental exposure to microbes and alteration of microbial communities represented in the GI microbiota are associated with an increased prevalence of allergic and some autoimmune disease (Nermes et al., 2013; McLean et al., 2015). *B. animalis* (Numico Research, Wageningen, the Netherlands) has been reported to regulate several immune parameters in a mouse model for respiratory allergy induced by ovalbumin, as well as in a rat model for experimental autoimmune encephalomyelitis (Enzendam et al., 2008). In addition, neonatal colonization of germ-free mice *Bifidobacterium longum* ssp. *longum* CCM 7952 reduced allergic sensitization to pollen allergens, in a response associated with increased levels of regulatory cytokines interleukin (IL)-10 and transforming growth factor (TGF)-β in serum (Schwarzer et al., 2013). Furthermore, *Bifidobacterium adolescentis* and *B. longum* (isolated from human fecal samples) may improve intestinal digestion and barrier function in the intestine with an increase in the height and the width of duodenal villi and increased levels of sIgA in the intestinal mucosa (Yang et al., 2009). Moreover, in a mouse model, maternal and postweaning probiotic dietary supplementation with a mix of probiotics (*L. acidophilus, Lactobacillus casei, B. bifidium*, and *Enterococcus faecium*; Primalac 454Feed Grade Microbials) appeared to provide immunological support by enhancing activated T helper cell, cytotoxic T cell, natural killer cell, and naturally occurring T regulatory cell populations. These changes may attenuate and regulate hypersensitivity responses to food allergens (Toomer et al., 2014).

In gnotobiotic pigs, supplementation with a combination of *L. rhamnosus* GG ATCC 53,103 and *B. lactis* Bb12 modulated the development of B cell response, which may affect the response to oral vaccines (Chatta et al., 2013). Moreover, in gnotobiotics pigs, *L. rhamnosus* GG ATCC 53,103 enhanced specific interferon (IFN)-γ–producing T cell responses to the human rotavirus vaccine (Wen et al., 2014).

Studies on the effects of probiotics appear to be strain dependent. For example, in a murine experimental autoimmune encephalomyelitis model *L. casei* 393 induced immunoregulatory cytokines and improved autoimmune encephalomyelitis, while *L. reuteri* ML1 induced proinflammatory cytokines and aggravated the disease (Maassen et al., 1998).

Most studies suggest that specific probiotics modulate the immune system associated with the intestinal mucosa. In addition, since the late 1990s it has been demonstrated in animal models that specific probiotics may stimulate enterocyte proliferation in a manner similar to the normal microbiome (Ichikawa et al., 1999; Di Giancamillo et al., 2008; Preidis et al., 2012), suggesting the ability to mediate the intestinal regeneration and rehabilitation in preterm, low birth weight infants.

Moreover, probiotics may impact mineral absorption in a beneficial manner when introduced in infant formula products containing prebiotics and probiotics together with a specific prebiotic compound selectively favoring the probiotic growth (Scholz-Ahrens et al., 2007). Some reports suggest that probiotic strains of *L. casei, L. reuteri*, and *Lactobacillus gasseri* (combined in a yogurt), *L. acidophilus* NCC90, and *Lactobacillus helveticus* 16H may increase calcium absorption in growing rats (Ghanem et al., 2004; Narva et al., 2004; Scholz-Ahrens et al., 2007). This effect is suggested to be mediated by increased solubility of minerals due to short chain fatty acids (SCFAs) and by promoting proliferation of enterocytes by bacterial fermentation products and increased expression of metal-binding proteins (Scholz-Ahrens et al., 2007).

3.2 PROBIOTICS PROVIDED TO MOTHERS

Studies in animal models have demonstrated a link between specific probiotic application to breeding mothers and changes in mammary gland microbiota. The administration of *L. rhamnosus* GG (obtained from Valio, Helsinki, Finland) and *L. gasseri* K7 (collection of Institute of Dairy Science and Probiotics, Biotechnical

Faculty, University of Ljubljana, Slovenia) increased bacterial translocation and lactic acid bacteria in the mammary gland of lactating mice (Treven et al., 2015). In the offspring of prenatally or perinatally treated mice, LGG (Valio, Helsinki, Finland) supplementation reduced allergic airway and peribronchial inflammation when compared with mice derived from nonsupplemented mothers (Blümer et al., 2007), demonstrating that maternal supplementation with probiotics affects the development of the offspring's immune response. This study suggests that the positive immunological effects of the use of probiotics in mothers are, at least in part, mediated via the placenta (Blümer et al., 2007). Moreover, in a mouse model of birch pollen allergy, perinatal administration of *L. paracasei* NCC 2461 to pregnant mothers, and with continued administration during lactation, protected against the development of airway inflammation in offspring (Schabussova et al., 2012).

Beyond the effect on the immune system, administration of *Lactobacillus plantarum* 299v, to lactating mothers improved GI tract–associated organ development of the pups, with an impact in growth and function of small intestine, pancreas, and liver and a decrease on GI permeability (Fåk et al., 2008).

Experiments in mice, rats, and pigs suggest that specific probiotics provided during pregnancy can colonize the neonatal GI tract during vaginal delivery (Buddington et al., 2009). In addition, the administration of one probiotic strain to the pregnant mother could exert changes in other bacterial strains in the intestinal tract of their offspring. For example, pregnant pigs fed *Enterococcus faecium* NCIMB10415 (SF68) 1 month before birth had increased *Lactobacillus amylovorus* and *L. acidophilus,* with increased lactobacilli composition of the microbiota in feces of the piglets (Starke et al., 2013).

These findings support the possibility that modulation of the maternal microbiota during gestation and the early postnatal period with specific probiotic strains may transfer beneficial microbiota to offspring and/or generate signals that induce changes on infant development, thereby providing protection from some diseases.

4. MICROBIOTA DURING THE PERINATAL PERIOD

The probiotic approach necessitates a profound understanding of the complex interactions among nutrition, the GI microbiota, the total genetic pool of the microbiota, and the answers provided by clinical intervention studies in humans. All these together may provide both the basis and the proof of causality for probiotic use.

Microbiota deviations during the stepwise developmental process may manifest as the emergence of noncommunicable diseases (NCDs) including allergies and obesity. The early colonizers coevolving during the immunological and metabolic maturation process during the critical stages of pregnancy, delivery, and breastfeeding confer the propensity to health and disease. There is a growing awareness that dietary and other environmental exposures impact GI microbiota development. Moreover, the age-appropriate composition appears to be fundamental to health Fig. 16.1.

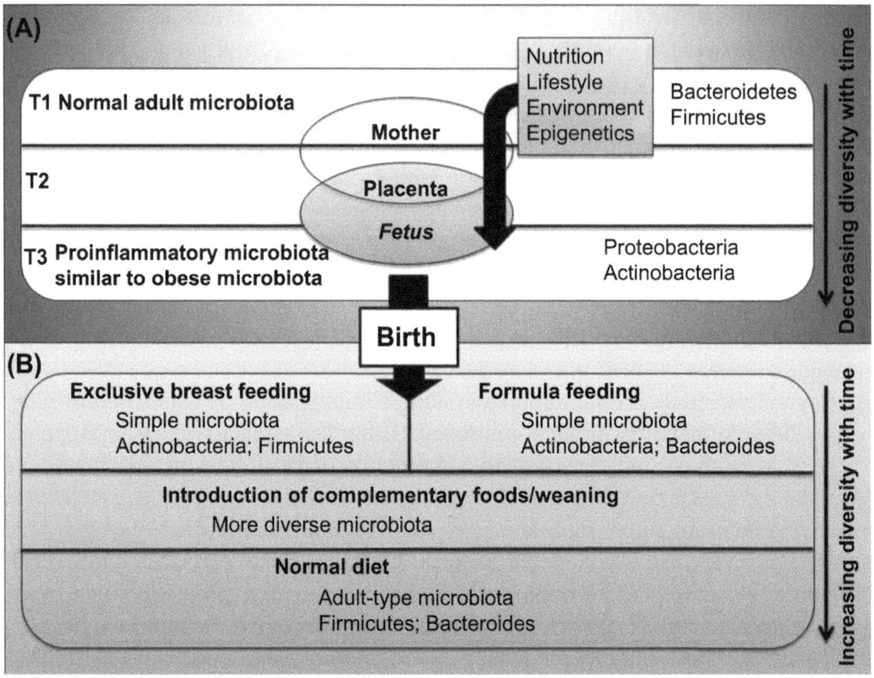

FIGURE 16.1

Microbial shifts and influences during pregnancy and infant GI tract maturation. (A) Maternal GI microbial community changes throughout pregnancy and is influenced by factors such as nutrition, lifestyle, environment, and epigenetics. The infant's GI tract colonization begins in utero via swallowing of amniotic fluid. Maternal GI microbiota changes from a normal adult microbiota, dominated by Bacteroidetes and Firmicutes in the first trimester (T1), through the second trimester (T2), and into the third trimester (T3), where it represents a proinflammatory microbiota, similar to that found in the obese GI tract with Proteobacteria and Actinobacteria predominating. The birth event acts as a bridge, continuing the transfer of maternal microbes (vaginal or skin) to the infant. Thereafter, (B) the infant's GI microbiota are shaped by mode of feeding (exclusive breastfeeding or formula-feeding), when and how complementary foods are introduced, finally normalizing to that of an adult microbiota between 3 and 5 years old.

4.1 HUMAN MILK MICROBIOTA

Human milk is considered as the optimal nutrition for infants and an important postnatal element in metabolic and immunological programming of health (Cabrera-Rubio et al., 2012). Human milk is a complex species-specific biological fluid able to satisfy all nutritional needs of a rapidly growing infant. The beneficial effects reflect synergistic action of many bioactive molecules present in colostrum and mature milk, which inactivate pathogens through different pathways. Human milk contains a complex mixture of proteins, lipids, human milk oligosaccharides (HMOs), and carbohydrates, all of which change in concentration during a single feed, as well as during the period of lactation. HMOs also act as substrates for specific bacteria within the infant GI microbial community.

Human milk is the main source of bacteria for the infant intestine, providing 1000 to 1 million live bacteria per mL of milk and about 1000 cells of bifidobacteria per mL of milk (Solís et al., 2010; Gueimonde et al., 2007). The presence of bacteria in human milk has been acknowledged for some time, but the origin of these bacteria is still debated. More than 200 different bacterial species belonging to 50 different genera have been isolated from human milk, and new members of this community and others are constantly being identified and characterized.

The human milk microbiome is dominated by staphyloccoci and streptococci and contains a "core" set of nine operational taxonomic units: streptococcci, staphylococci, *Serratia, Pseudomonas, Corynebacteria, Ralstonia, Propionibacterium, Sphingomonas,* and Bradyrhizobiaceae. Although traditionally skin associated, these bacteria are widespread in all human mucosal surfaces, reaching greatest abundances in mucosal layers of the digestive and genitourinary tracts. In addition, such bacteria have been detected in chorioamnion and amniotic fluid from pregnant women and in umbilical cord blood from healthy neonates born via vaginal or cesarean section birth. This suggests they may colonize fetal skin and the GI tract in utero (Rautava et al., 2012).

The acquisition and development of the human mammary microbiota start in the third trimester of pregnancy, reaching its highest complexity at the end of this period. It remains constant throughout lactation and declines sharply at weaning, rapidly disappearing when there is no more milk in mammary gland (Fernandez et al., 2013).

4.2 PERINATAL NUTRITION AND MICROBIOTA

Our appreciation of the complexity of host–microbe interactions in human health and disease is growing and evolving from viewing bacteria solely as potential pathogens (Rautava, 2015). The role of environmental and commensal microbes for host physiology and the development of noninfectious diseases are becoming apparent. The association between the composition of the GI microbiome and chronic noninfectious disease appears evident based on accumulating data from human studies, including atopy (Abrahamsson et al., 2012, 2014; Kalliomaki et al., 2001a), inflammatory bowel disease (IBD; Gevers et al., 2014), NEC in preterm infants (Mai et al., 2011), diabetes mellitus (Dunne et al., 2014; Kostic et al., 2015), obesity (Kalliomaki et al., 2008; Turnbaugh et al., 2009), and neurological conditions including autism (De Angelis et al., 2013) and Parkinson's disease (Scheperjans et al., 2015). Exposure to a wide range of environmental microbes has been shown to be necessary for normal development in early life (Rautava, 2015). The improvement of sanitation and the increased use of antibiotics and vaccines in Western society allowed for the management of disease (De Filippo et al., 2010). However, the unexpected side affect of this was the rise in new diseases, the so-called NCDs (Blaser, 2006; Rautava, 2015), giving rise to the hygiene hypothesis (Strachan, 1989). The hygiene hypothesis, originally proposed as a reason for the inverse correlation between family size and atopy, postulated an association between decreased microbial exposure and aberrant immune development leading to dysregulated immunity (Liu and Leung, 2006). In this light, the importance of this interaction has been termed "early microbial programming" and has recently been shown to begin in utero (Rautava et al., 2015) and to be modulated by maternal well-being, mode of birth, perinatal antibiotics, and breastfeeding, to mention a few. This critical process has been shown to have long-term health effects on the neonate, not only GI disease but also allergic, autoimmune, and metabolic disease.

4.3 MATERNAL GASTROINTESTINAL TRACT MICROBIOTA

During a normal, healthy pregnancy, the body undergoes substantial hormonal, immunological, and metabolic changes (Mor and Cardenas, 2010; Newbern and Freemark, 2011).

Collado et al. (2008) reported increasing total bacteria, *Bifidobacterium* spp., *Clostridium hystolyticum* group, *Bacteroides–Prevotella* group, *S. aureus*, and *Akkermansia muciniphila,* from the first trimester (T1) to the third trimester (T3). Koren et al. (2012), when analyzing a subset of the same study cohort by pyrosequencing, observed dramatic changes in microbiota composition, involving loss of diversity and increasing Proteobacteria and Actinobacteria populations from T1 to T3, which persisted 1 month postpartum. A study carried out on the GI tract microbiota of women during the perinatal period revealed that the predominant bacterial groups were Firmicutes, *Bacteroides*, and *Bifidobacterium*, without significant changes during this period (Jost et al., 2014). However, total fecal SCFA concentrations, especially isobutyrate and isovalerate, were higher in pregnant women compared to nonpregnant controls throughout the perinatal period. This suggests metabolic changes and increased energy extraction via proteolytic and saccharolytic fermentation, and based on fecal calprotectin levels, this fermentation was accompanied by low-grade inflammation (Jost et al., 2014). This low-grade inflammation may diminish epithelial barrier integrity (Turnbaugh et al., 2006), supporting the hypothesis of an increased bacterial translocation during pregnancy, and the existence of a bacterial enteromammary pathway as a novel way of mother–neonate communication via breastfeeding (Jost et al., 2013; Martin et al., 2004; Perez et al., 2007).

4.4 PERINATAL PROBIOTIC EXPOSURES, NUTRITION, AND PROGRAMMING

Early-life programming suggests that the environment during early development affects health and disease in adulthood, probably via epigenetic mechanisms (Nauta et al., 2013). Nutrition during pregnancy and early postnatal life is emerging as one of the most important environmental cues that programs microbiological, metabolic, and immunological development. Therefore, the use of nutritional strategies to program a beneficial microbiota composition and to support the development of the metabolic and immune systems may provide a good opportunity to prevent later health problems.

The "hygiene hypothesis" mentioned here has expanded to the "microbiota hypothesis" (Shreiner et al., 2008) and the developmental origins hypothesis for health and disease (DOHaD; Wadhwa et al., 2009). The DOHaD hypothesis proposes that environmental stimuli induce changes in developmental pathways during critical periods of prenatal and postnatal development that have long-term impact on later health and disease. These factors include parental lifestyle, well-being and diet, obesity, exposure to smoke, chemicals, and toxins.

Epigenetics, the root of the DOHaD hypothesis, involves the imprinting of environmental experiences on infant gene expression (Hanson et al., 2011). Epigenetic modifications affect gene expression without altering DNA sequence. There is strong evidence that early environmental exposures can activate or silence genes by altering DNA methylation, histone acetylation and methylation, and chromatin structure (Wadhwa et al., 2009).

Recently, amniotic fluid, previously thought to be sterile, has been shown to harbor bacteria, not only in the diseased state (DiGiulio 2012). These bacteria overlap with phyla common in oral bacteria such as Firmicutes, Bacteroidetes, and Actinobacteria. Thus, the intrauterine environment, which is protected by maternal barriers against pathogenic invaders, offers the embryo and fetus a controlled environment in which there is limited and selective exposure to microbes during the vulnerable periods of organogenesis and early development.

Meconium is also not sterile (Hu et al., 2013). This supports the notion that the fetus swallows the microbes in amniotic fluid possibly important in GI tract and immune system development. A recent study found most similarity in phyla between the meconium and amniotic fluid (Ardissone et al., 2014). Further, administration of *Enterococcus faecium* to pregnant rats allowed for isolation of the same bacteria from the meconium of term pups immediately after birth by caesarean section (Jimenez et al., 2008).

4.5 INFANT GASTROINTESTINAL TRACT MICROBIOTA

The "unhygienic" behavior of children in the first 3 years of life clearly promotes significant exposure to microbes: mouth contact with maternal skin, introduction of various objects to mouth, and contact of hands onto floor surfaces, especially during crawling and early walking stages (Arrieta et al., 2014). The microbiota in children under 3 years of age has been shown to change dramatically and is easily changed by environmental factors and contact with the enormous bacterial load of the extrauterine world during and after birth marks the beginning of massive bacterial colonization of mucosal surfaces (Rautava et al., 2012).

The stable individual GI microbiota are thought to develop according to modifications by dietary and environmental factors during infancy (Rautava et al., 2012). The first colonizers are Firmicutes such as aerobic or facultatively anaerobic bacteria *Staphylococcus, Streptococcus,* and Enterobacteriaceae. These are followed by Actinobacteria as well as more anaerobic bacteria, which typically include bifidobacteria especially in breastfed infants (Harmsen et al., 2000; Roger et al., 2010). Then an increase in the Bacteroidetes phylum of bacteria and other anaerobes, such as *Clostridia* and *Eubacteria*, appear after the increase in Bacteroidetes (Palmer et al., 2007; Koening et al., 2011). By 1 year of age, the infant GI tract microbiota are thought to begin to converge toward a profile that resembles that of adults.

Several factors can influence the composition of the infants GI tract microbiota, and some of these factors are discussed here.

Infant diet: Following birth, exclusive breastfeeding continues the "beneficial" transfer of maternal GI tract microbiota to infants, including increased colonization by Bifidobacteria and reduced prevalence and abundance of *C. difficile* compared with formula-fed infants (Penders et al., 2006). These benefits have been attributed to the prebiotic properties of HMOs or the transfer of intestinal bacteria from mother to infant through human milk (Fernandez et al., 2013). There is evidence suggesting that breastfeeding can protect against recurrent wheeze and asthma in later childhood; however, results are conflicting and may not apply when the nursing mother is atopic. This could be related to the microbiota, since human milk of allergic mothers has been reported to contain lower amounts of Bifidobacteria compared with nonallergic mothers, and their infants have concurrently lower counts of fecal Bifidobacteria (Gronlund et al., 2007).

The intestinal microbiota in the breastfed infant is considered as ideally healthy, seeming to have the most "beneficial" GI tract microbiota, with the highest numbers of bifidobacteria and lowest numbers of *C. difficile* and *E. coli* (Penders et al., 2006; Echarri et al., 2011). In humans, there is also evidence that infants who go on to develop allergic diseases have an altered pattern of GI microbiota in early life (Walker, 2013; Lee et al., 2015), indicating the importance of a balanced microbial colonization pattern in early programming.

Previous studies (Penders et al., 2006; Bezirtzoglou et al., 2011; Ly et al., 2011; Lee et al., 2015) showed that exclusively formula-fed newborns had a more diverse microbiota composed of more bacterial genera and dominated by *Bacteroides*, with high levels of Firmicutes and Proteobacteria, and being more often colonized with *E. coli, C. difficile, B. fragilis* group, and lactobacilli than those who were exclusively breastfed with a microbiota dominated by bifidobacteria and followed by *Bacteroides* and *Prevotella*. Furthermore, breastfed infants generally hold a more complex *Bifidobacterium* microbiota than formula-fed infants (Roger et al., 2010).

Due to the high variability that microbiota exert in early life, changes in infant formula composition (protein content and protein profile, nucleotides, oligosaccharides, probiotics, etc.) could have a large impact on microbial colonization of the infant's GI tract. For example, infants fed with a formula supplemented with oligosaccharides had higher counts of bifidobacteria and lactobacilli compared with infants fed a nonsupplemented formula (Penders et al., 2006). Moreover, it has been shown that artificially alimented newborns show a larger individual difference between *Bifidobacterium* and *Bacteroides* composition than do breastfed newborns (Penders et al., 2006; Lee et al., 2015).

Use of antibiotics: After human milk and other nutritional supplements, antibiotics are the next most commonly ingested substances by infants known to affect colonization of the intestine by suppressing commensal bacteria and causing the emergence of asthma-associated pathogens such as *C. difficile* (Torrazza and Neu, 2011). At birth, the use of antibiotics can severely alter GI microbiota in infants (Penders et al., 2006), potentially lasting months (Dethlefsen et al., 2008). Perinatal exposure also affects the infant, even though indirect, as GI microbial diversity is reduced in infants born to mothers who received antibiotics during pregnancy or while breastfeeding (Fallani et al., 2010).

Introduction to solid foods: The next shift in the infant's GI microbiota is found with the introduction of supplementary foods and, eventually, weaning (Arrieta et al., 2014). The introduction of a variety of nutrients, many of which are polysaccharides not digested by host enzymes, triggers an increase in abundance of *Bacteroides, Clostridium,* and *Ruminococcus* and a decrease in *Bifidobacterium* and Enterobacteriaceae (Koening et al., 2011). Additionally, changes in diet can shift the types and relative prevalence of microbial species in the GI tract, as certain microbial species may be better equipped to use specific substrates. Conversely, some bacterial phyla (e.g., Bacteroidetes) produce numerous carbohydrate-active enzymes that cover a large spectrum of substrates, allowing them to switch between energy sources depending on what is available to them (Thomas et al., 2011; Fig. 16.2).

The microbial community "signatures" associated with certain diseases do not appear until after 2–3 years, yet it is known that alterations to the early-life microbiota are closely associated the development of these diseases, suggesting that the microbial alterations observed after the disease manifests clinically may not be involved directly in disease pathogenesis and may in fact be, at least in part, a product of the disease manifestations and treatment. Interestingly, children do not develop a microbial community signature with either *Bacteroides* or *Prevotella* until after weaning (De Filippo et al., 2010). A longitudinal study on Danish infants revealed that a community structure signature was only detectable after 36 months of life, when the Bacteroidetes phylum, undetectable at 9 or 18 months, expanded in abundance (Bergstrom et al., 2014).

5. PROBIOTIC STUDIES DURING THE PERINATAL PERIOD

5.1 PROBIOTICS AND ALLERGY PREVENTION

Allergy prevention is one of the most studied areas of probiotic administration to at-risk infants where administration of specific probiotics has started either during pregnancy, delivery, during breastfeeding, or all of the previously mentioned phases even continuing through childhood. Studies include both randomized double-blinded and placebo-controlled trials as well as studies on different population groups using or not using defined probiotics (Fig. 16.3).

1. Prenatal probiotic administration

Boyle et al. (2011) examined whether prenatal treatment with LGG could influence the risk of eczema. They recruited 250 pregnant women to a randomized controlled trial of LGG supplementation (1.8×10^{10} colony forming units [CFU]/day) from 36 weeks' gestation until delivery. The study concluded that prenatal treatment with LGG was not sufficient for preventing eczema and the authors suggested both prenatal and postnatal treatment for prevention studies.

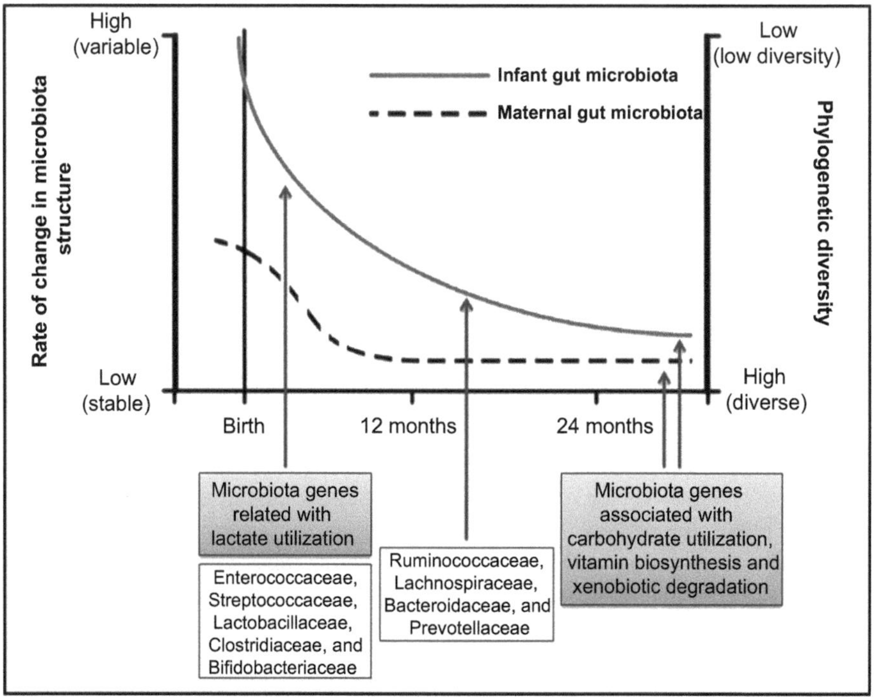

FIGURE 16.2

Rate of change in GI microbiota structure of both mother and child and phylogenetic diversity. The figure represents the changes of the main microbial groups present in the GI tract and the main function of genes found in the GI microbiome (Koening et al., 2011). In the first months of life, the rate of changes in bacterial composition decrease as gradually increases the grade of diversity of the microbiome. During the first few weeks, the microbial populations in the newborn GI tract resemble the first inoculum, however, this rapidly changes. During the next few months in exclusively milk-fed infants, the growth of lactic acid bacteria, such as *Bifidobacterium,* is favored. Maternal GI microbiota change during pregnancy and the first month postpartum, with the predominance of members of the Firmicutes, *Bacteroides,* and *Bifidobacterium,* which has been proposed as a way to promote transfer of bacterial strains to the infant. In the following months, the infant GI microbiota progress into an adult-like GI microbiota composed of relatively few bacterial phyla but with high species-level diversity. Once acquired, the majority of bacterial strains in a healthy adult are retained for long periods of time.

Adapted from Subramanian, S., Blanton, L.V., Frese, S.A., Charbonneau, M., Mills, D.A., Gordon, J.I., 2015. Cultivating healthy growth and nutrition through the gut microbiota. Cell 161 (1), 36–48.

2. Probiotic administration following delivery

A double-blind, placebo-controlled randomized clinical trial with 253 Asian infants with a family history of allergic disease was carried out in Singapore (Soh et al., 2009). Infants received commercial bovine milk-based formula that was supplemented with probiotic or placebo [*B. longum* (BL999) 1×10^7 CFU/g and *L. rhamnosus*

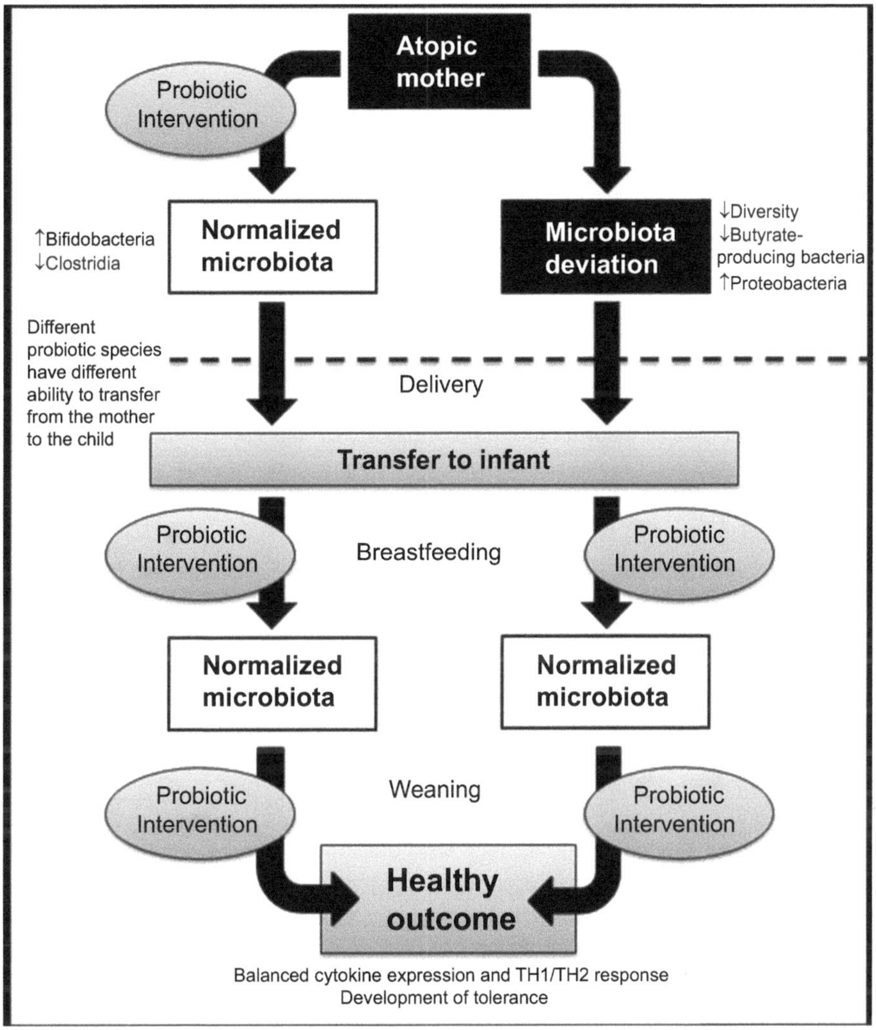

FIGURE 16.3

Timing and control of probiotic intervention. There are different stages to perform a probiotic intervention: (1) prenatal intervention of the mother during pregnancy; (2) postnatal intervention of the mother during breastfeeding; (3) postnatal intervention in infants during lactation; and (4) postnatal intervention after lactation. The probiotic intervention with the aim to reduce the risk of immune-related disorders such as atopic sensitization or eczema could be performed in each of these stages. There is increasing evidence that a comprehensive perinatal intervention of mother and infants may have better outcomes. It is important take into account all periods of intervention, that different probiotics strains could have different ability to transfer from the mother to the infant, and that difference in genetic and epigenetic background and the composition of the commensal microbiota could imply different responses to probiotic intervention.

(LPR) 2×10^7 CFU/g] daily for the first 6 months of life. The reported incidence of eczema in the probiotic group was similar to that in the placebo group at 1 year after administration (Soh et al., 2009).

3. Perinatal administration of probiotics

Kalliomäki et al. (2001a) first identified the dysbiosis or microbiota aberrancy preceding atopic eczema in at-risk infants. Kalliomäki et al. (2001b) administered in a double-blind, randomized placebo-controlled trial LGG prenatally to mothers who had at least one first-degree relative (or partner) with atopic eczema, allergic rhinitis, or asthma and postnatally for 6 months to their infants. Chronic recurring atopic eczema, which is the main sign of atopic disease in the first years of life, was the primary end point. They concluded that LGG was effective in prevention of early atopic disease in children at high risk. Thus, GI microbiota was for the first time suggested as source of natural immunomodulators, such as probiotics, for prevention of atopic disease (Kalliomäki et al., 2001b). Several studies have been published since suggesting that the atopic eczema can be prevented by LGG and other specific probiotic bacteria while not all probiotics do have the same effects (Nermes et al., 2013; Chang et al., 2016). In another study by Simpson et al. (2015), 415 pregnant women were randomized to receive probiotic or placebo milk in a double-blinded trial from 36 weeks gestation until 3 months postpartum. Probiotic milk contained LGG, *L. acidophilus* La-5, and *Bifidobacterium animalis* subsp. *lactis* Bb-12. At 6 years, children were reassessed for atopic disease, atopic sensitization, asthma, and allergic rhinoconjunctivitis (ARC).

5.1.1 Other Reports on Allergy Prevention

Bertelsen et al. (2014) examined associations between consumption of probiotic milk products during pregnancy and infancy with questionnaire-reported atopic eczema, ARC, and asthma in 40,614 children. In this population-based cohort, consumption of probiotic milk in pregnancy was associated with a slightly reduced relative risk (RR) of atopic eczema at 6 months (adjusted RR, 0.94; 95% confidence interval [CI], 0.89–0.99) and of ARC between 18 and 36 months (adjusted RR, 0.87; 95% CI, 0.78–0.98) compared with no consumption during pregnancy. When both the mother (during pregnancy) and infant (after 6 months of age) consumed probiotic milk, the adjusted RR of ARC was 0.80 (95% CI, 0.68–0.93) relative to no consumption by either.

5.1.2 Recommendations on Probiotics and Allergy Prevention

Several meta-analyses and comprehensive reviews have been conducted on probiotics and prevention of allergic disease. Conclusions earlier have been made on a strain-specific manner. However, in 2015 the World Allergy Organization (WAO) convened a guideline panel to develop evidence-based recommendations about the use of probiotics in the prevention of allergy (Fiocchi et al., 2015). They concluded that currently available evidence does not indicate that probiotic supplementation reduces the risk of developing allergy in children. However, considering all critical outcomes in this context, the WAO guideline panel determined that there is a likely net benefit from using probiotics resulting primarily from prevention of eczema. The WAO guideline panel (Fiocchi et al., 2015) suggested the following.

1. probiotics to pregnant women at high risk for having an allergic child,
2. probiotic use for women who breastfeed infants at high risk of developing allergy, and
3. probiotic use in infants at high risk of developing allergy.

The report also stated that recommendations about probiotic supplementation for prevention of allergy are intended to support both parents and clinicians as well as all health care professionals in their decisions on probiotic use during pregnancy and during breastfeeding, and whether to give them to infants. The report also states that all recommendations are conditional and supported by very-low-quality evidence. Further, strain-specific recommendations may occur at a later stage (Fiocchi et al., 2015).

5.2 MANAGEMENT OF GESTATIONAL DIABETES

Gestational diabetes (GDM) is a serious challenge during pregnancy, causing several different problems to the mother and the unborn child. Treatment of GDM improves pregnancy outcomes with significant reductions reported in serious perinatal outcomes including macrosomia, shoulder dystocia, and cesarean delivery (Crowther, 2005; Landon, 2009). Current management practices for GDM are expensive but also cost-effective for healthcare systems in the short term and longer term (Ohno et al., 2011). Primary prevention of GDM rather than treatment would, however, be ideal in preventing both the economic and health costs associated with GDM.

Efforts to prevent GDM have focused on lifestyle interventions (including diet and exercise) (Chuang, 2010). These interventions have proven challenging, both to perform and in the analysis of effect due to heterogeneity, small study size, limited patient adherence to the intervention, and methodological issues. Also, it is known that adherence to even simple measures such as folate supplementation is poor (Callaway, 2009). Recent systematic reviews have concluded that no firm statement on the utility of nutritional interventions in controlling excessive maternal weight gain or preventing GDM can be made (Dodd, 2010; Skouteris et al., 2010). A Cochrane Review (Tieu, 2008) examining the use of dietary advice in pregnancy for prevention of GDM has found that a low glycemic diet was beneficial for some outcomes including a reduced rate of large-for-gestational-age infants; but as only one study qualified for the analysis, further research is needed to confirm these findings. Therefore, even if complex lifestyle intervention strategies were shown to prevent GDM, compliance with these interventions for the general population would be low. On the other hand, if probiotic supplementation could be an effective method of reducing rates of GDM, there would be considerable benefits through improving maternal health and reducing pregnancy complications as well as a potential reduction in health service costs related to the management of GDM.

6. IMPACT OF PROBIOTICS ON THE HEALTH OF MOTHERS AND INFANTS

Taken together, the impact of microbiota is of great importance to both mothers and their infants. Early intervention to avoid or to reverse aberrancies may be a future tool to program infants for later health. Specific probiotics may provide an optimal tool for modification but further studies are required to identify safe and effective probiotics (individually or in combinations) for future use. At the same time, it is of great importance to continue long-term follow-up studies with currently used probiotics to verify that no detrimental effects are associated with their use in the long term. As many recommendations already suggest (Fiocchi et al., 2015; Szajewska et al., 2015), specific probiotics have a place in the treatment and prevention of acute gastroenteritis in infants and also prevention of antibiotic-associated side effects. Additionally, the effects against allergies are being verified, and first recommendations on probiotic use have been published (Fiocchi et al., 2015; Szajewska et al., 2015) focusing especially on the perinatal period. Further research into microbiome dysbiosis and its associations with NCDs needs to be done, including investigating new tools to measure these microbial changes.

6.1 IMPLICATIONS FOR HEALTH

The importance of microbial contact during fetal life, delivery, and infancy is becoming more apparent. Microbial exposure and its link to healthy immune and metabolic programming are hot topics currently and create new opportunities to improve infant health and therefore reduce the risk of disease in later life. The developmental origins of health and disease hypothesis proposes that nutrition and other environmental stimuli or insults can influence developmental pathways during critical periods of prenatal and postnatal development and subsequently induce permanent changes in metabolism and disease susceptibility (Wadhwa et al., 2009). A "critical window" exists early in life where interventions could have more of a profound, long-lasting, and irreversible impact on health. Supplementation with specific microbes with desirable effects on the host offers itself as a means of directly influencing early host–microbe interaction.

Modulation of the GI microbiome by early microbial contact during pregnancy and lactation with maternal probiotic supplementation could be effective in reducing the risk of immunoinflammatory and metabolic disease (Rautava, 2015). Still, it is not known whether particular probiotic bacteria administered to the mother are transferred to the amniotic cavity or the fetus despite experimental data suggesting that specific microbes introduced to the maternal GI tract during pregnancy may be recovered in the placenta in mice (Jimenez et al., 2008). As we gain a better understanding of shifts in the microbiota in relation to specific disease states, we could create interventions that rationally shift the microbiota to construct a healthy intestinal environment from a young age (Rautava, 2015). Nevertheless, the hypothesis of perinatal microbial programming stands strong in the long-lasting health effects of probiotic intervention (Grześkowiak et al., 2012; Schultz et al., 2004). When eaten by mothers during pregnancy, food products containing probiotic lactobacilli and bifidobacteria have been shown to decrease the risk of spontaneous preterm delivery (Myhre et al., 2011), preeclampsia (Brantsaeter et al., 2011) and increase levels of erythrocyte glutathione reductase in serum (Asemi et al., 2012). However, concerns exist about the overall safety of administering probiotics to high-risk patient groups, including pregnant women, preterm neonates, and infants (Neu, 2011). Infections caused by translocated probiotics into the blood stream have been reported in immunosuppressed patients or patients with GI tract mucosal barrier abnormalities (Boyle and Tang, 2006; Luong et al., 2010). There is also a risk of transfer of antibiotic resistance plasmids from some probiotic organisms (van Reenen and Dicks, 2011).

Several studies have shown that probiotic intervention is most effective if commenced prenatally (Abrahamssen et al., 2007; Kalliomaki et al., 2001a; Kukkonen et al., 2007). However, other studies have shown perinatal probiotic administration to be beneficial (Kim et al., 2010) and, postnatal via breastfeeding, to be most effective. A suggested mechanism for the postnatal protective effect of maternal probiotic supplementation is the increased concentration of TGF-β2 in milk (Rautava et al., 2002). These observations emphasize the importance of perinatal interaction between maternal gut microbes and infant immune systems.

Recent advances in experimental and human studies suggest that the GI microbiota may be involved in fat accumulation, enabling excessive harvest and storage of nutrients and hydrolysis of indigestible polysaccharides and activation of lipoprotein lipase with resulting excessive storage of liver-derived triglycerides (Collado et al., 2015; Turnbaugh et al., 2006, 2009). Specific probiotics may counteract this progress by modification of the GI microbiota composition. In this light, Rautava et al. (2005) observed altered innate immune gene expression in the placenta and fetal GI tract after prenatal maternal probiotic supplementation. In addition, the same intervention was found to moderate excessive weight gain especially among children who later became overweight during the first years of life, particularly at 4 years of age (Ilmonen et al., 2011). In combination with *Bifidobacterium lactis* Bb12 and dietary counseling, LGG has been shown to improve glucose homeostasis in healthy young females during and after pregnancy (Laitinen et al., 2009). This type of intervention also reduced the frequency of GDM and excessive weight gain (Luoto et al., 2010), reduced the proportion of infants with insulin resistance compared with control groups (Aaltonen et al., 2011) and increased placental concentration of phospholipid (exert immunomodulatory effects on the fetus later in pregnancy; Kaplas et al., 2007).

Preterm infants are endowed with lower microbial diversity compared with term neonates (Collado et al., 2015). Several clinical trials (Awad et al., 2010; Good et al., 2014; Khailova et al., 2009) have suggested that probiotic bacteria may reduce the incidence of NEC in preterm infants, and a recent meta-analysis (AlFaleh and Anabrees, 2014) of clinical studies concluded that probiotic interventions containing *Lactobacillus* spp. alone or together with *Bifidobacterium* spp. may have some positive effects in relation with overall mortality and NEC but did not influence the incidence of nosocomial sepsis. In addition, no side effects due to probiotic treatment were reported (AlFaleh and Anabrees, 2014). Routine administration of probiotics to all premature infants has been proposed and is common practice in many countries (Janvier et al., 2014; Ofek Shlomai et al., 2013). Interestingly, inactivated probiotics have also been shown to decrease the incidence of NEC in preterm babies (Awad et al., 2010).

When studying the effect of oral supplementation with LGG on pregnant mice, Blumer et al. (2007) reported an altered placental proinflammatory cytokine expression, with lower IL-4 and increased TNF-α gene expression levels. This was associated with reduced allergic airway inflammation in the offspring. In addition, maternal LGG supplementation was shown to increase cord blood and breast milk levels of anti-inflammatory cytokines, IFN-γ, and TGF-β1, in the first week compared with the placebo group (Prescott et al., 2008). A Finnish study also showed that maternal prenatal and postnatal supplementation with LGG reduced the frequency of eczema in the offspring but had no effect on atopic sensitization (Kim et al., 2010; Kalliomaki et al., 2001b; Wickens et al., 2008). Administration of LGG to mothers during pregnancy decreased plasma levels of IgE antibodies to a mixture of food allergens in infants up to 2 years of age (Abrahamsson et al., 2007). In a study by Salminen et al. (2009) and later by Laitinen et al. (2009), LGG treatment increased colonization by Bifidobacterium species but did not modulate the microbial diversity of 1-week-old infant GI tract (Ismail et al., 2012). In a human-like atopic dermatitis model in mice, perinatal administration of *L. rhamnosus* CGMCC also decreased clinical symptoms of dermatitis, scratching frequency, and plasma IgE levels and increased levels of IFN-γ in skin biopsies (Tanak et al., 2009).

In a later study, Rautava et al. (2012) demonstrated the efficacy of maternal probiotic supplementation in prevention of eczema in high-risk infants. The intervention was commenced 2 months before delivery and continued for 2 months after birth during exclusive breastfeeding with the probiotic combination of either *L. rhamnosus* LPR and *B. longum* BL999 or *L. paracasei* ST11 and *B. longum* BL999. A highly significant reduction in the risk of developing eczema was seen in both probiotic groups compared with placebo at the age of 2 years. A recent meta-analysis of probiotic studies concluded that both prenatal and postnatal probiotic intervention is needed to achieve reduction in eczema in children (Panduru et al., 2015).

Probiotics have shown promising immunomodulatory effects in animal studies, where perinatal maternal supplementation (Blumer et al., 2007) and direct supplementation of neonates (Feleszko et al., 2007) have been found to attenuate allergic airway responses. While there is some evidence that probiotics may be useful in the treatment or prevention of allergic rhinitis (Singh and Ranjan Das, 2010), there have been no conclusive studies for asthma to date (Sanz, 2011). Recent reports indicate that probiotics had no effect on asthma development (Dotterud et al., 2010), airway inflammation (Kukkonen et al., 2011), or asthma-related events (Rose et al., 2010).

An alternative to probiotics for the manipulation of the maternal GI tract microbiota may be the addition of prebiotics to the diet. Although published data regarding clinical efficacy of prebiotics in infancy are still sparse, it is known that oligosaccharides beneficially select and stimulate the growth and activity of beneficial bacteria such as bifidobacteria and lactobacilli (Roberfroid et al., 2010). Fujiwara et al. (2010) demonstrated that maternal dietary supplementation with fructo-oligosaccharide (FOS) modulated the GI tract microbiota of the offspring and reduced the severity of atopic dermatitis. However, a similar study by Shadid et al. (2007) showed that although galacto-oligosaccharide (GOS) and FOS supplementation changed the maternal microbiota, it did not have any effect on the offspring. Consumption of prebiotics by mothers may also increase the production of bacterial metabolites such as folate. A mother's diet supplemented with inulin and GOS increased the numbers of folate-synthesizing bacteria, and hence the levels of folate in the digesta of the large intestine and in the bloodstream (Aufreiter et al., 2011). Administration of a combination of GOS and FOS in infancy has been shown to modulate antibody production and reduce the incidence of allergic outcomes (Arslanoglu et al., 2008; van Hoffen et al., 2009). Following this, a larger multicenter trial of >800 infants demonstrated that an infant formula enriched with a specific mixture of neutral oligosaccharides and pectin-derived acidic oligosaccharides reduces the risk of eczema in low-risk infants (Grüber et al., 2010).

The synbiotic approach provides both the beneficial microbial stimulus (probiotics) and their growth factors (prebiotics). Although scarce, published data are available indicating that supplementation with synbiotics is associated with reduced incidence acute diarrheal disease (Passariello et al., 2012; Vandenplas and De Hert, 2011), whereas data on the effects of synbiotic combinations on the risk of eczema have been conflicting (Kukkonen et al., 2006; van der Aa et al., 2010).

Kukkonen et al. (2007, 2008) evaluated the treatment of pregnant women with synbiotics 2–4 weeks prior to delivery to assess the prevention of allergic diseases in infants at high risk of developing atopic dermatitis. After delivery, infants received the same treatment as the mother for up to 6 months. Symbiotic treatment showed no effect on the incidence of respiratory allergic diseases by 2 years of age but prevented atopic eczema, increased resistance to respiratory infections, and reduced IgE-associated atopic dermatitis. In the same study, the synbiotic treatment was able to improve the response to *Haemophilus influenzae* type b (Hib) immunization, increasing Hib antibody concentrations compared with the placebo group without impairing antibody responses to diphtheria, tetanus, or Hib.

A study by Maldonado et al. (2012) investigated the effect of adding 2×10^8 CFU/day *L. fermentum* (from human milk) to infant formula. A reduction in the incidence of GI tract and upper respiratory tracts infections in infants was observed.

Mastitis affects 30% of breastfeeding women and is usually caused by staphylococci or streptococci or corynebacteria (Arroyo et al., 2010). Mechanisms of immune evasion by staphylococci and streptococci and the use of antibiotics during late pregnancy and peripartum predispose the mother to this condition. Orally administered probiotics have proven to be an effective alternative to antibiotics to treat mastitis (Arroyo et al., 2010). Probiotic *L. salivarius* and *L. fermentum* modulated milk microbiome by decreasing total bacteria count by 2 log and by replacing mastitis-causing staphylococci with lactobacilli. Use of these probiotics prevented mothers from experiencing the side effects found with antibiotic use including vaginal infections and recurrent mastitis.

Most human intervention studies evaluating the effects of perinatal administration of probiotics and prebiotics to pregnant women and to infants after birth focus primarily on the prevention of atopic dermatitis (Sanz, 2011). The pregnant or breastfeeding mother is an emerging target for interventions aiming to support healthy microbial contact reducing the risk of chronic disease in the offspring (Rautava, 2015).

ACKNOWLEDGMENTS

C. Gómez-Gallego is a recipient of the Seneca Postdoctoral Grant from the Seneca Foundation, the Regional Agency of Science and Technology of the Region of Murcia (funded by the Education and Universities Council - Autonomous Community of the Region of Murcia).

REFERENCES

Aaltonen, J., Ojala, T., Laitinen, K., Poussa, T., Ozanne, S., Isolauri, E., 2011. Impact of maternal diet during pregnancy and breastfeeding on infant metabolic programming: a prospective randomized controlled study. European Journal of Clinical Nutrition 65, 10–19.

Abrahamsson, T.R., Jakobsson, H.E., Andersson, A.F., Björkstén, B., Engstrand, L., Jenmalm, M.C., 2012. Low diversity of the gut microbiota in infants with atopic eczema. Journal of Allergy and Clinical Immunology 129, 434–440.

Abrahamsson, T.R., Jakobsson, H.E., Andersson, A.F., Björkstén, B., Engstrand, L., Jenmalm, M.C., 2014. Low gut microbiota diversity in early infancy precedes asthma at school age. Clinical & Experimental Allergy 44 (6), 842–850.

Abrahamsson, T.R., Jakobsson, T., Böttcher, M.F., Fredrikson, M., Jenmalm, M.C., Björkstén, B., Oldaeus, G., 2007. Probiotics in prevention of IgE-associated eczema: a double-blind, randomized, placebo-controlled trial. Journal of Allergy and Clinical Immunology 119 (5), 1174–17780.

AlFaleh, K., Anabrees, J., 2014. Probiotics for prevention of necrotizing enterocolitis in preterm infants. Evidence-Based Child Health 9 (3), 584–671.

Ardissone, A.N., de la Cruz, D.M., Davis-Richardson, A.G., Rechcigel, K.T., Li, N., Drew, J.C., Murgas-Turrazza, R., Sharma, R., Hudak, M.L., Triplett, E.W., Neu, J., 2014. Meconium microbiome analysis identifies bacteria correlated with premature birth. PLoS One 9, 90784.

Arrieta, M.C., Stiemsma, L.T., Amenyogbe, N., Brown, E.M., Finlay, B., 2014. The intestinal microbiome in early life: health and disease. Frontiers in Immunology 5, 427.

Arroyo, R., Martín, V., Maldonado, A., Jiménez, E., Fernández, L., Rodríguez, J.M., 2010. Treatment of infectious mastitis during lactation: antibiotics versus oral administration of Lactobacilli isolated from breast milk. Clinical Infectious Diseases 50 (12), 1551–1558.

Arslanoglu, S., Moro, G.E., Schmitt, J., Tandoi, L., Rizzardi, S., Boehm, G., 2008. Early dietary intervention with a mixture of prebiotic oligosaccharides reduces the incidence of allergic manifestations and infections during the first two years of life. Journal of Nutrition 138 (6), 1091–1095.

Asemi, Z., Samimi, M., Tabasi, Z., Talebian, P., Azarbad, Z., Hydarzadeh, Z., Esmaillzadeh, A., 2012. Effect of daily consumption of probiotic yoghurt on lipid profiles in pregnant women: a randomized controlled clinical trial. Journal of Maternal-Fetal and Neonatal Medicine 25 (9), 1552–1556.

Aufreiter, S., Kim, J.H., O'Connor, D.L., 2011. Dietary oligosaccharides increase colonic weight and the amount but not concentration of bacterially synthesized folate in the colon of piglets. Journal of Nutrition 141 (3), 366–372.

Awad, H., Mokhtar, H., Imam, S.S., Gad, G.I., Hafez, H., Aboushady, N., 2010. Comparison between killed and living probiotic usage versus placebo for the prevention of necrotizing enterocolitis and sepsis in neonates. Pakistan Journal of Biological Sciences 94 (4), 486–494.

Bergstrom, A., Skov, T.H., Bahl, M.I., Roager, H.M., Christensen, L.B., Ejlerskov, K.T., Mølgaard, C., Michaelsen, K.F., Licht, T.R., 2014. Establishment of intestinal microbiota during early life: a longitudinal, explorative study of a large cohort of Danish infants. Applied and Environmental Microbiology 80, 2889–2900.

Bertelsen, R.J., Brantsæter, A.L., Magnus, M.C., Haugen, M., Myhre, R., Jacobsson, B., Longnecker, M.P., Meltzer, H.M., London, S.J., 2014. Probiotic milk consumption in pregnancy and infancy and subsequent childhood allergic diseases. Journal of Allergy and Clinical Immunology 133 (1), 165–171.

Bezirtzoglou, E., Tsiotsias, A., Welling, G.W., 2011. Microbiota profile in feces of breast- and formula-fed newborns by using fluorescence in situ hybridization (FISH). Anaerobe 17 (6), 478–482.

Blaser, M.J., 2006. Who are we? Indigenous microbes and the ecology of human diseases. EMBO Reports 7, 956–960.

Blümer, N., Sel, S., Virna, S., Patrascan, C.C., Zimmermann, S., Herz, U., Renz, H., Gran, H., 2007. Perinatal maternal application of *Lactobacillus rhamnosus* GG suppresses allergic airway inflammation in mouse offspring. Clinical and Experimental Allergy 37 (3), 348–357.

Boyle, R.J., Ismail, I.H., Kivivuori, S., Licciardi, P.V., Robins-Browne, R.M., Mah, L.J., Axelrad, C., Moore, S., Donath, S., Carlin, J.B., Lahtinen, S.J., Tang, M.L., 2011. *Lactobacillus GG* treatment during pregnancy for the prevention of eczema: a randomized controlled trial. Allergy 66 (4), 509–516.

Boyle, R.J., Tang, M.L., 2006. The role of probiotics in the management of allergic disease. Clinical and Experimental Allergy 36 (5), 568–576.

Brantsaeter, A.L., Myhre, R., Haugen, M., Myking, S., Sengpiel, V., Magnus, P., Jacobsson, B., Meltzer, H.M., 2011. Intake of probiotic food and risk of preeclampsia in primiparous women: the Norwegian Mother and Child Cohort Study. American Journal of Epidemiology 174 (7), 807–815.

Buddington, R.K., Williams, C.H., Kostek, B.M., Buddington, K.K., Kullen, M.J., 2009. Maternal-to-infant transmission of probiotics: concept validation in mice, rats, and pigs. Neonatology 97 (3), 250–256.

Cabrera-Rubio, R., Collado, M.C., Laitinen, K., Salminen, S., Isolauri, E., Mira, A., 2012. The human milk microbiome changes over lactation and is shaped by maternal weight and mode of delivery. The American Journal of Clinical Nutrition 96 (3), 544–551.

Callaway, L., Colditz, P.B., Fisk, N.M., 2009. Folic acid supplementation and spontaneous preterm birth: adding grist to the mill? PLOS Medicine 6 (5), e1000077.

Centre for Maternal and Child Enquiries, 2011. Saving Mothers' Lives: reviewing maternal deaths to make motherhood. BJOG: An International Journal of Obstetrics & Gynaecology 118, 1–203.

Chang, Y.S., Trivedi, M.K., Jha, A., Lin, Y.F., Dimaano, L., Garcia-Romero, M.T., 2016. Synbiotics for prevention and treatment of atomic dermatisis – a meta-analysis of randomized clinical trials. JAMA Paediatrics.

Chattha, K.S., Vlasova, A.N., Kandasamy, S., Esseili, M.A., Siegismund, C., Rajashekara, G., Saif, L.J., 2013. Probiotics and colostrum/milk differentially affect neonatal humoral immune responses to oral rotavirus vaccine. Vaccine 31 (15), 1916–1923.

Chuang, C.H., Velott, D.L., Weisman, C.S., 2010. Exploring knowledge and attitudes related to pregnancy and preconception health in women with chronic medical conditions. Maternal and Child Health Journal 14 (5), 713–719.

Collado, M.C., Cernada, M., Neu, J., Pérez-Martínez, G., Gormaz, M., Vento, M., 2015. Factors influencing gastrointestinal tract and microbiota immune interaction in preterm infants. Pediatric Research 77 (6), 726–731.

Collado, M.C., Isolauri, E., Laitinen, K., Salminen, S., 2008. Distinct composition of gut microbiota during pregnancy in overweight and normal-weight women. American Journal of Clinical Nutrition 88 (4), 894–899.

Crowther, C.A., Hiller, J.E., Moss, J.R., McPhee, A.J., Jeffries, W.S., Robinson, J.S., Australian Carbohydrate Intolerance Study in Pregnant Women (ACHOIS) Trial Group, 2005. Effect of treatment of gestational diabetes mellitus on pregnancy outcomes. New England Journal of Medicine 352 (24), 2477–2486.

De Angelis, M., Piccolo, M., Vannini, L., Siragusa, S., De Giacomo, A., Serrazzanetti, D.I., Cristofori, F., Guerzoni, M.E., Gobbetti, M., Francavilla, R., 2013. Fecal microbiota and metabolome of children with autism and pervasive developmental disorder not otherwise specified. PLoS One 8, 76993.

Dethlefsen, L., Huse, S., Sogin, M.L., Relman, D.A., 2008. The pervasive effects of an antibiotic on the human gut microbiota, as revealed by deep 16S rRNA sequencing. PLoS Biology 6 (11), 280.

DiGiulio, D.B., 2012. Diversity of microbes in amniotic fluid. In: Seminars in Fetal and Neonatal Medicine 17 (1), 2–11.

Dodd, J., Grivell, R., Crowther, C., Robinson, J., 2010. Antenatal interventions for overweight or obese pregnant women: a systematic review of randomised trials. International Journal of Obstetrics & Gynaecology 117, 1316–1326.

Dotterud, C.K., Storrø, O., Johnsen, R., Oien, T., 2010. Probiotics in pregnant women to prevent allergic disease: a randomized, double-blind trial. British Journal of Dermatology 163 (3), 616–623.

Dugoua, J.J., Machado, M., Zhu, X., Chen, X., Koren, G., Einarson, T.R., 2009. Probiotic safety in pregnancy: a systematic review and meta-analysis of randomized controlled trials of Lactobacillus, Bifidobacterium, and Saccharomyces spp. Journal of Obstetrics and Gynaecology Canada 31 (6), 542–552.

Dunne, J.L., Triplett, E.W., Gevers, D., Xavier, R., Insel, R., Danska, J., Atkinson, M.A., 2014. The intestinal microbiome in type 1 diabetes. Clinical and Experimental Immunology 177, 30–37.

Echarri, P.P., Graciá, C.M., Berruezo, G.R., Vives, I., Ballesta, M., Solís, G., Morillas, I.V., Reyes-Gavilán, C.G., Margolles, A., Gueimonde, M., 2011. Assessment of intestinal microbiota of full-term breast-fed infants from two different geographical locations. Early Human Development 87 (7), 511–513.

Ezendam, J., de Klerk, A., Gremmer, E.R., van Loveren, H., 2008. Effects of *Bifidobacterium animalis* administered during lactation on allergic and autoimmune responses in rodents. Clinical & Experimental Immunology 154 (3), 424–431.

De Filippo, C., Cavalieri, D., Di Paola, M., Ramazzotti, M., Poullet, J.B., Massart, S., Collini, S., Pieraccini, G., Lionetti, P., 2010. Impact of diet in shaping gut microbiota revealed by a comparative study in children from Europe and rural Africa. PNAS 107 (33), 14691–14696.

Fallani, M., Young, D., Scott, J., Norin, E., Amarri, S., Adam, R., Aguilera, M., Khanna, S., Gil, A., Edwards, C.A., Doré, J., INFABIO team, 2010. Intestinal microbiota of 6-week-old infants across Europe: geographic influence beyond delivery mode, breast-feeding, and antibiotics. Journal of Pediatric Gastroenterology and Nutrition 51 (1), 77–84.

Feleszko, W., Jaworska, J., Rha, R.D., Steinhausen, S., Avagyan, A., Jaudszus, A., Ahrens, B., Groneberg, D.A., Wahn, U., Hamelmann, E., 2007. Probiotic-induced suppression of allergic sensitization and airway inflammation is associated with an increase of T regulatory-dependent mechanisms in a murine model of asthma. Clinical and Experimental Allergy 37 (4), 498–505.

Fernández, L., Langa, S., Martín, V., Maldonado, A., Jiménez, E., Martín, R., Rodríguez, J.M., 2013. The human milk microbiota: origin and potential roles in health and disease. Pharmacological Research 69, 1–10.

Fiocchi, A., Pawankar, R., Cuello-Garcia, C., Ahn, K., Al-Hammadi, S., Agarwal, A., Beyer, K., Burks, W., Canonica, G.W., Ebisawa, M., Gandhi, S., Kamenwa, R., Lee, B.W., Li, H., Prescott, S., Riva, J.J., Rosenwasser, L., Sampson, H., Spigler, M., Terracciano, L., Vereda-Ortiz, A., Waserman, S., Yepes-Nuñez, J.J., Brożek, J.L., Schünemann, H.J., 2015. World allergy Organization-McMaster University guidelines for allergic disease prevention (GLAD-P): probiotics. World Allergy Organ 8, 4.

Food and Agricultural Organization of the United Nations and World Health Organization, 2001. Health and nutritional properties of probiotics in food including powder milk with live lactic acid bacteria. World Health Organization. Available at: http://www.who.int/foodsafety/publications/fs_management/en/probiotics.pdf.

Foye, O.T., Huang, I.F., Chiou, C.C., Walker, W.A., Shi, H.N., 2012. Early administration of probiotic *Lactobacillus acidophilus* and/or prebiotic inulin attenuates pathogen-mediated intestinal inflammation and Smad 7 cell signaling. FEMS Immunology and Medical Microbiology 65 (3), 467–480.

Fujiwara, R., Takemura, N., Watanabe, J., Sonoyama, K., 2010. Maternal consumption of fructo-oligosaccharide diminishes the severity of skin inflammation in offspring of NC/Nga mice. British Journal of Nutrition 103 (4), 530–538.

Fåk, F., Ahrné, S., Molin, G., Jeppsson, B., Weström, B.K., 2008. Maternal consumption of *Lactobacillus plantarum* 299v affects gastrointestinal growth and function in the suckling rat. British Journal of Nutrition 100 (2), 332–338.

Di Giancamillo, A., Vitari, F., Savoini, G., Bontempo, V., Bersani, C., Dell'Orto, V., Domeneghini, C., 2008. Effects of orally administered probiotic *Pediococcus acidilactici* on the small and large intestine of weaning piglets. A qualitative and quantitative micro-anatomical study. Journal of Histology & Histopathology 23 (6), 651–664.

Gevers, D., Kugathasan, S., Denson, L.A., Vázquez-Baeza, Y., Van Treuren, W., Ren, B., Schwager, E., Knights, D., Song, S.J., Yassour, M., Morgan, X.C., Kostic, A.D., Luo, C., González, A., McDonald, D., Haberman, Y., Walters, T., Baker, S., Rosh, J., Stephens, M., Heyman, M., Markowitz, J., Baldassano, R., Griffiths, A., Sylvester, F., Mack, D., Kim, S., Crandall, W., Hyams, J., Huttenhower, C., Knight, R., Xavier, R.J., 2014. The treatment-naive microbiome in new-onset Crohn's disease. Cell Host Microbe 15, 382–392.

Ghanem, K.Z., Badawy, I.H., Abdel-Samam, A.M., 2004. Influence of yoghurt and probiotic yoghurt on the absorption of calcium, magnesium, iron and bone mineralization in rats. Milk Science International 59, 472–475.

Good, M., Sodhi, C.P., Ozolek, J.A., Buck, R.H., Goehring, K.C., Thomas, D.L., Vikram, A., Bibby, K., Morowitz, M.J., Firek, B., Lu, P., Hackam, D.J., 2014. *Lactobacillus rhamnosus* HN001 decreases the severity of necrotizing enterocolitis in neonatal mice and preterm piglets: evidence in mice for a role of TLR9. American Journal of Physiology: Gastrointestinal and Liver Physiology 306 (11), G1021–G1032.

Grüber, C., van Stuijvenberg, M., Mosca, F., Moro, G., Chirico, G., Braegger, C.P., Riedler, J., Boehm, G., Wahn, U., Mips 1 working group, 2010. Reduced occurrence of early atopic dermatitis because of immunoactive prebiotics among low-atopy-risk infants. Journal of Allergy and Clinical Immunology 126 (4), 791–797.

Grönlund, M.M., Gueimonde, M., Laitinen, K., Kociubinski, G., Grönroos, T., Salminen, S., Isolauri, E., 2007. Maternal breast-milk and intestinal bifidobacteria guide the compositional development of the Bifidobacterium microbiota in infants at risk of allergic disease. Clinical and Experimental Allergy 37 (12), 1764–1772.

Gueimonde, M., Laitinen, K., Salminen, S., Isolauri, E., 2007. Breast milk: a source of bifidobacteria for infant gut development and maturation? Neonatology 92 (1), 64–66.

Grześkowiak, Ł., Grönlund, M.M., Beckmann, C., Salminen, S., von Berg, A., Isolauri, E., 2012. The impact of perinatal probiotic intervention on gut microbiota: double-blind placebo-controlled trials in Finland and Germany. Anaerobe 18 (1), 7–13.

Hanson, M., Godfrey, K.M., Lillycrop, K.A., Burdge, G.C., Gluckman, P.D., 2011. Developmental plasticity and developmental origins of non-communicable disease: theoretical considerations and epigenetic mechanisms. Progress in Biophysics and Molecular Biology 106 (1), 272–280.

Harmsen, H.J., Wildeboer–Veloo, A.C., Raangs, G.C., Wagendorp, A.A., Klijn, N., Bindels, J.G., Welling, G.W., 2000. Analysis of intestinal flora development in breast-fed and formula-fed infants by using molecular identification and detection methods. Journal of Pediatric Gastroenterology and Nutrition 30, 61–67.

Hill, C., Guarner, F., Reid, G., Gibson, G.R., Merenstein, D.J., Pot, B., Morelli, L., Canani, R.B., Flint, H.J., Salminen, S., Calder, P.C., Sanders, M.E., 2014. Expert consensus document. The International Scientific Association for Probiotics and Prebiotics consensus statement on the scope and appropriate use of the term probiotic. Nature Reviews Gastroenterology & Hepatology 11, 506–514.

Hu, J., Nomura, Y., Bashir, A., Fernandez-Hernandez, H., Itzkowitz, S., Pei, Z., Stone, J., Loudon, H., Peter, I., 2013. Diversified microbiota of meconium is affected by maternal diabetes status. PLoS One 9 (11).

Ichikawa, H., Kuroiwa, T., Inagaki, A., Shineha, R., Nishihira, T., Satomi, S., Sakata, T., 1999. Probiotic bacteria stimulate gut epithelial cell proliferation in rat. Digestive Diseases and Sciences 44 (10), 2119–2123.

Ilmonen, J., Isolauri, E., Poussa, T., Laitinen, K., 2011. Impact of dietary counselling and probiotic intervention on maternal anthropometric measurements during and after pregnancy: a randomized placebo-controlled trial. Clinical Nutrition 30 (2), 156–164.

Ismail, I.H., Oppedisano, F., Joseph, S.J., Boyle, R.J., Robins-Browne, R.M., Tang, M.L., 2012. Prenatal administration of *Lactobacillus rhamnosus* has no effect on the diversity of the early infant gut microbiota. Pediatric Allergy and Immunology 23 (3), 255–258.

Janvier, A., Malo, J., Barrington, K.J., 2014. Cohort study of probiotics in a North American neonatal intensive care unit. Journal of Pediatrics 164 (5), 980–985.

Jiménez, E., Marín, M.L., Martín, R., Odriozola, J.M., Olivares, M., Xaus, J., Rodríguez, J.M., 2008. Is meconium from healthy newborns actually sterile? Research in Microbiology 159 (3), 187–193.

Jost, T., Lacroix, C., Braegger, C., Chassard, C., 2014. Stability of the maternal gut microbiota during late pregnancy and early lactation. Current Microbiology 68 (4), 419–427.

Jost, T., Lacroix, C., Braegger, C., Chassard, C., 2013. Assessment of bacterial diversity in breast milk using culture-dependent and culture-independent approaches. British Journal of Nutrition 7, 1253–1262.

Kalliomäki, M., Collado, M.C., Salminen, S., Isolauri, E., 2008. Early differences in fecal microbiota composition in children may predict overweight. American Journal of Clinical Nutrition 87, 534–538.

Kalliomäki, M., Kirjavainen, P., Eerola, E., Kero, P., Salminen, S., Isolauri, E., 2001a. Distinct patterns of neonatal gut microflora in infants in whom atopy was and was not developing. Journal of Allergy and Clinical Immunology 107 (1), 129–134.

Kalliomäki, M., Salminen, S., Arvilommi, H., Kero, P., Koskinen, P., Isolauri, E., 2001b. Probiotics in primary prevention of atopic disease: a randomized placebo-controlled trial. Lancet 357 (9262), 1076–1079.

Kaplas, N., Isolauri, E., Lampi, A.M., Ojala, T., Laitinen, K., 2007. Dietary counseling and probiotic supplementation during pregnancy modify placental phospholipid fatty acids. Lipids 42 (9), 865–870.

Khailova, L., Dvorak, K., Arganbright, K.M., Halpern, M.D., Kinouchi, T., Yajima, M., Dvorak, B., 2009. *Bifidobacterium bifidum* improves intestinal integrity in a rat model of necrotizing enterocolitis. American Journal of Physiology: Gastrointestinal and Liver Physiology 297 (5), G940–G949.

Kim, J.Y., Kwon, J.H., Ahn, S.H., Lee, S.I., Han, Y.S., Choi, Y.O., Lee, S.Y., Ahn, K.M., Ji, G.E., 2010. Effect of probiotic mix (*Bifidobacterium bifidum, Bifidobacterium lactis, Lactobacillus acidophilus*) in the primary prevention of eczema: a double-blind, randomized, placebo-controlled trial. Pediatric Allergy and Immunology 21 (2 Pt 2), e386–93.

Koenig, J.E., Spor, A., Scalfone, N., Fricker, A.D., Stombaugh, J., Knight, R., Angenent, L.T., Ley, R.E., 2011. Succession of microbial consortia in the developing infant gut microbiome. Proceedings of the National Academy of Sciences of the United States of America 108, 4578–4585.

Koren, O., Goodrich, J.K., Cullender, T.C., Spor, A., Laitinen, K., Backhed, H.K., Gonzalez, A., Werner, J.J., Angenent, L.T., Knight, R., Backhed, F., Isolauri, E., Salminen, S., Ley, R.E., 2012. Host remodeling of the gut microbiome and metabolic changes during pregnancy. Cell 150 (3), 470–480.

Kostic, A.D., Gevers, D., Siljander, H., Vatanen, T., Hyötyläinen, T., Hämäläinen, A.M., DIABIMMUNE Study Group, 2015. The dynamics of the human infant gut microbiome in development and in progression toward type 1 diabetes. Cell Host Microbe 17, 260–273.

Kukkonen, A.K., Kuitunen, M., Savilahti, E., Pelkonen, A., Malmberg, P., Mäkelä, M., 2011. Airway inflammation in probiotic-treated children at 5 years. Pediatric Allergy and Immunology 22 (2), 249–251.

Kukkonen, K., Nieminen, T., Poussa, T., Savilahti, E., Kuitunen, M., 2006. Effect of probiotics on vaccine antibody responses in infancy-a randomized placebo-controlled double-blind trial. Pediatric Allergy and Immunology 17 (6), 416–421.

Kukkonen, K., Savilahti, E., Haahtela, T., Juntunen-Backman, K., Korpela, R., Poussa, T., Tuure, T., Kuitunen, M., 2007. Probiotics and prebiotic galacto-oligosaccharides in the prevention of allergic diseases: a randomized, double-blind, placebo-controlled trial. Journal of Allergy and Clinical Immunology 119 (1), 192–198.

Kukkonen, K., Savilahti, E., Haahtela, T., Juntunen-Backman, K., Korpela, R., Poussa, T., Tuure, T., Kuitunen, M., 2008. Long-term safety and impact on infection rates of postnatal probiotic and prebiotic (synbiotic) treatment: randomized, double-blind, placebo-controlled trial. Pediatrics 122 (1), 8–12.

Laitinen, K., Poussa, T., Isolauri, E., Nutrition, Allergy, Mucosal Immunology and Intestinal Microbiota Group, 2009. Probiotics and dietary counselling contribute to glucose regulation during and after pregnancy: a randomised controlled trial. British Journal of Nutrition 101 (11), 1679–1687.

Landon, M.B., Spong, C.Y., Thom, E., Carpenter, M.W., Ramin, S.M., Casey, B., Wapner, R.J., Varner, M.W., Rouse, D.J., Thorp Jr., J.M., Sciscione, A., Catalano, P., Harper, M., Saade, G., Lain, K.Y., Sorokin, Y., Peaceman, A.M., Tolosa, J.E., Anderson, G.B., Eunice Kennedy Shriver National Institute of Child Health and Human Development Maternal-Fetal Medicine Units Network, 2009. A multicenter, randomized trial of treatment for mild gestational diabetes. New England Journal of Medicine 361 (14), 1339–1348.

Lee, S.A., Lim, J.Y., Kim, B.S., Cho, S.J., Kim, N.Y., Kim, O.B., Kim, Y., 2015. Comparison of the gut microbiota profile in breast-fed and formula-fed Korean infants using pyrosequencing. Nutrition Research and Practice 9 (3), 242–248.

Liu, A.H., Leung, D.Y.M., 2006. Renaissance of the hygiene hypothesis. Journal of Allergy and Clinical Immunology 117, 1063–1066.

Liu, Y., Tran, D.Q., Fatheree, N.Y., Marc Rhoads, J., 2014. *Lactobacillus reuteri* DSM 17938 differentially modulates effector memory T cells and Foxp3+ regulatory T cells in a mouse model of necrotizing enterocolitis. American Journal of Physiology: Gastrointestinal and Liver Physiology 307 (2), G177–G186.

Luong, M.L., Sareyyupoglu, B., Nguyen, M.H., Silveira, F.P., Shields, R.K., Potoski, B.A., Pasculle, W.A., Clancy, C.J., Toyoda, Y., 2010. Lactobacillus probiotic use in cardiothoracic transplant recipients: a link to invasive Lactobacillus infection? Transplant Infectious Disease 12 (6), 561–564.

Luoto, R., Laitinen, K., Nermes, M., Isolauri, E., 2010. Impact of maternal probiotic-supplemented dietary counselling on pregnancy outcome and prenatal and postnatal growth: a double-blind, placebo-controlled study. British Journal of Nutrition 103 (12), 1792–1799.

Ly, N.P., Litonjua, A., Gold, D.R., Celedón, J.C., 2011. Gut microbiota, probiotics, and vitamin D: interrelated exposures influencing allergy, asthma, and obesity? Journal of Allergy and Clinical Immunology 127 (5), 1087–1094.

Maassen, C.B., van Holten, J.C., Balk, F., 1998. Orally administered Lactobacillus strains differentially affect the direction and efficacy of the immune response. Veterinary Quarterly 20 (3), S81–S83.

Marcobal, A., Underwood, M.A., Mills, D.A., 2008. Rapid determination of the bacterial composition of commercial probiotic products by terminal restriction fragment length polymorphism analysis. Journal of Pediatric of Gastroenterology and Nutrition 46 (5), 608–611.

Mai, V., Young, C.M., Ukhanova, M., Wang, X., Sun, Y., Casella, G., Neu, J., 2011. Fecal microbiota in premature infants prior to necrotizing enterocolitis. PLoS One 6, 20647.

Maldonado, J., Cañabate, F., Sempere, L., Vela, F., Sánchez, A.R., Narbona, E., López-Huertas, E., Geerlings, A., Valero, A.D., Olivares, M., Lara-Villoslada, F., 2012. Human milk probiotic *Lactobacillus fermentum* CECT5716 reduces the incidence of gastrointestinal and upper respiratory tract infections in infants. Journal of Pediatric Gastroenterology and Nutrition 54 (1), 55–61.

Martín, R., Langa, S., Reviriego, C., Jiménez, E., Marín, M.L., Olivares, M., Boza, J., Jiménez, J., Fernàndez, L., Xaus, J., Rodríguez, J.M., 2004. The commensal microflora of human milk: new perspectives for food bacteriotherapy and probiotics. Trends in Food Science and Technology 15 (3–4), 121–127.

McLean, M.H., Dieguez Jr., D., Miller, L.M., Young, H.A., 2015. Does the microbiota play a role in the pathogenesis of autoimmune diseases? Gut 64 (2), 332–341.

Meini, S., Laureano, R., Fani, L., Tascini, C., Galano, A., Antonelli, A., Rossolini, G.M., 2015. Breakthrough *Lactobacillus rhamnosus* GG bacteremia associated with probiotic use in an adult patient with severe active ulcerative colitis: case report and review of the literature. Infection 43 (6), 777–781.

Mor, G., Cardenas, I., 2010. The immune system in pregnancy: a unique complexity. American Journal of Reproductive Immunology 63, 425–433.

Myhre, R., Brantsæter, A.L., Myking, S., Gjessing, H.K., Sengpiel, V., Meltzer, H.M., Haugen, M., Jacobsson, B., 2011. Intake of probiotic food and risk of spontaneous preterm delivery. American Journal of Clinical Nutrition 93 (1), 151–157.

Narva, M., Collin, M., Lamberg-Allardt, C., Karkkainen, M., Poussa, T., Vapaatalo, H., Korpela, R., 2004. Effects of long-term intervention with *Lactobacillus helveticus*-fermented milk on bone mineral density and bone mineral content in growing rats. Annals of Nutrition and Metabolism 48, 228–234.

Nauta, A.J., Amor, K.B., Knol, J., Garssen, J., Van der Beek, E.M., 2013. Relevance of pre-and postnatal nutrition to development and interplay between the microbiota and metabolic and immune systems. American Journal of Clinical Nutrition 98 (2), 586–593.

Nermes, M., Salminen, S., Isolauri, E., 2013. Is there a role for probiotics in the prevention or treatment of food allergy? Current Allergy and Asthma 13 (6), 622–630.

Neu, J., 2011. Routine probiotics for premature infants: let's be careful! The Journal of pediatrics 158 (4), 672.

Newbern, D., Freemark, M., 2011. Placental hormones and the control of maternal metabolism and fetal growth. Current Opinion in Endocrinology, Diabetes and Obesity 18, 409–416.

Ofek Shlomai, N., Deshpande, G., Rao, S., Patole, S., 2013. Probiotics for preterm neonates: what will it take to change clinical practice? Neonatology 105, 64–70.

Ohno, M.S., Sparks, T.N., Cheng, Y.W., Caughey, A.B., 2011. Treating mild gestational diabetes mellitus: a cost-effectiveness analysis. American Journal of Obstetrics and Gynecology 205 (3) 282.e1–7.

Palmer, C., Bik, E.M., DiGiulio, D.B., Relman, D.A., Brown, P.O., 2007. Development of the human infant intestinal microbiota. PLoS Biology 5, 177.

Panduru, M., Panduru, N.M., Sălăvăstru, C.M., Tiplica, G.S., 2015. Probiotics and primary prevention of atopic dermatitis: a meta-analysis of randomized controlled studies. Journal of the European Academy of Dermatology and Venereology 29 (2), 232–242.

Passariello, A., Terrin, G., Cecere, G., Micillo, M., De Marco, G., Di Costanzo, M., Cosenza, L., Leone, L., Nocerino, R., Canani, R.B., 2012. Randomised clinical trial: efficacy of a new synbiotic formulation containing *Lactobacillus paraca*sei B21060 plus arabinogalactan and xilooligosaccharides in children with acute diarrhoea. Alimentary Pharmacology & Therapeutics 35 (7), 782–788.

Penders, J., Thijs, C., Vink, C., Stelma, F.F., Snijders, B., Kummeling, I., van den Brandt, P.A., Stobberingh, E.E., 2006. Factors influencing the composition of the intestinal microbiota in early infancy. Pediatrics 118 (2), 511–521.

Perez, P.F., Dore, J., Leclerc, M., Levenez, F., Benyacoub, J., Serrant, P., Segura-Roggero, I., Schiffrin, E.J., Donnet-Hughes, A., 2007. Bacterial imprinting of the neonatal immune system: lessons from maternal cells? Pediatrics 119 (3), 724–732.

Preidis, G.A., Saulnier, D.M., Blutt, S.E., Mistretta, T.A., Riehle, K.P., Major, A.M., Venable, S.F., Finegold, M.J., Petrosino, J.F., Conner, M.E., Versalovic, J., 2012. Probiotics stimulate enterocyte migration and microbial diversity in the neonatal mouse intestine. FASEB Journal 26 (5), 1960–1969.

Prescott, S.L., Wickens, K., Westcott, L., Jung, W., Currie, H., Black, P.N., Stanley, T.V., Mitchell, E.A., Fitzharris, P., Siebers, R., Wu, L., Crane, J., Probiotic study group, 2008. Supplementation with *Lactobacillus rhamnosus* or *Bifidobacterium lactis* probiotics in pregnancy increases cord blood interferon-gamma and breast milk transforming growth factor-beta and immunoglobin A detection. Clinical and Experimental Allergy 38 (10), 1606–1614.
Rautava, S., 2015. Early microbial contact, the breast milk microbiome and child health. Journal of Developmental Origins of Health and Disease 7 (1), 5–14.
Rautava, S., Kalliomäki, M., Isolauri, E., 2002. Probiotics during pregnancy and breast-feeding might confer immunomodulatory protection against atopic disease in the infant. Journal of Allergy and Clinical Immunology 109 (1), 119–121.
Rautava, S., Kalliomäki, M., Isolauri, E., 2005. New therapeutic strategy for combating the increasing burden of allergic disease: probiotics—a Nutrition, Allergy, Mucosal Immunology and Intestinal Microbiota (NAMI) Research Group report. Journal of allergy and clinical immunology 116 (1), 31–37.
Rautava, S., Luoto, R., Salminen, S., Isolauri, E., 2012. Microbial contact during pregnancy, intestinal colonization and human disease. Nature Reviews Gastroenterology and Hepatology 9 (10), 565–576.
Roberfroid, M., Gibson, G.R., Hoyles, L., McCartney, A.L., Rastall, R., Rowland, I., Wolvers, D., Watzl, B., Szajewska, H., Stahl, B., Guarner, F., Respondek, F., Whelan, K., Coxam, V., Davicco, M.J., Léotoing, L., Wittrant, Y., Delzenne, N.M., Cani, P.D., Neyrinck, A.M., Meheust, A., 2010. Prebiotic effects: metabolic and health benefits. British Journal of Nutrition 104 (Suppl. 2), S1–S63.
Robinson, J., 2014. Cochrane in context: probiotics for prevention of necrotizing enterocolitis in preterm infants. Evidence-Based Child Health 9 (3), 672–674.
Roger, L.C., Costabile, A., Holland, D.T., Hoyles, L., McCartney, A.L., 2010. Examination of faecal Bifidobacterium populations in breast- and formula-fed infants during the first 18 months of life. Microbiology 56, 3329–3341.
Rose, M.A., Stieglitz, F., Köksal, A., Schubert, R., Schulze, J., Zielen, S., 2010. Efficacy of probiotic Lactobacillus GG on allergic sensitization and asthma in infants at risk. Clinical and Experimental Allergy 40 (9), 1398–1405.
van Reenen, C.A., Dicks, L.M., 2011. Horizontal gene transfer amongst probiotic lactic acid bacteria and other intestinal microbiota: what are the possibilities. A review. Archives of Microbiology 193, 157–168.
Salminen, S., Collado, M.C., Isolauri, E., Gueimonde, M., 2009. Microbial–host Interactions: Selecting the Right Probiotics and Prebiotics for Infants, pp. 201–217.
Sanz, Y., 2011. Gut microbiota and probiotics in maternal and infant health. The American journal of clinical nutrition 94 (6), 2000S–2005S.
Schabussova, I., Hufnagl, K., Tang, M.L., Hoflehner, E., Wagner, A., Loupal, G., Nutten, S., Zuercher, A., Mercenier, A., Wiedermann, U., 2012. Perinatal maternal administration of *Lactobacillus paracasei* NCC 2461 prevents allergic inflammation in a mouse model of birch pollen allergy. PLoS One 7 (7), e40271.
Scheperjans, F., Aho, V., Pereira, P.A., Koskinen, K., Paulin, L., Pekkonen, E., Haapaniemi, E., Kaakkola, S., Eerola-Rautio, J., Pohja, M., Kinnunen, E., Murros, K., Auvinen, P., 2015. Gut microbiota are related to Parkinson's disease and clinical phenotype. Movement Disorders Journal 30, 350–358.
Scholz-Ahrens, K.E., Ade, P., Marten, B., Weber, P., Timm, W., Açil, Y., Glüer, C.C., Schrezenmeir, J., 2007. Prebiotics, probiotics, and synbiotics affect mineral absorption, bone mineral content, and bone structure. Journal of Nutrition 137 (3 Suppl. 2), 838S–846S.

Schultz, M., Gottl, C., Young, R.J., Iwen, P., Vanderhoof, J.A., 2004. Administration of oral probiotic bacteria to pregnant women causes temporary infantile colonization. Journal of Pediatric Gastroenterology and Nutrition 38, 293–297.

Schwarzer, M., Srutkova, D., Schabussova, I., Hudcovic, T., Akgün, J., Wiedermann, U., Kozakova, H., 2013. Neonatal colonization of germ-free mice with *Bifidobacterium longum* prevents allergic sensitization to major birch pollen allergen Bet v. 1. Vaccine 31 (46), 5405–5412.

Shadid, R., Haarman, M., Knol, J., Theis, W., Beermann, C., Rjosk-Dendorfer, D., Schendel, D.J., Koletzko, B.V., Krauss-Etschmann, S., 2007. Effects of galactooligosaccharide and long-chain fructooligosaccharide supplementation during pregnancy on maternal and neonatal microbiota and immunity–a randomized, double-blind, placebo-controlled study. American Journal of Clinical Nutrition 86 (5), 1426–1437.

Shreiner, A., Huffnagle, G.B., Noverr, M.C., 2008. The "micro-flora hypothesis" of allergic disease. Advances in Experimental Medicine and Biology 635, 113–134.

Simpson, M.R., Dotterud, C.K., Storrø, O., Johnsen, R., Øien, T., August 1, 2015. Perinatal probiotic supplementation in the prevention of allergy related disease: 6 year follow up of a randomised controlled trial. BMC Dermatology 15, 13.

Singh, M., Ranjan Das, R., 2010. Probiotics for allergic respiratory diseases–putting it into perspective. Pediatric Allergy and Immunology 21 (2 Pt 2), e368–e376.

Skouteris, H., Hartley-Clark, L., McCabe, M., Milgrom, J., Kent, B., Herring, S.J., Gale, J., 2010. Preventing excessive gestational weight gain: a systematic review of interventions. Obesity Reviews 11 (11), 757–768.

Smug, L.N., Salminen, S., Sanders, M.E., Ebner, S., 2014. Yoghurt and probiotic bacteria in dietary guidelines of the member states of the European Union. Beneficial Microbes 5 (1), 61–66.

Soh, S.E., Aw, M., Gerez, I., Chong, Y.S., Rauff, M., Ng, Y.P., Wong, H.B., Pai, N., Lee, B.W., Shek, L.P., 2009. Probiotic supplementation in the first 6 months of life in at risk Asian infants–effects on eczema and atopic sensitization at the age of 1 year. Clinical and Experimental Allergy 39 (4), 571–578.

Solís, G., de Los Reyes-Gavilan, C.G., Fernández, N., Margolles, A., Gueimonde, M., 2010. Establishment and development of lactic acid bacteria and bifidobacteria microbiota in breast-milk and the infant gut. Anaerobe 16 (3), 307–310.

Starke, I.C., Pieper, R., Neumann, K., Zentek, J., Vahjen, W., 2013. Individual responses of mother sows to a probiotic *Enterococcus faecium* strain lead to different microbiota composition in their offspring. Beneficial Microbes 4 (4), 345–356.

Strachan, D.P., 1989. Hay fever, hygiene, and household size. British Medical Journal 299, 1259–1260.

Subramanian, S., Blanton, L.V., Frese, S.A., Charbonneau, M., Mills, D.A., Gordon, J.I., 2015. Cultivating healthy growth and nutrition through the gut microbiota. Cell 161 (1), 36–48.

Szajewska, H., Guarino, A., Hojsak, I., Indrio, F., Kolacek, S., Shamir, R., Vandenplas, Y., Weizman, Z., 2014. European Society for Pediatric Gastroenterology, Hepatology, and Nutrition. Use of probiotics for management of acute gastroenteritis: a position paper by the ESPGHAN working group for probiotics and prebiotics. Journal of Pediatric Gastroenterology and Nutrition 58 (4), 531–539.

Szajewska, H., Kołodziej, M., 2015. Systematic review with meta-analysis: *Lactobacillus rhamnosus* GG in the prevention of antibiotic-associated diarrhoea in children and adults. Alimentary Pharmacology & Therapeutics 42 (10), 1149–1157.

Szajewska, H., Canani, R.B., Guarino, A., Hojsak, I., Indrio, F., Kolacek, S., Orel, R., Shamir, R., Vandenplas, Y., van Goudoever, J.B., Weizman, Z., ESPGHAN Working Group for Probiotics and Prebiotics, 2015. Probiotics for the prevention of antibiotic-associated diarrhea in children. Journal of Pediatric Gastroenterology and Nutrition (Epub ahead of print).

Tanaka, A., Jung, K., Benyacoub, J., Prioult, G., Okamoto, N., Ohmori, K., Blum, S., Mercenier, A., Matsuda, H., 2009. Oral supplementation with *Lactobacillus rhamnosus* CGMCC 1.3724 prevents development of atopic dermatitis in NC/NgaTnd mice possibly by modulating local production of IFN-γ. Experimental Dermatology 18 (12), 1022–1027.

Thomas, F., Hehemann, J.H., Rebuffet, E., Czjzek, M., Michel, G., 2011. Environmental and gut bacteroidetes: the food connection. Frontiers in Microbiology 2.

Tieu, J., Crowther, C.A., Middleton, P., 2008. Dietary advice in pregnancy for preventing gestational diabetes mellitus. Cochrane Database of Systematic Reviews 16 (2), CD006674.

Toomer, O.T., Ferguson, M., Pereira, M., Do, A., Bigley, E., Gaines, D., Williams, K., 2014. Maternal and postnatal dietary probiotic supplementation enhances splenic regulatory T helper cell population and reduces ovalbumin allergen-induced hypersensitivity responses in mice. Immunobiology 219 (5), 367–376.

Torrazza, R.M., Neu, J., 2011. The developing intestinal microbiome and its relationship to health and disease in the neonate. Journal of Perinatology 31, S29–S34.

Treven, P., Mrak, V., Bogovič Matijašić, B., Horvat, S., Rogelj, I., 2015. Administration of probiotics *Lactobacillus rhamnosus* GG and *Lactobacillus gasseri* K7 during pregnancy and lactation changes mouse mesenteric lymph nodes and mammary gland microbiota. Journal of Dairy Science 98 (4), 2114–2128.

Turnbaugh, P.J., Hamady, M., Yatsunenko, T., Cantarel, B.L., Duncan, A., Ley, R.E., Sogin, M.L., Jones, W.J., Roe, B.A., Affourtit, J.P., Egholm, M., Henrissat, B., Heath, A.C., Knight, R., Gordon, J.I., 2009. A core gut microbiome in obese and lean twins. Nature 457, 480–484.

Turnbaugh, P.J., Ley, R.E., Mahowald, M.A., Magrini, V., Mardis, E.R., Gordon, J.I., 2006. An obesity-associated gut microbiome with increased capacity for energy harvest. Nature 444 (7122), 1027–1031.

van der Aa, L.B., Heymans, H.S., van Aalderen, W.M., Sillevis, J.H., Smitt Knol, J., Ben Amor, K., Goossens, D.A., Sprikkelman, A.B., 2010. Effect of a new synbiotic mixture on atopic dermatitis in infants: a randomized-controlled trial. Clinical Experimental Allergy 40, 795–804.

Van Hoffen, E., Ruiter, B., Faber, J., M'Rabet, L., Knol, E.K., Stahl, B., Arslanoglu, S., Moro, G., Boehm, G., Garssen, J., 2009. A specific mixture of short-chain galacto-oligosaccharides and long-chain fructo-oligosaccharides induces a beneficial immunoglobulin profile in infants at high risk for allergy. Allergy 64 (3), 484–487.

Vallabhaneni, S., Walker, T.A., Lockhart, S.R., Ng, D., Chiller, T., Melchreit, R., Brandt, M.E., Smith, R.M., Centers for Disease Control and Prevention (CDC), 2014. Notes from the field: fatal gastrointestinal mucormycosis in a premature infant associated with a contaminated dietary supplement-Connecticut. Morbidity and Mortality Weekly Report 64, 155–156.

Vandenplas, Y., De Hert, S.G., PROBIOTICAL-study group, 2011. Randomised clinical trial: the synbiotic food supplement probiotical vs. placebo for acute gastroenteritis in children. Alimentary Pharmacology and Therapeutics 34, 862–867.

Wadhwa, D., Buss, C., Entringer, S., Swanson, J.M., 2009. Developmental origins of health and disease: brief history of the approach and current focus on epigenetic mechanisms. Seminars in Reproductive Medicine 27 (5), 358–368.

Walker, W.A., 2013. Initial intestinal colonization in the human infant and immune homeostasis. Annals of Nutrition and Metabolism 63 (2), 8–15.

Wang, W., Yang, S.F., Ren, L.H., Zhang, X.X., Yu, S.L., 2015. Effect of bifidobacterium on defensin-5 expression in intestinal injury of preweaning rats. World Journal of Gastroenterology 21 (9), 2638–2644.

Wen, K., Tin, C., Wang, H., Yang, X., Li, G., Giri-Rachman, E., Kocher, J., Bui, T., Clark-Deener, S., Yuan, L., 2014. Probiotic *Lactobacillus rhamnosus* GG enhanced Th1 cellular immunity but did not affect antibody responses in a human gut microbiota transplanted neonatal gnotobiotic pig model. PLoS One 9 (4), e94504.

Wickens, K., Ingham, T., Epton, M., Pattemore, P., Town, I., Fishwick, D., Crane, J., New Zealand Asthma and Allergy Cohort Study Group, 2008. The association of early life exposure to antibiotics and the development of asthma, eczema and atopy in a birth cohort: confounding or causality? Clinical and Experimental Allergy 38 (8), 1318–1324.

Yang, H., Liu, A., Zhang, M., Ibrahim, S.A., Pang, Z., Leng, X., Ren, F., 2009. Oral administration of live Bifidobacterium substrains isolated from centenarians enhances intestinal function in mice. Current Microbiology 59 (4), 439–445.

SECTION

Challenges and Opportunities

F

CHAPTER

Human Milk Microbes – Summary and Research Gaps

17

Mark A. McGuire[1], Michelle K. McGuire[2]
[1]*University of Idaho, Moscow, ID, United States;* [2]*Washington State University, Pullman, WA, United States*

1. INTRODUCTION

Whereas the previous chapters have systematically described what is known (and unknown) about various aspects of the human milk microbiome, here we pose and briefly discuss several overarching unanswered questions that tie together the current state of the science in this important field of research. Specifically, here we ask whether milk and/or mammary tissue are/is somehow ideal for supporting the growth of the bacteria found in milk; if there might exist a critical link between the external environment and milk via an "enteromammary pathway" for bacterial translocation, and if so whether it is selective; and if the mammary gland should be conceptualized as an organ with direct exposure to the external environment.

2. ARE THERE CHARACTERISTICS OF MAMMARY TISSUE AND/OR MILK THAT PROMOTE THE PRESENCE OR ABUNDANCE OF CERTAIN BACTERIA?

Despite the fact that humans have coexisted with microbes since the beginning of human existence, our appreciation of microbial ecology complexity is relatively rudimentary. Indeed, our understanding of the relationship between microbes and food—be it in terms of fermentation, preservation, infectious disease, or spoilage – is understood in substantially more detail than how the microbes in foods—particularly milk—positively impact physiologic health. Nonetheless, humans have taken advantage of microbes found in milk for millennia in terms of using them to produce fermented products such as cheese and yogurt. Although current methods rely mainly on the use of "starter cultures" to ferment such foods, it is likely that these bacteria were initially obtained from milk, itself. As such, one must wonder why milk has evolved to contain such bacteria, and whether there exist benefits of mammary-derived bacteria to both mother and recipient

Prebiotics and Probiotics in Human Milk. http://dx.doi.org/10.1016/B978-0-12-802725-7.00017-8

offspring. Furthermore, what is it about milk that supports the growth of these microorganisms?

Many of the bacteria found in bovine and human milk (determined using culture-dependent and -independent means) are shared, suggesting a common preference unique to the mammary gland and its product, milk (Jost et al., 2013; Quigley et al., 2013). For instance, common pathogens associated with mastitis such as staphylococci and streptococci are certainly found in both species using both methods of assessment. Although organisms found in bovine milk have long been used to create fermented dairy products, similar organisms such as lactobacilli and bifidobacteria have also been identified in and cultured from human milk (Jeurink et al., 2013; Martín et al., 2003, 2004, 2006, 2009). While the milk microbiome typically includes members found in other body sites, the profile of relative abundances of bacteria in milk is a somewhat unique community.

Intriguing recent work (Charbonneau et al., 2016) has also demonstrated that feeding sialylated bovine milk oligosaccharides to gnotobiotic mice or piglets alters the bacterial community of the recipient and increases growth. This supports associations found in human infants found by Alderete et al. (2015). Bifidobacteria represent the major taxa with the capacity to metabolize human milk oligosaccharides (HMOs) (Bode, 2012; Katayma, 2016). Thus, it is not surprising that the feeding of HMO-like complex carbohydrates may increase the abundance of bifidobacteria in the infant's gastrointestinal (GI) tract (Lewis et al., 2015; Wang et al., 2015). Additional work using rigorous human feeding trials will be needed to test this hypothesis further and determine short- and long-term health outcomes in both healthy and ill infants.

Furthermore, there is limited evidence that HMOs might influence the milk microbiome (and thus, indirectly, the infant's GI microbiome). For instance, Hunt et al. (2011) using culture-independent means demonstrated a positive relationship between total HMO concentration and relative abundance of staphylococci in human milk. Further in vitro experimentation (Hunt et al., 2012) supported the association found in vivo with stimulation of *Staphylococcus aureus* and *Staphylococcus epidermidis* growth by the addition of purified HMOs to a variety of media. Surprisingly, HMO was not reduced in the culture media but instead appeared to serve as a growth promotant to both *S. aureus* and *S. epidermidis*, which responded by metabolizing amino acids for adenosine triphosphate production. These results suggest that HMOs can influence the members of the bacterial community in milk; which HMO isotypes cause this effect are unknown.

Interestingly, since the concentrations of some isotypes of HMOs (e.g., 2-FL) are clearly driven, at least in part, by maternal genetics, it appears that the host genome could be one of the driving forces for shaping the milk microbiome. The GI microbiome has been shown to be heritable, but the extent is limited to a few bacterial taxa; environment (e.g., diet) is thought to represent a much more influential driving force (Davenport, 2016). Future work is needed to determine how significant the maternal genetic influence is on the milk microbiome.

3. DOES THE ENTEROMAMMARY PATHWAY OF MICROBIAL TRANSFER TO HUMAN MILK OCCUR FOR ALL BACTERIAL TAXA?

One of the most frequently asked (and reasonable) questions in this field is, "How do the bacteria in milk get there?" Seminal work from the Rodríguez group (see Chapter 13; Fernández et al., 2013; Martín et al., 2006) demonstrates that when certain bacteria are consumed by a lactating mother, they can be transferred into her milk. This amazing demonstration, coupled with additional studies of the transfer of bacteria from the GI tract to the lactating mammary gland, is incredible and strongly support an enteromammary pathway. Certain strains of lactobacilli and bifidobacteria have been tested; however, further work is necessary to determine if the pathway is discriminatory and/or acts like a gatekeeper for the milk microbiome.

Interestingly, maternal body composition (lean vs obese) may be related to variation in the human milk microbiome (Cabrera-Rubio et al., 2012). However, whether this association is related to body composition per se or differences in nutrient intake is not known. Whereas some work (e.g., Turnbaugh et al., 2009) demonstrates a relationship between body composition and the GI microbiome, research focused specifically on the lactating woman (Carrothers et al., 2015) does not. Nonetheless, Carrothers et al. (2015), using rigorous repeated 24-hour dietary recalls, reported that variation in the fecal microbiome profile of lactating women is related to the nutritional quality of her diet. Specifically, consumption of a more nutrient-rich diet appears to be associated with a fecal bacterial community with higher relative abundance of members of the Firmicutes phylum. This was true across nutrient categories, including vitamins, minerals, and essential amino acids. Consequently, future research will need to tease apart the independent and interactive influences (if indeed they exist) of maternal body composition (a gross indicator of chronic energy balance) and acute and chronic maternal nutrient intake on maternal fecal microbiome and milk microbiome. One critical question to consider in this regard is whether the milk microbiome from an obese mother creates a GI microbiome in her nursing infant that promotes future risk of obesity.

Understanding the biology of the translocation of living bacteria from the GI tract to the mammary gland may yield critical information for mammary health and food-borne illness. This will require prospective, longitudinal, human intervention trials ideally conducted in a broad range of women, including those differing in body composition, chronic dietary intakes, and environmental exposures.

4. SHOULD THE MAMMARY GLAND BE VIEWED AS AN EXTERIOR ORGAN (MUCH LIKE THE GASTROINTESTINAL TRACT) EXPOSED TO THE ENVIRONMENT?

Historically, the mammary gland has not been considered to be exposed directly to the external environment. However, emerging data suggest that this is not true; and if not, then milk composition (particularly its microbial component) may be directly influenced by environmental exposures. The bacterial community in human milk appears to be personalized to individuals with about half of the members shared (a "core" microbiome) and the remainder unique to the individual (Hunt et al., 2011). While variation in a portion of the community could be driven by maternal genetics, it is highly likely that the environment is influential. As such, could the identification of bacteria in human milk simply be due, at least in large part, to contamination of the milk during sample collection and/or storage? In order to address this concern, rigorous methods of milk collection, such as a surgical scrub of the breast before sampling using sterile containers, have been used in women (Hunt et al., 2011). However, use of these sampling methods does not negate the possibility that some of the bacteria found in milk is due to sampling protocol. Nonetheless, Urbaniak et al. (2014) have recently identified a mammary gland microbiome in biopsy samples taken from non-lactating women during surgery. Many of the bacterial taxa found in these tissue samples collected from Canadian and Irish women have also been found in human milk, suggesting a resident bacterial community in mammary tissue. In other words, the milk microbiome largely mirrors the mammary microbiome.

Furthermore, although surgical biopsy of the lactating human breast is rare, in dairy cows the biopsy of milk from within the mammary gland is possible. Indeed, our research group has biopsied bovine milk by needle aspiration through the wall of the teat after a surgical scrub of the teat wall (Reynolds et al., unpublished data). This work revealed that the bacterial community structure in the needle aspirate of bovine milk was largely similar to that of milk removed and collected via hand stripping with a sterile glove into a sterile tube immediately prior to the aspirate (Fig. 17.1). These results, combined with those of Urbaniak et al. (2014), support the presence of a commensal bacterial community in the mammary gland and its product, milk; this community is clearly not due entirely to environmental contamination.

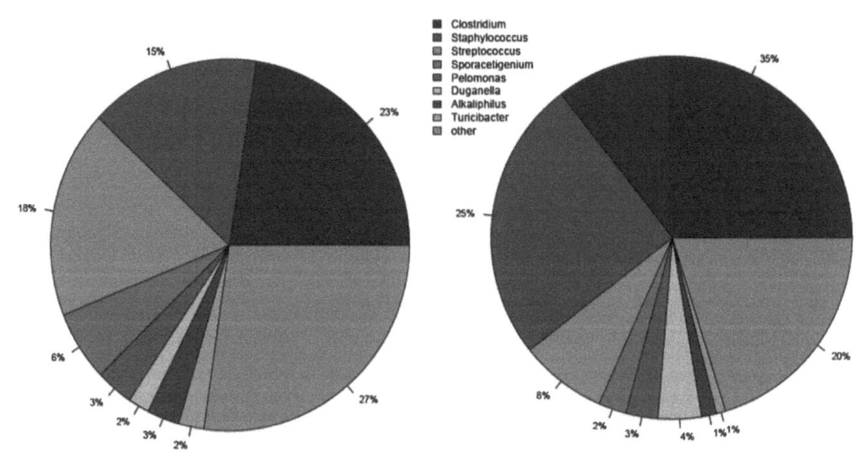

FIGURE 17.1

Bovine milk microbiome in a hand strip sample after cleaning (left piechart) and via aspiration by needle (right pie chart) through the teat wall.

Unpublished data from Reynolds, Yahvah, Williams, Fox, McGuire, and McGuire.

5. CONCLUSIONS

The long-held dogma that human milk is a sterile fluid has now clearly been disproved by many research groups which have, through both culture-dependent and -independent means, detected and characterized a rich community of bacteria in both carefully collected milk samples and mammary biopsies. The role that these bacteria play in the growth and development of the infant could be substantial—particularly in those at the highest risk of malnutrition, morbidity, and mortality. Possible effects on the infant include alteration of weight gain and nutrient partitioning during early life, immune sensitization and training, GI development, and even cognition and behavior. Resident bacteria in the mammary gland may also influence mammary health, for instance inflammation, and bacteria in milk may potentially work in concert with other milk components (e.g., HMOs) for many of these benefits. Thus, understanding independent and interactive effects of milk's microbiome and other milk constituents is both challenging and critical. In addition, delineating factors (e.g., maternal genetics, acute and chronic dietary intake, medications, environmental microbial exposures) that drive variation in the milk microbiome is also fundamental at this stage of research. In fact, basic research designed to understand the milk microbiome, and variability therein, in healthy women is a critical first step in understanding if and how its manipulation might impact both maternal and infant health. Clearly, we are currently only at the tip of the iceberg in terms of this entire new area of investigation.

REFERENCES

Alderete, T.L., Autran, C., Brekke, B.E., Knight, R., Bode, L., Goran, M.I., Fields, D.A., 2015. Associations between human milk oligosaccharides and infant body composition in the first 6 mo of life. American Journal of Clinical Nutrition 102, 1381–1388.

Bode, L., 2012. Human milk oligosaccharides: every baby needs a sugar mama. Glycobiology 22, 1147–1162.

Carrothers, J.M., York, M.A., Brooker, S.L., Lackey, K.A., Williams, J.E., Shafii, B., Price, W.J., Settles, M.L., McGuire, M.A., McGuire, M.K., 2015. Fecal microbial community structure is stable over time and related to variation in macronutrient and micronutrient intakes in lactating women. Journal of Nutrition 145, 2379–2388.

Cabrera-Rubio, R., Collado, M.C., Laitinen, K., Salminen, S., Isolauri, E., Mira, A., 2012. The human milk microbiome changes over lactation and is shaped by maternal weight and mode of delivery. American Journal of Clinical Nutrition 96, 544–551.

Charbonneau, M.R., O'Donnell, D., Blanton, L.V., Totten, S.M., Davis, J.C.C., Barratt, M.J., Cheng, J., Guruge, J., Talcott, M., Bain, J.R., Muehlbauer, M.J., Ilkayeva, O., Wu, C., Struckmeyer, T., Barile, D., Mangani, C., Jorgensen, J., Fan, Y.-M., Maleta, K., Dewey, K.G., Ashom, P., Newgard, C.B., Lebrilla, C., Mills, D.A., Gordon, J.I., 2016. Sialylated milk oligosaccharides promote microbiota-dependent growth in models of infant undernutrition. Cell 164, 859–871.

Davenport, E.R., 2016. Elucidating the role of the host genome in shaping microbiome composition. Gut Microbes 7, 178–184.

Fernández, L., Langa, S., Martín, V., Maldonado, A., Jiménez, E., Martín, R., Rodríguez, J.M., 2013. The human milk microbiota: origin and potential roles in health and disease. Pharmacological Research 59, 31–42.

Hunt, K.M., Foster, J.A., Forney, L.J., Schutte, U.M.E., Beck, D.L., Abdo, Z., Fox, L.K., Williams, J.E., McGuire, M.K., McGuire, M.A., 2011. Characterization of the diversity and temporal stability of bacterial communities in human milk. PLoS ONE 6, e21313. http://dx.doi.org/10.1371/journal.pone.0021313.

Hunt, K.M., Preuss, J., Nissan, C., Davlin, C.A., Williams, J.E., Shafii, B., Richardson, A.D., McGuire, M.K., Bode, L., McGuire, M.A., 2012. Human milk oligosaccharides promote the growth of staphylococci. Applied Environmental Microbiology 78, 4763–4770.

Jeurink, P.V., van Bergenhenegouwen, J., Jiménez, E., Knippels, L.M.J., Fernández, L., Garssen, J., Knol, J., Rodríguez, J.M., Martín, R., 2013. Human milk: a source of more life than we imagine. Beneficial Microbes 4, 17–30.

Jost, T., Lacroix, C., Braegger, C., Chassard, C., 2013. Assessment of bacterial diversity in breast milk using culture-dependent and culture-independent approaches. British Journal of Nutrition 14, 1–10.

Katayama, T., 2016. Host-derived glycans serve as selected nutrients for the gut microbe: human milk oligosaccharides and bifidobacteria. Bioscience, Biotechnology and Biochemistry 80, 621–632.

Lewis, Z.T., Totten, S.M., Smilowitz, J.T., Popovic, M., Parker, E., Lemay, D.G., Van Tassell, M.L., Miller, M.J., Jin, Y.S., German, J.B., Lebrilla, C.B., Mills, D.A., 2015. Maternal fucosyltransferase 2 status affects the gut bifidobacterial communities of breastfed infants. Microbiome 3, 13. http://dx.doi.org/10.1186/s40168-015-0071-z.

Martín, R., Jiménez, E., Heilig, H.G., Fernández, L., Marín, M.L., Zoetendal, E.G., Rodríguez, J.M., 2009. Isolation of bifidobacteria from breast milk and assessment of the bifidobacterial population by PCR-denaturing gradient gel electrophoresis and quantitative real-time PCR. Applied and Environmental Microbiology 75, 965–969.

Martín, R., Jiménez, E., Olivares, M., Marín, M.L., Fernández, L., Xaus, J., Rodríguez, J.M., 2006. *Lactobacillus salivarius* CECT 5713, a potential probiotic strain isolated from infant feces and breast milk of a mother-child pair. International Journal of Food Microbiology 112, 35–43.

Martín, R., Langa, S., Reviriego, C., Jiménez, E., Marín, M.L., Olivares, M., Boza, J., Jiménez, J., Fernández, L., Xaus, J., Rodríguez, J.M., 2004. The commensal microflora of human milk: new perspectives for food bacteriotherapy and probiotics. Trends in Food Science and Technology 15, 121–127.

Martín, R., Langa, S., Reviriego, C., Jiménez, E., Marín, M.L., Xaus, J., Fernández, L., Rodríguez, J.M., 2003. Human milk is a source of lactic acid bacteria for the infant gut. Journal of Pediatrics 143, 754–758.

Quigley, L., O'Sullivan, O., Stanton, C., Beresford, T.P., Ross, R.P., Fitzgerald, G.F., Cotter, P.D., 2013. The complex microbiota of raw milk. FEMS Microbiology Reviews 37, 664–698.

Turnbaugh, P.J., Hamady, M., Yatsunenko, T., Cantarel, B.L., Duncan, A., Ley, R.E., Sogin, M.L., Jones, W.J., Roe, B.A., Affourtit, J.P., Egholm, M., Henrissat, B., Heath, A.C., Knight, R., Gordon, J.I., 2009. A core gut microbiome in obese and lean twins. Nature 457, 480–484.

Urbaniak, C., Cummins, J., Brackstone, M., Macklaim, J.M., Gloor, G.B., Baban, C.K., Scott, L., O'Hanlon, D.M., Burton, J.P., Francis, K.P., Tangney, M., Reid, G., 2014. Microbiota of human breast tissue. Applied and Environmental Microbiology 80, 3007–3014.

Wang, M., Li, M., Wu, S., Lebrilla, C.B., Chapkin, R.S., Ivanov, I., Donovan, S.M., 2015. Fecal microbiota composition of breast-fed infants is correlated with human milk oligosaccharides consumed. Journal of Pediatric Gastroenterology and Nutrition 60, 825–833.

Index

'*Note*: Page numbers followed by "f" indicate figures and "t" indicate tables.'

C

D

G

H

I

M

N

O

P

T

U

Kolibri 360 GmbH
Ferdinand-Jühlke-Straße 7
99095 Erfurt, Deutschland
produktsicherheit@kolibri360.de